DATE DUE

APR 1 9 2001	
MAY 0 3 2001	
AUG 1 4 2001	
DEC 1 6 2001	
JAN 2 1 2003	
MAR 2 1 2003	
APR 1 8 2003	
NOV 0 6 2003	
NOV 2 0 2003	
FEB 1 2 2004	
NOV 3 0 2004	
FEB 0 7 2006	
MAR 1 9 2007	
NOV 0 9 2010	

TUBERCULOSIS

Current Concepts and Treatment

SECOND EDITION

TUBERCULOSIS
Current Concepts and Treatment
SECOND EDITION

EDITED BY

Lloyd N. Friedman, M.D.

CRC Press
Boca Raton   London   New York   Washington, D.C.

Library of Congress Cataloging-in-Publication Data

Tuberculosis : current concepts and treatment / edited by Lloyd N. Friedman.—2nd ed.
  p. cm.
  Includes bibliographical references and index.
  ISBN 0-8493-1565-4 (alk. paper)
  1. Tuberculosis. I. Friedman, Lloyd N.
  [DNLM: 1. Tuberculosis. WF 200 T88165 2000]
  RC311.T85 2000
  616.9'95—dc21
                                                                    00-025394
                                                                    CIP

No claim to original U.S. Government works
International Standard Book Number 0-8493-1565-4
Library of Congress Card Number 00-025394
Printed in the United States of America 1 2 3 4 5 6 7 8 9 0
Printed on acid-free paper

Preface

When the first edition of this book was published in 1994, there was a tuberculosis crisis in the U.S. The number of cases had reached a nadir of 22,201 in 1985, and then gradually had risen to 26,673 by 1992, reversing the usual trend towards a steady decline. There were hundreds of nosocomial drug-resistant cases reported from hospitals caring for AIDS patients. A unified nation-wide effort was directed to control this problem, with resources allocated toward case control and protection of patients and staff in hospitals. Directly observed therapy became standard in certain areas of the country. The effort was successful and the number of tuberculosis cases reported had decreased to 18,361 by 1998.

However, the "crisis" in the U.S. was not even a blip on the global screen. The entire number of new cases in the U.S. each year represents only 0.2% of the worldwide number. There are an estimated 30 million cases of active tuberculosis at any one time in the world, 10 million of which are new cases occurring each year, and there are 3 million annual deaths due to tuberculosis. Each year, foreign-born persons represent a higher and higher proportion of the total number of cases in the U.S. In 1998, there were 7591 cases in foreign-born persons, representing 41% of the total new case load. Thus, it is not enough to simply screen and treat foreign individuals when they enter the U.S. More resources must be made available to control tuberculosis worldwide, especially in underdeveloped countries.

There are approximately two billion people, one third of the world population, who are latently infected with tuberculosis. As much as 90% of new cases arise from this pool. We must develop a safe, effective, and inexpensive drug to treat infected persons so that positive skin tests can be treated in all individuals without worrying about toxic side effects. Unless we treat infection aggressively, new cases will always arise from this pool of individuals.

In this book, each chapter reflects a detailed review of a selected topic and a balanced account of the latest controversies. The reader will obtain a thorough understanding of the epidemiology, presentation, and treatment of sensitive and drug-resistant tuberculosis in normal and immunocom-promised hosts in the U.S. and the world, as well as environmental and public health issues. New diagnostic methods are discussed with an emphasis on molecular techniques. There are compre-hensive presentations of pulmonary and extrapulmonary tuberculosis as they occur in adults and children, as well as a special section on pregnancy, and a chapter on atypical mycobacteria. The global problem of tuberculosis is addressed, and there are more than 100 radiographs in a special chapter devoted solely to mycobacteriologic radiology. Included are summaries of the latest "Offi-cial Statements" on the Diagnostic Classification of Tuberculosis, and Targeted Tuberculin Screen-ing and Treatment of Latent Tuberculosis Infection, both published in April, 2000. Also, the controversies surrounding the use of BCG vaccine are addressed.

The reader will enjoy a current, practical, thorough, and balanced review of the literature from a group of outstanding contributors with vast clinical and research experience.

Editor

Lloyd N. Friedman, M.D., is an Associate Clinical Professor of Pulmonary and Critical Care Medicine at the Yale University School of Medicine, New Haven, CT. He is the Vice President of Medical Affairs and the Director of Intensive Care and Respiratory Therapy at Milford Hospital, Milford, CT.

Dr. Friedman graduated in 1975 from Columbia University, New York, with a B.A. degree in biochemistry and obtained his M.D. degree in 1979 from Yale University. He completed an internship in Internal Medicine at Beth Israel Medical Center in 1980, and residency training at Oregon Health Sciences University in 1983. He completed his fellowship training in Pulmonary and Critical Care Medicine at the Yale University School of Medicine in 1988, and received a National Institutes of Health Training Grant in Clinical Investigation.

Dr. Friedman began his work with tuberculosis in 1984 when he started evaluating welfare applicants who used drugs or alcohol in New York City. He has been following and publishing results of this cohort with respect to tuberculosis, AIDS, and death for the past 16 years. He also has conducted research in the development of a rapid immunologic test for tuberculosis, and has been examining various aspects of skin testing and chemoprophylaxis.

He is a member of the American Thoracic Society and a fellow of the American College of Chest Physicians, as well as a member of the Connecticut Tuberculosis Elimination Advisory Committee. Dr. Friedman is on the Program Committee of the Mycobacteriology and Infectious Disease Assembly of the American Thoracic Society. His current research interests include the epidemiology of AIDS and tuberculosis in the inner city, and the use of skin testing and chemoprophylaxis in the control of tuberculosis.

Contributors

Joseph H. Bates, M.D.
Professor of Medicine and Microbiology
University of Arkansas College of Medicine
  and
Director, Division of Tuberculosis Control
Arkansas Department of Health
Little Rock, Arkansas

Mercedes C. Becerra, Sc.D.
Program in Infectious Disease and Social
  Change Department of Social Medicine
Harvard Medical School
Boston, Massachusetts

George W. Comstock, M.D., Dr.P.H., F.A.C.E.
Alumni Centennial Professor of Epidemiology
Department of Epidemiology
School of Hygiene and Public Health
The Johns Hopkins University
Baltimore, Maryland

Amy B. Curtis, Ph.D., M.P.H.
Epidemiologist, Surveillance and
  Epidemiology Branch
Division of Tuberculosis Elimination
Centers for Disease Control and Prevention
Atlanta, Georgia

Anne McB. Curtis, M.D.
Professor of Diagnostic Radiology
Yale University School of Medicine
New Haven, Connecticut

Michael H. Cynamon, M.D.
Professor of Medicine
Infectious Disease Section
Department of Medicine
State University of New York Health Science
  Center
Veterans Affairs Medical Center
Syracuse, New York

Jerrold J. Ellner, M.D.
Professor of Medicine and
  Pathology
Case Western Reserve University School of
  Medicine
Chief, Division of Infectious Diseases
University Hospitals of Cleveland
Cleveland, Ohio

Paul E. Farmer, M.D., Ph.D.
Assoc. Professor of Medicine
Program in Infectious Disease and Social
  Change
Department of Social Medicine
Harvard Medical School
Boston, Massachusetts

Lloyd N. Friedman, M.D.
Vice President, Medical Affairs
Medical Director, Intensive Care and
  Respiratory Therapy
Milford Hospital
Milford, Connecticut
  and
Assoc. Clinical Professor of Medicine
Pulmonary and Critical Care Section
Yale University School of Medicine
New Haven, Connecticut

Marian Goble, M.D.
Clinical Professor of Medicine
University of Colorado Health Sciences Center
  and
Infectious Diseases Section
National Jewish Medical and Research Center
Denver, Colorado

James L. Hadler, M.D., M.P.H.
Director, Infectious Diseases
Department of Public Health
State of Connecticut
Hartford, Connecticut

Robin E. Huebner, Ph.D., M.P.H.
Infectious Disease Epidemiologist
Pneumococcal Diseases Research Unit
Medical Research Council/South Africa
  Institute for Medical Research
University of the Witwatersrand
Johannesburg, South Africa

John A. Jereb, M.D.
Medical Epidemiologist
Field Services Branch, Division of Tuberculosis
  Elimination
Centers for Disease Control and Prevention
Atlanta, Georgia

Ari Klapholz, M.D.
Chief, Division of Pulmonary/Critical Care
Cabrini Medical Center
  and
Associate Clinical Professor of Medicine
  (pending)
Mount Sinai School of Medicine
New York, New York

David L. Lakey, M.D.
Asst. Professor of Medicine
Division of Infectious Diseases
Center for Pulmonary Infection and Disease
  Control
University of Texas Health Center at Tyler
Tyler, Texas

Klaus-Dieter K. L. Lessnau, M.D.
Director, Respiratory Care Services
Division of Pulmonary/Critical Care Medicine
The Brooklyn Hospital Center
Brooklyn, New York

Eugene McCray, M.D.
Chief, Surveillance Section
Surveillance and Epidemiology Branch
Division of Tuberculosis Elimination
Centers for Disease Control and Prevention
Atlanta, Georgia

Rodolfo Miranda, M.D.
Fellow, Division of Pulmonary/Critical Care
  Medicine
Cabrini Medical Center
New York, New York

Edward A. Nardell, M.D.
Assoc. Professor of Medicine
Harvard Medical School
Director, Pulmonary Department
The Cambridge Hospital
Cambridge, Massachusetts
  and
Tuberculosis Control Officer
Massachusetts Department of Public
  Health
Boston, Massachusetts

Ida M. Onorato, M.D.
Chief, Surveillance and Epidemiology
  Branch
Division of Tuberculosis Elimination
Centers for Disease Control and
  Prevention
Atlanta, Georgia

Peter A. Selwyn, M.D., M.P.H.
Professor and Chairman
Department of Family Medicine
Albert Einstein College of Medicine
Montefiore Medical Center
Bronx, New York

Ronald W. Smithwick, M.S.
Senior Microbiologist
Tuberculosis/Mycobacteriology Branch
Division of AIDS, STD, and TB Lab.
  Research
Nation Center for Infectious Diseases
Centers for Disease Control and
  Prevention
Atlanta, Georgia

Jeffrey R. Starke, M.D.
Assoc. Professor of Pediatrics
Section of Infectious Diseases
Department of Pediatrics
Baylor College of Medicine
Houston, Texas
  and
Director, Children's Tuberculosis Clinic
Deputy Chief of Pediatrics
Ben Taub General Hospital
Houston, Texas

Wilfredo Talavera, M.D.
Director, Department of Medicine
Assoc. Chief, Division of Pulmonary and
  Critical Care Medicine
Cabrini Medical Center
New York, New York
  and
Clinical Professor of Medicine (pending)
Mount Sinai School of Medicine
New York, New York

Zahra Toossi, M.D.
Assoc. Professor of Medicine
Case Western Reserve University School of
  Medicine
Division of Infectious Diseases
University Hospitals of Cleveland
VA Medical Center
Cleveland, Ohio

Richard J. Wallace, Jr., M.D.
Chairman, Department of
  Microbiology
Professor of Medicine
John Chapman Professorship in Microbiology
University of Texas Health Center at Tyler
Tyler, Texas

David A. Walton
Program in Infectious Disease and Social
  Change
Department of Social Medicine
Harvard Medical School
Boston, Massachusetts

Paul W. Wright, M.D.
Professor of Family Medicine
University of Texas Health Center at Tyler
Tyler, Texas

Contents

Dedication

This book is dedicated to my wife, Kai, and my children, David, Jonathan, and Alexander, whose unceasing support allowed me to complete this volume. Also to Thomas J. Yang, D.V.M., Ph.D., who had the foresight to conceive this project.

In Memorium

We note with sadness the untimely passing of two authors of our first edition, Elizabeth A. Rich, M.D. (Pathogenesis of Tuberculosis) and Sandra Handwerger, M.D. (Extrapulmonary Tuberculosis), the promise of their lives only partially realized.

1 The Epidemiology of Tuberculosis in the U.S.

Amy B. Curtis, Ph.D., M.P.H., John A. Jereb, M.D., Eugene McCray, M.D., and Ida M. Onorato, M.D.

CONTENTS

I. INTRODUCTION

Tuberculosis (TB) is a disease that has affected man since the beginning of recorded history. TB is an infectious disease spread by airborne dispersal of droplet nuclei containing *Mycobacterium tuberculosis* from a contagious host who is coughing or sneezing (see Chapter 3). Incidence rates of TB in the U.S. were greater than 50 cases per 100,000 persons through the first half of the 20th century. In the late 1940s, antibiotics were discovered which led to effective cures for TB; streptomycin in 1947, para-aminosalicylic acid or PAS in 1949, and isoniazid in 1952. The rate of TB

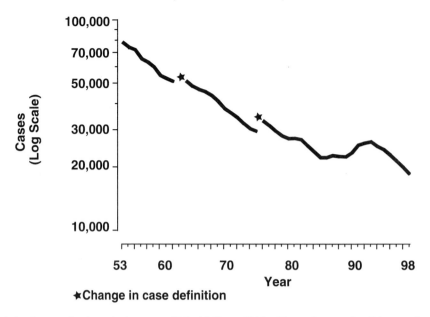

FIGURE 1.1   Reported tuberculosis cases, U.S. 1953 to 1998. (From Centers for Disease Control and Prevention, Atlanta, GA.)

steadily declined between the 1950s and 1980s due to a combination of improved standards of living, public health interventions designed to interrupt transmission, and treatments with the newly discovered anti-TB medications (Figure 1.1). However, beginning in 1985, the U.S. experienced a period of resurgence of TB. This period was characterized by an increase in TB in regions and demographic groups where human immunodeficiency virus (HIV) infection was prevalent, a decrease in the median age of persons who have TB, an increase of cases in foreign-born persons, extensive outbreaks of multidrug-resistant TB (MDR TB) in institutions housing HIV-infected persons, and a geographic dispersion of drug-resistant TB.[1-4] This resurgence lasted for 8 years, peaking in 1992 at 10.4 cases per 100,000 population (Figure 1.1). This chapter will describe the recent epidemiology of TB in the U.S. and address the reasons for the recently observed increase and subsequent decline in TB incidence.

II. TUBERCULOSIS SURVEILLANCE IN THE U.S.

TB is a reportable disease in all jurisdictions in the U.S. Fifty-nine reporting areas including the 50 states, the District of Columbia, New York City, and other U.S. jurisdictions in the Pacific and Caribbean (Puerto Rico, Guam, American Samoa, the Republic of the Marshall Islands, the Commonwealth of the Northern Mariana Islands, the Federated States of Micronesia, the Republic of Palau, and the U.S. Virgin Islands) report active cases of TB to the Centers for Disease Control and Prevention (CDC). For the purposes of this chapter, only data from the 50 states (including New York City) and the District of Columbia are included. From 1953 to 1985, aggregate-level TB surveillance data were reported. Beginning in 1985, individual, but anonymous, data were collected and reported to the CDC using the Report of a Verified Case of Tuberculosis (RVCT) form. In 1993, after the national increase in TB and the emergence of MDR TB, the CDC implemented an expanded surveillance system. Additional information on risk factors (e.g., HIV infection, drug use, homelessness, occupation, and residence in correctional and long-term care facilities) drug susceptibility, initial therapy, and treatment outcome (e.g., sputum culture conversion and completion of therapy) was added to the new expanded RVCT, and a computerized system was implemented to allow electronic transmission of data from the reporting areas to the national level.[5]

For surveillance purposes, a case of TB may be defined by laboratory or clinical criteria. The laboratory criteria requires *one* of the following: (1) isolation of *M. tuberculosis* from a clinical specimen, (2) demonstration of *M. tuberculosis* from a clinical specimen by nucleic acid amplification test,* or (3) demonstration of acid-fast bacilli in a clinical specimen when a culture has not been or cannot be obtained. Clinical criteria requires *all* of the following: (1) a positive tuberculin skin test; (2) other signs and symptoms compatible with TB, such as an abnormal, unstable chest x-ray, or clinical evidence of current disease; (3) treatment with two or more antituberculosis medications; and (4) a completed diagnostic evaluation.[6] In addition, reports of cases that are considered verified by the reporting areas but do not meet the published case definition (i.e., provider diagnoses) have also traditionally been included in the national surveillance system.[7]

A case may be counted only once within any consecutive 12-month period; however, a patient with TB may be counted more than once if he is discharged from supervision or lost to follow-up for more than 12 months and disease is verified again.[6]

III. RECENT TRENDS IN INCIDENCE RATES

Recent developments in the epidemiology of TB in the U.S. illustrate the importance of maintaining effective public health programs even for diseases whose incidence appears to be steadily decreasing. Effective cures for TB were developed in the mid 1950s and rates of TB in the U.S. steadily decreased until the mid 1980s. Starting in the 1960s, there was a decrease in the resources available to TB public health programs and the TB public health infrastructure deteriorated.[8-10] From 1985 through 1992, rates of TB increased 13% from 9.3 to 10.5 per 100,000 population (Figure 1.1). This resurgence has been largely ascribed to an increase in HIV/AIDS in several large urban centers combined with a deteriorated public health infrastructure and increased immigration from areas of the world with a high TB prevalence.[1,9,11] Between 1985 and 1992, California and New York, the two states with the largest number of cases in both years, accounted for 89% of the increased number of cases reported between those 2 years.

In 1993, the number of TB cases once again began to decrease, and this decrease has continued through 1998. In 1998, there were 18,361 cases of TB reported in the U.S.,[12] a reduction of 31% from the 26,673 cases reported in 1992 (Figure 1.1).[13] The 1998 case rate of 6.8 per 100,000[12] was 7% lower than the 1997 case rate of 7.4,[14] but remains above the year 2000 national goal of 3.5 per 100,000.[15] The decline in the overall number of reported TB cases has occurred with the strengthening of TB control programs nationwide. For example, the largest decreases in U.S.-born cases in 1993 to 1994 occurred in areas that reported greater increases in measures associated with effective TB control programs: completion of therapy, conversion of sputum, and number of contacts identified per case patient.[2] This strengthening of TB programs has occurred in the same urban centers that experienced the largest increases during the period of resurgence, leading to their large reduction in cases since 1992.[2] Although the overall number of TB cases continues to decrease, trends in the number of reported cases and TB incidence vary by geographic area and population characteristics.

IV. GEOGRAPHIC DISTRIBUTION

A. STATES

The number of reported TB cases is not evenly distributed throughout the U.S. Several states with large urban centers account for the majority of TB cases (Table 1.1). The states with the highest

---

* Nucleic acid amplification (NAA) tests must be accompanied by culture for mycobacteria species. However, for surveillance purposes, the CDC will accept results obtained from NAA tests approved by the Food and Drug Administration (FDA) and used according to the approved product labeling on the package insert. Current FDA-approved NAA tests are only approved for smear-positive respiratory specimens.

TABLE 1.1

Tuberculosis Cases and Case Rates Per 100,000 Population: U.S., 1992 and 1998

State	Cases		Rate	
	1992	1998	1992	1998
United States	26,673	18,361	10.5	6.8
Alabama	418	381	10.1	8.8
Alaska	57	55	9.7	9.0
Arizona	259	254	6.8	5.4
Arkansas	257	171	10.7	6.7
California	5382	3852	17.4	11.8
Colorado	104	79	3.0	2.0
Connecticut	156	128	4.8	3.9
Delaware	55	36	8.0	4.8
District of Columbia	146	107	24.8	20.5
Florida	1707	1302	12.7	8.7
Georgia	893	631	13.2	8.3
Hawaii	273	181	23.5	15.2
Idaho	26	14	2.4	1.1
Illinois	1270	850	10.9	7.1
Indiana	247	188	4.4	3.2
Iowa	49	55	1.7	1.9
Kansas	56	56	2.2	2.1
Kentucky	402	179	10.7	4.5
Louisiana	373	380	8.7	8.7
Maine	24	13	1.9	1.0
Maryland	442	324	9.0	6.3
Massachusetts	428	282	7.1	4.6
Michigan	495	385	5.2	3.9
Minnesota	165	161	3.7	3.4
Mississippi	281	225	10.7	8.2
Missouri	245	184	4.7	3.4
Montana	16	20	1.9	2.3
Nebraska	28	31	1.7	1.9
Nevada	99	128	7.5	7.3
New Hampshire	18	14	1.6	1.2
New Jersey	984	640	12.6	7.9
New Mexico	88	68	5.6	3.9
New York	4574	2000	25.2	11.0
North Carolina	604	498	8.8	6.6
North Dakota	11	10	1.7	1.6
Ohio	358	230	3.2	2.1
Oklahoma	216	198	6.7	5.9
Oregon	145	156	4.9	4.8
Pennsylvania	758	448	6.3	3.7
Rhode Island	54	63	5.4	6.4
South Carolina	387	286	10.7	7.5
South Dakota	32	23	4.5	3.1
Tennessee	527	439	10.5	8.1
Texas	2510	1820	14.2	9.2
Utah	78	52	4.3	2.5
Vermont	7	5	1.2	0.8
Virginia	457	339	7.2	5.0
Washington	306	265	6.0	4.7
West Virginia	92	42	5.1	2.3
Wisconsin	106	109	2.1	2.1
Wyoming	8	4	1.7	0.8

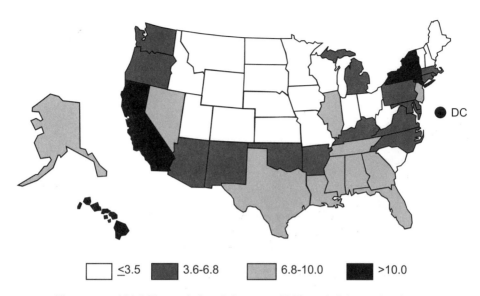

All rates per 100,000 population. 3.5 = year 2000 goal; 6.8 = national average

FIGURE 1.2   Reported incidence rate of tuberculosis by state, U.S., 1998. (From Centers for Disease Control and Prevention, Atlanta, GA.)

number of reported cases in 1998 were California, New York, Texas, Florida, and Illinois; these five states reported 54% of all 1998 TB cases. Each of these states had 1998 case rates above the national average of 6.8 cases per 100,000 and two of these states (California and New York) and one additional state (Hawaii) had case rates greater than 10.0 per 100,000 (Figure 1.2). TB incidence rates decreased in all three areas from 1992 to 1998 (Table 1.1). Since 1992 the five states with the highest number of cases (i.e., CA, NY, TX, FL, and IL) have experienced a marked decrease in the number of new cases, and the majority (68%) of the decrease in TB cases observed between 1992 and 1998 is accounted for by decreases in these states.

In 1998, 18 states reported less than 100 TB cases, 17 of which also reported less than 100 cases in 1992; 14 of these had no change or a decrease in the number of reported cases compared to 1992 (Table 1.1). The 1998 case rate in 19 states was lower than the year 2000 national goal of 3.5 cases per 100,000 population (Figure 1.2).[15]

B. CITIES

Several cities bear a substantial fraction of the TB burden in the U.S. The four cities with the greatest number of cases constitute 16% of 1998 cases. New York City reported 1558 cases in 1998, the most of any U.S. city, followed by Los Angeles, CA, (544 cases), Chicago, IL (473 cases), and Houston, TX (424 cases). All four cities experienced a decline in the number of reported cases during 1992 to 1998; the number of cases has decreased by 59% in New York City, 51% in Los Angeles, and 41% in both Chicago and Houston. Combined, these cities accounted for 41% of the observed decrease in the number of cases reported in the U.S. between 1992 and 1998.

C. COUNTIES

Among all states, the proportion of counties reporting no TB cases increased from 42% in 1992 to 49% in 1998 (Figure 1.3). Although this proportion is high, these counties represented only 11% of the total U.S. population in 1998.

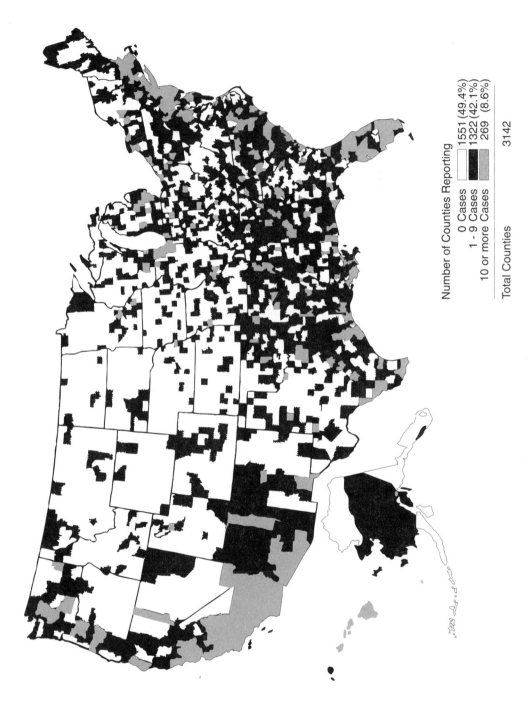

FIGURE 1.3 Reported tuberculosis cases by county, U.S., 1998. (From Centers for Disease Control and Prevention, Atlanta, GA.)

V. DEMOGRAPHICS

A. AGE

The age distribution of TB in the U.S. is affected by the incidence of TB, the HIV epidemic, and by the proportion of TB patients born in other countries. As rates of TB decrease, as they have in the U.S. throughout much of the 20th century, the age distribution shifts towards older ages. This likely occurs because most tuberculosis in the elderly represents reactivation of latent infection as a result of transmission which occurred earlier in life (at a time when the prevalence of TB was higher) rather than newly acquired infection. In contrast, TB in young children represents newly acquired disease. As transmission is reduced, the proportion of new TB cases caused by reactivated old disease increases, shifting the age distribution upward. This pattern was observed from the 1950s through the mid 1980s, when the age distribution of TB infection shifted increasingly into older groups and TB increasingly became a disease of the elderly. For instance, the percentage of new cases in patients over 65 years of age increased from 14 to 29% from 1953 to 1979, while the proportion of the population over 65 only increased from 9 to 11%.[16]

The resurgence of TB in the late 1980s and early 1990s affected younger populations disproportionately, causing the median age of TB patients in the U.S. to decrease.[1,17] The median age of TB patients reported to the national surveillance system was 49 years in 1985 and 43 years in 1992. Following the end of the TB resurgence, the median age of TB patients has increased again, to 45 years in 1998. The impact of HIV on the TB epidemic in the U.S. partly explains the shifting age distribution of TB cases over the past 13 years. Many of the large TB outbreaks that occurred in the late 1980s and early 1990s were among the HIV-infected populations.[18-21] Estimates from a 1993 to 1994 registry match between HIV/AIDS registries and national TB surveillance data found that among TB cases coinfected with HIV, 75% were 25 to 44 years old (the age group at highest risk for HIV), while only 32% of non-AIDS TB patients were 25 to 44 years old.[22] However, the shift toward an older age distribution has slowed because of an increasing percentage of persons born outside the U.S. (see Foreign-Born Persons in Section VI). The median age among foreign-born TB patients is younger (40 years old in 1998) than among the U.S.-born patients (48 years old in 1998).

B. GENDER

In the U.S., as in most countries, the differences in TB rates vary by gender as well as by age. Among persons < 20 years of age, rates of TB are similar for both sexes, with the lowest rates observed between 5 and 14 years of age. However, during adulthood, rates of TB are consistently higher for men than for women. Among adults, TB case rates for men are approximately twice that for women (Figure 1.4). Differences in exposure to sources of infection may account for some of the observed gender gap in the U.S.[23] In addition, biological differences also may contribute to these differences. For instance, it has been noted that iron overload can help increase the development of, and mortality from, TB.[24-26] U.S. women in their reproductive years are more likely than men to be iron deficient.[27]

C. RACE/ETHNICITY

Historically, nonwhite racial and ethnic groups have experienced 5 to 10 times the TB risk of whites.[1] Theories for the increased risk among minority groups have included biological, social, and economic explanations.[28-30] Recently, an analysis of 1987 to 1993 data from the national TB surveillance system examining causes for the racial/ethnic differences found that differences in indicators of socioeconomic status, especially crowding, accounted for approximately half of the racial/ethnic differences in case rates of TB among U.S. born blacks, Hispanics, and Native Americans.[1]

During the 1985 to 1992 resurgence, increases in tuberculosis cases were concentrated among racial/ethnic minorities;[1,31-33] however, all racial/ethnic groups observed a decreased number of

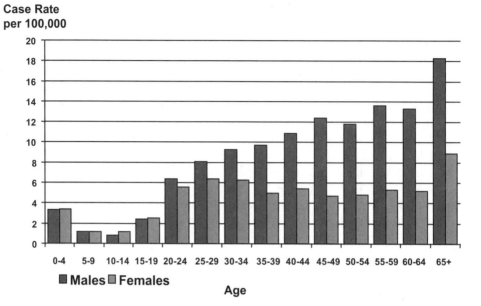

**Case Rate
per 100,000**

■ Males ▨ Females

Age

FIGURE 1.4   Tuberculosis incidence rates for men and women by age group, 1998. (From Centers for Disease Control and Prevention, Atlanta, GA.)

cases in 1998 compared to 1992. In both years, the greatest number of cases occurred among non-Hispanic Blacks; however, the greatest decrease in the number of cases during this period was for non-Hispanic blacks (39% decrease) and non-Hispanics whites (41% decrease). The decreases were smaller for Hispanics (25% decrease), Asians/Pacific Islanders (1% decrease), and Native Americans/Alaskans (15% decrease). Cases classified by race/ethnicity also varied by geographic region (Table 1.2). For instance, 8% of the 1998 cases in the South occurred among Asian/Pacific Islanders, while 38% of 1998 cases in the West were among Asian/Pacific Islanders. Such geographic concentration of cases supports the development of targeted tuberculosis control programs, but does not exclude the need for programmatic coverage throughout the U.S.

VI. SPECIAL HIGH-RISK POPULATIONS

A. Foreign-Born Persons

Human migration plays a large role in the epidemiology of tuberculosis. Historically, the impact of migration on tuberculosis has occurred through massive human displacement during wars and

**TABLE 1.2
Race/Ethnicity of TB Cases by Region, 1998**

	Northeast		South		Midwest		West	
	No.	%	No.	%	No.	%	No.	%
White, Non-Hispanic	788	21.9	2151	29.4	704	31.0	852	16.6
Black, Non-Hispanic	1251	34.8	3206	43.8	898	39.6	476	9.3
Hispanic	805	22.4	1346	18.4	252	11.1	1696	33.1
American Indian/Alaskan Native	1	0.0	56	0.8	41	1.8	155	3.0
Asian/Pacific Islander	746	20.8	559	7.6	375	16.5	1943	37.9

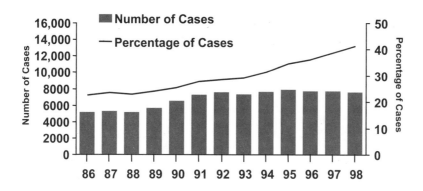

FIGURE 1.5 Trends in tuberculosis cases in foreign-born persons, U.S., 1986 to 1998. (From Centers for Disease Control and Prevention, Atlanta, GA.)

famines, and the results have been locally increased case rates and altered geographic distributions. However, in the 20th century, the emergence of convenient and affordable transportation has given TB global mobility, so that geopolitical boundaries mean less than ever in containing this disease. In this century, new patterns of worldwide epidemiology have been noted as people migrate for political or financial reasons, and routine travel has influenced local epidemiology in unusual ways, such as causing outbreaks in schools and universities.[34-35]

In the U.S., the proportion of TB cases that occur in foreign-born persons has steadily increased over the past decade. Between 1992 and 1998, the proportion of cases in foreign-born TB persons increased from 27 to 42%. Although foreign-born persons represent an increasingly greater proportion of U.S. TB patients, the number of cases in foreign-born persons has not increased substantially in the past 6 years (Figure 1.5). The overall decrease in TB cases over this period reflects a substantial decline of cases in U.S.-born persons. Over this time there has been a 44% decrease in the number of cases in U.S.-born persons, while the number of foreign-born cases has increased by 4%. In 1998, foreign-born cases spent a median of 6 years in the U.S. prior to diagnosis.

TB cases among foreign-born persons varies by race/ethnicity, country of origin, and geographic location. As shown in Table 1.3, the majority of foreign-born TB patients are Asian/Pacific Islanders or Hispanic. This reflects the high rates of TB occurring in the country of birth for many of these individuals. In 1998, the top five countries of birth accounted for 58% of the foreign-born TB patients; 23% (1757) of foreign-born cases came from Mexico, 13% (968 cases) from the Philippines, 10% (748 cases) from Vietnam, 7% (503 cases) from India, and 5% (373 cases) from the Republic of China.

The incidence of tuberculosis in foreign-born persons has great regional variation within the U.S. as well. The incidence among foreign-born persons is higher in states that have many immigrants from countries with higher tuberculosis incidence rates (parts of Asia, Central and South America, and Africa). In 1998, the greatest number of foreign-born cases were reported in California (2682 cases), New York (1067 cases), Texas (677 cases), Florida (397 cases), and New Jersey (321 cases). Thirteen states reported ≥50% of TB cases in foreign-born persons in 1998; Hawaii reported the largest proportion of cases in foreign-born persons, i.e., 72% (129 cases).

B. Persons Infected with HIV

Once infected with *M. tuberculosis,* HIV coinfection is the strongest risk factor for progression to active TB; the risk of developing active disease among HIV-infected persons with latent TB infection

TABLE 1.3
Number of Reported Cases and Percentage Change by
Race/Ethnicity and Country of Birth, 1992 to 1998

	Reported Cases		Change from 1992 to 1998
	1992[a]	1998[b]	(%)
U.S.-born			
White, non-Hispanic	7043	3918	−44.4
Black, non-Hispanic	9010	4973	−44.8
Hispanic	2530	1293	−48.9
Asian/Pacific Islander	319	215	−32.6
American Indian/Alaskan Native	298	246	−17.4
Foreign-born			
White, non-Hispanic	540	560	+3.7
Black, non-Hispanic	591	842	+42.5
Hispanic	2828	2774	−1.9
Asian/Pacific Islander	3296	3393	+2.9
American Indian/Alaskan Native	1	7	+600

[a] For 1992, 35 white, non-Hispanics; 22 black, non-Hispanics; 79 Hispanics; and 34 Asian/Pacific Islanders with unknown origin not included.
[b] For 1998, 17 white, non-Hispanics; 16 Black non-Hispanics; 30 Hispanics; and 18 Asian/Pacific Islanders with unknown origin not included.

has been estimated to be as great as 10% per year, compared to 5 to 10% lifetime risk among TB-infected persons without HIV infection.[36-38]

In the early 1990s several large TB outbreaks occurred among HIV-infected persons. These outbreaks have been characterized by rapid evolution, high attack rates, and severe morbidity, as well as high mortality rates. Most of the reported outbreaks in the U.S. in the early 1990s involved drug-resistant tuberculosis[18, 19, 39, 40] and occurred in healthcare facilities and other institutions where HIV-infected persons congregated (e.g., residential facilities, prisons).[41-44] These outbreaks were attributed to the congregation of HIV-infected patients, failure to detect and effectively treat tuberculosis, delayed detection of drug resistance, delayed isolation precautions, and inadequate facilities for effective isolation. The rapid evolution of these outbreaks — in some, secondary cases appeared as soon as a month after exposure to a source case — meant that several generations of transmission could take place before control measures were implemented. Because of the high attack rates and the rapid progression from infection to disease, these tuberculosis outbreaks among HIV-infected persons were larger and progressed faster than typical tuberculosis outbreaks among persons not infected with HIV. Increasing awareness as well as prevention and control measures taken at healthcare facilities and other institutional settings have helped decrease the number of large institutional TB outbreaks.[45]

Because of the impact of HIV on the recent TB resurgence, information about HIV status was incorporated into tuberculosis case reporting in the U.S. beginning in 1993. Information on the HIV status of reported TB cases is limited. In 1998, only 3509 (55%) of 6365 TB case reports for persons 25 to 44 years of age had information on HIV status, and only 22 states reported HIV test results for at least 75% of TB patients in this age group. Excluding California and Rhode Island, which do not report HIV test results on the TB case report form, 69% of 25- to 44-year-old TB patients had HIV test results reported, 6% refused HIV testing, 11% were not offered testing, 4% had a test done but results were unknown to the health department, and 10% had an unknown HIV status. Among the states with results for ≥75% of cases in this age group, the proportion of TB cases in HIV-infected persons ranged from 0% (Montana, North Dakota, Vermont, and Wyoming) to 47% (Florida).

Information regarding the prevalence of TB and HIV coinfection is also available from sources other than the national TB surveillance system. In the U.S., cross matches between local and state TB registries and AIDS registries conducted between 1981 and 1991 found that 4.3% of TB patients matched to an AIDS case in the AIDS registry. When examined by year of report, the percentage of TB cases that matched with an AIDS case increased from 0.1% in 1981 to 9.5% in 1990.[46] In the most recent match between TB and HIV–AIDS registries, 14% of reported TB cases were listed in the AIDS or HIV registries.[47] The proportion of TB cases varied by reporting area from 0 to 31%, with the highest percentage of TB-HIV coinfection found in Connecticut, Florida, New Jersey, New York City, and Puerto Rico.

C. HOMELESS PERSONS

Risk factors for the acquisition of *M. tuberculosis* infection and active disease are common among the homeless.[48] While crowded shelters with insufficient ventilation contribute to TB transmission,[49] HIV infection, malnutrition, and alcohol and drug use increase the risk of developing active disease among those infected.[50-52] Once identified, cases of active TB can be challenging to manage in this transient population, and relapse or reactivation of disease and emergence of drug resistance may occur as a result of incomplete treatment. In addition, exogenous reinfection, although generally believed to be uncommon in the U.S., has been documented.[53]

Although it is difficult to determine the number of homeless individuals living in the U.S., information is collected regarding the percent of TB patients who were homeless (i.e., persons who lack customary and regular access to a conventional dwelling or residence, including residents of welfare hotels, congregate shelters, and transitional housing for the mentally ill) within the year prior to diagnosis. In 1994, the first year homeless status was routinely reported by the majority of reporting areas, 6.4% (1227 patients) were homeless. In 1998, 6.3% (1125 cases) of reported TB cases were homeless, suggesting little change since 1994.

D. INSTITUTIONALIZED PERSONS

1. Residents of Correctional Facilities

Another group at risk for TB includes inmates of prisons and jails.[54,55] Prisons and jails may draw from groups for which tuberculosis incidence rates are greater than the national average, and they also draw from groups at risk for HIV infection.[56-60] The "closed" prison environment, inadequate ventilation, and prolonged contact between inmates promote tuberculosis outbreaks.[61-63] In 1991 an extensive outbreak of multidrug-resistant tuberculosis in the New York State correctional system was attributed to delayed detection of tuberculosis, the late recognition of drug resistance, the inadequate isolation of patients who had contagious tuberculosis, the interprison transfer of sick or newly infected inmates, and the high prevalence of HIV infection.[64] Jails are a special problem; inmates may stay in jails long enough to become infected but not long enough to progress to active disease, and the jail might not be suspected as the site of transmission.[65,66]

In 1998, 3.6% (656 cases) of all TB patients were inmates of correctional facilities at the time of their diagnosis. Of these, 59% were inmates of local jails, 28% were state prisoners, 5% were federal prisoners, 1% were in juvenile facilities, and the remaining 6% were in other types of correctional facilities. It is difficult to obtain estimates of the number of potentially exposed persons for jails; however, the TB incidence rate for state and federal prisoners has been estimated for the 4-year period from 1993 through 1997 as 25/100,000, and 27/100,000, respectively.

2. Residents of Long-Term Care Facilities

Residents of long-term care facilities are at high risk for exposure to *M. tuberculosis* and additionally, the elderly in nursing homes have elevated incidence rates of TB due to reactivation of latent tuberculous infection and relapse of prior disease.[55,67] Some persons residing in long-term care facilities have chronic conditions, such as diabetes and cancer, which predispose them to developing active TB. The extent of transmission can be increased by the delayed diagnosis of infectious TB and may lead to outbreaks.[68]

In 1998, 3.5% (640 cases) of TB cases were residents of long-term care facilities. Of the 1998 TB patients who were residents of long-term care facilities, 54% were residents of nursing homes, 18% were residents of hospital-based facilities, 12% were in residential facilities, 5% were in mental health facilities, 3.5% were residents of alcohol or drug rehabilitation centers, and 7% were in other long-term care facilities.

E. Migrant Farm Workers

Another group at high risk for TB is migrant farm workers (MFW).[69] As with the other populations at high risk for TB, it is difficult to obtain population data necessary to determine incidence rates of disease for the entire group. However, information on MFW was collected by the national TB surveillance system beginning in 1993. Since then, 1422 TB cases have occurred among MFW, 211 in 1998. From data collected in a 29-state survey in the 1980s, the risk of TB was estimated to be six times greater in MFW than in the general U.S. population of employed adults. Two studies of MFW in the eastern part of the U.S. found TB rates among MFW to be 18 and 3000 times higher than the U.S. case rate.[70,71] Poor access to healthcare, lack of continuity of medical care, crowded living conditions, and birth in countries with high rates of TB are all factors contributing to high rates of TB in MFW.[69,70,72,73] Furthermore, it is difficult to supervise a complete course of antituberculosis chemotherapy for MFW because the patients and their contacts move seasonally; 20% of MFW reported from 1993 through 1997 did not complete therapy because they moved or were lost to follow-up.

VII. DISEASE CHARACTERISTICS

A. Diagnostic Criteria

As mentioned, TB can be diagnosed by clinical or laboratory means. According to data collected from 1993 through 1998, 81% of the reported TB cases were diagnosed by a positive culture, 1% by a specimen positive for AFB (acid-fast bacilli) when culture was not available, 12% were diagnosed by clinical case definition, and 6% did not meet the published case definition but were considered verified cases by the reporting areas (i.e., provider diagnosis). Diagnostic criteria differed greatly by age of patient. Children < 15 years old are more than four times as likely as adults to have provider-defined diagnoses, while adults are almost four times as likely as children to be diagnosed by positive culture.

B. Site of Disease

M. tuberculosis can infect many sites in the body; however, pulmonary disease is the most common site. In 1993 to 1998, 83% of cases had pulmonary involvement. Of those with pulmonary disease, 8% had extrapulmonary disease as well. Among persons with extrapulmonary involvement, pleural (17%) and cervical lymph nodes (16%) were the most common extrapulmonary major sites of disease among adults (15+ years of age), while among children (<15 years of age) cervical lymph nodes (24%), intrathoracic lymph nodes (23%), and meningeal disease (8%) were most common.

Among those with pulmonary involvement, 84% had sputum smear results reported. Of those, 52% were sputum smear positive for acid-fast bacilli. Sputum smear results differed greatly by age. Among adults with pulmonary involvement, 88% had sputum smear results and 53% of those were positive. Twenty-eight percent of children had sputum smear results reported and only 14% of those were sputum smear positive for AFB.

C. Mortality

Using death certificate data, the National Center for Health Statistics has reported that the number of deaths due to TB has decreased dramatically since 1953. In 1953, there were 19,707 deaths from TB for a rate of 12.4 per 100,000 population; in 1997, the most recent year for which data are currently available, 1166 TB deaths occurred for a rate of 0.4/100,000. The number of TB deaths and the TB death rate increased slightly during the TB resurgence, reaching a high in 1989 of 1970 deaths and a rate of 0.8 deaths per 100,000 before decreasing again.

In addition to death certificate data, information regarding whether the TB patient is alive at diagnosis or stops TB therapy because they have died has been reported to the CDC since 1993. This information helps identify factors associated with mortality among TB patients. However, this information is limited as it only records mortality at those two periods of time and the cause of death is not recorded. In the U.S., the vast majority of cases are alive at the time of diagnosis; only 4% of the 1993 to 1998 reported TB cases were dead at the time of their diagnosis. Of those who were dead at diagnosis, the median age at diagnosis was 67 years, much older than the median age of 44 years for the 96% of TB patients alive at the time of diagnosis. Among those who were alive at time of diagnosis, 10% stopped therapy before completion because they died, including 23% of those TB patients 65 years old and greater. For those less than 65 years old, HIV infection is a major factor associated with increased mortality; 28% of HIV-infected TB patients died before completing therapy vs. 3% of those known to be HIV negative at the time of diagnosis.

D. Drug-Resistant Tuberculosis

Antimicrobial susceptibility patterns of tuberculosis were once the focus of systematic surveys in the U.S. When the prevalence of primary drug resistance became very low and continued to decrease, surveillance for drug susceptibility patterns ceased.[74-76] Large outbreaks of MDR TB in several institutions raised the possibility that the prevalence of resistance was increasing.[19-21,77-81] In 1993, drug susceptibility information was incorporated in the TB report form. During this first year, 8.9% were resistant to at least INH (isoniazid) and 2.8% were MDR TB. In 1998, initial isolates for 13,477 (93%) of the 14,830 culture-positive U.S. cases reported to the CDC had drug susceptibility testing to at least isoniazid and rifampin performed. Of the 13,477, 1086 (8.0%) were resistant to at least isoniazid; of these, 150 (1.1%) were considered to be MDR TB as they were resistant to at least isoniazid and rifampin, thus demonstrating a reduction in the incidence of drug resistance, particularly MDR TB, over the 6-year period. Over this same period, foreign-born cases represented a growing proportion of the MDR TB cases. In 1993, foreign-born TB cases represented 31% of all MDR TB cases; in 1998, this percent had grown to 61%. New York (38 cases) and California (34 cases) reported 49% of the 150 MDR TB cases in 1998. Between 1993 and 1998, 45 states and the District of Columbia reported at least one MDR TB case. Since 1993, only 5 states, Maine, Montana, South Dakota, Vermont, and Wyoming, have reported no cases of MDR TB.

VIII. CONCLUSION

These data highlight several important trends in reported cases of TB in the U.S. For the sixth consecutive year, the total number of reported cases has decreased; however, the case rate remains above the year 2000 goal for TB elimination in the U.S. Despite the overall decline in reported TB cases, the number of foreign-born cases has not decreased and represents an increasing proportion of the total U.S. cases. Reported rates of drug resistance, especially MDR TB, have decreased, but MDR TB cases have been reported from almost every state between 1993 and 1998. Finally, HIV reporting to the national TB surveillance system, while continuing to improve, still remains incomplete. Renewed TB prevention and control efforts in the 1990s have helped end the TB resurgence of the late 1980s and early 1990s which was caused by the HIV epidemic, the spread of MDR TB, an increase in immigrants from countries with a high TB prevalence, and a deteriorated public health infrastructure. To reach the U.S. goal of TB elimination, we need to sustain efforts aimed at promptly identifying and treating all persons with TB. These efforts should focus on populations identified as at high risk for TB, including persons born in countries with high rates of TB and persons infected with HIV.

REFERENCES

1. Cantwell, M.F., Snider, D.E., Cauthen, G.M., and Onorato, I.M., Epidemiology of tuberculosis in the United States, 1985 through 1992, *JAMA*, 272, 535, 1994.
2. McKenna, M.T., McCray, E., Jones, J.L., Onorato, I.M., and Castro, K.G., The fall after the rise: tuberculosis in the United States, 1991 through 1994, *Am. J. Publ. Health*, 88, 1059, 1998.
3. Moore, M., Onorato, I.M., McCray, E., and Castro, K.G., Trends in drug-resistant tuberculosis in the United States, 1993–1996, *JAMA*, 278, 833, 1997.
4. Zuber, P.L.F., McKenna, M.T., Binkin, N.J., Onorato, I.M., and Castro, K.G., Long-term risk of tuberculosis among foreign-born persons in the United States, *JAMA*, 278, 304, 1997.
5. Centers for Disease Control and Prevention, Expanded tuberculosis surveillance and tuberculosis mortality — United States, 1993, *Morb. Mortal Wkly. Rep.*, 43, 361, 1994.
6. Centers for Disease Control and Prevention, Case definitions for infectious conditions under public health surveillance, *Morb. Mortal Wkly. Rep.*, 46, (No. RR-10), 40, 1997.
7. McCombs, S.B., Onorato, I.M., McCray, E., and Castro, K.G., Tuberculosis surveillance in the United States: case definitions used by state health departments, *Am. J. Publ. Health*, 86, 728, 1996.
8. Binkin, N.J., Vernon, A.A., Simone, P.M., McCray, E., Miller, B.I., Schieffelbein, C.W., and Castro, K.G., Tuberculosis prevention and control activities in the United States: an overview of the organization of tuberculosis services, *Int. J. Tuberc. Lung Dis.*, 3, 663, 1999.
9. Bloom, B.R. and Murray, C.J.L., Tuberculosis: commentary on a reemergent killer, *Science*, 257, 1055, 1992.
10. Brudney, K. and Dobkin, J., Resurgent tuberculosis in New York City, *Am. Rev. Respir. Dis.*, 144, 745, 1991.
11. McKenna, M.T., McCray, E., and Onorato, I., The epidemiology of tuberculosis among foreign-born persons in the United States, 1986–1993, *N. Engl. J. Med.*, 332, 1071, 1995.
12. Centers for Disease Control and Prevention, Progress toward the elimination of tuberculosis — United States, 1998, *Morb. Mortal Wkly. Rep.*, 48, 732, 1999.
13. Centers for Disease Control and Prevention, Tuberculosis morbidity — United States, 1992, *Morb. Mortal Wkly. Rep.*, 42, 696, 1993.
14. Centers for Disease Control and Prevention, Tuberculosis morbidity — United States, 1997, *Morb. Mortal Wkly. Rep.*, 47, 253, 1998.
15. Centers for Disease Control, A strategic plan for the elimination of tuberculosis in the United States, *Morb. Mortal Wkly. Rep.*, 38 (No. S-3), 1989.
16. Powell, K.E. and Farerm, L.S., The rising age of the tuberculosis patient: a sign of success and failure, *J. Infect. Dis.*, 142, 946, 1980.
17. Ussery, X.T., Valway, S.E., McKenna, M., Cauthen, G.M., McCray, E., and Onorato, I.M., The epidemiology of tuberculosis among children in the United States, 1985–1994, *Pediatr. Infect. Dis. J.*, 15, 697, 1996.
18. Eldin, B.R., Tokars, J.I., Grieco, M.H., Crawford, J.T., Williams, J., Sordillo, E.M., Ong, K.R., Kilburn, J.O., Dooley, S.W., Castro, K.G., Jarvis, W.R., and Holmberg, S.D., An outbreak of multidrug-resistant tuberculosis among hospitalized patients with the acquired immunodeficiency syndrome, *N. Engl. J. Med.*, 326, 1514, 1992.
19. Beck-Sague, C., Dooley, S.W., Hutton, M.D., Otten, J., Breeden, A., Crawford, J.T., Pitchenik, T.M., Woodley, C., Cauthen, G., and Jarvis, W.R., Hospital outbreak of multi-drug resistant *Mycobacterium tuberculosis* infections. Factors in transmission to staff and HIV-infected patients, *JAMA*, 268, 1280, 1992.

20. Coronado, V.G., Beck-Sague, C.M., Hutton, M.D., Davis, B.J., Villareal, N.P., Woodley, C.L., Kilburn, J.O., Crawford, J.T., Frieden, T.R., Sinkowitz, R.L., and Jarvis, W.R., Transmission of multidrug-resistant *Mycobacterium tuberculosis* among persons with human immunodeficiency virus infection in an urban hospital: epidemiologic and restriction length polymorphism analysis, *J. Infect. Dis.,* 168, 1052, 1993.

21. Fischl, M.A., Uttamchandani, R.B., Daikos, G.L., Poblete, R.B., Moreno, J.N., Reyes, R.R., Boota, A.M., Thompson, L.M., Cleary, T.J., and Lai, S., An outbreak of tuberculosis caused by multiple-drug-resistant tubercle bacilli among patients with HIV infection, *Ann. Intern. Med.,* 117, 177, 1992.

23. Connolly, M. and Nunn, P., Women and tuberculosis, *World Health Stat. Q.,* 49, 115, 1996.

24. De Voss, J.J., Rutter, K., Schroeder, B.G., and Barry, C.E., Iron acquisition and metabolism by mycobacteria, *J. Bacteriol.,* 181, 4443, 1999.

25. Gordeuk, V.Y., McKaren, C.E., MacPhail, A.P., Deichsel, G., and Bothwell, T.H., Associations of iron overload in Africa with hepatocellular carcinoma and tuberculosis: Strachan's 1929 thesis revisited, *Blood,* 87, 3470, 1996.

26. Murray, M.J., Murray, A.B., Murray, M.B., and Murray, C.J., The adverse effect of iron repletion on the course of certain infections, *Br. Med. J.,* 2, 1113, 1978.

27. Looker, A.C., Dallman, P.R., Carroll, M.D., Gunter, E.W., and Johnson, C.L., Prevalence of iron deficiency in the United States, *JAMA,* 277, 973, 1997.

28. Long, E.R., Constitution and related factors in resistance to tuberculosis, *Arch. Pathol.,* 32, 122, 1941.

29. Stead, W.W., Senner, J.W., Reddick, W.T., and Lofgren, J.P., Racial differences in susceptibility to infection by *Mycobacterium tuberculosis, N. Engl. J. Med.,* 322, 422, 1990.

30. Torchia, M.M., Tuberculosis among American Negroes: medical research on a racial disease, *J. Hist. Med.,* 32, 252, 1977.

31. Bloch, A.B., Rieder, H.L., Kelly, G.D., Cauthen, G.M., Hayden, C.H., and Snider, D.E., The epidemiology of tuberculosis in the United States, *Sem. Respir. Infect.,* 4, 157, 1989.

32. Rieder, H.L., Cauthen, G.M., Kelly, G.D., Bloch, A.B., and Snider, D.E., Tuberculosis in the United States, *JAMA,* 262, 385, 1989.

33. Snider, D.E., Jr., Salinas, L., and Kelly, G.D., Tuberculosis: an increasing problem among minorities in the United States, *Publ. Health Rep.,* 104, 646, 1989.

34. Ridzon, R., Kent, J.H., Valway, S., Weismuller, P., Maxwell, R., Elcock, M., Meador, J., Royce, S., Shefer, A., Smith, P., Woodley, C., and Onorato, I., Outbreak of drug-resistant tuberculosis with second-generation transmission in a high school in California, *J. Pediatr.,* 131:863, 1997.

35. Hennessey, K.A., Schulte, J.M., Cook, L., Collins, M., Onorato, I.M., and Valway, S.E., Tuberculin skin test screening practices among U.S. colleges and universities, *JAMA,* 280, 2008, 1998.

36. Murray, J.F., Tuberculosis and human immunodeficiency virus infection during the 1990s. *Bull. Int. Union Tuberc. Lung Dis.,* 66, 21, 1991.

37. Selwyn, P.A., Hartel, D., Lewis, V.A., Schoenbaum, E.E., Vermund, S.H., Klein, R.S., Walker, A.T., and Friedland, G.H., A prospective study of the risk of tuberculosis among intravenous drug users with HIV infection, *N. Engl. J. Med.,* 320, 545, 1989.

38. Selwyn, P.A., Sckell, B.M., Alcabes, P., Friedland, G.H., Klein, R.S., and Schoenbaum, E.E., High risk of active tuberculosis in HIV-infected drug users with cutaneous anergy, *JAMA,* 268, 504, 1992.

39. Centers for Disease Control, Nosocomial transmission of multidrug-resistant tuberculosis among HIV-infected persons — Florida and New York, 1988–1991, *Morb. Mortal Wkly. Rep.,* 40, 585, 1991.

40. Dooley, S.W., Villarino, M.E., Lawrence, M., Salinas, L., Amil, S., Rullen, J.V., Jarvis, W.R., Bloch, A.B., and Cauthen, G.M., Nosocomial transmission of tuberculosis in a hospital unit for HIV-infected patients, *JAMA,* 267, 2632, 1992.

41. Centers for Disease Control, Transmission of multidrug-resistant tuberculosis from an HIV-positive client in a residential substance-abuse treatment facility — Michigan, *Morb. Mortal Wkly. Rep.,* 40, 129, 1991.

42. Daley, C.L., Small, P.M., Schecter, G.F., Schoolnik, G.K., McAdam, R.A., Jacobs, W.R., Jr., and Hopewell, P.C., An outbreak of tuberculosis with accelerated progression among persons infected with the human immunodeficiency virus, *N. Engl. J. Med.,* 326, 231, 1992.

43. Centers for Disease Control, Transmission of multidrug-resistant tuberculosis among immunocompromised persons in a correctional system — New York, 1991, *Morb. Mortal Wkly. Rep.,* 41, 507, 1992.

44. Centers for Disease Control, Crack cocaine use among persons with tuberculosis — Contra Costa County, California, 1987–1990, *Morb. Mortal Wkly. Rep.*, 40, 485, 1991.

45. Blumberg, H.M., Watkins, D.L., Berschling, J.D., Antle, A., Moore, P., White, N., Hunter, M., Green, B., Ray, S.M., and MCGowan, J.E., Preventing the nosocomial transmission of tuberculosis, *Ann. Intern. Med.*, 122, 658, 1995.

46. Burwen, D.R., Bloch, A.B., Griffin, L.D., Ciesielski, C.A., Stern, H.A., and Onorato, I.M., National trends in the concurrence of tuberculosis and acquired immunodeficiency syndrome, *Arch. Intern. Med.*, 155, 1281, 1995.

47. Moore, M., McCray, E., and Onorato, I.M., Cross matching TB and AIDS registries: TB patients with HIV coinfection, United States, 1993–1994, *Publ. Health Rep.*, 114, 269, 1999.

48. Gelberg, L., Panarites, C.J., Morgenstern, H., Leake, B., Andersen, R.M., and Koegel, P., Tuberculosis skin testing among homeless adults, *J. Gen. Intern. Med.*, 12, 25, 1997.

49. Nardell, E.A., Tuberculosis in homeless, residential care facilities, prisons, nursing homes, and other close communities, *Semin. Respir. Infect.*, 4, 206, 1989.

50. Zolopa, A.R., Hahn, J.A., Gorter, R., Miranda, J., Wlodarczyk, D., Peterson, J., Pilote, L., and Moss, A.R., HIV and tuberculosis infection in San Francisco's homeless adults, *JAMA*, 272, 455, 1994.

51. Fujiwara, P.I. and Frieden, T.R., Tuberculosis epidemiology and control in the inner city, *Tuberculosis*, 1st ed., Rom, W.N. and Garay, S.M., Eds., Little, Brown, Boston, 1996, 99.

52. Torres, R.A., Sridhar, M., Altholz, J., and Brickner, P.W., Human immunodeficiency virus infection among homeless men in a New York City shelter. Association with *Mycobacterium tuberculosis* infection, *Arch. Intern. Med.*, 150, 2030, 1990.

53. Nardell, E., McInnis, B., Thomas, B., and Weidhaas, S., Exogenous reinfection with tuberculosis in a shelter for the homeless, *N. Engl. J. Med.*, 315, 1570, 1986.

54. Centers for Disease Control and Prevention, Prevention and control of tuberculosis in correctional facilities, *Morb. Mortal Wkly. Rep.*, 45 (No. RR-8), 1, 1996.

55. Hutton, M.D., Cauthen, G.M., and Bloch, A.B., Tuberculosis in nursing homes and correctional facilities: results of a 29 state survey, *Publ. Health Rep.*, 108, 305, 1993.

56. Braun, M.M., Truman, B.I., Maquire, B., DiFerdinando, G.T., Jr., Wormser, G., Broaddus, R., and Morse, D.L., Increasing incidence of tuberculosis in a prison inmate population, association with HIV infection, *JAMA*, 261, 393, 1989.

57. Salive, M.E., Vlahov, D., and Brewer, T.F., Coinfection with tuberculosis and HIV-1 in male prison inmates, *Publ. Health Rep.*, 105, 307, 1990.

58. Snider, D.E., Jr. and Hutton, M.D., Tuberculosis in correctional facilities, *JAMA*, 261, 436, 1989.

59. Kendig, N., Tuberculosis control in prisons, *Int. J. Tuberc. Lung Dis.*, 2 (Suppl 1), S57, 1998.

60. Curtis, R., Friedman, S.R., Neaigus, A., Jose, B., Goldstein, M., and Des Jarlais, D.C., Implications of directly observed therapy in tuberculosis control measures among IDUs, *Publ. Health Rep.*, 109, 319, 1994.

61. Valway, S.E., Richards, S.B., Kovacovich, J., Greifinder, R.B., Crawford, J.T., and Dooley, S.W., Outbreak of multidrug-resistant tuberculosis in a New York State prison, 1991, *Am. J. Epidemiol.*, 140, 113, 1994.

62. Stead, W.W., Undetected tuberculosis in prison: source of infection for community at large, *JAMA*, 240, 2544, 1978.

63. Centers for Disease Control and Prevention, Tuberculosis outbreaks in prison housing units for HIV-infected inmates — California, 1995-1996, *Morb. Mortal Wkly. Rep.*, 48, 79, 1999.

64. Centers for Disease Control, Transmission of multidrug-resistant tuberculosis among immunocompromised persons in a correctional system — New York, 1991, *Morb. Mortal Wkly. Rep.*, 41, 507, 1992.

65. MacIntyre, C.R., Kendig, N., Kummer, L., Birago, S., and Graham, N.M.H., Impact of tuberculosis control measures and crowding on the incidence of tuberculosis infection in Maryland prisons, *Clin. Infect. Dis.*, 24, 1060, 1997.

66. Bellin, E.Y., Fletcher, D.D., and Safyer, S.M., Association of tuberculosis infection with increased time in or admission to the New York City jail system, *JAMA*, 269, 2228, 1993.

67. Centers for Disease Control, Prevention and control of tuberculosis in facilities providing long-term care to the elderly, *Morb. Mortal Wkly. Rep.*, 39(No. RR-10), 7, 1990.

68. Stead, W.W., Lofgren, J.P., Warren, E., and Thomas, C., Tuberculosis as an endemic and nosocomial infection among the elderly in nursing homes, *N. Engl. J. Med.*, 312, 1483, 1985.

69. Centers for Disease Control, Prevention and control of tuberculosis in migrant farm workers, *Morb. Mortal Wkly. Rep.,* 41 (No. RR-10), 1, 1992.
70. Ciesielski, S.D., Seed, J.R., Esposito, D.H., and Hunter, D.H., The epidemiology of tuberculosis among North Carolina migrant farm workers, *JAMA,* 265, 1715, 1991.
71. Jacobson, M.L., Mercer, M.A., Miller, L.K., and Simpson, T.W., Tuberculosis risk among migrant farm workers on the Delmarva Peninsula, *Am. J. Public Health,* 77, 29, 1987.
72. Rust, G.S., Health status of migrant farm workers: a literature review and commentary, *Am. J. Public Health,* 80, 1213, 1990.
73. Meister, J.S., The health of migrant farm workers. *Occup. Med.: State Art Rev.,* 6, 503, 1991.
74. Snider, D.E., Jr., Cauthen, G.M., Farer, L.S., Kelly, G.D., Kilburn, J.O., Good, R.C., and Dooley, S.W., Drug-resistant tuberculosis (letter), *Am. Rev. Respir. Dis.,* 144, 732, 1991.
75. Villarino, M.E., Geiter, L.J., and Simone, P.M., The multidrug-resistant tuberculosis challenge to public health efforts to control tuberculosis, *Publ. Health Rep.,* 107, 616, 1992.
76. Simone, P.M. and Iseman, M.D., Drug-resistant tuberculosis: a deadly — and growing — danger, *J. Respir. Dis.,* 13, 960, 1992.
77. Ikeda, R.M., Birkhead, G.S., DiFerdinando, G.T., Jr., Bornstein, D.L., Dooley, S.W., Kubica, G.P., and Morse, D.L., Nosocomial tuberculosis: an outbreak of a strain resistant to seven drugs, *Infect. Cont. Hosp. Epidemiol.,* 16, 152, 1995.
78. Pearson, M.L., Jereb, J.A., Frieden, T.R., Crawford, J.T., Davis, B.J., Dooley, S.W., and Jarvis, W.R., Nosocomial transmission of multidrug-resistant *Mycobacterium tuberculosis.* A risk to patients and health care workers, *Ann. Intern. Med.,* 117, 191, 1992.
79. Jereb, J.A., Klevens, R.M., Privett, T.D., Smith, P.J., Crawford, J.T., Sharp, V.L., Davis, B.J., Jarvis, W.R., and Dooley, S.W., Tuberculosis in health care workers at a hospital with an outbreak of multidrug-resistant *Mycobacterium tuberculosis,* *Arch. Intern. Med.,* 155, 854, 1995.
80. Valway, S.E., Greifinger, R.B., Papania, M., Kilburn, J.O., Woodley, C., DiFerdinando, G.T., and Dooley, S.W., Multidrug-resistant tuberculosis in the New York State Prison System, 1990–1991, *J. Infect. Dis.,* 170, 151, 1994.
81. Frieden, T.R., Sherman, L.F., Maw, K.L., Fujiwara, P.I., Crawford, J.T., Nivin, B., Sharp, V., Hewlett, D., Jr., Brudney, K., Alland, D., and Kreisworth, B.N., A multi-institutional outbreak of highly drug-resistant tuberculosis: epidemiology and clinical outcomes, *JAMA,* 276, 1229, 1996.

2 Pathogenesis of Tuberculosis

Zahra Toossi, M.D. and Jerrold J. Ellner, M.D.

CONTENTS

I. OVERVIEW

Tuberculosis (TB) continues to plague mankind.[1] Current understanding of the pathogenesis of TB derives from experimental observations in infected animals and clinical observations in humans; pathologic and immunologic studies of the blood and tissues of infected animals and humans with TB; and microbiologic, biochemical, and molecular genetic studies of *Mycobacterium tuberculosis* (MTB) and its molecular constituents. There are corresponding levels of complexity to the understanding of TB. No single approach to the elucidation of the pathogenesis of TB encompasses its entirety. Recent progress in the understanding of TB and MTB allow a more complete view of how this pathogen interacts with the host.

This chapter begins with a brief review of the natural history of TB and virulence factors, and then focuses on the major new developments in the pathogenesis of TB. Native resistance to MTB will be discussed from the standpoint of animal studies; from *in vitro* studies of phagocytosis and T-cell-independent growth inhibition of MTB by mononuclear phagocytes; and from host genetic influences on acquiring MTB infection and development of TB. Acquired resistance to MTB will include discussions of T-cell-dependent macrophage activation and the role of CD4 and CD8 T cells, TH-1 and TH-2 type responses and $\gamma\delta$ T-cells in the control of MTB infection. The role of cytokines in macrophage activation and deactivation, in the modulation of T-cell responses, and in tissue damage and granuloma formation will be considered. Class I- and II-restricted cytotoxicity and their role in protection and immunopathology will be considered. Immune responses in human TB will be reviewed in the blood, pleural, and lung compartments separately. Finally, the impact of the human immunodeficiency virus-1 (HIV) on the development of TB and the effect of TB on HIV disease will be considered.

II. NATURAL HISTORY AND IMMUNOPATHOLOGY

Exposure to an individual with active pulmonary TB carries a substantial risk of acquiring infection. In household contacts of TB cases this risk is approximately 25%, although it can be higher if exposure is more prolonged in sustained close quarters. Inhalation of microdroplets (droplet nuclei) containing MTB may result in infection. Whereas large droplets are deposited in the upper airways (trachea and bronchi) and removed by mucociliary clearance mechanisms, smaller droplets (approximately 1 to 5 μm) that contain three or fewer bacilli may reach the alveoli.[2-6] Thus, the first line of defense against MTB is the alveolar macrophages that line the alveoli. MTB organisms that are able to survive the intracellular host defenses may grow to a limited extent within alveolar macrophages. During the time required to develop cell-mediated immunity (CMI) to contain bacterial growth, MTB infection can spread by lymphohematogenous dissemination to other sites, including the upper lung fields. With the development of cellular immunity (4 to 6 weeks), small granulomas form at the sites of initial MTB inoculation and dissemination, and the PPD skin test converts to positive. Alternatively, and especially if anti-MTB immune responses do not develop in a timely manner, the bacilli may continue to replicate and manifest as progressive primary TB.

In the majority of infected individuals, the development of CMI leads either to local destruction of MTB or persistence of the organisms in a latent phase within tissue macrophages, often for a lifetime. Foci with latent MTB infection are the sites of the original dissemination and include the apices of the lungs, the cortices of the kidneys, and the growing ends of long bones. A characteristic common to these tissues is a high local concentration of oxygen. *In vitro* studies confirm that higher levels of ambient oxygen increase intracellular MTB growth within human macrophages.[7] Conversely, as oxygen is gradually depleted from MTB cultures, the bacilli become tolerant to anaerobic conditions and enter a phase of nonreplicating persistence.[8] The mechanism of this shift in MTB metabolism leading to MTB dormancy, and the factors that permit or interfere with latent MTB infection, are not known. However, in approximately 5 to 10% of cases, due to the failure of immunologic surveillance against MTB infection, bacillary multiplication resumes and manifests as clinical TB.The pathologic hallmark of TB is granuloma formation in various tissues.[9] Tuberculous granulomas are characterized by accumulations of blood-derived macrophages, epithelioid cells (i.e., differentiated macrophages), multinucleated giant cells (i.e., fused macrophages with nuclei around the periphery of the giant cell [Langhan's type of giant cells]), and T lymphocytes around the periphery of the granuloma. Thus, mononuclear phagocytes, a term referring to blood monocytes and tissue macrophages, are the main cellular constituents of tuberculoid granulomas. Whether the epithelioid cells and multinucleated giant cells are adapted for mycobacterial killing is not known, although activated macrophages may be more microbicidal than blood monocytes.[10] In tuberculous granulomas, acid fast bacilli (AFB) are found almost exclusively within the mononuclear phagocytes.[9]

Latent foci of MTB infection retain the ability to undergo reactivation, most commonly in the lung. Thus, pulmonary TB is the most common manifestation of TB in adults. Less commonly, reinfection of an immunocompromised patient by new exposure to MTB, may result in TB. Pulmonary TB generally is localized to the apical and posterior segments of the upper lobes or the superior segment of the lower lobes.[11] Caseous necrosis of granulomas is the pathologic hallmark of both primary and reactivation TB. In some granulomas, liquefaction of the caseous material occurs and it is believed that MTB thrives better in this liquefied material than in caseous material. Caseous necrosis and cavity formation likely result from sensitivity to MTB proteins, since cavity formation is prevented in rabbits by desensitizing the animals with a tuberculin-active peptide before infecting them.[12] Healing occurs by fibrosis and contraction of the affected structures. A characteristic feature of TB is the concurrent findings of caseation, liquefaction, cavity formation, and fibrosis in lungs and other organs of affected individuals. It is assumed that hydrolytic enzymes and oxygen radicals produced by macrophages and neutrophils mediate much of the tissue damage with resulting liquefaction of granulomas and cavity formation.[9] In addition, cytokines (see below) produced by mononuclear cells at sites of active MTB infection most likely contribute to the pathology. However, the cellular and molecular basis for the immunopathology of TB is not fully understood.

III. VIRULENCE FACTORS

MTB virulence factors have been the subject of intense study over the last decade. Previously, three major virulence factors from the outer layer of the complex mycobacterial cell wall have been characterized molecularly: MTB cord factor, mycobacterial sulfolipids (SL), and mycosides. Cord factor(s) are trehalose-6,6'-dimycolates,[13] which when coated onto *Bacillus subtilis*, inhibit the migration of blood leukocytes and result in the death of mice when injected intraperitoneally.[14] The toxic effects of cord factor have been attributed to an interaction with mitochondrial membranes resulting in reduction of the activity of NAD-dependent microsomal enzymes in various tissues (lung, liver, and spleen).[15,16] One problem with ascribing cord factor with a major role in virulence is its occurrence in nonpathogenic as well as pathogenic species of mycobacteria.[17]

SLs are trehalose 2'-sulfates acylated with pthioceranic, hydroxypthioceranic, or saturated straight-chain fatty acids.[22,23] SLs kill mice when injected intraperitoneally and enhance the toxicity of cord factor.[18,19] The production of SLs by MTB correlates with their virulence; avirulent strains are deficient and virulent strains produce SL abundantly.[20] Importantly, SLs inhibit the fusion of MTB phagosomes with lysosomes, thus allowing MTB to evade host microbicidal molecules,[21] although inhibition of phagosome-lysosome fusion also may be mediated by other molecules, such as ammonia produced by MTB.[22]

Mycosides are species-specific glycolipids and peptidoglycolipids of mycobacteria.[23] The complex chemical stucture of many of these compounds has been elucidated by Brennan et al.[24] The surface glycolipids of MTB consist of trehalose-containing lipooligosaccharides. Biochemical differences between surface mycosides of virulent MTB and nonpathogenic strains of MTB have been described.[24,25] Also, certain mycosides of mycobacteria induce formation of an electron transparent zone in bacilli phagocytized by macrophages.[26] The role of the electron-transparent zone in protecting MTB against intracellular killing has not been determined.

More recently, an abundant lipoglycan of the mycobacterial cell wall, lipoarabinomannan (LAM), has been ascribed virulence function(s).[24] LAM inactivates phagocytic cells, inhibits induction of cellular genes, and counteracts macrophage activation. By modulating the cytokine milieu toward one of deactivation, LAM may allow the persistence of MTB within tissues.[20,27]

Other virulence factors relate to MTB genes that allow the organism to survive during the stationary phase.[28] For example, sigma factors, which are small transcription factors, regulate the transcriptional activity of MTB during its adaptive states, and may be indispensable for its virulence.[29] Of note is the recent description of a small (16 kDa) heat shock protein, α-crystallin (acr), by Barry et al.,[30] which has a chaperoning function. Acr-knockout MTB mutants are able to grow normally, but are unable to persist *in vivo*, and therefore may not establish latent foci. With the recent discovery of the MTB genome, the understanding of MTB virulence factors may accelerate.

IV. CONTROL OF MTB INFECTION: INNATE MECHANISMS

With regard to understanding the innate responses of the host against MTB, animal models and, more recently, *in vitro* studies of human mononuclear cells have been most informative.

A. ANIMAL MODELS

In his classic studies, Lurie et al. followed the course of mycobacteria in the lung and in other tissues after inhalation of bacilli by inbred-resistant vs. inbred-susceptible rabbits.[5,6] In resistant rabbits, alveolar macrophages contained more mycobacteria than susceptible rabbits initially, and the drainage of bacilli to tracheobronchial nodes also was higher. However, 7 days after inhalation of bacilli (BCG), susceptible rabbits had 20- to 30-fold higher levels of bacilli in the lung than resistant rabbits,[31] and died sooner. Other histopathologic characteristics of resistant rabbits were increased differentiation of macrophages, enhanced interstitial inflammation, and faster progression through the caseous process. By contrast, the susceptible phenotype was associated with higher pneumonic inflammation, and increased number and size of tubercles in the lung. In this model, the native resistance of alveolar macrophages, conceivably through increased uptake and killing of mycobacteria by macrophages, was believed to underlie the differences between the two phenotypes. After this first stage of mycobacterial infection, both resistant and susceptible rabbits develop a state of symbiosis with the organism during which mycobacteria grow logarithmically within cells, but the cells are not lysed.[6,31] It appears that recently recruited monocyte-derived macrophages[11] of early granulomata contain more bacilli than differentiated tissue macrophages. This finding has been attributed to the efficiency of phagocytosis, to undeveloped microbicidal mechanisms, and to less MTB-induced cytotoxicity of immature macrophages.[6,30] Similar rates of logarithmic growth, in this stage and when MTB growth reaches a plateau with the development of CMI (after 3 weeks), was seen in both groups of animals. Interestingly, as compared to susceptible rabbits, the resistant animals developed a more robust acquired immunity to MTB after BCG vaccination.[5] Thus it appears that native resistance may be important to the development of antimycobacterial immunity.

Studies of murine tuberculosis have shown the relative resistance of this animal model to MTB. However, much important information regarding the development of the CMI response, and the role of T cells in CMI has been derived from this animal model.[32] Recent studies have shown the importance of the route of infection in mice, i.e., mice infected with MTB by aerosolization were predisposed to chronic MTB infection of the lung.[33] In fact, after the initial period of containment of MTB growth subsequent to aerosol infection, a chronic granulomatous inflammation developed, followed by resumption of MTB growth, and subsequently, death.

In a guinea pig model developed by Smith et al., 3 weeks after infection by the aerosal route, bacilli had disseminated hematogenously back to the lung in large numbers.[34] However, both in the lung and at distant sites, CMI finally controlled bacillary growth. In fact, of all animal models of MTB infection, the guinea pig model most closely resembles human infection. In this model, protein calorie malnutrition leads to an inability to control MTB growth, poor granuloma formation, and lack of development of CMI. However, data from this model are scarce due to lack of immunological reagents.

More recently, *in vitro* human studies have shown the ease with which mononuclear phagocytes can get parasitized with MTB, i.e., the capacity to develop bacteriostasis but not to kill MTB, and the relative superiority of alveolar macrophages compared to monocytes in MTB growth containment. The contribution of cytokines and various pathways to MTB infection and growth containment is described below.

B. MONONUCLEAR PHAGOCYTES

MTB, phagocytosed by mononuclear phagocytes, can evade intracellular bactericidal mechanisms and replicate within the cell. It is agreed generally that the degree of virulence of MTB depends on its relative capacity to multiply within host macrophages. There are three ways that the growth of MTB may be inhibited; each involves mononuclear phagocytes and two require both lymphocytes and mononuclear phagocytes. First, mononuclear phagocytes have a natural armamentarium against the bacillus known as natural resistance (see later in this section). Second, mononuclear phagocytes can be activated to kill MTB through cytokines or other mediators, and when such activation is conferred by sensitized T lymphocytes, acquired resistance has evolved, i.e., cell-mediated immunity in its strictest sense. Third, mononuclear phagocytes containing bacilli may be lysed by cytotoxic T cells, but the *in vivo* significance for the containment of MTB by this mechanism is still not clear; presumably, bacilli that are released when macrophages are lysed may be taken up by more activated macrophages which are better able to control their growth (these latter two mechanisms will be discussed in following sections).

1. Phagocytosis and MTB Growth Containment

Swartz et al. have observed that different species of mycobacteria vary in their extent of ingestion by blood monocytes.[35] *M. avium* complex was taken up by many monocytes, whereas MTB, *M. kansasii,* and other mycobacteria were taken up by fewer monocytes. Serum was found to be important for the uptake of *M. avium* complex and to a lesser extent for MTB. Complement played a major role in this effect of serum.[35] Complement receptor 1 (CR1) and CR3 mediate phagocytosis of virulent MTB by blood monocytes, and the C3 component of complement is the bacterial-bound ligand.[36] More recently, Schlesinger et al. have shown that avirulent and virulent MTB are comparable in adherence and phagocytosis by macrophages, and thus phagocytosis alone is not a determinant of virulence.[37] Other host molecules shown to have roles in phagocytosis of MTB are the mannose receptor and cell surface fibronectin (reviewed in Reference 38); the MTB ligands for these molecules are LAM and the cell wall 30 kDa antigen, respectively.

Recently, Hirsch et al.[39] assessed the phagocytosis and growth inhibition of MTB by human alveolar macrophages in comparison to blood monocytes. Alveolar macrophages from healthy subjects phagocytosed and inhibited the growth of this strain of MTB significantly better than blood monocytes. Phagocytosis by alveolar macrophages was mediated through CR4 to a greater extent than CR1 or CR3. In addition, pulmonary surfactant protein A mediated enhanced phagocytosis of MTB, possibly through mannose receptors.[40] In a study by Hirsch et al., the basis for improved growth inhibition of MTB by alveolar macrophages was attributed, in part, to increased expression of tumor necrosis factor α (TNF-α) by alveolar macrophages after phagocytosis of the organisms.[39] Previous studies have shown that Bacillus Calmette-Guérin (BCG) and purified protein derivative

(PPD) stimulate the production of the macrophage activating molecule, TNF-α, by human alveolar macrophages,[41] and that the capacity to produce TNF-α by alveolar macrophages exceeds that of blood monocytes.[42] Since healthy subjects were the source of alveolar macrophages in these studies, the growth inhibition by these cells is a reflection of the natural resistance of these cells. However, in addition to production of macrophage-activating cytokines, MTB and its PPD and secreted components induce the production of macrophage deactivating cytokines such as transforming growth factor β (TGF-β) and IL-10.[43,44]

2. Lysosomal Enzymes

The fusion of the MTB phagosomes with the lysosomes that contain lysosomal enzymes (including proteases, lysozyme, acid hydrolases, and cationic proteins) is critical to the containment of the intracellular growth of bacilli. Flesch and Kaufmann have demonstrated that chloroquine, a compound that increases fusion of phagosomes and lysosomes, increases growth inhibition of *M. bovis* in mouse bone marrow-derived macrophages.[45] However, whereas both normal and immune serum increased phagosome-lysosome fusion in mouse peritoneal macrophages, growth of MTB was unaffected by such treatment.[46] The capacity of virulent strains of MTB to disrupt the phagosomal membrane and multiply freely in the cytoplasm of rabbit alveolar macrophages,[47] recently has been shown in a mouse model,[47a] indicating that MTB may evade the lysosomal contents totally. In another study, Armstrong and d'Arcy Hart have shown that only after the phagocytosis of nonviable MTB, but not intact MTB, will mouse peritoneal macrophage phagosomes fuse with lysosomes.[46] Furthermore, metabolic products of MTB, such as ammonia, inhibit lysosome movement and thereby phagolysosomal fusion, and reduce the potency of lysosomal contents. Thus, a defect in phagosome-lysosome fusion and/or the function of lysosomal contents subsequent to phagocytosis of MTB by mononuclear cells is apparent.

Lurie and Dannenberg's histologic studies in rabbits showed an increase in lysosomal enzymes in activated macrophages that appeared to be killing tubercle bacilli; the macrophages in granulomas with fewer AFB contained high numbers of lysosomal granules.[6,31] Moreover, lysosomes from activated cells contained higher levels of lysosomal contents, such as cathepsins. Therefore, it appears that the digestion of MTB by the lysosomal enzymes of activated macrophages is important in the control of bacillary growth.

3. Oxygen Radicals

Mitchison et al. have found that resistance of MTB to hydrogen peroxide is associated with virulence.[48] Other studies have shown, in contrast, that although resistance to peroxide is necessary, it is not sufficient for virulence, and differences in susceptibility to peroxidative killing do not correlate with MTB virulence.[49,50] Furthermore, Douvas et al. have shown that the increased growth inhibition of MTB by monocyte-derived macrophages as compared to monocytes was not associated with increased release of reactive oxygen species.[50] Although mycobacteria are sensitive to oxygen radicals, scavengers of toxic oxygen metabolites failed to influence the capacity of IFN-γ-activated mouse bone marrow macrophages to inhibit the growth of *M. bovis*.[45] A number of MTB products, such as LAM and PGLs, interfere with the production of oxygen radicals; however, presently, the relevance of reactive oxygen intermediaries (ROI) to MTB growth containment by phagocytes is not clear.

4. Reactive Nitrogen Intermediaries (RNI)

The L-arginine-dependent pathway to produce nitric oxide (NO) and other nitrogen intermediaries is important in the control of intracellular microbes, including MTB. Compelling evidence for the role of RNIs as mediators of microbicidal activity first was shown in the mouse model.[51] Recently, it has been shown that in NO synthase (NOS) knockout mice, MTB replication is dramatically increased. Also, the inhibitors of inducible NOS (iNOS) increased the growth of MTB in wild-type mice.[52] We recently have shown that MTB induces the production of NO in human alveolar macrophages (but not monocytes). Levels of NO produced by alveolar macrophages from different donors varied, and correlated inversely with intracellular MTB growth.[53]

C. Neutrophils

MTB persists as a facultative intracellular pathogen within macrophages and chronically produces granulomatous inflammation. Neutrophils are, however, among the first cells to arrive at the site of a tuberculous infection in humans.[54] Moreover, the injection of mycobacteria or their products into tissues or the pleural space of animals produces an inflammatory response, initally dominated by neutrophils, that can persist for up to 48 hours.[55] Neutrophils stimulated by BCG can release chemokines which result in the recruitment of monocytes into the pleural spaces of rabbits.[56]

Brown et al. have demonstrated first that neutrophils from healthy humans are capable of killing MTB *in vitro*.[57] The mechanism of killing of MTB by neutrophils, however, is not clear. May et al. have found that MTB induces a respiratory burst in neutrophils.[58] However, neutrophils from patients with chronic granulomatous disease killed MTB as well as neutrophils from healthy subjects, suggesting nonoxidative mechanisms are involved in the mycobactericidal process.[57] Furthermore, inhibitors of oxygen radical formation do not neutralize the killing of MTB by human neutrophils.[59] These data suggest that oxygen radicals are unlikely to be important in the killing of MTB by neutrophils. However, activation of neutrophils by IFN-γ or phorbol myristate acetate increased mycobacterial killing.[57,60] Although arginine-like activity has been described in neutrophils (Ellner, J.J., unpublished data), it is not clear whether this finding indicates that neutrophils mediate their effect through the production of NO. In summary, neutrophils are present only early in the response to MTB in animals and humans but may, through release of chemokines in response to mycobacteria, participate in the initial influx of monocytes from the blood to the infected region (usually the lung). Neutrophils also can kill MTB *in vitro*. However, whether they contribute to intracellular and/or extracellular killing of MTB is not known.

D. Natural Killer Cells

A role for natural killer (NK) cells in MTB containment by mononuclear phagocytes has been suggested both in the mouse model and in human *in vitro* systems. NK cells mediate their effect by production of IFN-γ and thereby activation of MTB-parasitized phagocytes, or by direct cytotoxicity against infected cells. Recently, Yoneda et al. have shown comparable activity of NK cells and CD4 cells in the containment of MTB growth in infected monocytes.[61]

E. g and d T Cells

T cells bearing γ or δ T-cell receptors (TCR), which comprise up to 5% of circulating T cells, also are able to produce IFN-γ and mediate cytolysis of MTB-infected targets. δ cells do not require major histocompatibility (MHC) antigens for activation and effector function. Both murine and human *in vitro* studies indicate a possible role for γδ T cells in natural resistance to MTB infection. Since γδ T cells often are found in the lung and epithelia, it has been suggested that they may act as a first line of defense against foreign antigens. γδ T cells have been shown to be expanded in the lymph nodes and the lung following exposure to mycobacterial antigens.[62,63] Havlir et al. have found that live MTB, but not heat-killed organisms, ingested by monocytes, selectively induce the expansion of human peripheral blood γδ T cells.[64] The ability of other infectious pathogens such as *Salmonella, Listeria monocytogenes,* and *Staphylococcus aureus* to induce γδ T cells further suggests that this subpopulation has a general role in the primary immune response to infectious agents.[65] Whether γδ T cells ultimately will prove to be of major importance in protection against MTB remains to be determined.

V. IMMUNOGENETICS OF TB

Recently, a significant number of findings have accrued to define the role of host genetic make-up in the susceptibility to MTB infection. Overall, immunogenetics may affect three separate phenomena during MTB infection. Despite the obvious interdependence of these phenomena, they may be viewed as affecting MTB infection independently. The host genetic make-up may affect: (1) the susceptibility to MTB infection, (2) the susceptibility to develop TB, or (3) the clinical expression of TB.

In the murine model of BCG infection, resistance has been attributed to the natural resistance-associated macrophage protein (Nramp1) gene.[65] Mice with a functional deletion of this gene are susceptible to other intracellular pathogens, such as salmonella and leishmania. Nramp1 is a membrane component of macrophage cytoplasmic vesicles, which translocates to the phagosome subsequent to phagocytosis.[66] Nramp1 also was believed to confer susceptibility to *M. tuberculosis* infection in mice.[65] In recent studies, however, North et al. have shown unequivocally that Nramp1 plays no role in the determination of resistance against MTB infection in mice.[67] In humans, the homolog for Nramp1 is on chromosome 2q35, and polymorphisms have been shown to be associated with susceptibility to leprosy.[68] A small effect of Nramp1 has been observed in resistance to TB.[69] In another recent study looking at polymorphisms of Nramp1 in a Brazilian population,[70] an effect of this gene on susceptibility to TB was not observed. However, as the genetic approach and the Nramp1 loci studied were different in these two reports, it is hard to compare these findings.

In humans, evidence for a genetic predisposition to develop fatal mycobacterial infections has been established recently. Patients with severe recurrent atypical mycobacterial or salmonella infections have been shown to have mutations in their IFN-γ or IL-12 receptor genes.[71-73] Earlier studies have shown that blacks are more likely than whites to convert their tuberculin skin test to positive after exposure to a case of TB in an institutional setting.[74] Also, identical twins and blood relatives in a household with a case of TB are more likely to be concordant for disease than nonidentical twins and nonblood relatives.[75] Also, TB siblings in India demonstrate excess haplotype sharing.[76]

Several efforts have been made to show an association between HLA phenotype and TB; the results have been widely divergent. For example, expression of some HLA-B and HLA-DR2 antigens in various populations is associated with the development of TB. These antigens include B8, Bw15, Bw35, B27, and DR2.[77-82] The association of other Class I and Class II MHC phenotypes with TB have been reported in other populations.[82-86] Each of these studies was performed on unrelated subjects. Because there was no *a priori* hypothesis that a specific HLA type was associated with TB, the statistical analysis is questionable as it did not correct for the multiple alleles under study. The fact that different phenotypes identified in disparate populations are associated with TB is not discouraging in itself, since the HLA genes may be in linkage disequilibrium with one or a few genes that determines susceptibility to TB. Linkage studies of HLA phenotypes among multiple family members with or without TB or tuberculous infection, are required to confirm further the genetic predisposition for resistance or susceptibility to MTB in humans.

Cox et al. have assessed HLA-DR in a group of Mexican Americans with TB.[87] There was no association of a Class II MHC locus with disease or tuberculin skin test reactivity. Of interest, however, was a relationship between HLA-DR and *in vitro* lymphocyte responses to PPD. In fact the haplotype HLA-B14-DR1 was associated with low blastogenic responses. This is of considerable interest since this haplotype is associated with nonclassical adrenal 21-hydroxylase deficiency;[88] the gene for this abnormality maps to chromosome 6, within the Class II MHC, and is a trait that is associated with altered expression of HLA-DR1 such that there is failure to activate alloreactive or Class II restricted T-cell clones.

Pathologic studies show that TB is a more aggressive disease in blacks. TB also reportedly is more difficult to treat in black than in white people.[89-92] The incidence is higher among people of Asian origin than white people in the United Kingdom.[93] The basis for the epidemiologic and clinical observations of differences in susceptibility to TB among races of people, however, is far from understood. Crowle and Elkins addressed this issue by studying the growth of MTB in monocytes and monocyte-derived macrophages from black and white people.[94] Both monocytes and monocyte-derived macrophages from black people killed MTB better after phagocytosis, but significantly less well during culture thereafter, especially in the presence of black donor serum. Furthermore, the macrophage activating factor 1,25-(OH)-vitamin D3 provided less protection against the growth of tubercle bacilli in macrophages from black compared to white donors. Although these data implicate a genetic predisposition to the development of TB observed among black people, larger studies will be required to confirm this observation and to understand more fully the basis for the susceptibility.

An interesting link between genetic and environmental factors in the racial predisposition to TB was noted by Davies in an effort to explain the increased incidence of TB among Asians compared to white people in the United Kingdom.[93] Metabolites of vitamin D activate macrophages to kill MTB, but food in the United Kingdom is not supplemented with this vitamin. Thus, a dietary deficiency in vitamin D may predispose to the development of TB. Recently, polymorphisms in the vitamin D receptor gene were found to contribute to the susceptibility to TB in this population, particularly in combination with dietary deficiencies (Wilkinson, personal communication). This study, underscores the importance of the cumulative effect of genetic and environmental factors in the predisposition to TB.

In a recent study of Indians in the United Kingdom, we found that polymorphisms in the IL-1 receptor antagonist (IL-1Ra) were associated with the clinical expression of TB; IL-1Ra allele (A) A2 positive patients had a lower incidence of pleural and peritoneal TB, and reduced PPD skin test reactivity. This polymorphism, however, was similar in TB patients and their healthy household contacts, indicating that it did not have an effect on the development of TB.[95] Thus, a genetic basis for the development of clinical forms of TB exists.

VI. ACQUIRED RESISTANCE TO MTB

A. CELL-MEDIATED IMMUNITY

CMI is a consequence of the activation of macrophages by products of sensitized T lymphocytes such as IFN-γ. In general, cellular immune responses are initiated by exposure to a foreign antigen. The antigen is taken up, processed, and presented on the surface of antigen-presenting cells (accessory cells), such as macrophage and dendritic cells, to T lymphocytes.

Subsequently, T-cell activation and proliferation in response to the presented antigen occurs if such presentation is accompanied by HLA molecules on the surface of antigen-presenting cells as well as by amplifying cytokines such as IL-1 and IL-6. CD4 helper T cells react with Class II HLA molecules, whereas CD8 cytotoxic/suppressor T cells react with Class I HLA molecules. The interaction of antigen, T cells, and antigen-presenting cells results not only in the immediate proliferation of T cells and cytokine release but also in the development of sensitized or memory T cells that will respond to the antigen within 1 or 2 days of subsequent exposure. Cytotoxic effector cells are a second effector arm and may lyse overburdened macrophages.

Evidence for a definitive role for CMI in acquired resistance to MTB infection initially came from animal studies; specific antisera did not confer passive protection to mycobacterial antigens whereas protection was conferred by the transfer of T cells.[96-99] Over the last 2 decades, the occurence of TB in HIV-infected subjects has underscored the importance of CMI in resistance to MTB. Animal and human studies have continued to define the role of CMI in the host response to MTB.[100] However, no support of a role for the humoral immune response in the protection against MTB has been found. However, circulating levels of immunoglobulin G (IgG) generally increase during active tuberculosis[101,102] and, in fact, levels rise for 1 to 2 months during therapy, then fall, but remain detectable for 1 to several years.[103] IgM antibodies which are directed at polysaccharide antigens of MTB, do not correlate with active TB.[101] However, a role for humoral responses in the immunopathogenesis of tuberculosis still is possible.

Koch reported in 1891 that guinea pigs infected for 4 to 6 weeks with MTB and then challenged intracutaneously with a small number of virulent bacilli developed a localized area of induration and necrosis at the dermal inoculation site within 48 hrs.[104] The Koch phenomenon is the classical tuberculin delayed-type hypersensitivity reaction (DTH). A half-century later, Chase demonstrated that tuberculin DTH was transferred by lymphocytes.[105] Animal studies have indicated that CMI (protective immunity) and DTH are mediated by different T cell subsets, although they occur concurrently.[106] The argument that DTH and protective immunity are dissociable stems from studies demonstrating that animals can be desensitized without loss of protection; they can be rendered hypersensitive without causing an increase in protection; and certain fractions of tubercle bacilli incur resistance without producing cutaneous hypersensitivity.[107] Furthermore, Orme and Collins have demonstrated that DTH and protective antituberculous immunity are mediated by separate subpopulations of T lymphoctes in mice (Ly-1 for DTH and Ly-2 for protection).[106] In humans, protection and DTH are linked epidemiologically in that tuberculin skin test-positive subjects are relatively resistant to exogenous reinfection.[108]

Perhaps Rook summarized this issue of the relationship between protective immunity and DTH best by acknowledging their complexity.[109] Thus, it appears that DTH and CMI are dissociable yet overlapping and complex events, and are linked by mononuclear cells to the expression of an intricate network of suppressive and injurious vs. beneficial cytokines, with cross-modulatory capacity. This scenario is complicated further by the accumulating evidence that CMI is differentially expressed in various tissues. The following sections seek to summarize the knowledge to date about the functions of each of the major cellular players in response to MTB or its products *in vitro* and in patients with TB.

B. PROTECTIVE IMMUNITY AND T-LYMPHOCYTE-DEPENDENT MACROPHAGE ACTIVATION

1. Animal Studies

Immunization of mice with BCG results in the acquisition of the ability of splenic lymphocytes to transfer protective immunity adoptively after an aerogenic challenge with virulent MTB. Furthermore, immunization with live- but not heat-killed organisms generates protective immunity in mice.[110] Heat-killed organisms transfer nonspecific resistance and DTH. These data suggest that products of metabolically active mycobacteria may be particularly important in the protective response against MTB. Cooper et al. have shown that the memory immune response to MTB develops slowly in the lung following an aerosol challenge, but despite its strength, does not protect against the reestablishment of infection.[111]

2. CD4 AND CD8 SUBSETS

During the course of intravenous infection with MTB, protective CD4 lymphocytes appear early in the spleen, produce large quantities of IFN-γ, and are associated temporally with the onset of bacterial elimination; cytolytic T cells appear later and are less clearly associated with a role in protective immunity.[112] Depletion experiments using monoclonal antibodies against CD4 and CD8 cells in mice indicate that protection against mycobacteria can be conferred by both CD4[112-114] and by CD8[114] T lymphocytes. In mice, however, there is evidence of a functional separation of CD4 lymphocytes into IFN-γ secreting Type 1 (TH-1) and IL-4 (and IL-5, IL-10, and IL-13) secreting Type 2 cells.[115] TH-1 and TH-2 cytokines also are cross-modulatory. In mice, TH-1 CD4 cells confer protection against intracellular pathogens, including MTB.

Although the mechanism by which CD4 and CD8 T cells protect mice against subsequent challenge with MTB still is not totally clear, studies indicate that there are two potential mechanisms for protection. Secretion of macrophage-activating cytokines such as IFN-γ, and possibly other molecules such as granulocyte-macrophage colony stimulating factor, induce MTB growth inhibition within macrophages. Recent studies using mice with genetic disruption of IFN-γ, have shown the absolute necessity for this TH-1 cytokine in the control of MTB infection.[116,117] The other mechanism by which T cells may be protective is by cytotoxicity for mycobacterial-laden macrophages. Thus, Class I MHC dysfunctional mice were more susceptible to MTB infection.[118] However, mice with genetic disruption of perforin, a molecule involved in CD8 cytotoxicity, did not demonstrate enhanced susceptibility to MTB infection.[119]

3. Human Studies

a. T-Cell Responses of Healthy Subjects

MTB-infected persons are identified on the basis of a positive tuberculin PPD skin test. As noted, such infected individuals are relatively immune to exogenous reinfection and therefore protective T cells are likely to be present in their blood as well as in other compartments. Since the blood is the most accessible source in humans, the reactivity of blood T cells to mycobacterial antigens has been assessed most readily. Overall, these studies have shown the prominence of T cells in the production of cytokines, in particular IFN-γ, and cytotoxicity to MTB-infected mononuclear phagocytes.[120] However, as the antigenic repertoire of MTB is shared to a large extent with other mycobacteria, including environmental mycobacteria and BCG, these immunologic responses have to be understood in the context of the mycobacterial sensitization of the subjects recruited to these *in vitro* studies. In this regard, *in vitro* studies of household members of cases of tuberculosis may be most informative. In particular, studies of these households may allow analysis of responses over the spectrum of MTB infection, based on epidemiologic characterization. Preliminary results from one such study indicates a correlation of PPD skin test conversion with IFN-γ production in response to MTB culture filtrate (Whalen, personal communication). However, to date, T-cell responses of PPD skin test-reactive household contacts to a few MTB antigens have been used to understand the responses of TB patients (see below).

Bronchoalveolar lavage has allowed access to the immune cells that protect the alveoli. Studies of lung cells from healthy household members of TB cases may finally allow identification of important MTB protective mechanisms and antigens. Recently, Tan et al. have demonstrated that bronchoalveolar lymphocytes were prominent in the cytolytic lysis of MTB-infected alveolar macrophages.[121]

b. Pleural TB

Pleural TB generally is a self-limited process, suggesting that immune responses in this form of paucibacillary disease are highly protective.[122] However, 60% of patients with pleural TB present later with reactivation TB, indicating that the protection is compartmentalized to the pleural space alone. Pleural fluid from patients with pleural TB contains increased numbers of MTB-reactive CD4 T lymphocytes compared to blood,[122,123] and these cells are predominantly of the CD4+CDw29+ T-cell phenotype, which are thought to represent memory T cells.[124] Fujiwara et al. have shown that the frequency of antigen-reactive blood lymphocytes in patients with tuberculous pleurisy is normal, whereas the frequency is increased in pleural fluid.[125] Therefore, the increase in pleural fluid antigen-reactive CD4 T cells may be the result of *in situ* expansion rather than sequestration of such cells from the circulating pool. Despite adequate numbers of antigen-reactive T cells, however, the response of blood mononuclear cells to PPD in a third of patients is depressed relative to healthy tuberculin reactors and relative to the pleural fluid responses in the same patients.[126] This finding is due to the presence of suppressive monocytes (see below) in the blood but not the pleural fluid. Pleural fluid also contains several fold increased levels of IFN- γ, TNF-α, and 1-25-dihydroxycholecalciferol (vitamin D) relative to serum,[127] consistent with the vigorous and effective local immune response.

Since local protective mechanisms are effective in containing the pleural infection despite the inadequacy of the systemic response, Wallis et al. sought to identify potential protective antigens using cells from the pleural fluid.[128] Upon transformation with Epstein Barr virus, pleural fluid B lymphocytes from two subjects with pleural TB spontaneously elaborated immunoglobulins. The frequency of MTB-reactive clones was 54% and 9% in these two subjects. Most (83%) of the clones secreted IgM, and the remainder IgG, antibodies. Western blot analysis using these antibodies identified predominantly a 31.5 kDa band reactive to MTB culture filtrate. The 30 kDa alpha antigen (antigen 6) is a secreted mycobacterial protein, which has been shown to be protective (see below).

C. ANTIGENIC TARGETS OF THE T-CELL RESPONSE TO MTB

A number of mycobacterial antigens have been characterized molecularly that stimulate T cells in tuberculin reactors. Due to the complexity of MTB infection, and the enormous heterogeneity of the human immune response, antigens that are targets of protective immunity still are not fully identified. Host responses at different stages of MTB infection are likely to be directed at particular MTB antigens, which in turn may induce various degrees of anti-MTB immunity.[129] It also is possible that the heterogeneity in antigens recognized by T cells at least partly reflects the diversity of T-cell subpopulations and functions.

Initial studies identified human responses to highly conserved bacterial and eukaryotic heat-shock proteins, such as the 65 and 71 kDa proteins of MTB. Blastogenic responses of human blood T cells to these antigens have been reported in some, but not all studies.[130,131] Animal studies confirm that these antigens do not appear to be major targets of protective T-cell responses.[128] They are somatic antigens; murine T cells that confer protective immunity against tuberculosis do not recognize these molecules. However, the heat shock proteins may be involved in autoimmune processes targeted to peptides shared by mycobacteria and humans, and thereby in MTB-associated immunopathology. The 65 kDa heat-shock protein of BCG is a target molecule for CD4 cytotoxic T cells that in turn lyse human monocytes pulsed with this protein.[130] However, only 20% of BCG vaccinees respond to this 65 kDa protein.

Another approach to define targets of the T-cell response to MTB has been to separate lysates and filtrates of MTB by physicochemical techniques and assess the relative reactivity of T cells to the separated fractions. The most consistent finding has been heterogeneity of the targets of the human T-cell response. For example, we found that T cells from tuberculin-positive healthy donors showed peaks of reactivity to fractions of culture filtrate of MTB H37Rv of 30, 37, 44, 57, 71, and 88 kDa.[132] Western immunoblotting indicated that three of these fractions contained previously defined antigens (30, 64, and 71 kDa). This technique does not allow determination of whether these previously identified proteins account for the activity found in the respective fractions. Schoel et al. have found numerous and diverse responses to 400 fractions prepared by 2-D gel electro-phoresis of lysates of MTB, underscoring the extensive heterogeneity of the mycobacterial antigen targets of human T cells.[133]

As protective immunity is conferred by living MTB only, the search for a protective antigen has focused primarily on secreted, not somatic, MTB antigens. Of the wide variety of secreted mycobacterial proteins identified,[134] the 85 complex of MTB is the subject of intense interest. The 85 complex is a group of three major extracellular antigens of MTB encoded by separate genes and secreted by actively proliferating MTB cultures.[135-139] Two of these antigens, 85A and 85B, bind to fibronectin and are of molecular weights 30 to 32 kDa. Antigen 85B is identical to a previously recognized MTB antigen termed antigen 6, or the alpha antigen,[140] the gene of which has been cloned by Matsuo et al.[141] This protein, which will be designated 30 kDa here, contains specific and cross-reactive determinants, stimulates blastogenesis and IFN-γ production by T cells from healthy donors, and elicits DTH in sensitized guinea pigs. Immunization with 85 complex proteins confers protection against repiratory challenge with MTB in guinea pigs.[142] Also T-cell responses to the 30 and 32 kDa antigens are preserved in tuberculin reactors, but not in patients with active tuberculosis.[143] It is possible that the 30 kDa antigen is involved in virulence[144] and/or immunosuppressive circuits.[44] The 30 kDa alpha antigen recently has been identified as MTB mycolyl transferase.[145]

D. Cytokines in Resistance to MTB and Immunopathology of TB

MTB and its components are potent inducers of cytokine production by monocytes/macrophages. Initial studies have shown that PPD directly stimulates monocytes to produce IL-1,[146] TNF-α,[41] IL-2R,[147] and TGF-β.[148] Also, purified proteins of MTB culture filtrate, such as the 58 kDa antigen (identified as MTB glutamine synthetase[149,150]), are potent inducers of TNF-α. Binding of fibronectin by the 30 kDa antigen enhances cytokine production by monocytes[144] and, therefore, the interaction of MTB and the host may lead to further *in situ* amplification of cytokines. Furthermore, the 30 kDa antigen induces both IL-10[44] and TGF-β.[43] MTB and its cell wall component, LAM, also induce TGF-β.[27] Therefore, it appears that the cytokine milieu of the tuberculous lesion, containing mycobacteria and its constituents, may be particularly biased to excess expression of TGF-β. In fact, immunoreactive TGF-β was present both in Langhans' giant cells and epithelioid cells of tuberculous granulomas of patients with untreated tuberculosis.[151]

1. TNF-a and TGF-b in Resistance to MTB, Granuloma Formation, and Tissue Damage

Rook first suggested in 1983 that the secretory products of mononuclear phagocytes may induce the characteristic symptoms (fever, weight loss) and tissue necrosis of TB.[152] Whereas TNF-α is the most likely candidate, other cytokines such as TGF-β have also been associated with cachexia.[153] Although both TGF-β and TNF-α may be involved in tissue damage, stimulation of collagenase production by fibroblasts, activation of endothelial cells by TNF-α, and inhibition of endothelial growth by TGF-β have been reported. Additionally, TGF-β promotes fibrosis,[154] and excess TGF-β has been implicated in the pathogenesis of a number of diseases associated with fibrosis.[155]

TNF-α may have beneficial as well as detrimental effects. TNF-α leads to the inhibition of growth of *M. avium* in human monocytes and monocyte-derived macrophages. TNF-α activates macrophages through enhancement of both ROI and RNI.[156] Bermudez et al. have demonstrated that injection of TNF-α with or without IL-2 inhibits the growth of *M. avium* complex *in vivo*.[157] The role of TNF-α, however, in the intracellular growth containment of MTB by mononuclear phagocytes is not totally clear. The combination of IFN-γ, calcitriol, and TNF-α, however, decreased the growth of MTB in blood monocytes.[158] TNF-α is an important mediator of growth inhibition of MTB by human alveolar macrophages.[39] Together with the heightened production of TNF-α,[42] and the limitation of production of the macrophage-deactivating cytokine, TGF-β,[159] alveolar macrophages may be poised to inhibit initial MTB growth. Since IFN-γ enhances the production and effects of TNF-α, the MTB growth inhibitory effect of TNF-α may be even greater after the development of CMI. By contrast, pretreatment of human blood monocytes with TGF-β increases intracellular mycobacterial growth. As noted, MTB induces TGF-β, and through autoinduction, TGF-β may amplify its own production at sites of MTB infection.[43]

In addition, the local synthesis of TNF-α correlates with granuloma formation in mice infected with BCG, and injection of anti-TNF-α antibody has been shown to decrease the number and size of granulomas and the development of epithelioid cells, allowing for massive replication of BCG.[160] Granuloma formation is critical to the containment of mycobacteria. The effect of TGF-β on the formation of granulomas presently is not known. However, since TGF-β inhibits the production of a number of chemokines, its effect may be one of altering the cellularity of granulomas. Overall, the balance of production of deactivating and activating cytokines as well as other products of the cellular constituents of granulomas likely contributes to the fate of infecting mycobacteria within them and ultimately to the expression of disease.

2. Macrophage Activation by IFN-g at Sites of MTB Infection

Murine peritoneal macrophages respond to IFN-γ by increasing their control of the replication of MTB.[161,162] Murine bone marrow macrophages also are activated by IFN-γ for increased containment of MTB, but the response to IFN-γ is specific to the strain of MTB used; some are more affected than others. In contrast to these animal studies, Douvas et al. have reported that IFN-γ does not activate growth containment of MTB in human blood monocyte-derived macrophages and, in fact, enhances MTB growth.[163] Rook et al., however, have found that although IFN-γ has little effect on MTB growth inhibition in human blood monocytes, it enhances MTB growth inhibition by monocyte-derived macrophages.[164] We found a modest effect of IFN-γ on MTB growth inhibition by human monocytes.[165] The mechanism by which IFN-γ exerts its macrophage activation is partly through induction of the enzymes necessary for conversion of 25-hydroxyvitamin D3 to the active metabolite of vitamin D, i.e., 1,25-dihydroxyvitamin D3.[13266] This metabolite in turn induces the differentiation of monocytes into macrophages with increased capacity to contain MTB growth. In addition, IFN-γ induces the production of RNIs which have been found to be bacteriocidal against MTB.[51] Bermudez has shown that TGF-β produced by monocytes upon ingestion of *M. avium* blocks the activity of IFN-γ.[167] This effect of TGF-β may in part be secondary to inhibition of the expression of IFN-γ receptors or the IFN-γ response. In MTB-infected human monocytes, the modest growth inhibition by TNF-α and IFN-γ were mitigated by TGF-β.[165] In addition, neutralization of TGF-β activity enhanced MTB growth containment.[168] Inhibition of iNOS and, thereby, reduced production of NO, may in part be the basis for macrophage deactivation by TGF-β.[169]

In addition, TGF-β inhibits the production of IFN-γ by T cells in response to MTB and other stimuli.[170] This effect occurs in part by counteracting the TH-1 promoting cytokine, IL-12, which is necessary for induction of IFN-γ expression.

E. CLASS II-RESTRICTED CYTOTOXICITY — ROLE IN PROTECTION AND IMMUNOPATHOLOGY

As noted, cytolytic T lymphocytes (CTL) appear during the course of experimental MTB infections.[114] Most of the support for CTL as an effector mechanism in MTB are based on *in vitro* studies. Blood T lymphocytes from MTB or *M. leprae*-infected individuals are cytotoxic for monocytes pulsed with mycobacterial antigens. The cytotoxicity was found to be a property of CD4 T cells. Recently, Boom et al. demonstrated that CD4 T-cell clones from PPD-reactive individuals were cytotoxic to mycobacterial antigen-pulsed or MTB-infected monocytes.[171] The cytotoxicity was independent of the profile of cytokines released by these clones (IL-2 vs. IL-4) and was a common property of these T-cell clones.

CD4 blood lymphocytes and clones from BCG-vaccinated subjects have been shown to be cytotoxic to mycobacterial-antigen pulsed monocytes.[172] Interestingly, the cytotoxic CD4 clones also suppressed proliferation of BCG-specific T-cell clones in response to BCG. Whether the suppression of T-cell responses was a consequence of cytotoxicity for antigen-presenting cells or direct suppression of T-cell responses was not resolved by this study. Macrophages that have ingested MTB or have been pulsed with soluble products such as PPD are targets of the CTL response.[130,172] Recent studies have indicated that human alveolar lymphocytes that were expanded *in vitro* by IL-2 and PPD performed well both in Class I- and Class II-mediated cytotoxicity against MTB-pulsed target cells.

Most investigators have speculated that the cytotoxicity mediated by CD4 cells may be a default mechanism by which MTB is released from overburdened and, therefore, dysfunctional effector cells. Presumably, once the organisms are released, they will be ingested and killed by fresh monocytes drawn to the fray. Alternatively, CTL, by lysing host cells, must be considered a factor in immunopathology. Clearly, additional *in vivo* studies in experimental animals will be necessary to resolve the relative importance of these two diverse sequelae of CTL.

VII. IMMUNE RESPONSES IN HUMAN TUBERCULOSIS

A. ANERGY

From 17 to 25% of patients with active TB are unresponsive to PPD skin tests.[173-175] In a more recent population study in which TB was newly introduced into the community, the prevalence of

TB morbidity and mortality were high, and tuberculin anergy was present in as much as 50% of patients.[176] These data indicate that the expression of anergy in a population may depend upon the length of time that they are exposed to TB. In patients with pulmonary TB, tuberculin anergy correlates with the activity of TB; patients with far-advanced disease have a higher frequency of tuberculin anergy. Tuberculin anergy correlates with measurements of *in vitro* T-cell responses (see below).

B. T-Cell Responses

In vitro blastogenic responses of blood T cells to PPD are absent in approximately 40% of patients with active TB, including most skin test-nonreactors and some reactors.[177-181] Hyporesponsiveness to mycobacterial antigens has been described in various geographic areas and, therefore, seems to be relatively constant regardless of prior immunization with BCG, etc. Several studies have indicated that the responses to nonmycobacterial antigens and mitogens are intact, so that depression of tuberculin reactivity is relatively specific.[177-183] The basis for the lower mononuclear cell responsiveness during tuberculosis is due to functional suppression of T-cell production of the TH-1 cytokine, IL-2, and the expression of IL-2 receptors.[181,184] However, the relative number of the main T-cell subpopulations, namely CD4 and CD8 cells, are unaltered.[178,184] Moreover, the frequency of PPD-reactive T cells is not significantly lower than that of healthy skin test-reactive subjects.[185] In a recent study, both blastogenesis and IFN-γ production by blood mononuclear cells were decreased, but improved during treatment.[186] In another study, production of IFN-γ in response to PPD and the 30 kDa antigen of MTB were lower in mononuclear cells from TB patients compared to their healthy household contacts (Whalen, personal communication). Importantly, suppression of MTB-induced IFN-γ production correlates with the extent of pulmonary TB.[187]

However, lack of correction of low T-cell responses by IL-2, which has been observed in two of three studies,[181,183,187] may reflect low lymphocyte IL-2R expression.[181] However, the possibility of interference with the interaction of IL-2 and IL-2R by another mediator has been sought (see below). In parallel to the dysregulation of IL-2 and its receptor, other studies have shown that patients with tuberculosis have a defect in the production of IFN-γ to different antigens of *M. tuberculosis*.[187-190] Overall, the results of these *in vitro* experiments indicate that CD4 T cells from patients with tuberculosis are limited in their expression of the TH-1 cytokines, IL-2, and IFN-γ, in response to MTB antigens.

Evidence for involvement of TH-2 cytokines derives from studies of protozoal infections and leprosy.[191,192] The TH-2 cytokines, IL-4 and IL-10, are cross-modulatory in that they limit TH-1 responses and increase antibody production.[193] Both of these cytokines have been shown to have macrophage deactivating effects.[194,195] An increase in the frequency of IL-4 producing T cells in tuberculosis recently has been shown.[196] However, no correlation to low blastogenesis or IFN-γ production in response to mycobacterial antigens was found. In one (Hirsch, personal communication) of two[187] studies of patients with MTB infection, a modest increase in PPD-induced IL-10 production was observed.

C. Suppression by Monocytes

A predominant role for blood monocytes in the suppression of T-cell responses has been indicated by several studies examining immune responses of patients with tuberculosis. Depletion of adherent monocytes from peripheral blood mononuclear cells of patients caused enhanced T-cell blastogenesis,[177] and production of IL-2[181] and IFN-γ.[197] Conversely, small numbers of monocytes (2% of T cells) added back to T-cell cultures have been shown to suppress T-cell production of IL-2.[180] Blood monocytosis is a well-documented feature of active tuberculosis. DNA-labeling studies indicate that monocytes from patients appear to be less mature than those of healthy subjects.[198] Furthermore, monocytes from tuberculous subjects display stigmata of *in vivo* activation as they spontaneously express IL-2R mRNA, display surface IL-2R, and release IL-2R upon *in vitro* culture.[146] We have shown that in freshly obtained mononuclear cells from patients with active TB, nuclear factor kB (NFkB) is already activated.[199] The cytokine profile of monocytes from patients with tuberculosis also is consistent with the notion that these cells are activated *in vivo*. When compared to monocytes of healthy subjects, production of the proinflammatory cytokines, TNF-α,[73] IL-1,[32] and IL-6[55] are enhanced by tuberculous monocytes upon *in vitro* stimulation with PPD or lipopolysaccharide. As noted, expression of IL-2R is similarly increased.[146] The presence of NFkB-binding motifs in the promoters of these molecules links their transcriptional upregulation with activation of NFkB.

The mechanisms by which monocytes suppress T-cell responses in TB has been partially clarified. As noted, monocytes from TB patients express low numbers of IL-2R and shed IL-2R upon *in vitro* culture. When cultured with exogenous IL-2, monocytes from patients remove IL-2 from supernatants.[146] However, consumption of IL-2 by monocytes is not sufficient to explain lowered T-cell responses.[181] Other studies have indicated that upon isolation, monocytes from TB patients with active pulmonary tuberculosis contain immunoreactive TGF-β, and that the concentration of TGF-β in cultures of unstimulated and MTB-stimulated monocytes from TB patients is higher than in PPD skin test-reactive healthy subjects.[151] Importantly, neutralization of TGF-β enhanced both T-cell blastogenesis and production of IFN-γ in response to PPD in mononuclear cells of TB patients. Overall, excess production of TGF-β by monocytes may be central to low *in vitro* T-cell responses during TB. However, cytotoxic CD4 lymphocytes[130] and Fcγ-receptor-positive T cells[178] also may contribute to the suppression of T-cell responses during TB.

A critical and as yet unanswered question is the significance of the suppression of T-cell responses to mycobacterial antigens in patients with TB. Depressed T-cell responses may be a factor in the pathogenesis of reactivation TB. Alternatively, depressed T-cell responses may be an associated feature of active TB. Also, the relationship between suppressed responses in the blood and regulation of the immune response locally at the site of infection must be addressed.

D. Regulation by Monocyte-Stimulatory Antigens

The basis for the antigen specificity of suppression in TB has been studied intensively. As noted, PPD is a direct stimulus for monocytes to produce IL-1,[141] TNF-α,[41] IL-2R,[147] and TGF-β.[145] As noted, both the polysaccharide, LAM, and protein mycobacterial products also have the capacity to stimulate the production of TGF-β by monocytes.[43] The 30 kDa α antigen of MTB also has the capacity to stimulate the expression of TNF-α, TGF-β, and IL-10 by monocytes. Thus, the intense interaction of MTB with mononuclear phagocytes may create a cytokine milieu that is conducive to immunoprotection during latent MTB infection, and one of immunosuppression during active TB. The direct stimulatory properties of MTB components with the host mononuclear phagocytes most likely underlies the extensive tissue damage in TB.

E. Immunopathogenesis of TB; Bronchoalveolar Lavage Cells (BAC)

Studies indicate that alveolar cells and their functions reflect the pattern of activity found in the interstitium. A fundamental observation is that the cells from the lung do not represent the cells from the blood either phenotypically or functionally. Initially, Lenzini et al. analyzed the cellular pattern in the bronchoalveolar lavage fluid of several patients with various lung diseases.[200] One patient with acute TB had 53% lymphocytes and 45% alveolar macrophages (normal 6 to 10% lymphocytes, 90 to 95% macrophages). In another patient with chronic TB, there were 20% lymphocytes and 80% macrophages. Recent studies also have demonstrated a lymphocytic alveolitis.[201-206] Schwander et al. have demonstrated an alveolitis in TB-involved BAC, characterized by an abundance of immature macrophages (20 to 25%) and alveolar lymphocytes. However, the presence of memory (CD45RO+) alveolar lymphocytes and their state of activation were similar.[206]

Recently, Schwander et al. have found that BAC from TB patients have enhanced blastogenic responses to PPD, the 30 kDa antigen, and LAM, and an increased PPD-induced frequency of

IFN-γ producing cells.[207] The frequency of IL-4- and IL-10-producing cells were not expanded. Others have reported an enhanced production of IFN-γ and IL-12 by BAC of TB patients.[208]

VIII. HIV AND PATHOGENESIS OF TUBERCULOSIS

A. TB IN HIV INFECTION

HIV is the greatest known risk both for reactivation of latent MTB infection[209,210] and for the development of primary TB upon exposure to infectious persons.[210] However, the main impact of HIV on TB has occurred in developing countries where the prevalence of both MTB and HIV infection is high. The range of the median CD4 count at the time of diagnosis of TB varies widely,[211] and includes both normal and low CD4 counts. In the U.S., TB occurs relatively early in HIV infection; in 50 to 67% of cases, it occurs a mean of 6 to 9 months before another AIDS-defining condition.[212] The early onset of TB in HIV-infected individuals underscores the virulence of MTB, and suggests a strict requirement for a fully competent cell-mediated immune response for protection against MTB. HIV infection increases the likelihood of a negative tuberculin skin test in MTB-infected people,[213] which correlates with the number of CD4 cells.

Although anergy is common in HIV infection, HIV-infected patients with TB often have a positive cutaneous DTH response to PPD. Over two thirds of HIV-infected patients with active TB who do not have other AIDS-defining conditions are tuberculin reactive, whereas only one third are tuberculin reactive once another AIDS- defining condition has developed.[214] MTB-induced T-cell proliferation and cytokine production (IFN-γ and TNF-α) have been shown to be increased in symptomatic and asymptomatic tuberculin skin test-positive HIV-infected TB women who were studied as part of a mother-infant cohort.[215] These data support the concept that T-cell responses to MTB are boosted by active TB even in the presence of HIV-related immunosuppression. However, more subtle defects in cell-mediated immunity may be sufficient to increase susceptibility to TB. Also, defects in native resistance may account for some of the increase in predisposition to TB. The known abnormalities in T cell and mononuclear phagocyte function in HIV infection may provide clues.

1. T Lymphocytes

During infection with HIV, CD4 T helper cells are progressively depleted and profoundly impaired with respect to proliferation and production of TH-1 cytokines.[216] In contrast, B-lymphocyte activity increases during HIV infection resulting in a polyclonal hypergammaglobulinemia. The mechanisms of such progressive T-cell dysfunction include selective loss of memory T cells, immunoregulatory dysfunction of mononuclear phagocytes, active immunosuppression by products of HIV such as gp120 and tat, and excessive production of immunosuppressive cytokines.[217] Each of these mechanisms also may impact on susceptibility to TB in HIV infection. The production of immunoregulatory cytokines in HIV infection may be especially important with regard to TB. In a cohort of over 100 HIV-positive individuals, a selective loss of IL-2 and IFN-γ production in response to recall antigens correlated with an increase in phytohemagglutinin-stimulated IL-4 and IL-10 production,[210] indicating that a decline in TH-1 function and an increase in TH-2 function occur concurrently during HIV infection. However, Zhang et al. have shown that despite low TH-1 responses, IL-4 and IL-10 were comparable in HIV infected and uninfected TB patients.[218] Thus, the switch in the balance towards TH-2 function in HIV infection does not appear to contribute to the increased susceptibility to TB in HIV-infected persons.

2. Mononuclear Phagocytes

Mononuclear phagocytes, including blood monocytes and tissue macrophages, may be infected with HIV *in vitro* and *in vivo*.[219] Since MTB is an intracellular pathogen, mononuclear phagocytes may be affected particularly by dual infection with HIV and MTB. Cumulatively, studies indicate that the number of monocytes; expression of cytokines including IL-1 and TNF-α; production of oxygen radical production; expression of phenotypic markers such as Class II MHC, CR1, and CR3; and microbicidal activity against several pathogens are preserved.[219,220] Antigen presentation by monocytes, however, is decreased, whereas accessory cell function for T-cell responses to mitogens is normal.[221] Microbicidal activity of alveolar macrophages from subjects with AIDS is normal for *Toxoplasma gondii* and *Chlamydia psittaci* and killing is upregulated by IFN-γ.[222] However, these latter responses for MTB have not been studied fully.

Several immunologic and effector functions of alveolar macrophages from HIV-infected subjects are up-regulated, including the expression of markers of activation[223] and the expression of cytokines such as IL-1,[224] IL-6,[225] and TNF-α.[226] Whether these findings relate to the immuno-pathogenesis of TB in coinfected subjects is not clear. Furthermore, there is an expansion of CD8 lymphocytes in the lungs of patients with HIV infection. As noted, CD8 T cells lyse antigen-pulsed alveolar macrophages in a Class I-restricted manner.[227] Whether, CD8 cytotoxicity against MTB-infected alveolar macrophages is blunted in coinfected patients and/or contributes to pathology is unknown.

B. Impact of TB on HIV Infection

The impact of TB on the progression of HIV infection has been recognized widely. However, to date, this effect is most notable in Africa where 12 of the 15 million coinfected patients have originated.[228] Since the response of HIV-infected TB patients to antituberculous drugs is similar to HIV-uninfected TB patients, the increased morbidity[229] and mortality[229,230] in coinfected patients is attributable to worsening of HIV disease. For example, in Uganda, the mortality of TB in HIV-infected patients is 30%; this finding has been found to be due primarily to progressive HIV disease, and not to the tuberculosis disease.[231] Serum levels of β2 microglobulin, a marker of HIV disease progression, were twofold higher in HIV-infected Ugandan patients with pulmonary TB than in HIV-infected nontuberculous subjects and HIV-seronegative patients with TB.[215] Recent data from the U.S. have shown that HIV-infected patients with TB have reduced survival, more opportunistic infections, and a greater decrease in CD4 counts relative to CD4-matched controls.[229] In fact, the development of TB was associated with an increase in plasma HIV RNA.[232] Our data indicate that the increase in HIV load is particularly significant in HIV-infected TB patients with higher CD4 counts (Toossi, unpublished data).

Replication of HIV *in vitro* and presumably *in vivo* in both lymphocytes and monocytes requires activation by various stimuli such as antigens, mitogens, growth factors, and cytokines including TNF-α, IL-1, and IL-6. These stimuli initiate viral replication in part through activation of NFkB that, in turn, binds to the long terminal repeat (LTR) in the promoter region of HIV, thereby stimulating viral transcription. Blood monocytes from patients with TB release increased amounts of TNF-α, IL-1, and IL-6 upon stimulation,[43] and display spontaneous activation of NFkB.[199] Furthermore, mycobacteria, and protein and polysaccharide constituents of mycobacteria, enhance HIV replication in latently infected cell lines[233] and in HIV-infected monocytes (Toossi, unpublished). Finally, MTB and PPD induce HIV replication in alveolar macrophages from HIV-infected patients.[234] Recently, monocytes from patients with pulmonary TB have been found to be more susceptible to infection with HIV *in vitro* than monocytes from healthy subjects.[235] The increased susceptibility was not attributable to increased viral entry, reverse transcription, or the number of infected cells, suggesting that either integration or viral transcription was upregulated in these cells. The role of monocyte-derived cytokines in the enhanced replication of HIV in patients with TB is being examined. Other studies have indicated that TB generates a cytokine microenvironment (TNF-α, IL-6, IL-2) enhancing the infection of lymphocytes by HIV.[236] Cumulatively, these data indicate that the cytokines that may be relevant to protection against MTB may be deleterious for persons with HIV infection, and that anticytokine therapy may be effective in limiting HIV replication during the treatment of active TB in HIV-positive subjects.

NOTE:

This chapter is dedicated to the memory of our friend and colleague, Dr. E. A. Rich.

REFERENCES

1. Snider, D. E., Raviglione, M., and Kochi, A., Global burden of tuberculosis, in *Tuberculosis Pathogenesis, Protection, and Control*, (B. Bloom, Ed.), ASM Press, Materials Park, OH, 1994.
2. Wells, W. F., Wells, M. W., and Wilder, T. S., The environmental control of epidemic contagion: I. An epidemiologic study of radiant disinfection of air in day schools, *Am. J. Hyg.*, 35, 97, 1942.
3. Riley, R. L., Mills, C. C., O'Grady, F., Sultan, L. U., Wittstadt, F., and Shivpuri, D. N., Infectiousness of air from a tuberculosis Ward. Ultraviolet irradiation of infectiousness of different patients, *Am. Rev. Respir. Dis.*, 85, 511, 1962.
4. Smith, D. W., McMurray, D. N., Wiegeshaus, E. H., Grover, A. A., and Harding, G. E., Host-parasite relationships in experimental airborne tuberculosis. IV. Early events in the course of infection in vaccinated and nonvaccinated guinea pigs, *Am. Rev. Respir. Dis.*, 102, 937, 1970.
5. Lurie, M. B., *Resistance to Tuberculosis: Experimental Studies in Native and Acquired Defensive Mechanisms*, Harvard University Press, Cambridge, MA, 1964.
6. Lurie, M. B. and Dannenberg, A. M., Jr., Macrophage function in infectious disease with inbred rabbits, *Bact. Rev.*, 29, 466, 1965.
7. Meylan, P. R. A., Richman, D. D., and Kornbluth, R. S., Reduced intracellular growth of mycobacteria in human macrophages cultivated at physiologic oxygen pressure, *Am. Rev. Respir. Dis.*, 145, 947, 1992.
8. Wayne, L. G. and Hayes, L. G., An *in vitro* model for sequential study of shiftdown of mycrobacterium tuberculosis through two stages of nonreplicating persistence, *Infect. Immun.*, 64, 2062, 1996.
9. Dannenberg, A. M., Immune mechanisms in the pathogenesis of pulmonary tuberculosis, *Rev. Infect. Dis.*, 52, 369, 1989.
10. North, R. J., T-cell dependence of macrophage activation and mobilization during infection with *Mycobacterium tuberculosis*, *Infect. Immun.*, 10, 66, 1974.
11. Medlar, E. M., The behavior of pulmonary tuberculous lesions: a pathological study, *Am. Rev. Tuberc.*, 71, 1, 1955.
12. Yamamura, Y., Ogawa, Y., Maeda, H., and Yamamura, Y., Prevention of tuberculous cavity formation by desensitization with tuberculin-active peptide, *Am. Rev. Respir. Dis.*, 109, 594, 1974.
13. Noll, H., The chemistry of cord factor, a toxic glycolipid of *M. tuberculosis, Adv. Tuberc. Res.*, 7, 149, 1956.
14. Bloch, H., Studies on the virulence of tubercle bacilli, *J. Exp. Med.*, 91, 197, 1950.
15. Artman, M., Bekierkunst A., and Goldenberg, I., Tissue metabolism in infection: biochemical changes in mice treated with cord factor, *Arch. Biochem. Biophys.*, 105, 80, 1964.
16. Kato, M., Site II-Specific inhibition of mitochondial oxidative phosphorylation by trehalose-6,6'-dimycolate (cord factor) of *Mycobacterium tuberculosis, Arch. Biochem. Biophys.*, 140, 379, 1970.
17. Goren, M. B., In *Tuberculosis*, Youmans G. P., Ed., W.B. Saunders Co., Philadelphia, 1979.
18. Goren, M. B., Sulfolipid I of *Mycobacterium tuberculosis* strain H37Rv. II. Structural studies, *Biochem. Biophys. Acta*, 210, 127, 1970.
19. Kato, M. and Goren, M. B., Synergistic action of cord factor and mycobacterial sulfatides on mitochondria, *Infect. Immun.*, 10, 733, 1974.
20. Brennan, P. J. and Draper, P., Ultrastructure of *Mycobacterium tuberculosis*, In *Tuberculosis: Pathogenesis, Protection, and Control*, (B. Bloom, Ed.), ASM Press, Materials Park, OH, 1994.
21. Goren, M. B., D'Arcy Hart, P., Young, W. R., and Armstrong, J. A., Prevention of phagosome-lysosome fusion in cultured macrophages by sulfatides of *Mycobacterium tuberculosis, Proc. Nat. Acad. Sci. USA*, 73, 2510, 1976.
22. Gordon, A. H., D'Arcy Hart, P., and Young, M. R., Ammonia inhibits phagosome-lysosome fusion in macrophages. *Nature* (London), 286, 79, 1980.
23. Smith, D. W., Randall, H. M., Gaastambide-Odier, M. D., and Koevoet, A. L., Mycosides: a new class of type-specific glycolipids of mycobacteria, *Ann. N.Y. Acad. Sci.*, 69, 145, 1960.

24. Brennan, P. J., Hunter, S. W., McNeil, M., Chatterjee, D., and Daffe, M., Reappraisal of the chemistry of mycobacterial cell walls, with a view to understanding the roles of individual entities in disease processes, In *Microbial Determinants of Virulence and Host Response*, Ayoub, E. M., Cassell, G. H., Branch, W. C., Jr., and Henry, T. J., Eds., American Society for Microbiology, Washington, D.C., 1990.

25. Daffe, M., Lacave, C., Lanelle, M.-A., Gillois, M., and Lanelle, G., Polyphythinenacyl trehalose, glycolipids specific for virulent strains of the tubercule bacillus, *Eur. J. Biochem.*, 112, 579, 1988.

26. Rastogi, N., Recent observations concerning structure and function relationships in the mycobacterial cell envelope: elaboration of a model in terms of mycobacterial pathogenicity, virulence and drug-resistance, *Res. Microbiol.*, 142, 464, 1991.

27. Dahl, K. E., Shiratsuchi, H., Hamilton, B. D., Ellner, J. J., and Toossi, Z., Selective induction of TGF-β in human monocytes by lipoarabinomannan of *M. tuberculosis, Infect. Immun.*, 64, 399, 1996.

28. Parrish, N. and Bishai, W. R., Mechanisms of latency in Mycobacterium tuberculosis, *Trends Microbiol.*, 6, 107, 1998.

29. Gomez, J. E., Chen, J-M., and Bishai, W. R., Sigma factors of mycobacterium tuberculosis, *Tuberc. Lung Dis.*, 78, 175, 1997.

30. Yuan, Y., Crane, D. D., Simpson, R. M., Zhu, Y. Q., Hickey, M. J., Sherman, D. R., and Barry, C. E., III, The 16-kDa alpha-crystallin (Acr) protein of *Mycobacterium tuberculosis* is required for growth in macrophages, *Proc. Natl. Acad. Sci.*, 95, 9578, 1998.

31. Dannenberg, A. M., Jr., Review: delayed-type hypersensitivity and cell mediated immunity in the pathogenesis of tuberculosis, *Immunol. Today*, 12, 228, 1991.

32. Orme, I. and Collins, F. M., Mouse model of tuberculosis. In *Tuberculosis, Pathogenesis, Protection, and Control,* (B. Bloom, Ed.), ASM Press, Materials Park, OH, 1994.

33. Rhoades, E. R., Frank, A. A., and Orme, I. M., Progression of chronic pulmonary tuberculosis in mice aerogenically infected with virulent *Mycobacterium tuberculosis, Tuberc. Lung Dis.*, 78, 57, 1997.

34. Smith, D. W., McMurray, D. N., Wiegeshaus, E. H, Grover, A. A., and Harding, G. E., Host-parasite relationships in experimental airborne tuberculosis. IV. Early events in the course of infection in vaccinated and nonvaccinated guinea pigs, *Am. Rev. Resp. Dis.*, 102, 937, 1970.

35. Swartz, R. P., Naal, D., Vogel, C-W., and Yeager, H., Jr., Differences in uptake of mycobacteria by human monocytes: a role for complement, *Infect. Immun.*, 56, 2223, 1988.

36. Schlessinger, L., Bellinger-Kawahara, C. G., Payne, N. R., and Horwitz, M. A., Phagocytosis of *Mycobacterium tuberculosis* is mediated by human monocyte complement receptors and complement component C3, *J. Immunol.*, 144, 2771, 1990.

37. Schlesinger, L. S., Kaufman, T. M., Iyer, S., Hull, S. R., and Marchiando, L. K., Differences in mannose receptor-mediated uptake of lipoarabinomannan from virulent and attenuated strains of *Mycobacterium tuberculosis* by human macrophages, *J. Immunol.*, 157, 4568, 1996.

38. Schlesinger, L. S., Entry of *Mycobacterium tuberculosis* into mononuclear phagocytes, *Curr. Top Microbiol. Immunol.*, 215, 71, 1996.

39. Hirsch, C. S., Ellner, J. J., Russell, D. G., and Rich, E. A. Complement receptor mediated uptake and tumor necrosis-α-mediated growth inhibition of *Mycobacterium tuberculosis* by human alveolar macrophages, *J. Immunol.*, 152, 743, 1994.

40. Gaynor, C. D., McCormack, F. X., Voelker, D. R., McGowan, S. E., and Schlesinger, L. S., Pulmonary surfactant protein A mediates enhanced phagocytosis of *Mycobacterium tuberculosis* by a direct interaction with human macrophages, *J. Immunol.*, 55, 5343, 1995.

41. Valone, S. E., Rich, E. A., Wallis, R. R., and Ellner, J. J., Expression of tumor necrosis factor *in vitro* by human mononuclear phagocytes stimulated with BCF and mycobacterial antigens, *Infect. Immun.*, 56, 3313, 1988.

42. Rich, E. A., Panuska, J. R., Wallis, R. S., Wolf, C. B., and Ellner, J. J., Dyscoordinate expression of tumor necrosis factor-alpha by human blood monocytes and alveolar macrophages, *Am. Rev. Respir. Dis.*, 139, 1010, 1989.

43. Toossi, Z. and Ellner, J. J., The role of TGF-β in the pathogenesis of human tuberculosis, *Clin. Immunol. Immunopathol.*, 87, 107, 1998.

44. Torres, M., Herrera, T., Villareal, H., Rich, E. A., and Sada, E., Cytokine profiles for peripheral blood lymphocytes from patients with active pulmonary tuberculosis and healthy household contacts in response to the 30-kilodalton antigen of *Mycobacterium tuberculosis, Infect. Immun.*, 66, 176, 1998.

45. Flesch, I. E. A. and Kaufmann, S. N. E., Attempts to characterize the mechanisms involved in mycobacterial growth inhibition by gamma-interferon-activated bone marrow macrophages, *Infect. Immun.,* 56, 1464, 1988.

46. Armstrong, J. A. and d'Arcy Hart, P., Phagosome-lysosome interactions in cultured macrophages infected with virulent tubercle bacilli. Reversal of the usual nonfusion pattern and observations on bacterial survival, *J. Exp. Med.,* 142, 1, 1975.

47a. Myrvik, Q. N., Leake, E. E., and Wright, M. J., Disruption of phagosomal membranes of normal alveolar macrophages by the H37Rv strain of *Mycobacterium tuberculosis:* a correlate of virulence, *Am. Rev. Respir. Dis.,* 129, 322, 1984.

47b. McDonough, K. A., Kress, Y., and Bloom, B. R., Interaction of *Mycobacterium tuberculosis* with macrophages, *Infect. Immun.,* 61, 2763, 1993.

48. Mitchison, D. A., Selkon, J. B., and Lloyd, J., Virulence in the guinea-pig, susceptibility to hydrogen peroxide, and catalase activity of isoniazid-sensitive tubercle bacilli from South Indian and British patients, *J. Pathol. Bacteriol.,* 86, 377, 1963.

49. Jackett, P. S., Aber, V. R., and Lowrie, D. B., Virulence of *Mycobacterium tuberculosis* and susceptibility of peroxidative killing systems, *J. Gen. Microbiol.,* 106, 273, 1978.

50. Douvas, G. S., Berger, E. M., Repine, J. E., and Crowle, A. J., Natural mycobacteriostatic activity in human monocyte-derived adherent cells, *Am. Rev. Respir. Dis.,* 134, 44, 1986.

51. Chan, J., Tanaka, D., Caroll, D., Flynn, K. J., and Bloom, B. R., Effects of nitric oxide synthase inhibitors on murine infection with *Mycobacterium tuberculosis. Infect. Immun.,* 63, 736, 1995.

52. Macmicking, A. D., North, R. J., La Course, R., Mudgett, J. S., Shah, S. K., and Nathan, C. F., Identification of nitric oxide synthase as a protective locus against tuberculous. *Proc. Natl. Acad. Sci.,* 94, 5243, 1997.

53. Rich, E. A., Torres, M., Sada, E., Finegan, C. K., Hamilton, B. D., and Toossi, Z., Mycobacterium tuberculosis (MTB)-stimulated production of nitric oxide by human alveolar macrophages and relationship of nitric oxide production to growth inhibition of MTB, *Tuberc. Lung Dis.,* 78, 247, 1997.

54. Bloch, H., The relationship between phagocytic cells and human tubercle bacilli, *Am. Rev. Tuberc.,* 58, 662, 1948.

55. Martin, S. P., Pierce, C. H., Middlebrook, G., and Dubos, R. J., The effect of tubercle bacilli on the polymorphonuclear leukocytes of normal animals, *J. Exp. Med.,* 91, 381, 1950.

56. Antony, V. B., Sahn, S. A., Antony, A. C., and Repine, J. E., *Bacillus Calmette-Guerin*-stimulated neutrophils release chemotaxins for monocytes in rabbit pleural spaces and *in vitro, J. Clin. Invest.,* 76, 1514, 1985.

57. Brown, A. E., Holzer, T. J., and Andersen, B. R., Capacity of human neutrophils to kill *Mycobacterium tuberculosis, J. Infect. Dis.,* 156, 985, 1987.

58. May, M. E. and Spagnuolo, P. J., Evidence for activation of a respiratory burst in the interaction of human neutrophils with *Mycobacterium tuberculosis, Infect. Immun.,* 55, 2304, 1987.

59. Jones, G. S., Amirault, H. J., and Andersen, B. R., Killing of *Mycobacterium tuberculosis* by neutrophils: a nonoxidative process, *J. Infect. Dis.,* 162, 700, 1990.

60. Geertsman, M. F., Nibbering, P. H., Pos, O., and van Furth, R., Interferon-γ-activated human granulocytes kill ingested *Mycobacterium fortuitum* more efficiently than normal granulocytes, *Eur. J. Immunol.,* 20, 869, 1990.

61. Yoneda, T. and Ellner, J. J., CD4(+) T cell and natural killer cell-dependent killing of mycobacterium tuberculosis by human monocytes, *Am. J. Respir. Crit. Care Med.,* 158, 395, 1998.

62. Janis, E. M., Kaufmann, S. H. E., Schwartz, R. H., and Pardoll, D. M., Activation of γδ T-cells in the primary immune response to *Mycobacterium tuberculosis, Science,* 244, 2754, 1989.

63. Augustin, A., Kubo, R. T., and Sim, G., Resident pulmonary lymphocytes expressing the γδ T-cell receptor, *Nature,* 340, 239, 1989.

64. Havlir, D. V., Ellner, J. J., Chervenak, K. A., and Boom, W. H., Selective expansion of human γδ T-cells by monocytes infected by live *Mycobacterium tuberculosis, J. Clin. Invest.,* 87, 729, 1991.

65. Munk, M. E., Gatrill, A. J., and Kaufman, S. H. E., Target cell lysis and IL-2 secretion by γδ T-lymphocytes after activation with bacteria, *J. Immunol.,* 145, 2434, 1990.

66a. Skamene, E., Genetic control of susceptibility to mycobacterial infections, *Rev. Infect. Dis.,* 2, (Suppl. 1), S394, 1989.

66b. Vidal, S. M., Pinner, E., Lepage, P., Gauthier, S., and Gros, P., Natural resistance to intracellular infections: Nramp1 encodes a membrane phosphoglycoprotein absent in macrophages from susceptible mice, *J. Immunol.*, 157, 3559, 1996.

67. North, R. J. and Medina, E., How important is Nramp1 in tuberculosis? *Trends Microbiol.*, 6, 441, 1998.

68. Abel, L., Sanchez, F. O., Oberti, J., Thuc, N. V., Hoa, L. V., Lap, V. D., Skamene, E., Lagrange, P. H., and Schurr, E., Susceptibility to leprosy is linked to the human Nramp1 gene, *J. Infect. Dis.*, 177, 133, 1998.

69. Bellamy, R., Ruwende, C., Corrah, T., McAdam, K. P., Whittle, H. C., and Hill, A. V., Variations in the NRAMP1 gene and susceptibility to tuberculosis in West Africans, *N. Engl. J. Med.*, 338, 640, 1998.

70. Shaw, M. A., Collins, A., Peacock, C. S., Miller, E. N., Black, G. F., Sibthorpe, D., Lins-Lainson, Z., Shaw, J. J., Ramos, F., Silveira, F., and Blackwell, J. M., Evidence that genetic susceptibility to mycobacterium tuberculosis in a Brazilian population is under oligogenic control: linkage study of the candidate genes NRAMP1 and TNFA, *Tuberc. Lung Dis.*, 78, 35, 1997.

71. Newport, M. J., Huxley, C. M., Huston, S., Hawrylowicz, C. M., Oostra, B. A., Williamson, R., and Levin, M., A mutation in the interferon-g receptor gene and susceptibility to mycobacterial infection, *N. Engl. J. Med.*, 335, 1941, 1996.

72. Jong, R., Altare, F., Haagen, I. A., Elferink, D. G., Boer, T., van Breda Vriesman, P. J. C., Kabel, P. J., Draaisma, J. M. T., van Dissel, J. T., Kroon, F. P., Casanova, J. L., and Ottenhoff, T. H. M., Severe mycobacterial and salmonella infections in Interleukin-12 receptor-deficient patients, *Science*, 280, 1435, 1998.

73. Altare, F., Durandy, A., Lammas, D., Emile, J. F., Lamhamedi, S.,Le Deist, F., Drysdale, P., Jouanguy, E., Doffinger, R., Bernaudin, F., Jeppsson, O., Gollob, J. A., Meinl, E., Segal, A. W., Fischer, A., Kumararatne, D., and Casanova, J. L., Impairment of mycobacterial immunity in human Interleukin-12 receptor deficiency, *Science*, 280, 1432, 1998.

74. Stead, W. W., Racial differences in susceptibility to infection by *Mycobacterial tuberculosis*, *N. Engl. J. Med.*, 322, 422, 1990.

75. Comstock, G. W., Tuberculosis in twins: a re-analysis of the prophit survey, *Am. Rev. Respir. Dis.*, 117, 621, 1978.

76. Singh, S. P. N., Mehra, N. K., Dingley, H. B., Pande, J. N., and Vaidya, M. C., HLA haplotype segregation study in multiple case families of pulmonary tuberculosis, *Tissue Antigens*, 23, 84, 1984.

77. Selby, R., Barnard, J. M., Buehler, S. K., Crumley, J., Larsen, B., and Marshall, W. H., Tuberculosis associated with HLA-B8, BfS in a Newfoundland community study, *Tissue Antigens*, 11, 403, 1978.

78. Al-Arif, L. I., Goldstein, R. A., Affronti, L. F., and Janicki, J. W., HLA Bw15 and tuberculosis in a North American black population, *Am. Rev. Respir Dis.*, 120, 1275, 1979.

79. Jian, Z. F., An, J. B., Sun, Y. P, Mittal, K. K., and Lee, T. D., Association of HLA-BW35 with tuberculosis in the Chinese, *Tissue Antigen*, 22, 86, 1983.

80. Khomenko, A. G., Litvinov, V. I., Chukanova, V. P., and Pospelov, L. E., Tuberculosis in patients with various HLA phenotypes, *Tubercle*, 71, 187, 1990.

81. Bothamley, G. H., Beck, J. S., Schreuder, G. M. Th., D'Amaro, J., deVries, R. R. P., Kardjito, T., and Ivanyi, J., Association of tuberculosis and MTB-specific antibody levels with HLA, *J. Infect. Dis.*, 159, 549, 1989.

82. Hwange, C. H., Khan, S., Ende, N., Mangura, B. T., Reichman, L. B., and Chou, J., The HLA-A, -B, and -DR phenotypes and tuberculosis, *Am. Rev. Respir. Dis.*, 132, 382, 1985.

83. Hafez, M., El-Salab, S. H., El-Shennawy, F., and Bassiony, M. R., HLA-antigens and tuberculosis in the Egyptian population, *Tubercle*, 66, 35, 1985.

84. Zervas, J., Castantopoulos, C., Toubis, M., Anagnostopoulos, D., and Cotsovoulou, V., HLA-A and B antigens and pulmonary tuberculosis in Greeks, *Br. J. Dis. Chest*, 81, 147, 1987.

85. Cox, R. A., Arnold, D. R., Cook, D., and Lundberg, D. I., HLA phenotypes in Mexican Americans with tuberculosis, *Am. Rev. Respir. Dis.*, 126, 653, 1982.

86. Singh, S. P. N., Mehra, N. K., Dingley, H. B., Pande, J. N., and Vaidya, M. C., HLA-A, -B, -C, and -DR antigen profile in pulmonary tuberculosis in North India, *Tissue Antigens*, 21, 380, 1983.

87. Cox, R. A., Downs, M., Neimes, R. E., Ognibene, A. J., Yamashita, T. S., and Ellner, J. J., Immunogenetic analysis of human tuberculosis, *J. Infect. Dis.*, 158, 1302, 1988.

88. Davis, J. E., Rich, R. R., Van, M., Le, M. V., Pollach, M. S., and Cook, R. G., Defective antigen presentation and novel structural properties of DR1 from an HLA haplotype associated with 21-hydroxylase deficiency, *J. Clin. Invest.*, 80, 898, 1987.

89. Centers for Disease Control, A strategic plan for the elimination of tuberculosis in the United States, *J. Am. Med. Assoc.*, 261, 2929, 1989.

90. Rook, G. A. W., The role of vitamin D in tuberculosis, *Am. Rev. Respir. Dis.*, 138, 768, 1988.

91. Snider, D. E., Reorientation of tuberculosis control programs in the USA, *Bull. Int. Union Tuberc.*, 64, 25, 1989.

92. Snider, D. E. and Hutton, M. D., Tuberculosis in correctional institutions, *J. Am. Med. Assoc.*, 261, 436, 1989.

93. Davies, P. D. O., A possible link between vitamin D deficiency and impaired host defence to *Mycobacterium tuberculosis*, *Tubercle*, 66, 301, 1985.

94. Crowle, A. and Elkines, N., Relative permissiveness of macrophages from black and white people for virulent tubercle bacilli, *Infect. Immun.*, 58, 632, 1990.

95. Wilkinson, R., Patel, P., Llewlyn, M., Hirsh, C. S., Passoval, G., Snounou, G., Davidson, R. N., and Toossi, Z., Influence of polymorphism in the genes for Interleukin (IL)-1 beta and IL-1 receptor antagonist on tuberculosis, *J. Exp. Med.*, 189, 1863, 1999.

96. North, R. J., Importance of thymus-derived lymphocytes in cell-mediated immunity to infection, *Cell. Immunol.*, 7, 166, 1973.

97. Lefford, M. J., Transfer of adoptive immunity to tuberculosis in mice, *Infect. Immun.*, 11, 1174, 1975.

98. Orme, I. M. and Collins, F. M., Passive transfer of tuberculin sensitivity from anergic mice, *Infect. Immun.*, 46, 850, 1984.

99. Orme, I. M. and Collins F. M., Protection against *Mycobacterium tuberculosis* infection by adoptive immunotherapy, *J. Exp. Med.*, 158, 74, 1983.

100. Orme, I., Andersen, P., and Boom, W. H., T-cell responses to *Mycobacterium tuberculosis, J. Infect. Dis.*, 167, 1481, 1993.

101. Daniel, T. M. and Debanne, S. M., State of the art: the serodiagnosis of tuberculosis and other mycobacterial diseases by enzyme-linked immunosorbent assay, *Am. Rev. Respir. Dis.*, 135, 1137, 1987.

102. Chan, S. L, Reggiardo, Z., Daniel, T. M., Girling, D. J., and Mitchison, D. A., Serodiagnosis of tuberculosis using an enzyme-linked immunosorbent assay (ELISA) with antigen 5 and a hemagglutination assay with glycolipid antigens. Results in patients with newly diagnosed pulmonary tuberculosis ranging in extent of disease from minimal to extensive, *Am. Rev. Respir. Dis.*, 142, 385, 1990.

103. Daniel, T. M., Debanne, S. M., and van der Kuyp, F., Enzyme-linked immunoabsorbent assay using *Mycobacterium tuberculosis* antigen 5 and PPD for serodiagnosis of tuberculosis, *Chest*, 88, 388, 1985.

104. Koch, R., Weitere mitteilungen uber ein heilmittel gegen tuberculose, *Dtsch. Med. Wschr.*, 17, 101, 1891.

105. Chase, M. W., The cellular transfer of cutaneous hypersensitivity to tuberculin, *Proc. Soc. Exper. Biol. Med.*, 59, 134, 1945.

106. Orme, I. M. and Collins, F. M., Adoptive protection of the *Mycobacterium tuberculosis*-infected lung; dissociation between cells that passively transfer protective immunity and those that transfer delayed-type hypersensitivity to tuberculin, *Cell Immunol.*, 84, 113, 1984.

107. Boom, W. H., Wallis, R. S., and Chervenak, K. A., Human MTB-reactive CD4+ T-cell clones: heterogeneity in antigen recognition, cytokine production, and cytotoxicity for mononuclear phagocytes, *Infect. Immun.*, 59, 2737, 1991.

108. Lanier, L. L., Ruitenberg, J. J., and Phillips, J. H., Human CD3+ T-lymphocytes that express neither CD4+ nor CD8+ antigens, *J. Exp. Med.*, 164, 339, 1986.

109. Rook, G. A. W., Immunity and hypersensitivity, *Practitioner*, 227, iv, 1983.

110. Orme, I. M., Induction of nonspecific acquired resistance and delayed type hypersensitivity, but not specific acquired resistance, in mice inoculated with killed mycobacterial vaccines, *Infect. Immun.*, 56, 3310, 1988.

111. Cooper, A. M., Callahan, J. E., Keen, M., Belisle, J. T., and Orme, I. M., Expression of memory immunity in the lung following re-exposure to *Mycobacterium tuberculosis, Tuberc. Lung Dis.*, 78, 67, 1997.

112. Orme, I. M., Miller, E. S., Roberts, A. D., Furney, S. K., Griffin, J. P., Dobos, E. M., Chi, D., Rivoire, B., and Brennan, P. J., T-lymphocytes mediating protection and cellular cytolysis during the course of *Mycobacterium tuberculosis, J. Immunol.,* 148, 189, 1992.

113. Orme, I. M., Characteristics and specificity of acquired immunologic memory to MTB infection, *J. Immunol.,* 140, 3589, 1988.

114. Muller, I. Cobbold, S., Waldmann, H., and Kaufmann, S. M. E., Impaired resistance to MTB after selective *in vivo* depletion of L3T4+ and Lyt -2+ T-cells, *Infect. Immun.,* 55, 2037, 1987.

115. Fiorentino, D. F., Bond, M. W., and Mosmann, T. R., Two types of mouse T helper cell IV. TH-2 clones secrete a factor that inhibits cytokine production by TH-1 clones, *J. Exp. Med.,* 170, 2081, 1989.

116. Cooper, M. A., Dalton, D. K., Stewart, T. A., Griffin, J. P., Russell, D. G., and Orme, I. M., Disseminated tuberculosis in interferon-g gene-disrupted mice, *J. Exp. Med.,* 178, 2243, 1993.

117. Flynn, J. L., Chan, J., Triebold, K. J., Dalton, D. K., Stewart, T. A., and Bloom, B. R., An essential role for interferon-g in resistance to *Mycobacterium tuberculosis. J. Exp. Med.,* 178, 2249, 1993.

118. Flynn, J. L., Goldstein, M. M., Triebold, K. J., Koller, B., and Bloom, B. R., Major histocompatibility complex class I-restricted T cells are required for resistance to *Mycobacterium tuberculosis* infection. *Proc. Natl. Acad. Sci. USA,* 89, 12013, 1992.

119. Cooper, A. M., D'Souza, C., Frank, A. A., and Orme, I. M., The course of *Mycobacterium tuberculosis* infection in the lungs of mice lacking expression of either Perforin- or Granzyme-mediated cytolytic mechanisms, *Infect. Immun.,* 65, 1317, 1997.

120. Boom, W. H., Wallis, R. S., and Chervenak, K. A., Human MTB-reactive CD4+ T-cell clones: heterogeneity in antigen recognition, cytokine production, and cytotoxicity for mononuclear phago-cytes., *Infect. Immun.,* 59, 2737, 1991.

121. Tan, J. S., Canaday, D. H., Boom, W. H., Balaji, K. N., Schwander, S. K., and Rich, E. A., Human alveolar T lymphocyte responses to *Mycobacterium tuberculosis* antigens, *J. Immunol.,* 159, 290, 1997.

122. Berger, H. W. and Mejia, E., Tuberculous pleurisy, *Chest,* 63, 88, 1973.

123. Fujiwara, H., Okuda, Y., Fukukawa, T., and Tsuyuguchi, I., *In vitro* tuberculin reactivity of lymphocytes from patients with tuberculous pleurisy, *Infect. Immun.,* 35, 402, 1982.

124. Barnes, P. F., Mistry, S. D., Cooper, C. L., Pirmez, C., Rea, T. H., and Modlin, R. L., Compartmen-talization of a CD4+ T-lymphocyte subpopulation in tuberculous pleuritis, *J. Immunol.,* 142, 1114, 1989.

125. Fujiwara, H. and Tsuyuguchi, I., Frequency of tuberculin-reactive T-lymphocytes in pleural fluid and blood from patients with tuberculous pleurisy, *Chest,* 89, 530, 1984.

126. Ellner, J. J., Pleural fluid and peripheral blood lymphocyte function in tuberculosis, *Ann. Int. Med.,* 89, 932, 1978.

127. Barnes, P. F., Fong, S. J., Brennan, P. J., Twomey, P. E., Mazumder, A., and Modlin, R. L., Local production of tumor necrosis factor and interferon-g in tuberculous pleuritis, *J. Immunol.,* 145, 149, 1990.

128. Wallis, R. S., Alde, S. L., Havlir, D. V., Amir-Tahmasseb, H., Daniel, T. M., and Ellner, J. J., Identification of antigens of *Mycobacterium tuberculosis* using human monoclonal antibodies, *J. Clin. Invest.,* 84, 214, 1989.

129. Anderseen, P., Host responses and antigens involved in protective immunity to *Mycobacterium tuber-culosis, Scand. J. Immunol.,* 45, 115, 1997.

130. Ottenhoff, T. H. M., Kale, B., van Embden, J. D. A., Thole, J. E. R., and Kiessling, R., The recombinant 65 kD heat shock protein of *Mycobacterium bovis Bacillus Calmette Guérin*/MTB is a target molecule for CD4+ cytotoxic T-lymphocytes that lyse human monocytes, *J. Exp. Med.,* 168, 1947, 1988.

131. Munk, M. E., Schoel, B., and Kaufmann, S. H. E., T. cell responses of normal individuals towards recombinant protein antigens of MTB, *Eur. J. Immunol.,* 18, 1835, 1988.

132. Havlir, D. V., Wallis, R. S., Boom, W. H., Daniel, T. M., Chervenak, K., and Ellner, J. J., Human immune response to MTB antigens, *Infect. Immun.,* 59, 665, 1991.

133. Schoel, B., Gulle, M., and Kaufmann, S. H. E., Heterogeneity of the repertoire of T cells of tuberculosis patients and healthy contacts to MTB antigens separated by high resolution techniques, *Infect. Immun.,* 60, 1717, 1992.

134. Young, D. B., Kaufmann, S. H. E., Hermans, P. W. M., and Thole, J. E. R., Mycobacterial proteins, a compilation, *Mol. Micro.,* 6, 133, 1992.

135. Wiker, H. G., Sletten, K., Nagai, S., and Harboe, M., Evidence for three separate genes encoding the proteins of the mycobacterial antigen 85 complex, *Infect. Immun.,* 58, 272, 1990.

136. Rambukkhan, A., Das, P. K., Chand, A., Baas, J. G., Grothuis, D. G., and Kold, A. H. J., Subcellular distribution of monoclonal antibody-defined epitopes on immunuo dominant 33-kilodalton proteins of MTB: identification and localization of 29/33 kilodalton doublet proteins in mycobacterial cell walls, *Scand. J. Immunol.*, 33, 763, 1991.

137. Abou-Zeid, C., Ratliff, T. L., Wiker, H. G., Harboe, M., Bennedsen, J., and Rook, G. A. W., Characterization of fibronectin-binding antigens released by MTB and *M. bovis* BCG, *Infect. Immun.*, 56, 3046, 1988.

138. Abou-Zeid, C., Smith, I., Grange, J. M., Ratliff, T. L., Steele, J., and Rook, G. A. W., The secreted antigens of MTB and their relationship to those recognized by the available antibodies, *J. Gen. Microbiol.*, 134, 531, 1988.

139. Wiker, H. G., Harboe, M., and Lea, T. E., Purification and characterization of two protein antigens from the heterogenous BCG85 complex in *M. bovis* BCG, *Int. Arch. Allerg. Appl. Immunol.*, 81, 298, 1986.

140. Salata, R. A., Sanson, A. J., Malhotra, I. J., Wiker, H. G., Harboe, H. G., Phillips, N. B., and Daniel, T. M., Purification and characterization of the 30,000 dalton native antigen of *Mycobacterium tuberculosis* and characterization of six monoclonal antibodies reactive with a major epitope of this antigen, *J. Lab. Clin. Med.*, 118, 589, 1991.

141. Matsuo, K., Yamaguchi, R., Yamakazi, A., Tasaka, H., and Yamada, T., Cloning and expression of the *M. bovis* BCG gene for extracellular alpha antigen, *J. Bacteriol.*, 160, 3847, 1988.

142. Pal, P. G. and Horowitz, M. A., Immunization with extracellular proteins of *M. tuberculosis* induces cell-mediated immune responses with substantial protective immunity in a guinea pig model of pulmonary tuberculosis, *Infect. Immun.*, 60, 4782, 1992.

143. Huygen, K., van Vooren, J. P., Turneer, M., Bosmans, R., Dierckx, P., and De Bruyn, J., Specific lymphoproliferation, gamma interferon production, and serum immunoglobulin G directed against a purified 32 kDA mycobacterial protein antigen (P32) in patients with active tuberculosis, *Scand. J. Immunol.*, 27, 187, 1988.

144. Abou-Zeid, C., Ratliff, T. L., Wiker, H. G., Harboe, M., Bennedsen, J., and Rook, G. A. W., Characterization of fibronectin-binding antigens released by MTB and *M. bovis* BCG, *Infect. Immun.*, 56, 3046, 1988.

145. Yuan, Y., Lee, R. E., Besra, G. S., Belisle, J. T., and Barry, C. E., III, Identification of a gene involved in the biosynthesis of cyclopropanated mycolic acids in *Mycobacterium tuberculosis. Proc. Natl. Acad. Sci. (USA)*, 92, 6630, 1995.

146. Wallis, R. S., Fujiwara, H., and Ellner, J. J., Direct stimulation of monocyte release of Interleukin-1 by mycobacterial protein antigens, *J. Immunol.*, 36, 193, 1986.

147. Toossi, Z., Lapurga, J. P., Ondash, R., Sedor, J. R., and Ellner, J. J., Expression of functional Interleukin-2 receptors by peripheral blood monocytes from patients with active pulmonary tuberculosis, *J. Clin. Invest.*, 85, 1777, 1990.

148. Toossi, Z., Young, T. G., Averill, L. E., Hamilton, B. D., Shiratsuchi, H., and Ellner, J. J., Induction of transforming growth factor-β (TGF-β) by purified protein derivative (PPD) of *Mycobacterium tuberculosis*, *Infect. Immun.*, 63, 224, 1995.

149. Harth, G., Clemens, D. L., and Horwitz, M. A., Glutamine synthetase of *Mycobacterium tuberculosis:* extracellular release and characterization of itsenzymatic activity, *Proc. Natl. Acad. Sci. USA*, 91, 9342, 1994.

150. Wallis, R. S., Raranjape, R., and Phillips, M., Identification of 2-D gel electrophonesis of a 58 kD TNF-α-reducing protein of MTB, *J. Immun.*, 61, 627, 1993.

151. Toossi, Z., Gogate, P., Shiratsuchi, H., Young, T., and Ellner, J. J., Enhanced production of TGF-β by blood monocytes from patients with active tuberculosis and presence of TGF-β in tuberculosis granulomatous lung lesions, *J. Immunol.*, 154, 465, 1995.

152. Rook, G. A. W., Importance of recent advances in our understanding of antimicrobial cell-mediated immunity to the International Union for the Prevention of Tuberculosis, *Bull. Int. Union Tuberc.*, 58, 60, 1983.

153. Zugmaier, G., Paik, S., Wilding, G., et al., Transforming growth factor β1 induces cachexia and systemic fibrosis without an antitumor effect in nude mice, *Cancer Res.*, 51, 3590, 1991.

154. Broekelmann, T. J., Limper, A. H., Colby, T. V., and McDonald, J. A., Transforming growth factor β is present at sites of extracellular matrix gene expression in human pulmonary fibrosis, *Proc. Natl. Acad. Sci. USA*, 88, 6642, 1991.

155. Border, W. A. and Noble, N. A., Transforming growth factor β in tissue fibrosis, *N. Engl. J. Med.*, 331, 1286, 1994.

156. Denis, M., Tumor necrosis factor and granulocyte macrophage-colony stimulating factor stimulates human macrophages to restrict growth of virulent *Mycobacterium avium* and to kill avirulent *M. avium*. Killing effector mechanism depends on the generation of reactive nitrogen intermediates, *J. Leuk. Biol.*, 49, 380, 1991.

157. Bermudez, L. E. M. and Young, L. S., Tumor necrosis factor alone or in combination with IL-2 but not IFN-g-;gg, is associated with macrophage killing of *Mycobacterium avium* complex, *J. Immunol.*, 140, 3006, 1988.

158. Rook, G. A. W., Steele, J., Fraber, L., Barker, S., Karmali, R., O'Riordan, J., and Standford, J., Vitamin D3, gamma interferon and control of proliferation of *Mycobacterium tuberculosis* by human monocytes, *Immunol.*, 56, 159, 1986.

159. Toossi, Z., Hirsch, C. S., Hamilton, B. D., Kunuth, C. K., Friedlander, M. A., and Rich, E. A., Decreased production of transforming growth factor β1 (TGF-β1) in human alveolar macrophages. *J. Immunol.*, 156, 3461, 1996.

160. Kindler, V., Sappino, A. P., Grau, G. E., Piquet, P. I., and Vassali, P., The reducing role of tumor necrosis factor in the development of bactericidal granulomas during BCG infection, *Cell*, 56, 731, 1989.

161. Flesch, I. and Kaufmann, S. H. E., Mycobacterial growth inhibition by interferon-;gg activated bone marrow macrophages and differential susceptibility among strains of MTB, *J. Immunol.*, 138, 4408, 1987.

162. Flesch, I. E. and Kaufmann, S. H. E., Mechanisms involved in mycobacterial growth inhibition by gamma interferon-activated bone marrow macrophages: role of reactive nitrogen intermediates, *Infect. Immun.*, 59, 3213, 1991.

163. Douvas, G. S., Looker, D. L., Vatter, A., E., and Crowle, A. J., Gamma interferon activates human macrophages to become tumoricidal and leishmanicidal but enhances replication of macrophage-associated mycobacteria, *Infect. Immun.*, 50, 1, 1985.

164. Rook, G. A. W., Steele, J., Fraher, L., Barker, S., Karmali, R., O'Riordan, J., and Stanfor, J., Vitamin D3, gamma interferon, and control of proliferation of *Mycobacterium tuberculosis* by human monocytes, *Immunol.*, 57, 159, 1986.

165. Hirsch, C. S., Yoneda, T., Ellner, J. J., Averill, L. E., and Toossi, Z., Enhancement of intracellular growth of *M. tuberculosis* in human monocytes by transforming growth factor beta, *J. Infect. Dis.*, 170, 1229, 1994.

166. Rook, G. A., Steele, J., Fraher, L., Barker, S., O'Riordan, J., Stanford, J., Vitamin D3, gamma interferon, and control of proliferation of *Mycobacterium tuberculosis* by human monocytes, *Immunology*, 57, 159, 1986.

167. Bermudez, L. E., Production of transforming growth factor-β by *Mycobacterium avium*-infected human macrophages is associated with unresponsiveness to IFN-γ, *J. Immunol.*, 150, 1838, 1993.

168. Hirsch, C. S., Jerrold, J. E., Blinkhorn, R., and Toossi, Z., *In vitro* restoration of T-cell responses in tuberculosis and augmentation of monocyte effector function against *Mycobacterium tuberculosis* by natural inhibitors of transforming growth factor-β, *Proc. Natl. Acad. Sci. USA*, 94, 3926, 1997.

169. Ding, A., Nathan, C., and Srimal, S., Macrophage deactivating factor and TGF-β inhibit of macrophage nitrogen oxide synthesis by IFN-γ, *J. Immunol.*, 145, 940, 1990.

170. Toossi, Z., Mincek, M., Seeholtzer, E., Fulton, S. A., Hamilton, B. D., and Hirsch, C. S., Modulation of IL-12 by transforming growth factor-β (TGF-β) in *Mycobacterium tuberculosis*-infected mononuclear phagocytes and in patients with active tuberculosis, *J. Clin. Lab. Immunol.*, 49, 59, 1997.

171. Boom, W. H., Wallis, R. S., and Chervenak, K. A., Human MTB-reactive CD4+ T-cell clones: heterogeneity in antigen recognition, cytokine production, and cytotoxicity for mononuclear phagocytes, *Infect. Immun.*, 59, 2737, 1991.

172. Mustafa, A. S. and Godal, T., BCG-induced CD4+ cytotoxic T cells from BCG vaccinated healthy subjects: relation between cytotoxicity and suppression *in vitro*, *Clin. Exp. Immunol.*, 69, 255, 1987.

173. Daniel, T. M., Oxtoby, M. J., Pinto, E., and Moreno, E., The immune spectrum in patients with pulmonary tuberculosis, *Am. Rev. Respir. Dis.*, 123, 556, 1981.

174. Nash, D. R. and Douglass, J. E., Anergy in pulmonary tuberculosis: comparison between positive and negative reactors and an evaluation of 5TU and 250 TU skin test doses, *Chest*, 77, 32, 1980.

175. Rooney, J. J., Crocco, J. A., Kramer, S., and Lyons, H. A., Further observations on tuberculin reactions in tuberculosis, *Am. J. Med.*, 60, 517, 1976.

176. Sousa, A. O., Salem, J. I., Lee, F. K., Vercosa, M. C., Cruad, P., Bloom, B. R., Lagrange, P. H., and David, H. L., An epidemic of tuberculosis with a high rate of tuberculin anergy among a population previously unexposed to tuberculosis, the Yanomami Indians of the Brazilian Amazon, *Proc. Natl. Acad. Sci. USA*, 94, 13227, 1997.

177. Ellner, J. J., Suppressor adherent cells in human tuberculosis, *J. Immunol.*, 121, 2573, 1978.

178. Kleinhenz, M. E. and Ellner, J. J., Antigen responsiveness during tuberculosis: regulatory interaction of T-cell subpopulations and adherent cells, *J. Lab. Clin. Med.*, 110, 31, 1987.

179. Kleinhenz, M. E. and Ellner, J. J., Immunoregulatory adherent cells in human tuberculosis: radiation-sensitive antigen-specific suppression by monocytes, *J. Infect. Dis.*, 152, 171, 1985.

180. Toossi, Z., Edmonds, K. L., Tomford, W. J., and Ellner, J. J., Suppression of PPD-induced interleukin-2 production by interaction of Leu-22 (CD16) lymphocytes and adherent mononuclear cells in tuberculosis, *J. Infect. Dis.*, 159, 352, 1989.

181. Toossi, Z., Kleinhenz, M. E., and Ellner, J. J., Defective Interleukin-2 production and responsiveness in human pulmonary tuberculosis, *J. Exp. Med.*, 163, 1162, 1986.

182. Hussain, R., Dawood, G., Obaid, M., Toossi, Z., Wallis, R. S., Minai, A., Dojki, M., Sturm, A. W., and Ellner, J. J., Depressed cellular and augmented humoral responses in patients with active tuberculosis from Pakistan, *Clin. Diag. Lab. Immunol.*, 2, 726, 1995.

183. Andrade-Arzabe, R., Machado, I. V., Fernandez, B., Blanca, I., Ramirez, R., and Bianco, N. E., Cellular immunity in current active pulmonary tuberculosis, *Am. Rev. Respir. Dis.*, 143, 496, 1991.

184. Vanham, G., Edmonds, K., Qing, L., Hom, D., Toossi, Z., Jones, B., Daley, C. L., Huebner, R., Kestens, L., Gigase, P., and Ellner, J. J., Generalized immune activation in pulmonary tuberculosis: co-activation with HIV infection, *Clin. Exp. Immunol.*, 103, 30, 1996.

185. Fujiwara, H. and Tsuyuguchi, I., Frequency of tuberculin-reactive T-lymphocytes in pleural fluid and blood from patients with tuberculous pleuritis, *Chest,* 89, 530, 1984.

186. Carlucci, S., Beschin, A., Tuosto, L., Ameglio, F., Gandolfo, G., Cocito, C., Fiorucci, F., Saltini, C., and Piccolella, E., Mycobacterial antigen complex A60-specific T-cell repertoire during the course of pulmonary tuberculosis, *Infect. Immmun.*, 61, 439, 1993.

187. Hirsch, C. S., Hussain, R., Toossi, Z., Dawood, G., Shahid, F., and Ellner, J. J., Cross modulation by transforming growth factor β in human tuberculosis: suppression of antigen-driven blastogenesis and interferon γ production, *Proc. Natl. Acad. Sci. (USA)*, 93, 3193, 1995.

188. Shiratsuchi, H., Okuda, Y., and Tsuyuguchi, I., Recombinant human Interleukin-2 reverses *in vitro*-deficient cell-mediated immune responses to tuberculin purified protein derivative by lymphocytes of tuberculous patients, *Infect. Immun.*, 55, 2126, 1987.

189. Huygen, K., van Vooren, J. P., Turneer, M., Bosmans, R., Dierckx, P., and De Bruyn, J., Specific lymphoproliferation, gamma interferon production, and serum immunoglobulin G directed against a purified 32 kDA mycobacterial protein antigen (P32) in patients with active tuberculosis, *Scand. J. Immunol.*, 27, 187, 1988.

190. Vilcek, J., Klion, A., Henriksen-DeStefano, D., Zemtsov, A., Davidson, D. M., Davidson, M., and Friedman-Kien, A., Defective gamma-interferon production in peripheral blood leukocytes of patients with acute tuberculosis, *J. Clin. Immunol.*, 6, 146, 1986.

191. Gazzinelli, R. T., Hieny, S., Wynn, T. A., Wolf, S., and Sher, A., Interleukin 12 is required for the T-lymphocyte-independent induction of interferon γ by an intracellular parasite and induces resistance in T-cell-deficient hosts. *Proc. Natl. Acad. Sci.*, 90, 6115, 1993.

192. Sieling, P. A., Abrams, J. S., Yamamura, M., Salgame, P., Bloom, B. R., Rea, T. H., and Modlin, R. L., Immunosuppressive roles for IL-10 and IL-4 in human infection. *J. Immunol.*, 150, 5501, 1993.

193. Street, N. E. and Mossman, T. R., Functional diversity of T lymphocytes due to secretion of different cytokine patterns, *FASB J.*, 5, 171, 1991.

194. Bogdan, C., Vodovotz, Y., and Nathan, C., Macrophage deactivation by Interleukin 10, *J. Exp. Med.*, 174, 1549, 1991.

195. Lehn, M. W., Weisner, W. Y., Engelhorn, S., Gillis, S., and Remold, H. G., IL-4 inhibits H2O2 production and antileishmanial capacity of human cultured monocytes mediated by IFN gamma, *J. Immunol.*, 143, 3020, 1989.

196. Sucrel, H. M., Tory-Blomberg, M., Paulie, S., Anderson, G., Moreno, C., Pasvol, G., and Ivanyi, J., TH-1/TH-2 profiles in tuberculosis, based on the proliferation and cytokine response of blood lymphocytes to mycobacterial antigens, *Immunology,* 81, 171, 1994.

197. Hirsch, C. S., Toossi, Z., Hussain, R., and Ellner, J. J., Suppression of T-cell responses by TGF-β in tuberculosis, *J. Invest. Med.,* 43, 365A, 1995.

198. Schmitt, E., Meuret, G., and Stix, L., Monocyte recruitment in tuberculosis and sarcoidosis, *Brit. J. Hematol.,* 35, 11, 1977.

199. Toossi, Z., Hamilton, B. D., Phillips, M. H., Averill, L. E., Ellner, J. J., and Salvekar, A., Regulation of nuclear factor-kB and its inhibitor IkB-a/ MAD-3 in monocytes by *Mycobacterium tuberculosis* and during human tuberculosis, *J. Immunol.,* 159, 4109, 1997.

200. Lenzini, L., Heather, C. J., Rottoli, L., and Rottoli, P., Studies on bronchoalveolar cells in humans. I. Preliminary morphological studies in various respiratory diseases, *Respir.,* 36, 145, 1978.

201. Venet, A., Niaudet, P., Bach, J. F., and Even, P., Study of alveolar lymphocytes obtained by bronchoalveolar lavage, *Ann. Anest. Franc.,* 6, 634, 1980.

202. Sharma, S. K., Pande, J. N., and Verma, K., Bronchoalveolar lavage (BAL) in miliary tuberculosis, *Tubercle,* 69, 175, 1988.

203. Dhank R., De, A., Ganguly, N. K., Gupta, N., Jaswal, S., Malik, S. K., and Kohli, K. K., Factors influencing the cellular response in bronchoalveolar lavage and peripheral blood of patients with pulmonary tuberculosis, *Tubercle,* 69, 161, 1988.

204. Baughman, R. P., Dohn M. N., Loudon, R. G., and Trame, P. T., Bronchoscopy with bronchoalveolar lavage in tuberculosis and fungal infections, *Chest,* 99, 92, 1991.

205. Ozaki, T., Nakahira, S., Tani, K., Ogushi, F., Yasuoka, S., and Ogura, T., Differential cell analysis in bronchoalveolar lavage fluid from pulmonary lesions of patients with tuberculosis, *Chest,* 102, 54, 1992.

206. Schwander, S. K., Sada, E., Torres, M., Escobedo, D., Sierra, J. G., Alt, S., and Rich, E. A., T lymphocytic and immature macrophage alveolitis in active pulmonary tuberculosis, *J. Infect. Dis.,* 176, 1267, 1996.

207. Schwander, S. K., Torres, M., Sada, E., Carranza, C., Ramos, E., Tary-Lehmann, M., Wallis, R. S., Sierra, J., and Rich, E. A., Enhanced responses to *Mycobacterium tuberculosis* antigens by human alveolar lymphocytes during active pulmonary tuberculosis, *J. Infect. Dis.,* 178, 1434, 1998.

208. Taha, R. A., Kotsimbos, T. C., Song, Y-L., Menzies, D., and Hamid, Q., IFN-γ and IL-12 are increased in active compared with inactive tuberculosis, *Am. J. Respir. Crit. Care Med.,* 155, 1135, 1997.

209. Reider, H. L., Cauthen, G. M., Bloch, A. B., Cole, C. H., Holtzman, D., Snider D. E., Bigler, W. J., and Witte, J. J., Tuberculosis and AIDS: Florida, *Arch. Intern. Med.,* 149, 1268, 1989.

210. Daley, C. L., Small, G. F., Schecter, G. K., Schoolnik, G. K., McAdam, R. A., Jacobs, W. R., and Hopewell, P. C., An out- break of tuberculosis with accelerated progression among persons infected with HIV, *N. Engl. J. Med.,* 326, 2131, 1992.

211. Lucas, S. and Nelson, A. M., Pathogenesis of tuberculosis in human immunodeficiency virus-infected people. In *Tuberculosis Pathogenesis, Protection, and Control,* (B. Bloom, Ed.), ASM Press, Materials Park, OH, 1994.

212. Ellner, J. J., [Editorial] Tuberculosis in the time of AIDS: the facts and the message, *Chest,* 98, 1051, 1990.

213. Okwera, A., Eriki, P. P., Guay, L. A., Ball, P., and Daniel, T. M., Tuberculin reactions in HIV-seropositive and HIV-seronegative healthy women in Uganda, *MMWR,* 39, 638, 1990.

214. Johnson, J. L., Vjecha, M. J., Okwera, A., Hatanga, E., Byekwaso, F., Wolski, K., Aisu, T., Whalen, C. C., Huebner, R., Mugerwa, R. D., and Ellner, J. J., Impact of human immunodeficiency virus type-1 infection on the initial bacteriologic and radiographic manifestations of pulmonary tuberculosis in Uganda (Makerere University-Case Western Reserve Research Collaboration), *Int. J. Tuberc. Lung Dis.,* 2, 397, 1998.

215. Wallis, R. S., Vjecha, M., Amir-Tahmasseb, M. Okwera, A., Byekwaso, F., Nyole, J., Kabengera, J., Mugerwa, R. D., and Ellner, J. J., Influence of tuberculosis on HIV: enhanced cytokine expression and elevated B2 microglobulin in HIV-1 associated tuberculosis, *J. Infect. Dis.,* 167, 43, 1992.

216. Cohen, O. J., Kinter, A., and Fauci, A. S., Host factors in the pathogenesis of HIV disease, *Immunol. Rev.,* 159, 31, 1997.

217. Clerici, M. and Shearer, G. M., A TH-1/TH-2 switch is a critical step in the etiology of HIV infection, *Immunol. Today,* 14, 107, 1993.

218. Zhang, M., Gong, J., Iyer, D., Jones, B. E., Modlin, R. L., and Barnes, P. F., T-cell cytokine responses in persons with tuberculosis and human immunodeficiency virus infection, *J. Clin. Invest.*, 94, 2435, 1994.

219. Orenstein, J. M., Fox, C., and Wahl, M. S., Macrophages as a source of HIV during opportunistic infections, *Science*, 276, 1857, 1997.

220. Meltzer, M. S., Skillman, D. R., Gomatos, P. J., Kalter, D. C., and Gendelman, H. E., Role of mononuclear phagocytes in the pathogenesis of human immunodeficiency virus infection, *Ann. Rev. Immunol.*, 8, 169, 1990.

221. Twigg, H. L., Lipscomb, M. F., Yoffe, B., Barbaro, D. J., and Weissler, J. C., Enhanced accessory cell function by alveolar macrophages from patients infected with the human immunodeficiency virus: potential role for depletion of CD4+ cells in the lung, *Am. J. Respir. Cell Mol. Biol.*, 1, 391, 1989.

222. Murray, H. W., Gellene, R. A., Libby, D. M., Roth, E., Armmel, C. D., and Rubin, B. Y., Activation of tissue macrophages from AIDS patients: *in vitro* responses of AIDS alveolar macrophages to lymphokines and interferon-γ, *J. Immunol.*, 135, 2374, 1985.

223. Buhl, R., Jaffe, H. A., Holroyd, K. J., Borok, Z., Roum, J. H., Mastrangeli, A., Wells, F. B., Kirby, M., Saltini, C., and Crystal, R. G., Activation of alveolar macrophages in asymptomatic HIV-infected individuals, *J. Immunol.*, 150, 1019, 1993.

224. Twigg, H. L., Iwamoto, G. K., and Soliman, D. M., Role of cytokines in alveolar macrophage accessory cell function in HIV-infected individuals, *J. Immunol.*, 149, 1462, 1992.

225. Trentin, L., Barbisa, S., Zambello, R., Agostini, C., Caenazzo, C., di Francesco, C., Cipriani, A., Francavalla, E., and Semenzato, G., Spontaneous production of IL-6 by alveolar macrophages form human immunodeficiency virus type 1-infected patients, *J. Infect. Dis.*, 166, 731, 1992.

226. Agostini, C., Zambello, R., Trentin, L., Garbisa, S., DiCelle, P. F., Bulian, P., Onisto, M., Poletti, V., Spiga, L., Raise, E., Foa, R., and Semenzato, G., Alveolar macrophages from patients with AIDS and AIDS-related complex constitutively synthesize and release tumor necrosis factor alpha, *Am. Rev. Respir. Dis.*, 144, 195, 1991.

227. Plata, F., Autran, B., Pedroza Martins, L., Wain-Hobson, S., Raphael, M., Mayaud, C., Denis, M., Guillon, J. M., and Debre, P., AIDS virus-specific cytotoxic T-lymphocytes in lung disorders, *Nature* (London), 328, 348, 1987.

228. De Cock, K. M., Soro, B., Coulibaly, I. M., and Lucas, S. B., Tuberculosis and HIV infection in sub-Saharan Africa, *JAMA*, 268, 1581, 1992.

229. Whalen, C., Horsburgh, C. R., Hom, D., Lahart, C., Simberkoff, M., and Ellner, J. J., Accelerated course of human immunodeficiency virus infection after tuberculosis, *Am. J. Respir. Crit. Care. Med.*, 151, 129, 1995.

230. Braun, M. M., Nsanga B., and Ryder, R. W., A retrospective cohort study of the risks of tuberculosis among women of childbearing age with HIV infection in Zaire, *Am. Rev. Respir. Dis.*, 143, 501, 1991.

231. Vjecha, M., Okwera, A., Byekwaso, F., Nakibali, J., Nyole, F., Okot-nwang, M., Aisu, T., Eriki, P., Mugerwa, R., Daniel, T., Heubner, R., and Ellner, J. J., Predictors of mortality and drug toxicity in HIV-infected patients from Uganda treated for pulmonary tuberculosis, 8th International Conference on AIDS/3rd STD World Congress, Amsterdam, Netherlands, July 1992.

232. Goletti, D., Weissman, D., Jackson, R. W., Graham, N. M., Vlahov, D., Klein, R. S., Munsiff, S. S., Ortona, L., Cauda, R., and Fauci, A. S., Effect of *Mycobacterium tuberculosis* on HIV replication: role of immune activation, *J. Immunol.*, 157, 1271, 1996.

233. Lederman, M. M., Georges, D.L., Kusner, D. J., Mudido, P., Giam, C-Z., and Toossi, Z., *Mycobacterium tuberculosis* and its purified protein derivative activate expression of the human immunodeficiency virus, *J. Acq. Immune Defic. Synd.*, 7, 727, 1994.

234. Toossi, Z., Nicolacakis, K., Xia, L., Ferrari, N. A., and Rich, E. A., Activation of latent HIV-1 by *Mycobacterium tuberculosis* and its purified protein derivative in alveolar macrophages from HIV-infected individuals *in vitro, J. Acq. Immune Defic. Synd. Human Retrovirol.*, 15, 325, 1997.

235. Toossi, Z., Sierra-Madero, J. G., Blinkhorn, R. A., Mettler, M. A., and Rich, E. A., Enhanced susceptibility of blood monocytes from patients with pulmonary tuberculosis to productive infection with human immunodeficiency virus-1 (HIV-1), *J. Exp. Med.*, 177, 1511, 1993.

236. Garrait, C. J., Esvant, H., Henry, I., Morinet, P., Mayaud, C., and Israel-Biet, D., Tuberculosis generates a microenvironment enhancing the productive infection of local lymphocytes by HIV, *J. Immunol.*, 159, 2824, 1997.

3 Transmission and Safety Issues

Edward A. Nardell, M.D.

CONTENTS

0-8493-1565-4/97/$0.00+$.50
© 2000 by CRC Press LLC

I. INTRODUCTION

In the early part of this century, when tuberculosis was the major cause of death and misery in the U.S. and Europe, control of airborne spread, then a theory of growing popularity, became an important component of evolving scientific strategies to combat the disease. Isolation of contagious patients was in part the rationale for sanatorium treatment, although at times only early cases were admitted in hope of cure while advanced, more infectious cases were sent home to die, thereby undoing the benefits of isolation.[1] In 1934 William Firth Wells proposed a clear distinction between true airborne infections (e.g., TB, measles) transmitted by droplet nuclei, the buoyant, dried residue of aerosolized respiratory droplets, and infections spread by the larger respiratory droplets themselves (e.g., staphylococci, streptococci).[2] Unlike droplet nuclei that disperse widely, large respiratory droplets remain within the immediate vicinity of their source, carrying infection as an extension of direct person to person contact.

During the next 4 decades airborne infection was the subject of intensive research, with the ultimate goal of better environmental control — a strategy analogous to the hygienic control of waterborne infections such as cholera.[3] Unlike the disinfection of public water supplies, however, disinfection of air in the many environments where TB transmission occurs was not a feasible goal. Moreover, with the accelerated decline in tuberculosis in developed countries after the introduction of chemotherapy, and the prospect of immunizations against many of the common respiratory viruses, research on airborne infection and environmental control all but ended. Transmission has continued since the advent of chemotherapy, of course, before the diagnosis is made and in cases where therapy fails, increasingly facilitated in tightly constructed buildings by central heating, ventilating, and air conditioning (HVAC) systems, and by the growing pool of previously uninfected, fully susceptible persons. In the U.S. in the mid-1980s, an increase in homelessness and the advent of HIV infection, at a time when the public health systems were unable to assure the completion of tuberculosis treatment, led to outbreaks of accelerated tuberculosis transmission in congregate settings such as healthcare facilities, homeless shelters, prisons, and drug treatment centers, once again underscoring the importance of airborne transmission and the need for air disinfection as an adjunct to prompt diagnosis and effective treatment.[4,5]

Although tuberculosis infection for an individual is considered an all or nothing event, the probability of infection resulting from a given exposure depends on the interaction of a limited number of host and environmental factors, the relative importance of which have been examined epidemiologically, experimentally, and theoretically.[6] However, recent discussions of tuberculosis transmission and its control have often ignored important quantitative concepts and the substantial experimental data upon which they are based. Instead, environmental control recommendations have been based largely on tradition, intuition, and strategies used to control such indoor air pollutants as odors or industrial toxins. The premise of this discussion is that a quantitative approach to understanding tuberculosis transmission leads to emphasis on somewhat different control strategies than have been currently recommended.[4] Important differences between factories and healthcare facilities that limit the application of industrial respirators as personal protection against TB also will be emphasized.

II. EXPERIMENTAL BASIS FOR UNDERSTANDING TB TRANSMISSION

A. EXPERIMENTAL TRANSMISSION TO ANIMALS

Although decades of careful clinical and epidemiologic observations had provided important insights into TB transmission and pathogenesis, early experiments in which rabbits were infected with bovine tuberculosis or guinea pigs with human tuberculosis, organisms to which each species is exquisitely susceptible, provided the foundation for a new level of understanding, much of which remains valid today. Inhalation experiments using dilute aerosols where droplets contained mostly single organisms, for example, resulted in infection in a predictable percentage of exposed animals, depending on the airborne concentration and the volume of air breathed.[7-9] Infections were detected several weeks after inhalation by tuberculin skin test conversion, and this correlated with the finding of single, discrete tubercles visible in the lungs of animals sacrificed 5 to 6 weeks after infection.

As already noted, the size of airborne particles is a critical determinant of infection. In experiments using concentrated aerosols of cultured organisms, Wells et al. found 16 times as many tubercles in the lungs of rabbits breathing equal numbers of fine (2 μm) droplets compared to coarse aerosol suspensions (12 to 15 μm).[8] Fine droplets (droplet nuclei) were carried with air into ✷ the vulnerable alveoli, whereas larger droplets were much more likely to impact on the upper airways which are highly resistant to infection. Such quantitative inhalation experiments in animals established the fundamental principle that the probability of infection is proportional to the concentration of infectious droplet nuclei in air, and the volume of air breathed over the exposure time.[9] Within the limits of the experimental methods, complete parity was established between the number of bacilli aerosolized into air as determined by colony counts on air centrifuge culture tubes, and the numbers of tubercles in the lungs of exposed animals. The minimum infective dose for highly susceptible experimental animals was a single droplet nucleus containing one or at most several tubercle bacilli. Rabbits and guinea pigs, therefore, have been used as nearly ideal quantitative samplers for infectious droplet nuclei in air.

B. Transmission from Humans

The ultimate use of animals as samplers of airborne tubercle bacilli was a remarkable experiment conceived by Wells to demonstrate convincingly that airborne contagion was sufficient to transmit human tuberculosis, and to quantify the infectiousness of patients under hospital conditions. The experiment was carried out between 1956 and 1961 by Riley and colleagues with the cooperation of the Baltimore Veterans Administration Hospital.[10-12] A unique six-bed experimental ward for tuberculosis patients was constructed so that all exhaust air passed through a chamber designed by Wells to uniformly expose more than 100 guinea pigs simultaneously. The six rooms were occupied continuously by newly diagnosed patients about to begin chemotherapy, and by chronic tuberculosis patients, many with drug resistant disease. During the first 2 years, 71 of an average 156 exposed animals were infected, having breathed approximately 1 million cubic feet (cf) of ward air, yielding a calculated average concentration of 1 infectious unit in 14,000 cf of air.[13] During the second 2 years, under slightly modified conditions (to be discussed), 63 of an average 120 exposed animals were infected, for an average concentration of 1 infectious unit in 11,000 cf of ward air.[12] Careful correlation of the presence of individual patients on the ward, guinea pig conversions, and drug resistance patterns of organisms recovered from the animals permitted further analysis of factors associated with infectiousness.[14]

C. Source Factors

Clinical, epidemiologic, and experimental observations indicate that some patients with tuberculosis are much more contagious than others. Factors generally associated with greater contagiousness ✷ include more extensive lung involvement, especially lung cavitation, laryngeal or endobronchial disease, more frequent cough, greater numbers of tubercle bacilli in sputum, less viscous sputum, and an indolent rather than a fulminant clinical course, allowing more time for transmission.[6,15] In contrast, noncavitary pulmonary tuberculosis, including primary and pediatric disease, generally has been less contagious. However, cases of pulmonary tuberculosis associated with HIV infection have been infectious in the absence of lung cavitation, presumably because lung tissues contain unusually large numbers of organisms.[16] Although extrapulmonary tuberculosis usually is not very contagious, a hip abscess containing large numbers of tubercle bacilli was responsible for extensive transmission in a hospital, in part because high pressure wound irrigation generated infectious droplet nuclei.[17] In the Baltimore VA Hospital study, great variability in infectivity of cases was observed, with 35 of 48 bacteriologically traceable guinea pig infections caused by just 3 of 77 patients on the ward during the initial 2 years.[14] Effective disseminators were noted to have had more violent coughing, to have been less likely to have covered their mouths while coughing, and were more likely to have had drug-resistant tuberculosis, thereby not receiving effective treatment as did the drug-susceptible cases. In recent outbreaks of multidrug-resistant TB in institutions, some of the same transmission factors have been identified, most notably, unrecognized drug resistance.[18]

D. MECHANICAL AIR SAMPLING

Although the lungs of highly susceptible animals proved to be nearly ideal selective air samplers for tuberculosis, their use under clinical conditions was cumbersome to say the least. Mechanical air sampling methods using culture techniques are simpler to use by comparison, and have been used to detect and quantify a variety of airborne microorganisms. Unfortunately, technical limitations prevent the application of mechanical air sampling for tubercle bacilli in clinical settings. At the very low average concentrations of tubercle bacilli found in the air of Riley's experimental TB ward, detection would require prolonged sampling time (5 to 10 h) at extremely high sampling rates (1000 lpm), whereas the concentration of background environmental microorganisms would likely exceed 1000/l.[19] Moreover, the slow growth rate of tubercle bacilli compared to most other microorganisms makes their detection doubly difficult. Using the Wells air centrifuge for sampling, First was unable to detect airborne tubercle bacilli during bronchoscopies performed at a Detroit tuberculosis hospital in the pre-chemotherapeutic era.[20] Polymerase chain reaction (PCR) techniques that selectively amplify identifying segments of mycobacterial nucleic acids amid a soup of other organisms have the potential to detect even rare airborne tubercle bacilli, living or dead, and this application of PCR has recently been reported.[21] Unfortunately, at its current stage of development, because PCR cannot distinguish living from dead organisms and results have not been correlated with infectivity, its application is limited at best and potentially misleading.

E. TRANSMISSION TO HUMANS

The infecting dose for humans is harder to estimate than for inbred rabbits and guinea pigs. Tubercles in peripheral lung tissue comparable to those found in experimental animals are seen in humans, suggesting that single droplet nuclei are also sufficient to infect.[22] However, while the number of inhalations of viable tubercle bacilli required before infection occurs in humans is uncertain, the very low average concentrations of droplet nuclei estimated under clinical conditions makes multiple inhalations statistically unlikely under most circumstances. Assuming susceptibility to 1 to 3 inhalations, the estimated concentrations of infectious droplet nuclei in the air of Riley's experimental tuberculosis ward (1 in 11,000 to 14,000 cf) was sufficient to explain the rate of skin test conversion of student nurses (6 to 18 months) working 40 h per week on general medical wards in the prechemotherapy era.[11]

Not knowing how many droplet nuclei were required to infect humans, Wells coined the term "quanta" to represent an infectious unit of droplet nuclei, whatever the number.[3,23] Quanta, symbolized by "q" will appear in the mathematical analysis of TB transmission, representing an infecting dose of one or at most a few droplet nuclei — containing one or at most a few viable tubercle bacilli.

Recent epidemiologic data suggest that there may be as much as a twofold difference in the initial rate of tuberculosis infection between blacks and whites under conditions of approximately equal exposure, a finding attributed to greater inherited resistance among whites, resulting from generations of selective genetic pressure, whereas blacks in central Africa historically had been geographically isolated from the disease.[24,25] Individual variation in susceptibility based on innate resistance and concomitant medical conditions is also likely.

Under low prevalence conditions among otherwise healthy persons, previous infection with tuberculosis appears to convey almost complete immunity to exogenous reinfection. Under conditions of repeated exposure and decreased host immunity, however, true exogenous reinfection occurs, and although often difficult to prove, may be an important pathogenic pathway in high prevalence countries and among high-risk persons in congregate settings.[26-29] Furthermore, HIV immunosuppression clearly predisposes persons with new TB infection to progress rapidly to active disease, and persons with old foci of infection to reactivate. There also is a strong suggestion, but as yet no proof, that HIV infection predisposes individuals to acquire TB infection, an event believed to be determined locally by the innate microbicidal capacity of resident alveolar macrophages, not by cell-mediated immunity (CMI).[16,30] However, restriction fragment-length polymorphism (RFLP), a technique for genetic fingerprinting of tubercle bacilli, has shown exogenous reinfection with tuberculosis to be prevalent among persons with advanced HIV immunosuppression, strongly suggesting impairment of innate macrophage killing, as well as of CMI.[16] Increased susceptibility to new infection together with rapid progression to active, communicable disease probably explains the accelerated rate of propagation observed among HIV-infected persons in congregate settings.[26]

Whether the infecting dose is one or several droplet nuclei for a given individual, clearly there is no safe level of exposure for tuberculosis comparable to a TLV (threshold limit value) for chemical and physical agents. When concentrations are extremely low, infection remains possible, but statistically unlikely. The absence of a TLV distinguishes tuberculosis and certain other infectious agents from indoor air pollutants where exposure concentration more often correlates with symptoms or disease, rather than the probability of an all or nothing event.

F. Microbial Factors

Tuberculosis is transmitted from person to person with no important intermediary hosts or reservoirs in nature. Whereas buildings can contribute substantially to TB transmission, unlike true building-associated infections like legionellosis, buildings are never the source of infection, and cannot harbor the organism in an infectious state for very long after the source case leaves. Although the half-life of airborne tubercle bacilli of the H37Rv strain was approximately 6 h under controlled conditions of temperature and humidity, dilution with infection-free air through ventilation limits the long-term potential for infection far more than does viability.[31] Only 1% of airborne droplet nuclei persist for an hour in a room with five air changes (AC) per hour (infection-free air), assuming complete mixing. If droplet nuclei were not being continuously produced by an active case, even relatively poor ventilation would be expected to greatly reduce their concentration (and the probability of infection) within several hours. Although a large fraction of tubercle bacilli in larger respiratory droplets settle onto surfaces, becoming part of room dust, residual viable bacilli pose no threat of infection unless they are resuspended as airborne particles of a respirable size (1 to 5 μm).[6] Aerosolization from the surface of the respiratory tract requires a thin fluid layer and the high velocity air flow rates generated by coughs and other respiratory maneuvers — conditions not easily reproduced in the environment. The possibility of an environmental source was examined in the Byrd study of shipboard transmission, but no convincing evidence was found.[32] Tuberculosis transmission, therefore, depends heavily on the simultaneous presence both of a contagious source and a potential victim under conditions supportive of transmission.

Virulence of human tubercle bacilli appears to vary somewhat around the world, based on experimental and epidemiologic evidence.[33] The basis for increased virulence appears to be ill-defined microbial factors which allow the organisms to evade macrophage-mediated host defenses. Clinically, virulence is manifest as a relatively high rate of clinical disease for a given level of infection. Experimentally, pathogenicity for guinea pigs has been used to distinguish fully virulent strains from strains of less virulence. Reduced virulence may be a microbial accommodation ("balanced pathogenicity") to endemic infection among highly susceptible persons, a situation where full virulence eventually might adversely affect microbial propagation and survival.[34]

Although it's harder to infect guinea pigs with drug-resistant tuberculosis, a large number of outbreaks with such organisms has discredited the notion that drug resistance correlates with decreased virulence for humans.[35] In fact, there is a popular misconception that the multidrug resistant (MDR) tuberculosis responsible for recent outbreaks in congregate settings must be a supervirulent strain. Although there is no standard biological assay for increased virulence, there is no reason to believe that MDR TB is more virulent than susceptible strains. The accelerated propagation and high fatality rate among HIV-infected persons appears to be explained by rapid progression from infection to active disease, by environmental factors favoring wide transmission, and by a high rate of dissemination outside the lungs.[36] An episode of extensive transmission in the workplace has been reported where increased microbial virulence may have been responsible.[37] More rapid growth in the mouse model suggests evasion of host immune defenses as a possible mechanism. Not yet explored is the possibility that greater transmission potential may involve greater viability during airborne transport as droplet nuclei. The isolate responsible for this outbreak has been selected along with a less virulent laboratory strain for complete DNA decoding.[38] Differences in genetic material between the two organisms may lead to a better understanding of mycobacterial virulence.

G. Environmental Factors

In low prevalence countries, tuberculosis spreads almost exclusively within buildings because droplet nuclei are diluted outside to concentrations so low that transmission becomes statistically unlikely. The hostility of outdoor environments for tubercle bacilli, including the germicidal effects of the ultraviolet irradiation in sunlight, may be another important factor. The effects of environmental stresses on *E. coli, Serratia,* and other test airborne pathogens have been studied extensively under laboratory conditions, but similar research has not been done on slower growing mycobacteria which are more difficult to study.[39] It is likely, for example, that high humidity, by preventing dehydration, protects tubercle bacilli from ultraviolet irradiation.[40]

Within buildings, droplet nuclei become less concentrated as they disperse from the source, diffusing within the available space, moved by convection currents and forced air movement. Mechanical ventilation redistributes droplet nuclei within buildings, lowering their local concentration by dilution within a larger volume of air, and by dilution with a variable fraction of infection-free, outside air. Outside air replaces a variable volume of mixed room air which is exhausted to the outside, and it is the exhaust air together with air leakage from buildings that actually removes droplet nuclei.

In small, poorly ventilated indoor spaces, droplet nuclei reach relatively high concentrations quickly compared to larger, well-ventilated spaces. If small spaces are crowded, a common condition for the economically disadvantaged, the potential for TB transmission is increased, accounting in part for the high prevalence of TB among the poor.

H. Patterns of TB Outbreaks Within Buildings

Airborne TB transmission within buildings occurs by two routes: (1) within rooms and adjacent spaces and (2) to nonadjacent spaces through a mechanical ventilation system. In unventilated spaces, transmission occurs predominantly by spread within contiguous spaces, with greater infection rates closer to the source case and lower rates at greater distances, presumably the result of the dilution of droplet nuclei as they disperse.[17,41] In buildings with ventilation systems, infections may occur throughout buildings, not clustered around the source case or specific high-risk activities, suggesting the recirculation of infectious droplet nuclei.[32,42,43] Recirculation mixes, dilutes, and distributes droplet nuclei, producing a relatively uniform exposure within the entire ventilation circuit, as if the exposure occurred in one common breathing space. Mobility of the source case and of susceptible persons within buildings also tends to distribute exposure more evenly. One of the best studied episodes of tuberculosis transmission occurred in the confines of a ship, an epidemic on the SS Byrd where the source case resided in one of two separate living compartments.[32] The infection rate was high in the compartment where the source case resided and worked, where the air was largely recirculated. Infections in the other compartment were proportional to the percentage of air mixing between the two compartments.

III. MATHEMATICAL MODEL OF AIRBORNE INFECTION

A. THE WELLS-RILEY MODEL OF AIRBORNE INFECTION

While it is not possible to consider all of the transmission factors involved in a given TB exposure, a mathematical model has been developed which accounts for the major determinants, including the statistical probability of escaping infection.[44] The model assumes steady-state conditions, complete air mixing, equal susceptibility to a quanta of infection (assumed to be a single droplet nucleus — as discussed above under Section E, "Transmission to Humans"), and other conditions which may not be entirely valid for each exposure, but which have permitted insights not otherwise possible into the relative importance of ventilation and various other factors.[12,41,42]

If infectious droplet nuclei suspended in air were evenly distributed, the number of quanta inhaled by susceptible hosts, N, would be equal to the concentration of quanta in the air times the volume of air breathed. In the steady-state, the concentration of quanta would equal Iq/Q: the number of infectious sources, I, times the rate of production of quanta per source, q, divided by the volume of infection-free air (i.e., ventilation) into which the quanta are distributed, Q. The volume of air breathed by susceptible hosts would equal Stp: the number of susceptible hosts, S, times the pulmonary ventilation per susceptible, p, times the duration of exposure, t.

$$N = \text{concentration} \times \text{volume}$$

$$= (Iq/Q) \times Stp \tag{3.1}$$

$$= S(Iqpt/Q)$$

For simplicity in further developing this mathematical model, consider a hypothetical, high-exposure situation where the combination of transmission factors $(Iqpt/Q) = 1$, in which case $N = S$; that is, all susceptible hosts would become infected. Cases this infectious occur rarely, although the situation was approximated during a bronchoscopy and intubation in which 10 of 13 exposed persons were infected.[41] Under more commonly encountered conditions, droplet nuclei appear to be separated by large volumes of infection-free air, an average of 10,000 to 14,000 cf of air in the experimental TB ward already discussed, and the distribution of droplet nuclei tends to be random rather than even.[11]

Under random conditions, if $(Iqpt/Q) = 1$ and $N = S$, some susceptibles would, by chance, escape infection, while others would inhale more than one quantum. According to Poisson's law of small chances, the probability of escaping infection under the hypothetical circumstance where $(Iqpt/Q) = 1$ would be approximately e^{-1}, or 0.37, where e is the base of natural logarithms, with a value of approximately 2.7. The probability of infection under the above circumstances would be $S(1 - e^{-1})$, or 63%. Thus, in the hypothetical case where $(Iqpt/Q) = 1$ and the distribution of droplet nuclei is random, 63% of susceptible persons would be infected compared to 100% with even distribution. The general mathematical expression, referred to as the "Wells-Riley Model for Airborne Infection," describing the interaction of transmission factors, therefore, is

$$C = S(1 - e^{-Iqpt/Q}) \tag{3.2}$$

where C = the number of new infections. This modified form of Equation 3.1 was derived by E. C. Riley for use in airborne infection.[44] Further mathematical refinements have been introduced recently, but their value is questionable, given the assumptions required to model airborne infection in the first place.[45] The relationship has been used to analyze measles as well as TB transmission, and a similar mass balance equation has been successfully used to predict the effects of ventilation and filtration on the concentration of aeroallergens in animal quarters.[42,44,46] More recently, the equation has been modified to analyze the relative contribution of ventilation and personal respiratory protection in the intensive care unit.[47]

B. Application of the Wells-Riley Model

The model has been applied to TB transmission under circumstances where the quantifiable transmission factors have been known or could be estimated. Knowing all other factors, q, the generation rate of quanta, the infecting dose of droplet nuclei, has been calculated for several infectious TB cases. Estimates for q range from approximately 1 quanta per hour (i.e., 1 qph) for the treated patients transmitting TB to guinea pigs on the Baltimore experimental ward, to 13 qph for a highly infectious office worker, to 60 qph for a case of laryngeal TB on the experimental ward, to approximately 250 qph for the bronchoscopy case already mentioned.[12,14,41,42] Even the highest reported level for TB infectivity pales in comparison to a highly infectious measles case where, from the first generation of secondary cases, q was estimated to be more than 5000 qph.[44] The calculated q value should be considered a crude index of infectivity, recognizing that patients probably generate droplet nuclei sporadically, in bursts related to coughing, sneezing, and other respiratory maneuvers, not continuously as the average figures would suggest. Local air concentrations of droplet nuclei presumably vary greatly, depending on production rate, dilution rate, and the other transmission factors discussed. However, air recirculation and personal mobility tend to dampen exposure fluctuations over time. Over a period of years, the true exposure for healthcare workers serving high-risk populations is probably a mixture of rare, brief exposures to relatively high concentrations, and longer exposures to much lower concentrations. For most individuals, infection is ordinarily a low-probability, random event. Table 3.1 lists the transmission factors for several exposures where the Wells-Riley model has been applied.

C. Limited Protection of Building Ventilation

In an office outbreak, 27 of 67 (40%) workers became infected during a 4-week exposure to a coworker with active TB.[42] The office building had been the subject of chronic air quality complaints, and the Wells-Riley model was applied to assess the importance of outdoor air ventilation as a transmission factor. Infections occurred throughout both floors of the office building, and a case-control analysis failed to reveal risk factors other than being in the building during the 4-week exposure. For analytical purposes, therefore, the office building was considered a single exposure chamber with an average outdoor air ventilation (Q) of approximately 15 cubic feet per minute per person (cfm/person), or a total of 1395 cfm based on air quality measurements made before and after the exposure. Knowing all other transmission factors, q was calculated at 13 qph (see Table 3.1). It was then possible to estimate the infection rate at ventilation rates greater and less than that actually determined for the building, assuming other factors remained unchanged. The results of that analysis are represented in Figure 3.1 (curve marked "Nardell") where infection rate is plotted as a function of ventilation. For comparison, a similar analysis was plotted for the bronchoscopy case where 10 of 13 exposed persons were infected during a 150 min. exposure (curve marked "Catanzaro" — see also Table 3.1).[41] In both cases poor outside air ventilation had contributed to the extent of transmission observed, and in both cases increased ventilation was predicted to greatly reduce, but not eliminate, transmission. The curves show that increasing ventilation of an area that is below the level recommended for comfort achieves the greatest increment in protection. Similar

TABLE 3.1
Airborne Transmission Factors[a]: Three Different Exposures

Factors	VA Hospital[12]	Office Building[42]	Bronchoscopy[41]
Source (I)	6 pts.	1 pt.	1 pt.
Exposure time (t)	730 days	6.7 days	150 min.
Susceptibles (S)	120 guinea pigs	67 people	13 people
Air sampled (Spt)	693,000 cf	230,000 cf	688 cf
Infected (C)	63/120 (52%)	27/67 (40%)	10/13 (77%)
Ventilation (Q)	38 cfm/person	15 cfm/person	11.5 cfm/person
Infectivity (q)	1.25 qph	13 qph	249 qph
Concentration	1/11,000 cf	1/8,500 cf	1/70 cf

[a] See text for further discussion of transmission factors and exposure conditions.

Source: Friedman, L. N., Ed., *Tuberculosis: Current Concepts and Treatment,* 1st ed., CRC Press LLC, Boca Raton, FL, 1994. With permission.

increases when ventilation already meets comfort levels is predicted to result in much smaller improvements in protection. In the office exposure, going from 15 cfm to a generous 35 cfm of outside air per occupant (3255 cfm total outside air) would be expected to reduce the infection rate only by half, with 13 infections still predicted.

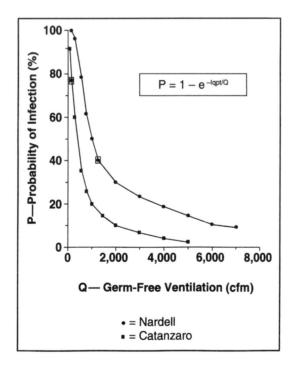

$$P = 1 - e^{-Iqpt/Q}$$

P—Probability of Infection (%)

Q— Germ-Free Ventilation (cfm)

• = Nardell
■ = Catanzaro

FIGURE 3.1 Probability of infection (*P*) as a function of germfree ventilation (*Q*), based on actual outbreaks published by Cantanzaro[41] and Nardell et al.,[42] using the equation of airborne infection shown, where *I* is the number of infectors, *p* is the ventilation rate of those exposed, *q* is the rate of production of quanta per source, and *t* is the exposure time. (From Riley R. L. and Nardell, E. A., Controlling transmission of tuberculosis in healthcare facilities: ventilation, filtration, and ultraviolet air disinfection. Plant, Technology, and Safety Management Series, Joint Commission on Accreditation of Healthcare Organizations, Number 1, PTSM Series, 1993. With permission.)

The logarithmic curve of infection and ventilation can be better understood if one considers the low concentrations of infectious quanta calculated for the office exposure, or measured on the Baltimore VA Hospital experimental TB ward: 1 in 8500 to 1 in 11,000 cf of air, respectively (Table 3.1). Under either conditions, approximately 10,000 cf of air would need to be exhausted on average to remove a single droplet nucleus. If ventilation were to successfully remove droplet nuclei faster than they were being added by the source case, reducing their concentration, for example, by half, then 20,000 cf of air would have to be vented to remove a single droplet nucleus. Ventilation becomes less and less efficient at removing droplet nuclei as their concentration falls. When the concentration of airborne droplet nuclei is much higher, as in the bronchoscopy case (Table 3.1, Figure 3.1), each cf of air exhausted removes many more droplet nuclei, but unfortunately, many more remain behind, and occupants remain at higher risk than under dilute conditions. Ventilation, indeed all approaches to air disinfection, are inherently limited in their ability to protect occupants from airborne infection, especially where concentrations of infectious droplet nuclei are low, where exposures are potentially long, and where a single inhaled droplet nucleus may be all that is required for infection.

The Wells-Riley model, and other calculations of clearance rates for building contaminants, assume complete air mixing, a condition rarely achieved in reality. Air supply diffusers, for example, are often located too close to exhaust grills, allowing air to enter and leave the room with little effect on air composition (i.e., short-circuiting). Ideally, when the volume of infection-free air entering a room and the volume of well-mixed air leaving a room equals the volume of the room, one air change (AC) is said to have occurred and approximately 63% of airborne organisms are flushed out. After five ideal room air changes, approximately 1% of the original airborne organisms remain. Such calculations, presumably, are the basis for recommending six room air changes per hour for isolation rooms, although such simple clearance calculations do not account for incomplete air mixing, and the ongoing generation of droplet nuclei. There are no clinical trials demonstrating protection from airborne infection with six room air changes, or any other ventilation rate.

IV. PRACTICAL APPROACHES TO CONTROLLING TB TRANSMISSION IN BUILDINGS

A. SURVEILLANCE, TREATMENT, PREVENTION, AND ADMINISTRATIVE APPROACHES

1. Patient Isolation Procedures

As stated earlier, because the most important factor in TB transmission is the prolonged presence of the infectious case in the same indoor space with susceptible persons, detection of cases, isolation, and effective therapy are the most important control strategies.[5] This often is far easier said than done. Despite growing awareness of tuberculosis, infectious cases will continue to be missed, or the diagnosis delayed, because of healthcare access problems, nonspecific symptoms, inadequate tests, and human error.[48] After diagnosis, the single best way to reduce the chance of transmission is through prompt, continuous, and effective treatment.[5] With less effective, older treatment regimens, epidemiologic observations suggested that patients started on effective therapy became rapidly noninfectious, even though tubercle bacilli persisted on sputum smear.[49] However, there also is evidence that sputum samples that remain culture positive will infect guinea pigs regardless of the duration of treatment.[50] With current, more potent, multidrug regimens, it has been assumed that noninfectiousness is achieved earlier, but there are little recent data.[51] However, the rising prevalence of drug resistant tuberculosis in some regions of the country now requires that the infectiousness of TB cases be assessed individually. Parameters for estimating infectiousness include the transmission factors already discussed: cough frequency, cavitation, sputum smear and culture results, as well as the history of past adherence with therapy and the probability of drug-resistant organisms.[5,15]

Patients who are responding clinically to therapy, as evidenced by decreasing cough, diminished fever, and fewer organisms in sputum are less likely to be infectious. In a setting where there is the potential for transmission to highly susceptible persons, such as on a hospital floor with HIV-infected patients, evidence of response to therapy should be compelling before the patient is permitted out of isolation and in contact with other patients and providers. Under these high-risk conditions, there should be a clear and consistent clinical response to therapy, and at least three separate sputum specimens should be negative for acid fast bacilli (AFB) on smear. Negative cultures constitute even stronger evidence against infectiousness, but the time required for culture results is usually too long to be of practical use in the day-to-day decisions on isolation in acute care hospitals. Molecular amplification tests for *M. tuberculosis* are faster than culture, but currently available tests have an unacceptable false-negative rate in smear-negative specimens, and treated patients may test positive many months after cultures become negative due to the presence of nucleic acids from dead or dying organisms. Because many newly diagnosed TB patients in developed countries are not now hospitalized, it follows that patients need not be considered noninfectious prior to discharge, depending on who would be exposed when they leave the hospital. Most household contacts would have been exposed for months before diagnosis and treatment, after which infectiousness is greatly reduced. Of greatest concern are very young children at home, and persons sharing congregate living space such as shelters, prisons, residential care facilities, especially those with HIV infection. Before a patient is released to such a high-risk setting, a high degree of certainty is required that the patient is noninfectious, and that effective therapy will continue to be fully supervised after discharge. Because of the serious consequences of transmission of multidrug-resistant tuberculosis, it is essential that such cases be rendered noninfectious before isolation is broken in hospitals, and before discharge, especially to congregate settings. The potential for transmission of multidrug-resistant tuberculosis among HIV-infected persons in congregate living situations is a powerful argument for the necessity of long-term treatment facilities for selected cases.[52]

2. Facemasks on Patients

The subject of particulate respirators for healthcare workers is discussed in a later section, but the use of facemasks for patients deserves mention here, where the subject of patient isolation is discussed. The use of surgical masks on TB patients is more widespread than reason would dictate. No surgical mask or particulate respirator can contain the volume and force of air expelled by vigorous coughing, and leakage must occur around the mask. Surgical masks are designed to keep large respiratory droplets from falling onto surgical fields — not to contain droplet nuclei. The problem is not the pore size, although droplet nuclei can pass through as well as around most surgical masks. Surgical masks serve to stop many large particles that would become droplet nuclei, thereby reducing their number. However, a hand or a tissue held over the mouth serves the same purpose and is far less stigmatizing. If a patient can and will cooperate with this simple hygienic practice, the use of a facemask is unnecessary and undesirable both for social reasons and because a wet facemask may itself become an effective atomizer of droplet nuclei when the patient coughs vigorously. Although they offer some protection, there are few circumstances where even the short-term use of masks on patients is warranted, for example, in transporting infectious patients who cannot or will not cooperate with instructions, or infectious prisoners whose hands are restrained.

3. Administrative Controls

Administrative policies such as TB surveillance, triage of potentially infectious cases, patient isolation, testing of healthcare workers, treatment of latent infection, and the logistics of patient flow and scheduling may help prevent nosocomial tuberculosis as much or more than engineering controls. For example, potential transmission may be avoided by scheduling a TB clinic, an HIV clinic, and a high-risk neonatal clinic in separate clinic locations, or at different times. Another policy decision is the administration of pentamidine aerosol treatments or sputum inductions only in booths designed for those purposes, in areas and at times that expose as few others as possible.

In the outpatient setting, administrative controls deserve further consideration, especially the subject of the waiting room. In primary care clinics and emergency waiting rooms, patients with chronic coughs of unknown cause sit together for hours with other patients, some with increased susceptibility to tuberculosis. Pediatricians recognized the problem of airborne infection in common waiting rooms many years ago, and many private offices and clinics have separate sick and well child waiting areas. Although that strategy might protect some otherwise healthy adults from airborne infection, it still leaves the sick with the sick, the potential infector with the vulnerable patient. For control of tuberculosis and other airborne infections, it is the patient with a cough of several weeks duration who should be promptly identified, asked to wait in a separate, environmentally controlled area, or escorted to a special examination room for prompt evaluation. For the reasons mentioned above, masking coughing patients in a waiting area is not a satisfactory alternative solution. Simple triage questions need to be developed and tested to allow a trained desk clerk to identify and separate certain patients with unexplained, chronic cough within minutes of arrival — not 45 minutes later when interviewed by the triage nurse. A number of clinical prediction models have been developed and validated in order to reduce the number of patients over-isolated, or reduce the duration of isolation.[53-55] Most patients with cough of 2 or more weeks duration will have chronic bronchitis, asthma, viral infections, or lung cancer — not tuberculosis. However, influenza transmission in waiting rooms also is a serious health risk for the elderly and the infirm, and the triaging of chronically coughing patients may add to the protection afforded by influenza immunization and treatment.

4. Surveillance and Prevention

Early detection of potentially infectious tuberculosis through vigilance and appropriate screening procedures is a highly desirable goal in theory, but often is difficult to achieve in practice. Symptoms and signs of tuberculosis are nonspecific, and tests are neither uniformly sensitive nor rapid. Acute, more critical medical problems often predominate, delaying consideration of chronic problems like tuberculosis.[48] Among immunocompromised patients, respiratory infections are common, and active tuberculosis may present itself with skin test anergy, nonspecific symptoms, and atypical radiographic findings. Skin testing protocols can often detect TB infection, but positive tuberculin tests rarely are the first clue to active disease. Ideally, positive skin tests lead to treatment of latent infection and fewer future active tuberculosis cases in long-term facilities, but routine testing of patients is likely to have little effect on TB transmission in acute care settings. Baseline and periodic skin testing of employees potentially exposed to patients with tuberculosis should help detect recent transmission and lead to therapy for latent infection, and is an important epidemiologic tool for institutions serving high-risk populations.

B. Environmental Control Measures

1. Source Control: Negative Pressure Isolation Rooms

Given the inherent difficulty of removing infectious droplet nuclei from the air once they are dispersed, control at the source is an important preventive strategy. As discussed, effective treatment is the best form of source control. However, for suspected and newly diagnosed cases in institutions, physical isolation is necessary until patients become noninfectious. Source control also makes sense for high-risk procedures such as bronchoscopy and sputum induction. For sputum induction and the administration of cough-inducing aerosols, such as pentamidine, isolation booths are available to protect the therapist and other building occupants.

The 1994 Centers for Disease Control (CDC) Guidelines to reduce the risk of TB transmission in healthcare facilities emphasizes the importance of negative pressure isolation as an environmental strategy.[56] While isolation is necessary, it assumes that all or most source cases of tuberculosis transmission are known or suspected, whereas it is the undiagnosed case that often is the most dangerous in the healthcare setting.

The four walls of the isolation room or sputum induction booth are its most important feature, physically limiting dispersion of droplet nuclei. In order to prevent the egress of contaminated air around the door, however, it is recommended that room exhaust exceed intake at a rate sufficient to draw air into the room from the corridor.[57] The isolation room is then under slightly negative pressure relative to adjacent areas, but the pressure difference is so small that it is difficult to measure. It is the direction of airflow into the isolation room, not the pressure difference, which is important, and direction is readily determined by holding a wisp of cotton or a special smoke stick near the bottom, side, and top of the door.[56]

Directional airflow into isolation rooms can be difficult to achieve if sufficient exhaust capacity is not available. Adding exhaust capacity may require extensive renovations to the central HVAC system and to the building. Operating costs also are high because air must be exhausted directly outside and not recirculated elsewhere in the building.[56,57] Moreover, once established, directional airflow readily changes as ventilation systems become unbalanced over time, and as airflow in adjacent areas changes due to opening and closing of doors and windows, and countless other variables.[58] In some areas of the country, fire codes require that patient rooms be neutral, or be under positive pressure relative to corridors, to avoid drawing smoke into the room in case of fire elsewhere in the vicinity. Although both fire safety and protection from TB infection are legitimate goals of ventilation, apparent conflicts may require hard choices and revisions of existing codes.

2. VENTILATION: NUMBERS OF ROOM AIR CHANGES — OUTSIDE AIR MIX

Four walls and directional airflow into isolation rooms protect other building occupants from airborne tuberculosis. Within an isolation room the probability of infection for healthcare workers depends on the transmission factors already discussed; most importantly, the volume of infection-free air that dilutes, removes, or inactivates the infectious droplet nuclei generated by the patient. Six room air changes per hour are recommended for isolation rooms, at least two of which are outside air.[56] Using the Wells-Riley model already discussed, it is possible to estimate the infection risk for hypothetical exposures of various durations.

A large isolation room, 10 by 20 ft with an 8-ft ceiling, contains 1600 cf of air, and 6 room air changes per hour is a ventilation rate of 9600 cf per hour or 160 cfm, assuming that all supply air is infection free. The risks of infection have been calculated for cumulative exposures of 1 h and 8 h, assuming the patient in the room is as infectious as the case in the office building discussed earlier (13 qph on average), approximately 10 times more infectious than the 6 treated patients on Riley's experimental ward, but much less infectious than the most infectious recorded TB cases (Table 3.2).[41,42] This moderately infectious case was chosen because such infectious patients probably are not unusual, and because such cases present a substantial risk of transmission — one that any environmental intervention must address.

These infection risks seem somewhat high compared to the anecdotal experience of most hospitals, although very little broad-based data on hospital worker conversions are available. The relatively high predicted infection rates may indicate that cases as infectious as that of the office building exposure are really not common, that droplet nuclei are actually generated in bursts, episodically, not continuously as the model assumes, and that some innately resistant persons may inhale more than one droplet nucleus without infection. The point of the calculation is to illustrate that, in theory at least, six room air changes would not be expected to fully protect a healthcare worker in an isolation room with an active case of tuberculosis. The calculation favors maximum benefit by assuming that all six air changes are nonrecirculated, infection-free air, and that there is complete mixing within the room. Current recommendations are for two outside air changes per hour, and four recirculated, presumably from low-risk areas.[56]

3. High-Efficiency Particle Air (HEPA) Filtration

HEPA filters remove 99.97% of airborne particles over 0.3 µ in diameter and have long been used to remove airborne microorganisms in laboratory, pharmaceutical, and medical settings. A number of devices are being marketed in which a fan or blower is combined with a HEPA filter in a portable air filtration machine designed to supplement the air disinfection provided by ventilation. Given the cost of ventilation renovations, the ability to disinfect air with portable filtration units is attractive. Moreover, there are large potential cost savings in recirculating air within an isolation room rather than exhausting six room changes per hour of conditioned air to the outside as is currently recommended. Depending on the region of the country, the annual energy savings from heating or cooling for one isolation room ranges from approximately $1000 to $7000, using standard engineering energy consumption formulas.[59] HEPA filtration also is being used in central ventilation ducts to remove droplet nuclei from recirculated air, and to disinfect air being exhausted to the outside in congested areas. Unfortunately, there are a number of problems, both practical and theoretical, with this otherwise attractive approach to air disinfection.

The fundamental problem with HEPA filtration is the potential for a single droplet nucleus to cause infection, the enormous dilution of droplet nuclei in air, already discussed, and the necessity to move large volumes of air to remove or further dilute droplet nuclei. The relationship between ventilation and risk of infection in Figure 3.1 and in Table 3.2 applies as well to HEPA-filtered air. Mathematical modeling indicates that it is extremely difficult to move enough air through a filter to substantially reduce the risk of infection unless ambient ventilation is grossly inadequate, and the task gets progressively harder as the concentration of droplet nuclei falls. Because HEPA filters offer considerable resistance to airflow, larger, noisier blowers are required to move large volumes of air compared to ordinary HVAC specifications. Air mixing within the room is another problem, especially when air supply and exhaust ducts are located in close proximity, as in most portable fan-filter units. A variable portion of the air that was just filtered is likely to be entrained again by the intake (i.e., "short-circuiting"), whereas other air in the room may not be filtered at all. Room furnishings and other obstructions may preclude optimal air circulation patterns.

TABLE 3.2
Risk of Infection in an Isolation Room with Variable Ventilation[a]

Air Changes (AC/h)	Ventilation (CFM)	Cumulative Exposure	
		1 h	8 h
6	160	2.8%	20%
10	267	1.7%	13%
15	400	1.1%	9%
25	667	0.7%	5%

[a] Assumptions: Room volume, 1600 cf; all infection-free supply air; infectivity of hypothetical source case (q), 13 qph. See text for additional details.

Source: Friedman, L. N., Ed., *Tuberculosis: Current Concepts and Treatment,* 1st ed., CRC Press LLC, Boca Raton, FL, 1994. With permission.

Effective room air changes may be far fewer than the advertised high flow rates through the machine would suggest. Leakage around filters is an inherent problem with HEPA filtration, requiring great care to assure filters are sealed within their housings, and regular testing for leaks both at the manufacturing stage, and periodically after delivery, since movement of the device may break seals. Filter seals also must be retested whenever filters are replaced. Leakage around HEPA filters in duct installations is harder to detect. In-place filter testing routines should precisely follow the procedures established for biological safely cabinets (available from NSF International, P.O. Box 130140, Ann Arbor, MI 48113).

Ultimately, the efficacy of all HEPA filtration devices (and ventilation) should be tested in room experiments in which airborne particulates of a respirable size are removed. Air should be sampled in various room locations over time to produce clearance curves under controlled conditions designed to approximate the conditions where the devices will be used. Such testing has been performed with a number of filtration devices.[60] In one study, the best clearance rates were obtained using a ceiling-mounted air filtration unit. In theory, air filtration should work best in relatively small volume rooms whereas upper room air disinfection (see below) is better suited to large volume spaces. However, there are high-risk situations not suitable for other interventions where any improvement would be welcome. There is no doubt that HEPA filters remove droplet nuclei; the issue is effectiveness, efficiency, and acceptability to occupants compared to the alternative methods of air disinfection.

4. Ultraviolet Germicidal Irradiation (UVGI)

William Firth Wells not only pioneered the scientific study of droplet nuclei transmission, he also explored the use of ultraviolet germicidal irradiation (UVGI) to halt transmission of tuberculosis and the common epidemic respiratory viral infections, such as measles.[61] More than 40 years after the publication of his landmark monograph on air hygiene, however, the full potential of upper room UVGI in halting airborne transmission has yet to be realized.[3] The advent of effective treatment for tuberculosis, and of immunizations for some of the epidemic viral infections accounts in part for the decline in interest in UVGI. However, disillusionment also followed the failure of UVGI to prevent common colds in offices, and measles in several clinical trials where infections occurred outside of irradiated classrooms, on school buses, and in crowded urban tenements.[62-64] Wells had raised expectations by demonstrating UVGI efficacy in halting measles transmission in a carefully conducted field trial in suburban Philadelphia schools under conditions where infection outside of school was unlikely.[3] McLean later used the same technology to effectively prevent influenza transmission on a ward for respiratory patients.[65] Through these and other successes and failures it is now understood that air disinfection can only work for infections that are predominantly spread as droplet nuclei — not by direct contact or as larger respiratory droplets — and where the site of air disinfection is the principal site of transmission, thereby excluding some common infections even though the pathogenic agents are highly susceptible to UVGI. The use of UVGI to reduce tuberculosis transmission in a number of high-risk areas should be effective, but wide application is hampered by several longstanding obstacles: (1) general misconceptions about the application of UVGI, (2) specific concerns about radiation injury, (3) the lack of technical expertise to plan UV installations, and (4) the absence of controlled clinical trials to support its use for tuberculosis. The general lack of information about UVGI, and the personal interest of the author, are the reasons for its disproportionate discussion in this chapter.

a. UV Misconceptions

The most common misconceptions regarding UVGI are that it is dangerous and of unproven efficacy, requiring extensive maintenance, i.e., regular cleaning. Although there is minimal basis for each of these concerns, in the aggregate they reflect widespread unfamiliarity with the technology and its application. These concerns are discussed below.

b. UVGI Safety

UVGI utilizes a narrow-band (95% output at 253.7 nm wavelength) of the ultraviolet portion of the electromagnetic spectrum (200 to 400 nm) to inactivate airborne pathogens. Short wavelength UV irradiation (253.7 nm, UV-C) is rapidly lethal for airborne bacteria at intensity levels easily achieved in the upper room, above people's heads, but it is safe for occupants at the much lower intensity levels permitted in the occupied part of the room.[66] Longer wavelength UV-B has a much greater penetrating capacity than does UV-C, and chronic exposure to the intensive UV-B in sunlight has been associated with skin cancer and cataracts. UV-C has more energy than UV-B, and might be more damaging to tissues than UV-B were it not almost completely (95%) absorbed by the outer, dead layer of the stratum corneum.[67] Accidental direct exposure to high intensity UV-C can cause temporary, painful, but superficial irritation of eyes (photokeratoconjuctivitis) or skin erythema. Eye irritation is transient due to the normally rapid turnover of the corneal epithelium.[68] Painters and maintenance personnel have experienced photokeratoconjunctivitis due to accidental direct UV-C exposure after working in the upper room without first turning off UV fixtures. Because UV-C does not penetrate the cornea, it does not reach the lens to cause cataracts.[68] Intensive, direct skin exposure can cause erythema, and could cause a mild to moderate "sunburn" in sensitive individuals. Prolonged high-intensity irradiation of hairless mice with UV-C has produced skin cancers, but at the low level exposures permitted for people in the lower room (6 mJ/cm2), Urbach has estimated that human skin cancer would require more than 300 years of exposure.[69-72]

Although systemic immunosuppression has been induced by UV-B irradiation of mice, the UV dosage required was relatively large compared to potential UVGI exposures in the lower room.[73] Moreover, the immunosuppressive effect presumably requires UV penetration to the cellular level — readily achieved with more penetrating UV-B in mice, due to their relatively thin epidermis, but unlikely in thicker skinned humans with low-intensity, low-penetrating UV-C exposure. There is no evidence of systemic immunosuppression in humans from UV-C exposure. Activation of HIV virus in cell cultures exposed to UV-B or UV-C has been reported, and concerns were raised a decade ago that PUVA therapy and sunbathing could be an important activating factor for HIV-infected persons.[74] If true, the effect should be discernible epidemiologically given the large number of HIV-infected persons under observation, and the wide range of sun exposure, geographically, among individuals. However, a recent report from the Multicenter AIDS Cohort Study found no correlation between sun exposure or sun sensitivity and progression to AIDS among HIV-infected men, or in the rate of decrease in their CD4 count.[75] Ironically, individuals purposefully seeking the sun had slower CD4 declines, probably reflecting an activity of healthier individuals. In another study, UV-B phototherapy had no effect on plasma HIV type 1 RNA viral levels in HIV-infected persons with UV-responsive skin conditions.[76] By comparison to the more intense and penetrating UV-B in sunlight, or UV-B phototherapy, the low levels of UV-C permitted in the lower room should pose no significant added risk, while it should offer substantial protection from TB infection, a well-established hazard for HIV-infected persons.[77]

Current exposure safety guidelines for UV-C are based on a combination of animal data and voluntary human exposures using eye irritation as the end-point.[78] The daily 8 h UV exposure limit is 6 mJ.[79] The exposure limit derived for 254 nm UV of 0.2 μW/cm^2 over 8 h already incorporates a margin of safety and, furthermore, assumes continuous eye exposure at the maximum level detected by a meter aimed at the fixture (i.e., stare time). Occupant movement within rooms, angles of incidence of UV rays reflected from ceilings, and shielding by brows and eyelids all greatly reduce true UV exposure to the cornea — the same factors that ordinarily prevent photokeratocon-juctivitis outside from exposure to the more dangerous UV-A and UV-B in sunlight.

For over 50 years, upper room UVGI has been used safely in hospitals, clinics, jails, and shelters around the country without injuries more serious than an occasional, transient photokeratoconjuc-tivitis from accidental direct exposure.[80] Until recently, however, little attention has been paid to the measurement of UV in the lower room, and to the design of fixtures intended for upper room UV air disinfection. In contemporary, low-ceiling rooms equipped with some common UVGI fixtures of older design, UV intensity at eye level has been measured at well over the 0.2 µW/cm², as high as 6.0 µW/cm² in one installation. Fortunately, such fixtures have been used for years in most cases without photokeratitis, a fact attributable to the safety margin built into the exposure standard, which, as noted, was based on "stare time" rather than the relatively brief, indirect exposures common in real life. To meet the somewhat arbitrary 0.2 µW/cm² interpretation of the 6 mJ standard, newer louvered fixtures are designed to effectively confine irradiation to the space above people's heads.[81] In the process of meeting the 0.2 µW/cm² intensity, these tightly louvered fixtures also greatly reduce the radiation output into the upper room, potentially compromising efficacy. Common sense dictates that UV-C exposure in occupied spaces should be kept as low as possible while still achieving effective upper room air disinfection. Efforts now are underway to develop personal monitors for UV that, like radiation badges, would permit more flexible application of UV in the varied settings where it is indicated. In the meantime, designers of UV installations should not be concerned with point measurements in excess of 0.2 µW/cm² in situations where prolonged eye exposure is unlikely and where there have been no eye complaints.

c. Technical Expertise

The application of UVGI in healthcare facilities falls into no established area of technical expertise. While building engineers are expert at HVAC systems, most are unfamiliar with the use of UVGI, and often are biased in their views on UVGI by rumors of health hazards, unproven efficacy, and high maintenance requirements. Manufacturers have traditionally sold fixtures, but neither have planned installations nor checked UV fixture post-installation with a sensitive UV meter before use. Federal agencies have offered little guidance and often have contributed some of the misconceptions, lumping UVGI (UV-C) together with more hazardous forms of UV (UV-B) found in the workplace.[82] As demand for practical environmental interventions rises, however, engineers and other technically qualified consultants undoubtedly will acquire the skills needed to assist institutions wanting to apply UVGI and other environmental interventions safely and effectively. Recent engineering guidelines on the use of upper room UVGI have been published.[83,84] These guidelines are still based primarily on experience and older studies and should be considered preliminary. They will be revised based on the results of ongoing research.

d. Absence of Clinical Trials

Although a large body of credible basic research supports the use of UVGI and the lethal UV dose for various airborne pathogens has been established, there are no clinical field trials demonstrating UVGI efficacy in protecting workers from nosocomial tuberculosis.[66] The major problem preventing the performance of clinical trials has been the highly variable nature of TB transmission, as demonstrated by Riley and colleagues.[85] Infection rates among hospital staff, for example, are heavily influenced by the number and infectiousness of TB patients who happen to be under their care, the duration of exposure before detection and effective treatment, environmental conditions, and the variable susceptibility to infection of those exposed. One highly infectious undiagnosed TB patient could badly skew even a large clinical trial. The lack of clinical trials applies as well to triage and isolation policies, isolation rooms, ventilation, HEPA filtration, and the use of particulate respirators to prevent TB transmission. However, there is reluctance to question the protection attributed to administrative controls, negative pressure isolation rooms and respirators, all time-honored and relatively risk-free methods of infection control, the underlying principles of which seem intuitive. Fortunately, a number of new research initiatives in the U.S. and abroad are striving to fill in missing gaps in the science and application of ultraviolet air disinfection. The global resurgence of tuberculosis and the emergence of multidrug resistant strains as a threat to both institutional workers and residents, heightens the need for effective and inexpensive air disinfection for resource-poor countries.

e. Upper Room UVGI: Theory and Experimental Basis

Using culture techniques to determine viability, the relative and absolute susceptibility of a variety of airborne microbes, including both virulent tuberculosis and avirulent BCG strains, has been determined under controlled experimental conditions.[66,85,86] Mycobacteria were approximately seven times harder to kill than aerosolized *E. coli* or *S. marcescens*, but easier to kill than common fungal spores. For virulent tubercle bacilli and for BCG, exposure to 10 μW/cm^2 for 60 s or 50 μW/cm^2 for 12 s killed 90% of airborne organisms. That a powerfully germicidal dose was achievable within ventilation ducts under hospital conditions was convincingly demonstrated on Riley's experimental tuberculosis ward where UVGI completely protected an average of 120 guinea pigs exposed to patient-generated contagion over a 2-year period.[12] An equal number of guinea pigs breathing nonirradiated air from the same ward became infected at approximately the same rate as during the first 2 years of the experiment, already discussed. Drug-resistant organisms infected many of the control animals breathing nonirradiated air, demonstrating that organisms resistant to chemotherapy were quite susceptible to UVGI.

Despite this highly successful demonstration of efficacy when UVGI is used between the infectious source and the susceptibles, the main limitation to using UVGI in ventilation ducts remains exactly that described for HEPA filters, and that of outdoor air ventilation itself — the need to move large volumes of air to substantially reduce the risk of infection for occupants of the same room as an infectious case. Compared to HEPA filters, UVGI in ducts requires less maintenance and offers less airflow resistance, permitting the use of smaller, quieter blowers to achieve a given air flow. According to Riley, no routine maintenance of the duct UV lamps occurred during the guinea pig experiments, yet they performed flawlessly for 2 years. While dust accumulation can diminish UV output, within ducts it is possible to overcome any anticipated fall-off with higher initial UV intensity. Despite the theoretical limitations of duct irradiation, the National Jewish Center for Immunology and Respiratory Medicine in Denver has long used UVGI within air-recirculating units (mounted above the ceiling) in isolation rooms on the inpatient unit for drug-resistant tuberculosis.[87] Air flow through the units is said to be equivalent to 12 to 15 room air changes per hour. Although there had been several infections among staff before the room units were installed, there have been only two infections over the past 10 years. The air-moving UVGI units are more costly than upper room UV fixtures, which have produced the equivalent of 20 added room air changes under experimental conditions, as described below, and which are more suitable for larger spaces such as waiting areas, emergency rooms, and shelters for the homeless.

Room air disinfection through upper air UVGI is achieved through the surprisingly rapid, but imperceptible dilution of contaminated lower room air with germ-free, irradiated upper room air.[88-90] Effective mixing within the room occurs as a result of natural convection currents, mechanical ventilation, radiant heat, agitation of air due to the opening of doors, and the movement of occupants within the room. Rather than forcing room air rapidly through a relatively small duct for disinfection, upper room UVGI uses the entire cross-sectional area of a room as the duct and irradiation chamber, permitting high volume, low velocity mixing of disinfected upper with contaminated lower room air. Although the susceptibility of tubercle bacilli is known, given the many variables within a room, it was not possible to predict the air disinfection achievable in the lower room by upper room UV without actual room experiments. Riley and colleagues aerosolized test organisms into sealed rooms, mixed and distributed airborne droplet nuclei with a fan, then sampled and cultured lower room air quantitatively over time, with and without upper room irradiation.[86]

Because of the hazard of aerosolizing virulent tubercle bacilli into a room, it was necessary to perform room experiments using safer surrogate organisms, the UV susceptibility of which had been established relative to virulent TB by previous controlled experiments, as noted above. The results of one experiment using aerosolized BCG are shown in Figure 3.2. A single 17-W UV tube irradiating the upper 2 feet of a 200 ft^2 room inactivated airborne organisms at a rate equivalent to adding 10 air changes to the existing 2 air changes of the room. Many more room experiments were performed using aerosolized *S. marcescens* under a variety of conditions intended to increase mixing between the upper and lower room, thereby increasing air disinfection in the lower room. Results in an unventilated room using Serratia confirmed the findings of the BCG experiments, allowing for a sevenfold greater susceptibility to UV irradiation.[88-90]

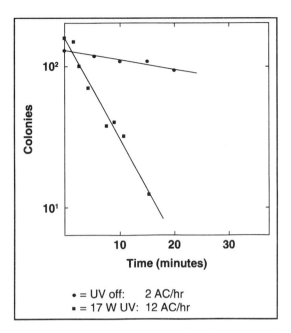

FIGURE 3.2 Disappearance of Bacillus Calmette-Guérin (BCG) from a naturally ventilated, sealed room, with and without upper room ultraviolet air disinfection, using one 17-W tube; AC/h = air changes per hour. (From Riley, R. et al., Ultraviolet susceptibility of BCG and virulent tubercle bacilli, *Am. Rev. Resp. Dis.*, 113, 413, 1976. With permission.)

Despite these successful experiments, the inability to readily predict or measure the air disinfection produced in an occupied lower room by an upper room UVGI installation under actual conditions may be the main reason why many engineers are reluctant to embrace this technology. By comparison, it is easier to measure the removal of inert airborne test particles by ventilation or filtration, although it is not done routinely. Room experiments and computer simulations at several universities are attempting to better define the interactions of upper room UV, ventilation, and room air mixing. The goal of these efforts is to be able to predict the effect of UV installations under a variety of actual room conditions.

f. Application of UVGI: Practical Considerations

Based on the above room experiments, and on the remarkable ability of UVGI in ducts to protect guinea pigs from patient-generated droplet nuclei, upper room UVGI has long been used in a variety of indoor environments where TB transmission has been a problem. The criteria for applying UVGI are (1) a demonstrably high-risk indoor environment for TB transmission; (2) a comparatively low risk of infection outside of the proposed area; (3) sufficient unobstructed ceiling height (i.e., 8 ft or more) to install fixtures at 7 ft (to avoid direct or reflected eye overexposure), with at least 1 additional foot for air disinfection; and (4) understanding and acceptance by room occupants or those responsible for their well being.

Although the planning of an upper room UV installation is not difficult, some experience, and access to a 254 nm wavelength UV radiometer sensitive down to 0.1 µW/cm², are required. The objective is to flood the upper room (above 7.5 ft) with UV irradiation at the highest intensity possible (at least 50 µW/cm² at a distance of 3 ft from the fixture, 10 to 15 µW/cm² at 10 ft) while maintaining safe exposure levels in the lower room, depending on the estimated true duration of exposure (as discussed above). New, multilouvered fixture designs have made safe upper room UV installations possible in rooms with ceilings as low as 8 ft, but at the expense of reduced intensity.[81] UV radiometers measure radiation unidirectionally and cannot accurately quantify the additive exposure from multiple fixtures and reflected UV experienced by airborne microbes. Using a spherical actinometer, however, Rahn et al. have more accurately demonstrated the spatial distribution of UV in a test room with multiple fixtures.[91] One 30-W wall fixture (Riley design) generally is used for an average size (150 to 200 ft²) single hospital room, depending on its configuration.[83,84] Air disinfection equivalent to approximately 20 room air changes is anticipated, without noise, drafts, reconstruction, or excessive energy costs. Actual air disinfection achieved in a given room depends on room air mixing and is not easily predicted or measured. The placement of UVGI in corridors as well as rooms has been shown to prevent transfer of airborne test organisms, and has been suggested as an alternative to negative pressure isolation when the latter cannot be achieved.[92,93] The estimated protection predicted for 25 room air changes, 20 equivalent air changes added by UVGI, plus 5 produced by mechanical ventilation, is listed in Table 3.2. Compared to major ventilation renovations, high-volume ventilation, and self-contained air disinfecting units (HEPA filter or UV), upper room UVGI is likely to be more effective, much less costly to install and operate, and more applicable to shelters, emergency rooms, waiting rooms, and other large spaces.

Operating room have high levels of ventilation, but are under positive pressure by design in order to prevent wound infections. TB transmission has been associated with operating room procedures, and rooms used for necessary procedures on patients known or suspected of having TB, including certain cases of extrapulmonary TB, should be equipped with upper room germicidal UV.

Ideally, an engineering consultant or industrial hygienist thoroughly familiar with ventilation, filtration, UV air disinfection, and personal respirators should evaluate buildings in consultation with infection control staff and recommend the appropriate environmental control interventions for each potential exposure situation.

g. Air Recirculation

As noted, outbreaks of tuberculosis have been documented where recirculation of infectious droplet nuclei was thought to have played an important role.[32,42,94] Under those circumstances, air disinfection centrally, through HEPA filtration or UVGI, should be highly effective. However, central air disinfection does little to protect the health worker in the same room with an infectious case, whereas room-by-room air disinfection does reduce the chance that droplet nuclei will be recirculated. Under most circumstances, therefore, central air disinfection should be a second tier defense against transmission, to be employed after source control and room control measures are in place.

5. Personal Respirators

In the traditional hierarchy of controls for environmental hazards, source control, environmental controls, and administrative controls all precede the use of personal protective devices; in this case, personal respirators (PRs) to prevent the inhalation of droplet nuclei. In the current terminology, "masks" refer to mouth and nose covers designed to protect the patient from the wearer's large respiratory droplets (e.g., surgical masks). PRs can appear similar to masks, but are designed to protect the wearer from a variety of hazards, depending on the design. Personal protective devices are employed when control by the other three tiers is considered inadequate. Although it is unlikely that 100% protection from TB infection can be achieved in healthcare settings, PRs, however technically sophisticated, may not play a major role for the following reasons:

1. Except in unusual circumstances, PRs are applicable for healthcare workers only, whereas patients and their visitors also must be protected (different from industrial applications where everyone in a high-risk area can be required to comply).
2. Cooperation and training are required for the proper use of PRs, and failures through lapses in technique are inevitable.
3. Simple, inexpensive masks are least intrusive, most acceptable to workers, but offer the least protection because of leaks between the face and the PR.

4. Sophisticated PRs designed to prevent leaks are expensive, cumbersome, impair verbal communication, and are least acceptable to workers and their patients. However, there are high-risk settings, e.g., bronchoscopies and autopsies (see below), where some form of effective PR is warranted.

5. A PR strategy assumes that most potential transmitters are identified, whereas unsuspected cases in emergency rooms, intensive care units, and other clinical settings are important. Healthcare workers cannot function wearing respirators all day.

Respiratory protection that is both reasonably effective and inexpensive has become available as a result of a new testing and classification scheme introduced by National Institute of Occupational Safety and Health (NIOSH), stimulated by the inappropriateness of the older industrial classification for medical use.[95] Details on respirator certification are available through the NIOSH homepage on the World Wide Web (*www.cdc.gov/niosh/homepage.html*). Two reports have modeled the relative role of respiratory protection and other infection control strategies.[47,96]

C. TRANSMISSION ASSOCIATED WITH BRONCHOSCOPY AND AUTOPSY

1. Tuberculosis Transmission Associated with Bronchoscopy

There are two distinct ways that bronchoscopy has been associated with the transmission of tuberculosis and other mycobacterial diseases. First, bronchoscopy as a cough-inducing procedure, often performed in a relatively small room, has been associated with airborne transmission from patient to healthcare workers, as exemplified by the intensive care unit exposure analyzed above in detail.[41] The second type of TB risk is mycobacterial contamination of the instrument from patients or from environmental sources. The airborne transmission problem associated with bronchoscopy is closely related to the main theme of this chapter and is not considered here in detail, whereas the contamination problem requires greater discussion.

No systematic data have been published on the TB transmission risk of bronchoscopy. One survey of pulmonary and infectious disease specialists in training showed much higher TB skin test conversions among pulmonary fellows even though both groups consulted on patients with known or suspected tuberculosis.[97] The survey concluded that the difference was likely to be due to bronchoscopy performed by pulmonary but not infectious disease fellows. Bronchoscopy should be considered a high-risk procedure for TB transmission regardless of the level of suspicion for the disease. It is invariably the case bronchoscoped for suspected lung cancer, for example, where no precautions are taken, that turns out to be tuberculosis and results in transmission. While universal precautions for bronchoscopy are recommended, local experience should dictate the level of protection that is appropriate in each institution. In an institution where MDR TB is relatively common, for example, powered air-purifying respirators (PAPRs) would be highly recommended; whereas in an institution where MDR is rare, they might not be worth the extra expense, inconvenience, and potential operator impairment during bronchoscopy. In 1998, for example, just one MDR TB case was identified among a total of 283 Massachusetts cases. While bronchoscopy in Massachusetts hospitals represents a potential TB risk, the risk is clearly less than in higher incidence areas and in institutions where MDR occurs more often. In addition to personal respiratory protection, air disinfection through increased ventilation, air filtration, or upper room UV irradiation have been recommended.[56] Perhaps the most important precautions against nosocomial TB transmission from bronchoscopy are (1) the judicious use of the procedure and (2) considering the possibility of tuberculosis in persons with risk factors, regardless of the working diagnosis. Although bronchoscopy is an effective way to diagnose TB, it is not often required.[98] Sputum induction using hypertonic saline can be done in an isolation booth with much less potential exposure for workers. It has been my practice not to routinely bronchoscope suspected TB patients for a bacteriologic diagnosis because of the risk to coworkers. Possible exceptions have included the unusual circumstance where sputum induction has not yielded a satisfactory sample, and tuberculosis is strongly suspected. For more information on these matters, see Chapter 6.

a. Bronchoscope Contamination, Pseudoinfection, and True Transmission

Contamination of bronchoscopes can cause any of several clinical problems. True tuberculosis infection has been spread from one patient to another, and false-positive cultures from contaminated instruments have resulted in potential misdiagnoses (pseudoinfection). It also is possible that true infection with nontuberculous mycobacteria might result from contaminated bronchoscopes, but this has yet to be reported. The solution to all three potential problems is effective cleaning and decontamination of the instruments between patients.

It has been estimated that if 1 to 5% of the approximately 500,000 bronchoscopies performed each year are on persons with active TB, and if just 10% of the instruments used become contaminated, as many as 500 to 2500 other patients would be exposed to TB.[99] Just how often transmission occurs by this route, however, is difficult to know given our inability to routinely detect latent TB infection or trace secondary active cases of TB to the source of infection months to years prior to the onset of symptoms. A number of convincing case reports suggest that the problem can be serious, even life-threatening.[100,101] In one report, inadequate cleaning and disinfection of the bronchoscope between patients led to false-positive tuberculosis cultures in two patients, transmission of infection (without disease) to a third patient, and active multidrug resistant TB in a fourth patient, who died despite therapy.[100] In another report, DNA fingerprinting of two isolates showing identical patterns prompted an epidemiologic investigation that revealed that both patients had been bronchoscoped within 2 days of each other with the same instrument.[101] The secondary case developed TB symptoms 6 months after the bronchoscopy, having had chemotherapy and radiation therapy for lung cancer.

Over a 12-month period, one hospital reported contamination of 13 bronchial washings with *M. gordonae*.[102] None of the patients met the American Thoracic Society criteria for disease due to environmental mycobacteria, and none received treatment. The source of the organism was traced to an automatic bronchoscope disinfection machine.

b. Guidelines to Prevent Transmission

Authoratative guidelines for bronchoscope decontamination have been published.[103] Readers are referred to the most current versions of APIC's guidelines. The published reports of transmission and contamination make it clear that at least a 20-min exposure to 2% glutaraldehyde is adequate for mycobacteria only after a thorough cleaning. However, even a 60-min exposure to 2% gluteraldehyde, or 10 cycles, may not sterilize a contaminated valve that is not clean. Thorough cleaning of the instrument, including mechanical valves, is an essential first step. Recent bronchoscope models have replaced many reusable parts, including valves, with single-use disposable parts. Nondisposable valves should be heat disinfected, if possible. The instrument should be leak tested for tears in the cover that could harbor bacteria. All surfaces should be rinsed with 70% alcohol and the surface should be stored hanging, not coiled. Once established, decontamination protocols require continual monitoring for quality assurance. Transmission recently has been associated with an automated bronchoscope cleaning system. Investigation revealed inconsistencies between the disinfection procedures recommended by the automated cleaning system and those of various bronchoscope manufacturers. Better coordination and other remedial recommendations were made, including a color-coded connector system.

Episodes of nosomial transmission associated with bronchoscopy are reportable to the FDA under the Safe Medical Devices Act of 1990 (301 827-4570), to the FDA's MedWatch program (*http://www.fda.gov/medwatch*), and to the CDC's Hospital Infections Program ((404) 639-6413).

2. Tuberculosis Transmission Associated with Autopsy and Other Aerosol Generating Procedures

Surgery, autopsy, and embalming are associated with cutaneous tuberculosis from cuts and punctures, but aerosol generation associated with these procedures appear to be a much more effective mode of transmission.[104] In a population-based survey of occupational risks associated with tuberculosis, morticians had the highest rates of any profession.[105] There are multiple reports of tuberculosis transmission associated with autopsy.[106-109] In the episode reported by Templeton, all five nonreactors present during a 3-hr autopsy converted their skin tests, and two had positive sputum 8 weeks later.[108] During life, however, the same patient infected none of 40 skin test-negative healthcare workers who cared for him over 3 weeks on a general medical ward before tuberculosis was suspected. High velocity reciprocal bone saws used in autopsies, and high-pressure jets used in surgery and other procedures appear to be highly effective aerosol generators. A high-pressure jet used on a patient to irrigate a large hip and thigh abscess, not initially known to be tuberculous, was responsible for 9 secondary cases and 59 skin test conversions in a surgical suite, intensive care unit, and general medical floor.[17]

Like bronchoscopy, aerosols generated during surgery, autopsies, and embalming can be controlled by precautions similar to those applied to infectious patients. Like other exposures, most reported bronchoscopy transmissions have involved source patients where tuberculosis was not suspected before the procedure was performed. These procedures are generally done in specialized rooms where precautions can be universally applied, regardless of the perceived risk. Especially important is the use of effective air disinfection and personal respiratory protection. Depending on the risk of TB in the population served, and on the risk of MDR TB, recommended respiratory protection may range from simple N-95 disposable respirators to full or half-mask powered air purifying respirators (PAPRs), as discussed earlier.

REFERENCES

1. Bates, B., *Bargaining for Life: A Social History of Tuberculosis 1876–1938,* University of Pennsylvania, Philadelphia, 1992.
2. Wells, W., On air-borne infection: II. Droplets and droplet nuclei, *Am. J. Hyg.,* 20, 611, 1934.
3. Wells, W., *Airborne Contagion and Air Hygiene,* Harvard University Press, Cambridge, MA, 1955.
4. Centers for Disease Control and Prevention, Guidelines for preventing the transmission of *Mycobacterium tuberculosis* in health care facilities, *MMWR,* 43 (RR-13), 1, 1994.
5. American Thoracic Society, Control of tuberculosis in the United States, *Am. Rev. Respir. Dis.,* 146, 1623, 1992.
6. Riley, R. and O'Grady, F., *Airborne Infection,* The Macmillan Company, New York, 1961.
7. Ratcliff, H., Tuberculosis induced by droplet nuclei infection: pulmonary tuberculosis of predetermined initial intensity in mammals, *Am. J. Hyg.,* 55, 36, 1952.
8. Wells, W., Ratcliff, H., and Crumb, C., On the mechanism of droplet nuclei infection, II: quantitative experimental airborne infection in rabbits, *Am. J. Hyg.,* 47, 11, 1948.
9. Lurie, M., Heppleston, A., Abramson, S., and Swartz, I., An evaluation of the method of quantitative airborne infection and its use in the study of the pathogenesis of tuberculosis, *Am. Rev. Tuberc.,* 61, 765, 1950.
10. Riley, R., Wells, W., Mills, C., Nyka, W., and McLean, R., Air hygiene in tuberclosis: quantitative studies of infectivity and control in a pilot ward, *Am. Rev. Tuberc. Pulmon. Dis.,* 75, 420, 1957.
11. Riley, R., Aerial dissemination of pulmonary tuberculosis — the Burns Amberson Lecture, *Am. Rev. Tuberc. Pulmon. Dis.,* 76, 931, 1957.
12. Riley, R., Mills, C., and O'Grady, F., Infectiousness of air from a tuberculosis ward — ultraviolet irradiation of infected air: comparative infectiousness of different patients, *Am. Rev. Resp. Dis.,* 84, 511, 1962.

13. Riley, R., Mills, C., and Nyka, W., Aerial dissemination of pulmonary tuberculosis — a two-year study of contagion in a tuberculosis ward, *Am. J. Hyg.*, 70, 185, 1959.

14. Sultan, L., Nyka, C., Mills, C., O'Grady, F., and Riley, R., Tuberculosis disseminators — a study of variability of aerial infectivity of tuberculosis patients, *Am. Rev. Respir. Dis.*, 82, 358, 1960.

15. Loudon, R. and Spohn, S., Cough frequency and infectivity in patients with pulmonary tuberculosis, *Am. Rev. Resp. Dis.*, 99, 109, 1969.

16. Barnes, P. F., Bloch, A. B., Davidson, P. T., and Snider, D. E., Jr., Tuberculosis in patients with human immunodeficiency virus infection, *N. Engl. J. Med.*, 324, 1644, 1991.

17. Hutton, M. D., Stead, W. W., Cauthen, G. M., and Block, A. B., Nosocomial transmission with tuberculosis associated with a draining abcess, *J. Infect. Dis.*, 161, 286, 1990.

18. Edlin, B. R., Tokars, J. I., Grieco, M. H., Crawford, J. T., Williams, J., Sordillo, E. M., Ong, K. R., Kilburn, J. O., Dooley, S. W., Castro, K. G., et al., An outbreak of multidrug-resistant tuberculosis among hospitalized patients with the acquired immunodeficiency syndrome, *N. Engl. J. Med.*, 326, 1514, 1992.

19. American Conference of Governmental and Industrial Hygienists, Guidelines for the assessment of bioaerosols in the indoor environment, Cincinnati, OH, 1989.

20. First, M., personal communication, 1993.

21. Mastorides, S. M., Oehler, R. L., Greene, J. N., Sinnot, J. T., Kranik, M. K., and Sandin, R. L., The detection of airborne *Mycobacterium tuberculosis* using micropore membrane air sampling and polymerase chain reaction, *Chest*, 115, 19, 1999.

22. Dannenberg, A., Delayed-type hypersensitivity and cell mediated immunity in the pathogenesis of tuberculosis, *Immunol. Today*, 12, 228, 1991.

23. Wells, W., *Response and Reaction to Inhaled Droplet Nuclei, Airborne Infection and Air Hygiene*, Harvard University, Cambridge, MA, 1955.

24. Stead, W. W., Senner, J. W., Reddick, W. T., and Lofgren, J. P., Racial differences in susceptibility to infection by *Mycobacterium tuberculosis*, *N. Engl. J. Med.*, 322, 422, 1990.

25. Stead, W. W., Genetics and resistance to tuberculosis. Could resistance be enhanced by genetic engineering? *Ann. Intern. Med.*, 116, 937, 1992.

26. Nardell, E., McInnis, B., Thomas, B., and Weidhaas, S., Exogenous reinfection with tuberculosis in a shelter for the homeless, *N. Engl. J. Med.*, 315, 1570, 1986.

27. Small, P. M., Shafer, R. W., Hopewell, P. C., Singh, S. P., Murphy, M. J., Desmond, E., Sierra, M. F., and Schoolnik, G. K., Exogenous reinfection with multidrug-resistant *Mycobacterium tuberculosis* in patients with advanced HIV infection, *N. Engl. J. Med.*, 328, 1137, 1993.

28. van Rie, A., Warren, R., Richardson, M., Victor, T. C., Gie, R. P., Enarson, D. A., Beyers, N., and van Helden, P. D., Exogenous reinfection as a cause of recurrent tuberculosis after curative treatment, *N. Engl. J. Med.*, 341, 1174, 1999.

29. Fine, P. E. M. and Small, P. M., Exogenous reinfection in tuberculosis (editorial), *N. Engl. J. Med.*, 341, 1226, 1999.

30. Nardell, E., Pathogenesis of tuberculosis, in Reichman, L. and Hershfield, E., eds., *Tuberculosis*, Marcel Dekker, New York, 1993, Chap 5.

31. Loudon, R., Bumbarner, L., Lacy, J., and Coffman, G., Aerial transmission of mycobacteria, *Am. Rev. Resp. Dis.*, 100, 165, 1969.

32. Houk, V., Kent, D., Baker, J., and Sorensen, K., The epidemiology of tuberculosis transmission in a closed environment, *Arch. Environ. Health*, 16, 26, 1968.

33. Myrvik, Q., Leake, E., and Goren, M., Mechanisms of toxicity of tubercle bacilli for macrophages, in Bendinelli, M. and Friedman, H., eds., *Mycobacterium Tuberculosis: Interactions with the Immune System*, Plenum Press, New York, 1988, Chap 14.

34. Mims, C., *The Pathogenesis of Infectious Disease*, 3rd ed., Academic Press, London, 1987, Chap 1.

35. Dooley, S. W., Jarvis, W. R., Martone, W. J., and Snider, D. E., Jr., Multidrug-resistant tuberculosis (editorial), *Ann. Intern. Med.*, 117, 257, 1992.

36. Daley, C. L., Small, P. M., Schecter, G. F., Schoolnik, G. K., McAdam, R. A., Jacobs, W. R., Jr., and Hopewell, P. C., An outbreak of tuberculosis with accelerated progression among persons infected with the human immunodeficiency virus. An analysis using restriction-fragment-length polymorphisms, *N. Engl. J. Med.*, 326, 231, 1992.

37. Valway, S. E., Sanchez, M. P., Shinnick, T. F., Orme, I., Agerton, T., Hoy, D., Jones, J. S., Westmoreland, H., and Onorato, I. M., An outbreak involving extensive transmission of a virulent strain of *Mycobacterium tuberculosis, N. Engl. J. Med.*, 338, 633, 1998. (Published erratum appears in *N. Engl. J. Med.*, 338, 1783, 1998.)

38. Cole, S. T., Brosch, R., Parkhill, J., Garnier, T., Churcher, C., Harris, D., Gordon, S. V., Eiglmeier, K., Gas, S., Barry, C. E., et al., Deciphering the biology of *Mycobacterium tuberculosis* from the complete genome sequence, *Nature*, 393, 537, 1998. (Published erratum appears in *Nature*, 396, 190, 1998.)

39. Cox, C., *The Aerobiological Pathway of Microorganisms,* John Wiley & Sons, Chichester, 1987.

40. Ko, G., First, M. W., and Burge, H. A., Influence of relative humidity on particle size and UV sensitivity of Serratia marcescens and BCG aerosols, Conference Proc. 41st Annual Biological Safety Conference, Oct 17–20, 1999, St. Louis.

41. Catanzaro, A., Nosocomial tuberculosis, *Am. Rev. Resp. Dis.*, 123, 559, 1982.

42. Nardell, E., Keegan, J., Cheney, S., and Etkind, S., Airborne infection: theoretical limits of protection achievable by building ventilation, *Am. Rev. Resp. Dis.* 144, 302, 1991.

43. Centers for Disease Control and Prevention, *Mycobacterium tuberculosis* transmission in a health clinic — Florida, *MMWR*, 38, 256, 1989.

44. Riley, E., Murphy, G., and Riley, R., Airborne spread of measles in a suburban elementary school, *Am. J. Epidemiol.,* 107, 421, 1978.

45. Gammaitoni, L. and Nucci, M. C., Using a mathematical model to evaluate the efficacy of TB control measures, *Emerg. Infect. Dis.,* 3, 335, 1997.

46. Swanson, M., Campbell, A., O'Hallaren, M., and Reed, C., Role of ventilation, air filtration, and allergen production rate in determining concentrations of rat allergens in the air of animal quarters, *Am. Rev. Resp. Dis.,* 141, 1578, 1990.

47. Fennelly, K. and Nardell, E., The relative efficacy of respirators and room ventilation in preventing occupational tuberculosis, *Inf. Cont. Hosp. Epidemiol.,* 19, 754, 1998.

48. Lin-Greenberg, A. and Anez, T., Delays in respiratory isolation of patients with pulmonary tuberculosis and human immunodeficiency virus infection, *Am. J. Infect. Cont.,* 20, 16, 1992.

49. Gunnels, J., Bates, J., and Swindoll, H., Infectivity of sputum positive tuberculosis patients on chemotherapy, *Am. Rev. Resp. Dis.*, 109, 323, 1974.

50. Clancy, L., Kelly, P., O'Reilly, L., Byrne, C., and Costello, E., The pathogenicity of *Mycobacterium tuberculosis* during chemotherapy, *Eur. Respir. J.,* 3, 399, 1990.

51. Noble, R., Infectiousness of pulmonary tuberculosis after starting chemotherapy: review of available data on an unresolved question, *Am. J. Infect. Cont.,* 9, 6, 1981.

52. Etkind, S., Boutotte, J., Ford, J., Singleton, L., and Nardell, E. A., Treating hard-to-treat tuberculosis patients in Massachusetts, *Sem. Respir. Infect.,* 6, 273, 1991.

53. Mylotte, J., Rodgers, J., Fassl, M., Seibel, K., and Vacanti, A., Derivation and validation of a pulmonary tuberculosis prediction model, *Infect. Cont. Hosp. Epidemiol.,* 18, 554, 1997.

54. Tattevin, P., Casalino, E., Fleury, L., Egmann, G., Ruel, M., and Bouvet, E., The validity of medical history, classic symptoms, and chest radiographs in predicting pulmonary tuberculosis: derivation of a pulmonary tuberculosis prediction model, *Chest*, 115, 1248, 1999.

55. Knirsch, C. A., Jain, N. L., Pablos-Mendez, A., Friedman, C., and Hripcsak, G., Respiratory isolation of tuberculosis patients using clinical guidelines and an automated clinical decision support system, *Infect. Cont. Hosp. Epidemiol.,* 19, 94, 1998.

56. Centers for Disease Control, Guideline for preventing the transmission of *Mycobacterium tuberculosis* in health-care facilities, 1994, *MMWR*, 43(RR-13), 1, 1994.

57. Lindberg, P., Improving hospital ventilation systems for tuberculosis infection control. *Joint Commission: 1993 Plant Technology and Safety Management (PTSM) Series,* No. 1, 19, 1993.

58. Keene, J. and Sansone, E., Airborne transport of contaminants in ventilated spaces, *Lab. Anim. Sci.,* 34, 453, 1984.

59. Nelson, T., Recirculating air from respiratory isolation rooms: evaluation of energy loss due to exterior venting. Unpublished promotional material distributed by Component Systems, Inc., Cleveland, OH, 1992.

60. Miller-Leiden, S., Lobascio, C., Nazaroff, W. W., and Macher, J. M., Effectiveness of in-room air filtration and dilution ventilation for tuberculosis infection control, *J. Air Waste Manage. Assoc.,* 46, 869, 1996.

61. Wells, W. F., Wells, M. F., and Wilder, T. S., The envioronmental control of epidemic contagion. I. An epidemiologic study of radiant disinfection of air in day schools, *Am. J. Hyg.,* 35, 97, 1942.
62. Medical Research Council, *Disinfection with Ultraviolet Irradiation of Classrooms — Its Effects on Illness in School Children,* Special Report Series No. 283, London, 1954.
63. Kingston, D., Lidwell, O., and Williams, R., The epidemiology of the common cold. III. The effects of ventilation, air disinfection, air disinfection and room size, *J. Hyg. London,* 60, 341, 1962.
64. Perkins, J. E., Bahlke, A. M., and Silverman, H. F., Effects of ultraviolet irradiation of classrooms on the spread of measles in large rural central schools, *Am. J. Public Health,* 37, 529, 1947.
65. McLean, R., The effects of ultraviolet radiation upon the transmission of epidemic influenza in long-term hospital patients, International Conference on Asian Influenza, Feb 17-19, 1960, Bethesda, MD, *Am. Rev. Resp. Dis.,* 83(suppl.), 36, 1961.
66. Riley, R. and Nardell, E., Clearing the air: the theory and application of ultraviolet air disinfection, *Am. Rev. Resp. Dis.,* 139, 286, 1989.
67. Bruls, W., Transmission of human epidermis and stratum corneum as a function of thickness in the ultravilolet and visible wavelengths, *Photochem. Photobiol.,* 40, 485, 1984.
68. Sliney, D., Ultraviolet radiation and the eye, in Grandolfo, M., ed., *Light, Lasers and Synchrotron Radiation,* Plenum Press, New York, 1990, 237.
69. Blum, H. and Lippincott, S., Carcinogenic effects of ultraviolet radiation of wavelength 2537A, *J. Natl. Cancer Inst.,* 1, 211, 1942.
70. Forbes, P. and Urbach, F., Experimental modifications of carcinogenesis. I. Fluorescent whitening agents and shortwave ultraviolet irradiation, *Food Cosmet. Toxicol.,* 13, 335, 1974.
71. Urbach, F., Potential carcinogenic effects for human skin of ultraviolet radiation of 253.7 nm wavelength, Centers for Disease Control, Consultants Meeting on Ultraviolet Germicidal Irradiation, Atlanta, GA, December 10–11, 1991. Unpublished presentation.
72. Sterenborg, H., The dose-response relationship of tumorgenesis by ultraviolet radiation of 254 nm, *Photochem. Photobiol.,* 47, 245, 1988.
73. Jeevan, A. and Kripke, M., Alteration of the immune response to *M. bovis* BCG in mice exposed chronically to low dose of UV irradiation, *Cell. Immunol.,* 130, 32, 1990.
74. Zmudzka, B. and Beer, J., Activation of human immunodeficiency virus by ultraviolet radiation, *Photochem. Photobiol.,* 52, 1153, 1990.
75. Saah, A., Horn, T., Hoover, D., Chen, C., Whitmore, S., Flynn, C., Wesch, J., Detels, R., and Anderson, R., Solar ultraviolet radiation exposure does not appear to exacerbate HIV infection in homosexual men, *AIDS,* 15, 1773, 1997.
76. Gefand, J., Rudikoff, D., Lebwohl, M., and Klotman, M., Effect of UV-B phototheapy on plasma HIV type 1 RNA viral level: a self-controlled prospective study, *Arch. Dermatol.,* 134, 940, 1998.
77. Zmudzka, B., Miller, S., Jacobs, M., and Beer, J., Medical UV exposures and HIV activation, *Photochem. Photobiol.,* 64, 246, 1996.
78. National Institute for Occupational Safety and Health, Criteria for a recommended standard for occupational exposure to ultraviolet radiation, NIOSH, Cincinnati, OH, 1972.
79. American Conference of Governmental Industrial Hygienists, TLVs and BEIs, ACGIH, Cincinnati, OH, 1999, 181.
80. Rose, R. and Parker, R., Erythema and conjunctivitis: outbreaks caused by inadvertent exposure to ultraviolet light, *JAMA,* 242, 1155, 1979.
81. Nardell, E. and Riley, R., A new ultraviolet germicidal irradiation (UVGI) fixture design for upper room air disinfection with low ceilings, in *Program and Abstracts of the World Congress on Tuberculosis,* Bethesda, MD, 1992, 38.
82. Moss, C. and Seitz, T., Ultraviolet irradiation exposure to health care workers from germicidal lamps, *Appl. Occup. Environ. Hyg.,* 6, 168, 1991.
83. First, M., Nardell, E., Chaission, W., and Riley, R., Guidelines for the application of upper-room ultraviolet germicidal irradiation for preventing transmission of airborne contagion. Part I: Basic Principles, *ASHRAE Transact.,* 105, 1999. (In press)
84. First, M., Nardell, E., Chaission, W., and Riley, R., Guidelines for the application of upper-room ultraviolet germicidal irradiation for preventing transmission of airborne contagion. Part II: Design and operations guidance, *ASRAE Transact.,* 105, 1999. (In press.)

85. Riley, R. and Kaufman, J., Effect of relative humidity on the inactivation of airborne *Serratia marcescens* by ultraviolet irradiation, *Appl. Microbiol.*, 23, 1113, 1972.

86. Riley, R., Knight, M., and Middlebrook, G., Ultraviolet susceptibility of BCG and virulent tubercle bacilli, *Am. Rev. Respir. Dis.*, 113, 413, 1976.

87. Iseman, M. D., A leap of faith. What can we do to curtail intrainstitutional transmission of tuberculosis? *Ann. Intern. Med.*, 117, 251, 1992.

88. Riley, R., Permutt, S., and Kaufman, J., Convection, air mixing, and ultraviolet air disinfection in rooms, *Arch. Environ. Health*, 22, 200, 1971.

89. Riley, R. and Permutt, S., Room air disinfection by ultraviolet irradiation of upper air — air mixing and germicidal effectiveness, *Arch. Environ. Health*, 22, 208, 1971.

90. Riley, R., Permutt, S., and Kaufman, J., Room air disinfection by ultraviolet irradiation of upper room air, *Arch. Environ. Health*, 23, 35, 1971.

91. Rahn, R., Peng, X., and Miller, S., Dosimetry of room-air germicidal (254 nm) radiation using spherical actinometry, *Photochem. Photobiol.*, 70, 314, 1999.

92. Riley, R. and Kaufman, J., Air disinfection in corridors by upper air irradiation with ultraviolet, *Arch. Environ. Health*, 22, 551, 1971.

93. Nardell, E. A., Iseman, M. D., Kubica, G., Riley, R. L., Stead, W. W., and Urbach, F., Multidrug-resistant tuberculosis (letter), *N. Engl. J. Med.*, 327, 1173, 1992.

94. Calder, R. A., Duclos, P., Wilder, M. H., Pryor, V. L., and Scheel, W. J., *Mycobacterium tuberculosis* transmission in a health clinic, *Bull. Int. Union Tuberc. Lung Dis.*, 66, 103, 1991.

95. Fennelly, K. P., Personal respiratory protection against *Mycobacterium tuberculosis, Clin. Chest Med.*, 18, 1, 1997.

96. Barnhart, S., Sheppard, L., Beaudet, N., Stover, B., and Balmes, J., Tuberculosis in health care settings and the estimated benefits of engineering controls and respiratory protection, *J. Occup. Environ. Med.*, 39, 849, 1997.

97. Malasky, C., Jordan, T., Potulski, F., and Reichman, L. B., Occupational tuberculous infections among pulmonary physicians in training, *Am. Rev. Respir. Dis.*, 142, 505, 1990.

98. Neff, T. A., Bronchoscopy and Bactec for the diagnosis of tuberculosis: state of the art, or a brief dissertation on the efficient search for the tubercle bacillus? (Editorial), *Am. Rev. Respir. Dis.*, 133, 962, 1986.

99. Wenzel, R. P. and Edmond, M. B., Tuberculosis infection after bronchoscopy, *JAMA*, 278, 1111, 1997.

100. Agerton, T., Valway, S., Gore, B., Pozsik, C., Plikaytis, B., Woodley, C., and Onorato, I., Transmission of a highly drug-resistant strain (strain W1) of *Mycobacterium tuberculosis:* community outbreak and nosocomial transmission via a contaminated bronchoscope, *JAMA*, 278, 1073, 1997.

101. Michele, T. M., Cronin, W. A., Graham, N. M., Dwyer, D. M., Pope, D. S., Harrington, S., Chaisson, R. E., and Bishai, W. R., Transmission of *Mycobacterium tuberculosis* by a fiberoptic bronchoscope: identification by DNA fingerprinting, *JAMA*, 278, 1093, 1997.

102. Ramirez, J., Ahmed, Z., Gutierrez, C. L., Byrd, R. P., Roy, T. M., and Sarrubi, F. A., Impact of atypical mycobacterial contamination of bronchoscopy on patient care: report of an outbreak and reveiw of the literature, *Infect. Dis. Clin. Pract.*, 7, 281, 1998.

103. Martin, M. and Reichelderfer, M., APIC guidelines for infection prevention and control in flexible endoscopies, *Am. J. Infect. Cont.*, 22, 19, 1994.

104. Goette, D., Jacobson, K., and Doty, R., Primary inoculation tuberculosis of the skin: prosector's paronychia, *Arch. Dermatol.*, 114, 567, 1978.

105. McKenna, M. T., Cauthen, G., and Onorato, I. M., The association between occupation and tuberculosis: a population-based survey, *Am. J. Resp. Crit. Care Med.*, 154, 587, 1996.

106. Lundgren, R., Norrman, E., and Asberg, I., Tuberculosis infection transmitted by autopsy, *Tubercle*, 68, 147, 1987.

107. Ussery, X. T., Bierman, J. A., Valway, S. E., Seitz, T. A., DiFerdinando, G. T., Jr., and Ostroff, S. M., Transmission of multidrug-resistant *Mycobacterium tuberculosis* among persons exposed in a medical examiner's office, New York, *Infect. Control Hosp. Epidemiol.*, 16, 160, 1995.

108. Templeton, G., Illing, L., Young, L., Cave, D., Stead, W., and Bates, J., The risk of transmission of *Mycobacterium tuberculosis* at the bedside and during autopsy, *Ann. Intern. Med.*, 15, 955, 1995.

109. Collins, C. and Grange, J., Tuberculosis acquired in laboratory and necropsy rooms, *Commun. Dis. Publ. Health*, 2, 161, 1999.

4 The Working Mycobacteriology Laboratory

Ronald W. Smithwick, M.S.

CONTENTS

I. INTRODUCTION

Mycobacteriology is the field of science dedicated to the study of microorganisms in the genus *Mycobacterium*, which includes the species *tuberculosis* and more than 80 other described species. These microorganisms have features similar to both fungi and bacteria, thus the genus name *Mycobacterium*.

The role of the diagnostic mycobacteriology laboratory is to examine clinical specimens to confirm a clinician's diagnosis of tuberculosis or other mycobacterioses, to test mycobacterial isolates for susceptibility to antimicrobial drugs, to monitor therapy with bacteriologic tests, to support epidemiologic investigations, and to identify isolates from mycobacterioses.

Microscopically, mycobacteria vary in appearance from spherical to short filaments, which may be branched. Although tubercle bacilli from clinical specimens usually appear as short to moderately long rods, they can be curved and frequently are seen in a closely bound mass or clump. Individual bacilli generally are 0.5 to 1.0 µm in diameter and 1.5 to 10 µm long.[1,2]

One of the distinguishing characteristics of mycobacteria is their ability to retain dyes within the bacilli that usually are removed from other microorganisms by alcohols and dilute solutions of strong mineral acids such as hydrochloric acid. Consequently, mycobacteria are termed acid-fast and are called acid-fast bacilli or just AFB. This ability to resist destaining by acids and alcohols has been attributed to a wax-like layer composed of long-chain fatty acids, the mycolic acids, in their cell wall.[1]

The detection of tubercle bacilli in specimens from tuberculosis patients begins with specimen collection. Both the quality of the specimen and the conditions for transport to the laboratory can affect how accurately the laboratory report reflects the status of the patient. Good quality laboratory work cannot compensate for a poor quality specimen.

Acid-fast microscopy usually is the first and most rapid diagnostic test. Subsequently, the specimen is processed in an attempt to grow the AFB on artificial media. This growth is used to perform tests for antimicrobial susceptibility, species identification, and any other required testing.

II. LABORATORY SAFETY

Since tuberculosis is transmitted primarily by the airborne route, protecting laboratory workers against infection should be a primary consideration in a mycobacteriology laboratory. Moreover, an increase in cases of multidrug-resistant tuberculosis has made safety even more critical to laboratory operation.

Most laboratory manipulations of clinical specimens and cultures of microorganisms create aerosols that can be infectious. Breaking the surface tension of a liquid almost always creates an aerosol. In the laboratory, aerosols are created by bursting bubbles, by removing an instrument from a liquid or moist surface, or by a drop leaving a pipet or landing on a medium surface. These aerosols then dry to form droplet nuclei, which remain suspended in the air and may contain infectious microorganisms, such as tubercle bacilli. Although preventing aerosol production and the resultant droplet nuclei is impossible, aerosol formation can be minimized and those aerosols that are produced can be contained. Procedures that avoid both bubble production and agitation of liquids or moist materials help to minimize aerosol production. The control of airflow, such as one-pass air in conjunction with negative-pressure containment laboratories and the use of biological safety cabinets, helps isolate and eliminate any droplet nuclei created by laboratory-generated aerosols. The use of protective clothing, autoclave sterilization, ultraviolet light, and effective disinfectants all contribute to protecting laboratory workers and others from infection in the laboratory.

III. SPECIMEN COLLECTION

Proper specimen collection and transport are critical to producing a laboratory report that reflects the microbiological condition of the patient. To assure the best sputum for mycobacteriology, the specimen collector must be properly trained, the patient must be given explicit instructions and must understand them. The patient then must be supervised, at least during the first sputum collection. Frequently, collecting a good sputum specimen is not easy. Collectors must manage some patients who are uncooperative, very young, very old, or debilitated. They must attempt to collect only sputum. Saliva and nasopharyngeal discharge are not acceptable specimens. Also, it is important for the collector to evaluate a patient's effort to produce sputum. Not all patients sent for sputum collection will have tuberculosis, and they may not be able to produce purulent sputum and/or a satisfactory volume. After evaluating a patient's effort as good, the collector may accept a 1 to 2 ml sample of even nonpurulent sputum as satisfactory. Because the collection was properly supervised, laboratory workers may consider this the best sputum that the patient can produce and do not need to reject it as appearing unsatisfactory.

Three single sputa should be collected on different days within 1 week, usually on 3 consecutive days. Because a tuberculous lesion in the lungs may drain intermittently into the bronchial tree, a specimen taken on any particular day may be AFB negative, while a specimen taken the next day may be positive. Therefore, any AFB-positive specimen in a series should be considered to be diagnostic for that patient. A patient should not be asked to expectorate multiple specimens in one container to be submitted for laboratory evaluation because AFB isolations frequently are lost due to overgrowth by contaminating microorganisms that multiply in these specimens during the extended collection period.[3]

Unsupervised sputum collection should be avoided. Sputum collection by unsupervised patients allows not only for the submission of unacceptable sputum but for substitution as well.

Since coughing, sneezing, and talking all create aerosols, precautions must be taken to protect workers and patients from infection. Transmission of tuberculosis in the sputum collection area can be avoided by the use of efficient directional airflow exhausted to the outside and away from public areas, by the use of well-ventilated sputum collection booths, and by the proper use of NIOSH (National Institute for Occupational Safety and Health)-approved respirators (N95, HEPA, or PAPR). NIOSH regulations for respirator use require annual fit testing, use training, and medical evaluation. Although some N95 respirators look like surgical masks, they are not. Surgical masks are not designed to protect the wearer from respiratory infection and must not be used as substitutes for approved respirators.

The sputum collection area should be well organized to create a smooth flow of patients who are supervised by the sputum collectors. A waiting area with sufficient seating should be provided for patients. All materials should be prepared beforehand with adequate supplies to last throughout the collection period. Sputum collection containers must be clean, sterile, and new, and must have a 2 to 5-cm opening and a tight-fitting lid. The lid should seal well enough to prevent leaks and, for transported specimens, should be strong enough to withstand air pressure changes during air transport. Fifty-milliliter, screw-capped, plastic centrifuge tubes frequently are recommended for sputum collection and subsequent processing in the laboratory. There must be a label on the *side* of the container with the patient's name and/or identification number and the date.

The sputum collector should not collect sputum specimens from more patients than can be effectively supervised at one time; usually no more than three and frequently only one. The immediate area of sputum collection should be free of onlookers. Easily-read instructions illustrated with photographs or drawings, should be posted in the waiting area to prepare the patient, and in the collection area to reinforce the sputum collector's verbal instructions.

Before collecting a sputum it is advisable to have the patient rinse food particles and unwanted bacteria from the mouth with water, as well as to clear the throat of postnasal discharge. Although water can contain saprophytic mycobacteria, these organisms are rarely isolated and present less of a problem for the laboratory than the food and other material that could contaminate the sputum.

To collect sputum, the collector should instruct the patient to take four deep breaths: the first two times to inhale deeply, hold the breath for a few seconds, then exhale slowly; the third time, to forcefully blow the air out; and the fourth time, to inhale deeply and cough. The patient may have to cough several times before producing sputum. The sputum collector may need to use back-percussion to supplement the patient's efforts. The patient should rest after coughing three or four times or when appearing stressed.

The patient should hold the sputum container to the lower lip and gently release the specimen into the container. An adequate specimen is 5 to 10 ml of sputum. More than 10 ml may be too much for laboratory processing. If attempts to collect the minimum of 5 ml are unsuccessful, the specimen should be submitted to the laboratory with a brief explanation for the small amount.

A nebulizer may be used for sputum induction but should not be considered the method of choice. Naturally produced sputum is preferred to the diluted watery sputum obtained by nebulizer induction. Also, nebulizer sputum induction may cause a patient unnecessary respiratory distress for several hours after use. Nebulizer maintenance and parts replacement create additional expenses.

A throat swab should be considered inadequate or the least acceptable type of specimen. Throat swabs should be done only if sputum cannot be collected because of the patient's inability to cooperate or if collecting a specimen by other means is impractical or impossible. AFB-positive reports are diagnostic but negative reports are unreliable because reflex swallowing can clear AFB from the throat before the swabbing is done.

Other specimens that may be submitted to the laboratory for mycobacteria isolation are specimens collected during bronchoscopy, gastric washings, body fluids, tissue, urine, and feces.[4] Collecting feces to isolate mycobacteria should be limited to immunocompromised patients.

Instructions for storing and transporting specimens must be obtained from the receiving laboratory; specimens can become useless when improperly stored or transported. Some general rules are (1) always use sterile collection containers, even for feces; (2) use aseptic collection techniques if possible; (3) do not freeze specimens; (4) refrigerate specimens when possible; and (5) obtain regulations and instructions from your local or state health department for packaging and shipping clinical specimens.

IV. ACID-FAST MICROSCOPY

Acid-fast microscopy is a rapid, inexpensive, and simple method to detect the presence of myco-bacteria in a clinical specimen. It usually is the first bacteriologic test to confirm the clinical diagnosis of tuberculosis. Microscopy also identifies potentially infectious patients, helps to monitor the effects of therapy, and helps the laboratory staff to determine inoculum adjustments for tests. However, the method has limitations. *Mycobacterium* species cannot be differentiated by acid-fast microscopy. It is relatively insensitive compared with isolation by culture because only a small portion of sputum is used to prepare a smear and only a portion of the smear is examined by microscopy. It has been estimated that a milliliter of sputum must contain approximately 6000 AFB to have a 50% chance of finding 3 AFB and reporting the smear as positive for AFB.[5] Another estimate indicates that at least 10,000 AFB must be present in a milliliter of sputum to consistently find 3 AFB by microscopy.[1] This means that a smear could be reported negative for AFB even though as many as 600 to 1000 colonies might grow in culture if 0.1 ml of this material were used to inoculate a tube of isolation medium. This assumes that all AFB in this theoretical specimen are viable; usually, they are not.

Because aerosols are generated during smear preparation, the smears must be prepared in a biological safety cabinet or other measures must be taken to prevent respiratory infection, such as proper use of N95 or HEPA respirators.

A smear is prepared by spreading 0.01 to 0.03 ml of specimen or specimen concentrate over an area approximately 1×2 cm on a new, labeled, glass microscope slide. Smears then are dried at ambient temperature and heat-fixed at approximately 75°C for 2 hours or over a flame for 2 to 3 sec. The smears then are stained with specific dyes and searched by microscopy to find AFB. Heat- fixing kills many but not all AFB in a smear. The infection hazard from any tubercle bacilli that remain viable in a smear is very small because it is unlikely (1) that the bacilli would be rubbed off the slide in particles smaller than 5 μm, or (2) that they might be inhaled or enter the skin by puncture from a broken slide. The phenol in acid-fast staining solutions will kill any AFB on the slide during staining, so staining smears soon after preparation is best.[6]

Usually, only 5 to 15% of clinical specimens submitted for acid-fast microscopy are positive for AFB. Therefore, a microscopist will see very few AFB-positive smears if less than 15 specimens are examined each week. This lack of experience, in addition to the problems of deterioration of staining reagents that are used infrequently, makes it difficult to maintain proficiency. It is recom-mended that unless a microscopist does at least 15 acid-fast microscopic examinations per week, all specimens should be sent to a more qualified laboratory to confirm results.[5]

A smear prepared from a specimen without initial processing usually is referred to as a direct smear. Concentrated specimen smears usually are prepared from the sediments of specimens cen-trifuged for isolating AFB by culture. A smear from a concentrated specimen also can be made by mixing sputum with an equal volume of 5% sodium hypochlorite (household bleach), waiting for 10 min, centrifuging at 3000 to 3500 × g for 15 min, and then preparing a smear from the sediment.

There are a number of acid-fast staining techniques. The standard technique is the 1883 Neelsen modification of the 1882 Ziehl method.[5] This Ziehl-Neelsen method requires moderate heat for optimum AFB staining. The Kinyoun cold staining method uses a higher concentration of dye and stains AFB just as well as the Ziehl-Neelsen method. The dye used in these staining solutions is the phenyl methane dye, basic fuchsin, also known as magenta, which stains AFB red. After the initial specific staining, the smear is destained with an acid-alcohol solution, leaving only the stained

AFB. The background tissue debris may be lightly stained a contrasting blue, green, or yellow through which the microscopist searches for the red-stained AFB.

For fluorescence acid-fast microscopy, the fluorescent dye auramine or a combination of auramine and rhodamine is used. The staining process is similar to the Ziehl-Neelsen method. Fluorescence acid-fast staining is not a fluorescent antibody (FA) technique but frequently and incorrectly is referred to as FA. When stained with auramine alone and observed with a fluorescence microscope, the AFB fluorescence appears white to yellow-green. Fluorescence appears pink or orange when stained with the auramine and rhodamine combination.

An AFB-positive control smear should be stained with each group of smears being stained. This assures that the reagents are staining properly, the staining procedure is done correctly, and the microscope is functioning; it also reminds the microscopist of what to look for. AFB-negative control smears are used to detect conditions that may cause false-positive smears, such as saprophytic mycobacteria in the water or the stains. In the U.S., the use of both AFB-positive and -negative control smears is required by federal regulations.

Phenol is a primary ingredient in acid-fast staining solutions. Its function is to accelerate dye penetration of the mycolic acid layer of the AFB cell envelope. The phenol must be pure, colorless crystals or a clear, colorless solid. Any yellow or brown discoloration indicates deterioration of the phenol, and such phenol must not be used. Phenol kept tightly sealed at about 4°C will not deteriorate as rapidly as it will at room temperature.

Smears should be scanned in an orderly fashion, usually in successive horizontal sweeps across the smear. For Ziehl-Neelsen or Kinyoun stained smears using bright-field microscopy, a magnification of 1000× commonly is used. In fluorescence microscopy, the fluorescing AFB appear as bright points of light in a dark background and are more easily detected than the fuchsin- stained bacilli seen by standard, visible-light microscopy. Therefore, for fluorescence microscopy, a lower magnification of 200× to 250× is used to observe smears, and AFB morphology is then confirmed at 400× to 600×. The area of a 250× field usually is more than 10 times larger than that of a field at 1000×. An observation of 300 microscopic fields of view is recommended before reporting a smear negative for AFB for fuchsin-stained smears, whereas observing only 30 fields at 200× to 250× is required for fluorescence microscopy. This saving in work time usually justifies the additional cost of a fluorescence microscope.[5]

There are several methods for reporting the results of acid- fast microscopy. Table 4.1 displays the method recommended currently.[5,7]

The tenfold increments for reporting microscopy results can be easily charted to help the physician follow the effect of therapy and give laboratory workers the information needed to prepare inocula for direct drug susceptibility tests.

Distinctive cell morphology and staining characteristics have been described for some species of mycobacteria but are not seen consistently and are shared by more than one species. Although these clues are helpful for species identification, *Mycobacterium* species cannot be differentiated by microscopy alone.

Although mycobacteria are considered Gram-stain positive, this test has no real meaning in defining mycobacteria and, therefore, has no useful purpose in mycobacteriology.

Several reports on FA tests for mycobacteria have been published. However, reliable commercial FA conjugates to identify mycobacteria have not been produced, and the test is not available.[8]

V. ISOLATION BY CULTURE

Sputa contain many different microorganisms, most of which reproduce much faster than tubercle bacilli. The goal in the laboratory is to kill or inhibit the growth of these unwanted microorganisms while promoting the growth of mycobacteria. Sodium hydroxide has been the most widely used substance to decontaminate sputa and other clinical specimens for isolating mycobacteria.

TABLE 4.1
Recommended Method for Reporting Acid-Fast
Microscopy Results on Smears Scanned at 1000×[a]

Number of AFB Seen	Preferred Report	Alternate Report
0	Negative for AFB	—
1–2/300 fields	Number/smear	+/–
1–9/100 fields	Number/100 fields	1+
1–9/10 fields	Number/10 fields	2+
1–9/field	Number/field	3+
>9/field	>9/field	4+

[a] Reports for Ziehl-Neelsen-stained smears usually are based on magnifications of approximately 1000×. Fluorochrome-stained smears may be scanned at 200× to 250×, but usually are evaluated at 400× or 600×. The area of a 400× field is approximately four times the area of a 1000× field; the area of a 600× field is approximately twice that of a 1000× field. These area differences may be considered when comparing results of the two methods of acid-fast microscopy. A report of one or two AFB per smear is not considered positive because of a possible observation error or contamination with AFB from the environment. The microscopist should review the results of companion specimens or request a replacement specimen.

Source: Friedman, L. N., Ed., *Tuberculosis: Current Concepts and Treatment,* 1st ed., CRC Press LLC, Boca Raton, FL, 1994. With permission.

Trisodium phosphate is another strong and often used base. Acids such as sulfuric and oxalic are used for special specimen decontamination applications.[7]

Mycobacteria are resistant to many of the quaternary ammonium detergents. Benzalkonium chloride and cetylpyridinium chloride are two such compounds used to decontaminate specimens to isolate mycobacteria.[9,10]

The ideal decontaminant works rapidly, is inexpensive, eliminates all unwanted microorganisms, and does not kill any mycobacteria present in the specimen. Unfortunately, no decontaminant is ideal; most will kill or inhibit some of the mycobacteria in the specimen.

Because mycobacteria are resistant to many of the common antibiotics, several antibiotics have been incorporated into media to inhibit contaminant growth and still allow mycobacterial growth. Penicillin derivatives, cycloheximide, trimethoprim, amphotericin B, and nalidixic acid have been used.[11,12]

The mucus in sputum must be liquefied for effective decontamination to take place. This liquefaction process is called digestion. The entire process often is referred to as "digestion and decontamination." Four percent sodium hydroxide will both digest and decontaminate sputa. If mucolytic substances such as N-acetyl-L-cysteine or dithiothreitol are used, the concentration of sodium hydroxide can be lowered and still attain good decontamination with more mycobacteria surviving.[13]

Immediately after decontamination, sterile buffer or distilled water is added to the specimen either to neutralize or to dilute the decontaminant and to balance the centrifuge load. Solid material and any AFB are concentrated at the bottom of the tube by centrifugation at a relative centrifugal force (RCF) of 3000 to 3500× g. The supernatant is decanted into a pan of disinfectant, and the sediment is resuspended in 1 or 2 ml of sterile buffer solution, distilled water, or bovine serum albumin solution. Media are inoculated and smears are prepared from this suspension.

An RCF of 3000 to 3500× g is necessary to attain adequate sedimentation of tubercle bacilli during centrifugation.[14] Although a higher RCF might be more efficient, some plastic centrifuge tubes may fail and additional frictional heat could kill tubercle bacilli.[7] Using a refrigerated centrifuge is advisable since frictional heating at 3000× g can reduce the number of viable tubercle bacilli in centrifuged specimens.[7]

There are many formulations of growth media for mycobacteria; they can be characterized as three basic types. The first type of medium is coagulated egg represented by the well-known Lowenstein-Jensen (L-J) medium. It is composed of whole eggs, glycerol, other nutrients and trace elements, plus a dye, usually malachite green, which inhibits contaminant growth. This medium is prepared as a liquid and, after being dispensed in screw-capped glass containers and placed in the desired position, the liquid is solidified by coagulation at 85°C for 45 min. Several other egg-based media, such as the American Thoracic Society (ATS) medium, frequently are used for mycobacteriology.

The second type of medium also is solid and is composed of soluble nutrients and trace elements, with agar as a solidified substrate. The most common examples are Middlebrook 7H10 and 7H11. These media have several advantages over the egg-based media. Colonies are more distinct on the transparent agar media than on the opaque egg media, some tubercle bacilli prefer it to other media, and drugs for susceptibility testing tend to be more stable in it than in egg media.[15] Two disadvantages are that exposure to heat and light cause formaldehyde production, which inhibits mycobacterial growth,[16] and that growth of tubercle bacilli from specimens requires an atmosphere containing 5 to 10% carbon dioxide.[17]

The third type of medium is a clear liquid and is egg free. The most common example is Middlebrook 7H9. This medium is used primarily to produce cultures of suspended, single cells and very small clumps. These easily diluted cultures are used to prepare inocula to produce isolated colonies on solid media for antimicrobial-drug-susceptibility tests and identification tests. Modifications of Middlebrook 7H9 are used as isolation media in several commercially available systems. When used to isolate tubercle bacilli from specimens, Middlebrook 7H9 and its modifications also require a 5 to 10% carbon dioxide atmosphere.

Compared with other microorganisms, tubercle bacilli grow very slowly. Cell doubling time is 15 to 24 hours, depending on growth conditions,[2] compared with approximately 20 min for some of the common bacteria. Colonies can be seen on solid media in 2 to 3 weeks for some strains, but visible growth can take as long as 8 weeks for other strains. This slow growth has been a perpetual problem for laboratory confirmation of tuberculosis and the timely reporting of drug-susceptibility test results. Tubercle bacilli from specimens usually do not produce visible colonies on solid media until approximately 3 weeks after inoculation, and may take 6 weeks or more if only a few colonies are present. Growth can be detected earlier in modified 7H9 media, especially if the specimen contains a relatively large number of viable AFB.[18-20]

There are several different commercial systems available that use modified 7H9 liquid medium. On average, mycobacterial growth can be detected earlier with these systems than when observing for growth of colonies on solid media. Growth is detected either by measuring the increase in metabolic products (radioactive carbon dioxide), by noting a decrease in oxygen, or by an increase in turbidity.[21-24] Not only is the time required to detect initial growth usually decreased, but the time required to do antibiotic susceptibility tests is decreased. The greater the number of AFB in the inoculum, the earlier growth is detected. However, if the inoculum contains few AFB, then growth detection may take as long as the detection of visible colonies on solid media. At least one solid medium should be used in conjunction with a modified 7H9 because some strains will grow on one medium and not in/on the other. These systems usually incorporate common antibiotics in the medium to inhibit contaminants while allowing mycobacteria to grow. When growth is detected in the liquid medium, the presence of AFB and absence of contamination are confirmed by acid-fast microscopy.

Occasionally, isolation by culture fails with a patient whose symptoms, medical history, or AFB positive smears indicate tuberculosis or other mycobacterioses. This can occur for many reasons, including effective therapy, poor specimen collection, specimen mix-up, overheating or freezing specimens during storage or shipment, misdiagnosis, overdecontamination, collecting specimens shortly after beginning antibiotic therapy, toxic substances in specimens, and improper specimen processing. Unusual growth requirements are an infrequent cause of missed isolation as well. Some rare strains of *M. tuberculosis* are carbon dioxide dependent. *M. bovis* may not grow in the presence of glycerol. *M. africanum* prefers a medium supplemented with pyruvic acid or its salt. Mycobacteria other than tubercle bacilli may prefer temperatures higher or lower than 37°C or, in the case of *M. haemophilum,* require a medium rich in iron. It is important that the physician give the laboratory staff information about the patient and source of a specimen to help determine if any unusual processing or growth conditions are necessary.

False-positive reports may be caused by a mix-up in specimens during collection or processing; this is best avoided by good organization and careful attention to detail. Other factors can also cause misleading AFB-positive reports. Mycobacteria other than tubercle bacilli are present in most water supplies, even in nonsterile distilled water.[25,26] These potential troublemakers can be introduced into the specimen during collection or during processing in the laboratory. If they are not recognized as contaminants, they may be mistakenly implicated in disease. As a general rule, when five or fewer colonies of AFB not appearing to be tubercle bacilli are isolated from only one specimen in a series, a laboratory may choose not to do additional testing unless the physician is convinced the isolate is causing disease. The expensive identification of AFB contaminants seldom serves any useful medical purpose. Such isolates from immunocompromised patients should be considered an exception to this recommendation.

VI. DRUG SUSCEPTIBILITY TESTING

Drug-resistant mutants occur spontaneously in actively growing populations of tubercle bacilli. For any one drug, the rate of spontaneous mutation in a population is relatively constant, but the rate varies from drug to drug. The rate of drug-resistant mutations in a susceptible population may range from 1 per 10^5 to 1 per 10^8 bacilli, depending on the drug and its concentration.[27,28] Since the mutations are spontaneous and not induced, the drug need not be present for the mutations to occur. Treatment with only a single drug can then select the mutants resistant to that drug, and they will become the replacement population of tubercle bacilli.

In the past, unless the patient was from a population in which drug-resistant tuberculosis was common, testing initial *M. tuberculosis* isolates for drug susceptibility was considered impractical. Because of the emergence of multidrug-resistant *M. tuberculosis,* this practice has changed. All initial isolates of tubercle bacilli should be tested for drug susceptibility.[29] As in the past, susceptibility testing is indicated for apparent drug treatment failures, retreatment cases, and isolates from close contacts of patients with known drug-resistant tuberculosis.[4] In a drug-resistance surveillance investigation, drug susceptibility tests are done on isolates from patients not previously treated for tuberculosis to determine the level of primary drug resistance in specified populations.

Drug susceptibility tests detect growth of drug-resistant tubercle bacilli on drug-containing media. Of the several methods for determining drug resistance, the proportion method is the most widely accepted and recommended.[30] Colonies are counted on the drug-containing medium and compared with the number of colonies on the control medium without drugs. Growth in the presence of drugs is reported as a percentage of the growth on the control, i.e., the proportion of drug-resistant growth compared to control growth.

The critical concentration of each drug must be determined for each medium before routine use because drugs are affected differently by each type of medium used for testing (Table 4.2).[7,30,31] Critical concentration has been defined as "the weakest concentration at which susceptible bacilli are unable to grow in the presence of the drug." [32] Minimal inhibitory concentration (MIC) is not the same as critical concentration. MIC is based on the test results of a single strain with multiple concentrations of a drug to determine the lowest concentration to which it is susceptible. Critical

TABLE 4.2

Examples of Critical Concentrations of Five Primary Antituberculosis Drugs in Three Common Media

Drugs	Media Critical Concentrations (μg/ml)		
	L–J	7H10	BACTEC 12B
Isoniazid	0.2	0.2	0.1
Rifampin	40.0	1.0	2.0
Streptomycin	4.0	2.0	2.0
Ethambutol	2.0	5.0	2.5
Pyrazinamide	100.0	25.0	100.0

Source: Centers for Disease Control and Prevention, Atlanta.

concentration is determined to be the highest MIC in a large group of susceptible strains. Initially, the MIC of a drug must be determined for many susceptible strains to establish the critical concentration of a drug for a particular medium. The critical concentrations of tuberculosis drugs has been established for Middlebrook 7H10 and has been used extensively in the U.S. The critical concentration has not been established for all tuberculosis drugs in the modified 7H9 medium at this time.

The inoculum for the test medium must contain a selection of bacilli that represents the population in the patient: the inoculum must contain only single cells or only very small clumps of bacilli and it must contain the appropriate number of colony-forming units to achieve valid test results. For the direct drug susceptibility test, the microbiologist first must observe an acid-fast-stained smear prepared from the decontaminated specimen concentrate. If the smear is positive for AFB, the bacilli are enumerated for a report to the physician, and dilutions of the centrifuge concentrate are calculated for the drug-testing inoculum. The inoculum theoretically contains a representative sample of the patient's *M. tuberculosis* population. The dilutions are prepared to produce the desired number of colonies on the control medium, and the susceptibility test media are inoculated.

Direct-drug susceptibility tests can be performed only on AFB-smear-positive specimens because the testing of specimens not containing tubercle bacilli is wasteful and because knowing the approximate number of AFB in the inoculum is necessary to assure useful numbers of colonies on the drug test and control media.

Indirect susceptibility tests are performed on isolated cultures of *M. tuberculosis*. The inoculum is prepared by scraping or rubbing the surface of the medium to dislodge portions of all of the colonies, thereby obtaining a representative sample of the patient's *M. tuberculosis* population; this is important. These clumps of colonies either are used to inoculate a tube of liquid medium or they are placed in a sterile glass tube containing glass beads and a buffer solution which is vortex-mixed to grind the clumps to produce a fine suspension of single cells and very small clumps. The ground clumps are used to prepare inocula to immediately inoculate the test media. The inoculated liquid medium is incubated at 37°C for a week and the growth of single cells and small clumps is used to prepare inocula for drug susceptibility test media.

Plates containing 7H10 drug susceptibility test media are inoculated with appropriate dilutions of the resuspended specimen sediment, the ground culture, or the liquid medium culture grown for 1 week at 37°C. The plates are sealed in carbon dioxide-permeable plastic bags and incubated at 37°C. An atmosphere of 5 to 10% carbon dioxide is required for the direct susceptibility tests but not for the indirect tests. After 3 weeks, colonies are counted on both the control and drug media and the percent of resistance is calculated for the growth seen on the drug-containing medium.

Microcolonies seen on drug susceptibility test media are considered evidence of drug resistance. Therefore, the surfaces of the media are scanned at 10× to 20× to assure that all colonies are counted.

A calculated proportion of resistance of 1% or greater at the critical concentration is considered to be clinically significant resistance, and the tested drug probably will no longer be effective for antituberculosis therapy.[30] Although concentrations higher than the critical concentration may be reported, only the report at the critical concentration is to be used to determine resistance. Typically, the lowest concentration of the drug in the tested media is the critical concentration.

Drug susceptibility tests using modified 7H9 media systems may be completed within 5 to 10 days.[31,33,34] The inoculum is prepared from an *M. tuberculosis*-positive liquid-medium isolation vial or from other culture media, just as in the solid-media susceptibility tests. The control vial is inoculated with a 100-fold dilution of the inoculum used for the test medium. The rate of growth in a test vial, if any, is compared to the rate of growth in the control vial. A greater rate of growth in the test vial indicates more than 1% resistance, and is as valid an indicator of drug resistance as results from solid media.

Most of the slowly growing species of mycobacteria other than tubercle bacilli are resistant to many of the antituberculosis drugs, and testing them for drug susceptibility has not been officially recommended. The exception is *M. kansasii,* which usually is susceptible to some of the antituberculosis drugs.

A drug susceptibility testing procedure has been developed for the rapidly growing mycobacteria and several laboratories offer this service.

VII. IDENTIFICATION TESTS

Species identification refers to the act of differentiating a particular life form, or a pure culture in the field of microbiology, from others to determine its species name among the classified species. The term "speciation" refers to the evolutionary production of new species. Speciation or speciate are not used in the context of species identification in this text.

From the 1950s to the late 1980s, a series of tests using growth characteristics, specific enzyme activity, and growth inhibition were used to identify *M. tuberculosis* and differentiate the other *Mycobacterium* species. These tests require a large number of test media and reagents and some can take several weeks to complete. Some newer methods are more efficient and more discriminating and, therefore, are making many of the older tests all but obsolete.

In the mid-1980s, genetic probes were introduced to identify *M. tuberculosis, M. avium,* and *M. intracellulare,* the three species that most often cause pulmonary mycobacterioses. Since then, genetic probes have been developed for *M. gordonae,* a frequent contaminant from the environment, and *M. kansasii,* which also causes pulmonary mycobacterioses (Gen-Probe, Inc., San Diego, CA).[35]

The target for the probe can be either DNA or RNA. Ribosomal RNA (rRNA) was the first target for the probes developed for *Mycobacterium* species because, in part, there are many more rRNA molecules per cell than chromosomes. There are several procedures in which probes are used. The basic steps in each procedure are

1. Place cells for testing in a container and then rupture them to release the DNA or rRNA.
2. React the DNA or rRNA with the probe, i.e., *hybridization.*
3. Remove the unhybridized probe or inactivate the label on the unhybridized probe.
4. Use a detection system to determine positive or negative reactions for identification reports (see Chapter 5).

A method to identify *Mycobacterium* species using high-performance liquid chromatography (HPLC) also was introduced in the mid-1980s.[36] This is the identification method used in many mycobacteriology reference laboratories in North America. As mentioned earlier, mycobacteria and related genera produce long-chain fatty acids, the mycolic acids. Mycolic acids, produced by the

Mycobacterium genus, are 60 to 90 carbons long, which is much longer than the fatty acids produced by other microorganisms. The amount of each chain length produced varies from one species to another. HPLC is used to determine the amount of each of the mycolic acids produced by a culture of a particular strain of mycobacteria. The relative amounts of each mycolic acid are displayed as a pattern on a chart. The culture is identified as a particular *Mycobacterium* species by matching its HPLC pattern to previously determined and standardized species pattern.[37]

Gas chromatography (GC) is used in another identification system for mycobacteria (MIDI, 115 Barksdale Prof. Center, Newark, DE). In this system, patterns of shorter chained fatty acids are produced to identify *Mycobacterium* species.[38]

Restriction fragment length polymorphism (RFLP) is a method used most often to determine strain relatedness within a species. RFLP compares electrophoretic patterns of different sized segments of DNA. This method, whimsically called DNA fingerprinting, has replaced phage typing in tuberculosis epidemiology investigations and is used to investigate cross-contamination problems in mycobacteriology laboratories (see Chapter 5).

Several nucleic acid amplification tests have been developed to identify tubercle bacilli rapidly and directly from clinical specimens (see also Chapter 5). Although they have shown promise as rapid identification tests, the results require critical interpretation. One study has shown a general lack of sensitivity of these amplification tests, and not all laboratories in the study used sufficient quality controls to provide reliable results.[39,40] These tests have not replaced the need to do standard isolation and identification tests, and a culture still is required to perform drug susceptibility testing.

VIII. LABORATORY OPERATION

The function of a clinical laboratory is to receive clinical specimens, evaluate the information provided with the specimens, perform appropriate specimen tests, and provide understandable and accurate reports in a timely manner. A report should give the clinician the necessary specimen information to help provide effective healthcare for a patient.

Specimens sent to the laboratory for diagnostic evaluation should be the best possible specimens for the required testing. In addition, these specimens and requested tests should be only those necessary to provide good patient care. Specimens should be transported from the collection site to the testing laboratory in a manner sufficient to maintain specimen quality and to assure the health safety of the general population and laboratory staff. The testing laboratory staff should be given enough information about the patient and specimen to assure that all appropriate testing methods are used.

Quality assurance is an essential part of the operation of a clinical laboratory. Quality control is the use of known positive and negative controls for tests to assure that the testing system is functioning properly. This part of laboratory testing is essential to quality assurance, but quality assurance has other aspects.

The Clinical Laboratory Improvement Amendment (CLIA), 1988 (PL 100-578), requires laboratories to participate in proficiency testing programs. Central laboratories or outside agencies send "unknown" samples to the tested clinical laboratory for evaluation. The tested laboratory is graded on its ability to evaluate the samples properly and return a correct report within a specified time. This system provides an unbiased evaluation of the tested laboratory's ability to give an accurate and timely report.

On-site evaluations by licensing agencies also are part of this quality assurance process. Laboratories may be evaluated for effective safety programs and equipment, personnel qualifications, equipment maintenance, reagent quality, testing controls, recordkeeping, and reports. These evaluations assure safe, correct, and efficient laboratory operation. An evaluator should have extensive experience in the type of laboratory work being evaluated, or should be able to provide a list of recognized consultants to the evaluated laboratory to assure that any noted deficiencies will be quickly and properly corrected.

A training program is essential for a proficient laboratory. Training should include specimen collection, laboratory safety, and quality assurance, as well as testing methods.

In conclusion, to provide high-quality healthcare, it is important that good quality specimens and information be provided to the laboratory and that the laboratory provide easily understood, accurate reports. The physician must give adequate specimen information and request clarification of unfamiliar test reports. The testing laboratory should specify the characteristics of a good quality specimen to be submitted for evaluation. The laboratory staff should be free to request additional specimen information to avoid improper or inadequate testing and to request replacements for unsatisfactory specimens. Laboratory reports should be informative and useful, and should provide information about normal parameters, cut-off levels, and should avoid or define such ambiguous terms as "2+" or "few."

Open, clear communication between the healthcare providers and clinical laboratory staff must exist so that each person understands the needs, abilities, and limitations of the others. This is both a responsibility and a benefit.

REFERENCES

1. Barksdale, L. and Kim, K. S., *Mycobacterium, Bacteriol. Rev.,* 41, 217, 1977.
2. Darzins, E., *The Bacteriology of Tuberculosis,* University of Minnesota Press, Minneapolis, MN, 1958.
3. Kestle, D. G. and Kubica, G. P., Sputum collection for cultivation of mycobacteria — an early morning specimen or the 24- to 72-hour pool? *Tech. Bull. Reg. Med. Tech.,* 37, 347, 1967.
4. Bass, J. B., Farer, L. S., Hopewell, P. C., Jacobs, R. F., and Snider, D. E., Diagnostic standards and classification of tuberculosis, *Am. Rev. Respir. Dis.,* 142, 725, 1990.
5. Smithwick, R. W., Laboratory Manual for Acid-Fast Microscopy, Department of Health and Human Services, Public Health Service, Centers for Disease Control and Prevention, Atlanta, GA, 1976.
6. Allen, B. W., Survival of tubercle bacilli in heat-fixed sputum smears, *J. Clin. Pathol.,* 34, 719, 1981.
7. Kent, P. T. and Kubica, G. P., Public Health Mycobacteriology — A Guide for the Level III Laboratory, U.S. Department of Health and Human Services, Public Health Service, Centers for Disease Control and Prevention, Atlanta, GA, 1985.
8. Nassau, E., Parsons, E. R., and Johnson, G. D., Detection of antibodies to *Mycobacterium tuberculosis* by solid phase radioimmunoassay, *J. Immunol. Methods,* 6, 261, 1975.
9. Wayne, L. G., Krasnow, I., and Kidd, G., Finding the "hidden positive" in tuberculosis eradication programs. The role of the sensitive trisodium phosphate-benzalkonium (Zephiran) culture techniques, *Am. Rev. Respir. Dis.,* 86, 537, 1962
10. Smithwick, R. W., Stratigos, C. B., and David, H. L., Use of cetylpyridinium chloride and sodium chloride for decontamination of sputum specimens that are transported to the laboratory for the isolation of *Mycobacterium tuberculosis, J. Clin. Microbiol.,* 1, 411, 1975.
11. Gruft, H., Isolation of acid-fast bacilli from contaminated specimens, *Health Lab. Sci.,* 8, 79, 1971.
12. Mitchison, D. A., Allen, B. W., Carrol, L., Dickinson, J. M., and Aber, V. R., A selective oleic acid albumin agar medium for tubercle bacilli, *J. Med. Microbiol.,* 5, 165, 1972.
13. Kubica, G. P., Dye, W. E., Cohn, M. L., and Middlebrook, G., Sputum digestion and decontamination with N-acetyl-L-cysteine-sodium hydroxide for culture of mycobacteria, *Am. Rev. Respir. Dis.,* 87, 775, 1963.
14. Rickman, T. W. and Moyer, N. P., Increased sensitivity of acid-fast smears, *J. Clin. Microbiol.,* 11, 618, 1980.
15. Kubica, G. P. and Dye, W. E., Laboratory Methods for Clinical and Public Health Mycobacteriology, Public Health Service Publication No. 1547, U.S. Government Printing Office, Washington, D.C., 1967.
16. Miliner, R. A., Stottmeier, K. D., and Kubica, G. P., Formaldehyde: a photothermal activated toxic substance produced in Middlebrook 7H10 medium, *Am. Rev. Respir. Dis.,* 99, 603, 1969.
17. Beam, R. E. and Kubica, G. P., Stimulatory effect of carbon dioxide on the primary isolation of tubercle bacilli on agar-containing medium, *Am. J. Clin. Pathol.,* 50, 395, 1968.

18. Stager, C. E., Libonati, J. P., Siddiqi, S. H., Davis, J. R., Hooper, N. M., Baker, J. F., and Carter, M. E., Role of solid media when used in conjunction with the BACTEC system for mycobacterial isolation and identification, *J. Clin. Microbiol.,* 29, 154, 1991.
19. Abe, C., Hosojima, S., Fukasawa, Y., Kazumi, Y., Takahashi, M., Hirano, K., and Mori, T., Comparison of MB-Check, BACTEC, and egg-based media for recovery of mycobacteria, *J. Clin. Microbiol.,* 30, 878, 1992.
20. Isenberg, H. D., D'Amato, R. F., Heifets, L., Murray, P. R., Scardamaglia, M., Jacobs, M. C., Aperstein, P., and Niles, A., Collaborative feasibility study of a biphasic system (Roche Septi-Chek AFB) for rapid detection and isolation of mycobacteria, *J. Clin. Microbiol.,* 29, 1719, 1991.
21. Pfyffer, G. E., Welscher, H., Kissling, P., Cieslak, C., Casal, M. J., Gutterrez, J., and Rusch-Gerdes, S., Comparison of the mycobacteria growth indicator tube (MGIT) with radiometric and solid culture for recovery of acid-fast bacilli, *J. Clin. Microbiol.,* 35, 364, 1997.
22. Benjamin, W. H., Jr., Waites, K. B., Beverly, A., Waller, M., Nix, S., Moser, S. A., and Willert, M., Comparison of the MB/BacT System with a revised antibiotic supplement kit to the BACTEC 460 system for detection of mycobacteria in clinical specimens, *J. Clin. Microbiol.,* 36, 3234, 1998.
23. Tortoli, E., Cichero, P., Chirillo, M. G., Gismondo, M. R., Bono, L., Gesu, G., Simonetti, M. T., Volpe, G., Nardi, G., and Marone, P., Multicenter comparison of ESP Culture System II with BACTEC 460TB and with Lowenstein-Jensen medium for recovery of mycobacteria from different clinical specimens, including blood, *J. Clin. Microbiol.,* 36, 1378, 1998.
24. Pfyffer, G., Cieslak, C., Welscher, H., Kissling, P., and Rusch-Gerdes, S., Rapid detection of mycobacteria in clinical specimens by using the automaated BACTEC 9000 MB system and comparison with radiometric and solid-culture systems, *J. Clin. Microbiol.,* 35, 2229, 1997.
25. Wright, E. P., Collins, C. H., and Yates, M. D., *Mycobacterium xenopi* and *Mycobacterium kansasii* in a hospital water supply, *J. Hosp. Infect.,* 6, 175, 1985.
26. Wenger, J. D., Spika, J. S., Smithwick, R. W., Pryor, V., Dodson, D. W., Carden, G. A., and Klontz, K. C., Outbreak of *Mycobacterium chelonae* infection associated with use of jet injectors, *J. Am. Med. Assn.,* 264, 373, 1990.
27. David, H. L., Probability distribution of drug-resistant mutants in unselected populations of *Mycobacterium tuberculosis*, *Appl. Microbiol.,* 20, 810, 1970.
28. Canetti, G., Present aspects of bacterial resistance in tuberculosis, *Am. Rev. Respir. Dis.,* 92, 687, 1965.
29. Centers for Disease Control, National Action Plan to Combat Multidrug-Resistant Tuberculosis, *MMWR*, 41(RR-11), 1992.
30. Canetti, G., Fox, W., Khomenko, A., Mahler, H. T., Menon, N. K., Mitchison, D. A., Rist, N., and Smelev, N. A., Advances in techniques of testing mycobacterial drug sensitivity, and the use of sensitivity tests in tuberculosis control programmes, *Bull. World Health Org.,* 41, 21, 1969.
31. Siddiqi, S., *BACTEC 460TB System Product and Procedure Manual,* Becton Dickinson and Company, Sparks, MD, 1995.
32. Canetti, G., Froman, S., Grosset, J., Hauduroy, P., Langerova, M., Mahler H. T., Meissner, G., Mitchison, D. A., and Sula, L., Mycobacteria: laboratory methods for testing drug sensitivity and resistance, *Bull. World Health Org.,* 29, 565, 1963.
33. Rusch-Gerdes, S., Domehl, C., Nardi, G., Gismondo, M. R., Welscher, H., and Pfyffer, G., Multicenter evaluation of the mycobacteria growth indicator tube for testing susceptibility of *Mycobacterium tuberculosis* to first-line drugs, *J. Clin. Microbiol.,* 37, 45, 1999.
34. Bergmann, J. S. and Woods, G. L., Evaluation of the ESP Culture System II for testing susceptibilities of *Mycobacterium tuberculosis* isolates to four primary antituberculosis drugs, *J. Clin. Microbiol.,* 36, 2940, 1998.
35. Lebrun, L., Espinasse, F., Poveda, J. D., and Vincent-Levy- Frebault, V., Evaluation of nonradioactive DNA probes for identification of mycobacteria, *J. Clin. Microbiol.,* 30, 2476, 1992.
36. Butler, W. R., Ahern, D. G., and Kilburn, J. O., High-performance liquid chromatography of mycolic acids as a tool in the identification of *Corynebacterium, Nocardia, Rhodococcus,* and *Mycobacterium* species, *J. Clin. Microbiol.,* 23, 182, 1986.
37. Butler, W. R., Cage, G., Desmond, E., Duffey, P. S., Guthertz, L. S., Gross, W. M., Jost, K. C., Ramos, L. S., Thibert, L., and Warren, N., Standardized Method for HPLC Identification of Mycobacteria, Centers for Disease Control and Prevention, PHS, U.S. Department of Health and Human Services, 1996.

38. Lambert, M. A., Moss, C. W., Silcox, V. A., and Good, R. C., Analysis of mycolic acid cleavage products and cellular fatty acids of *Mycobacterium* species by capillary gas chromatography, *J. Clin. Microbiol.*, 23, 731, 1986.

39. Noordhoek, G. T., van Embden, J. D. A., and Kolk, A. H. J., Reliability of nucleic acid amplification for detection of *Mycobacterium tuberculosis*: an international collaborative quality control study among 30 laboratories, *J. Clin. Microbiol.*, 34, 2522, 1996.

40. Centers for Disease Control and Prevention, Nucleic acid amplification tests for tuberculosis, *MMWR*, 45, 950, 1996.

5 New Diagnostic Methods

Joseph H. Bates, M.D.

CONTENTS

I. INTRODUCTION

The laboratory techniques most commonly employed in the U.S. and around the world for the diagnosis of tuberculosis were developed in the last century and have been only slightly modified over the past decades. The tubercle bacillus replicates slowly, dividing only once every 18 to 21 h, and efforts to reduce the time required for its division have been unsuccessful. This has meant that reports of positive culture growth from clinical specimens have required several weeks and sometimes up to 2 months. In addition, dependence on the stained smear of sputum or other clinical specimens has marked limitations. Although the smear report can be returned quickly from the laboratory, the sensitivity is poor because many thousands of organisms per ml must be present in the sample for the microscopist to detect their presence. Thus, the laboratory diagnosis of tuberculosis has remained little changed and rather unsatisfactory by modern medicine standards for many years. Now there is promise for improvement. New laboratory techniques using advances in immunology, molecular biology, and instrumentation provide a framework for significant change. This chapter will review recent developments in this regard.

II. SEROLOGICAL METHODS

A. IMMUNOASSAYS FOR MYCOBACTERIAL ANTIBODIES

Serological methods have been applied widely for the diagnosis of a variety of infectious diseases and it was only in 1898, a few years after Koch's identification of the tubercle bacillus, that Arloing published the first report of the value of a serological method for the diagnosis of tuberculosis.[1] He developed an agglutination test and noted that 57% of sera from tuberculosis patients showed an agglutinating antibody; healthy controls and persons ill with other diseases showed positive reactions in 11%. Over the years, many serological tests have been put forward as showing promise, but each failed to find wide acceptance. When Engvall and Perlmann described the sensitive and relatively simple enzyme-linked immunosorbent assay (ELISA) in 1972, it opened the way for a new approach to the serodiagnosis of tuberculosis and since that time many different antigens and antibodies have been studied.[2]

The largest single problem in the serodiagnosis of tuberculosis has turned on the antigen employed. A detailed description of more than 50 of these antigens has been published by Young et al.[3] Many workers have referred to mycobacterial antigens on the basis of approximate subunit molecular weights as judged by sodium dodecyl sulfate/polyacrylamide gel electrophoresis. The development of mycobacterial genes in *Escherichia coli* have allowed the demonstration of immunological activity associated with a particular polypeptide, and sequence analysis have given insight into the biochemical function of the native protein. As this methodology improves, the ultimate mycobacterial antigens used for serodiagnosis will be cloned and sequenced and the events regarding expression of its gene will be understood. Currently, knowledge of this type is very fragmentary for all mycobacterial antigens.

At present most mycobacterial antigens are nonspecific because these proteins are shared widely among species and genera.[4] Since humans and most animals have repeated contacts with environmental mycobacteria that may have little or no capacity to cause disease but do provoke an antibody response, a test subject infected or diseased by *Mycobacterium tuberculosis* may demonstrate antibody production that is a combination of both present and past antigenic stimuli. The development of a simple and rapid test to sort out this complex immunological pattern has proven to be a demanding task with great potential for error.

Nassau, Parsons, and Johnson were the first to use ELISA techniques for the diagnosis of tuberculosis.[5] They used as antigen a filtrate of *M. tuberculosis* H37RV and studied healthy controls together with diseased subjects and reported a sensitivity of 56% and a specificity of 98%. Few workers have been able to improve on these initial results. Grange and Kardjito published a series of studies with ELISA assays using sonicates of *M. bovis* BCG as the antigen.[6] They measured IgG, IgM, and IgA antibody levels and obtained the best results with IgG antibody. Tuberculin status did not influence the IgM and IgA antibody levels. Their best sensitivity was 68% and their best specificity was 98%. Other reports using unheated culture filtrates of *M. tuberculosis* H37Ra, as well as saline extracts and sonicates, have failed to improve on these initial reports.

The use of tuberculin purified protein derivative (PPD) as an antigen has been studied extensively in ELISA serodiagnostic tests. The most complete report using PPD is that of Kalish et al., who found a sensitivity of 67% and a specificity of only 79% with IgG antibody providing the best results, although IgA antibody also correlated with the diagnosis of tuberculosis.[7] Daniel and his coworkers have published several reports testing PPD as the antigen with the ELISA technique. PPD was found to rank below antigen 5, but ahead of antigen 6 and crude filtrates in terms of sensitivity and specificity.[8-10]

False-positive results with ELISA probably result from antibodies induced by mycobacteria that come from the environment or from normal flora that share common antigens with *M. tuberculosis*. To avoid these nonspecific results, efforts have been made to use purified or semipurified antigens that might be unique to the tubercle bacillus. The most commonly used protein for this purpose has been designated by Daniel and Anderson as antigen 5, but this antigen also contains nonspecific epitopes found in other mycobacteria.[11] In a study of South and North American patients, antigen 5 gave a sensitivity of 84% for serum obtained from bacteriologically positive patients in Bolivia and a sensitivity of 68% for patients in Ohio.[12] Approximately one third of the patients with atypical mycobacterial infections were also positive.

A significant disadvantage of antigen 5 is its instability under conditions of storage and shipping, whereas antigen 6 can be lyophilized without loss of activity.[13] In general, antigen 6 has been found to be a less satisfactory antigen for ELISA serodiagnosis than either antigen 5 or PPD.[14]

Reggiardo and Vazques described three serologically active mycobacterial glycolipids and tested their value in the serodiagnosis of tuberculosis.[15] These antigens, when compared with antigen 5, give the same efficiency of prediction for disease.[16]

Lipoarabinomannan (LAM) is a component of the cell wall of many, if not all, mycobacteria including *M. leprae*. Hunter et al. have purified it in its native acylated state and this product has been tested for use as an antigen in the serodiagnosis of tuberculosis.[17] Sada et al. evaluated sera from 66 patients with pulmonary or extrapulmonary tuberculosis using LAM with an ELISA technique and found 91% specificity and 72% sensitivity.[18] Subsequently they tested the serum of patients with tuberculosis for the presence of LAM antigenemia.[19] The antigen was detected using a coagglutination method and the test was able to detect as little as 50 ng/ml of LAM in a test sample. The sensitivity for patients having pulmonary tuberculosis who had no acid-fast bacilli present on stained sputum smears was 67% and the specificity was 100%.

Charpin et al. evaluated an ELISA method using an antigen designated as A60 obtained from *M. bovis* BCG.[20] The patients studied were suspected of having pulmonary tuberculosis, but had negative sputum stains. Both IgM and IgG antibody activity were measured and, combining the results of IgG and IgM, the sensitivity was 68%, the specificity was 100%, and the positive predictive value was 100%.

In an effort to simplify the technical aspects of ELISA serodiagnosis, McDonough et al. evaluated a dot enzyme immunoassay using nitrocellulose strips to which had been added a *M. tuberculosis* antigen of 30,000 dalton molecular weight.[21] This method was compared using an ELISA procedure for measuring IgG antibody. The dot assay results were less satisfactory than the ELISA, but it was suggested that this simple technique might be useful as a screening test in areas with limited technical support.

A study of the role of ELISA serodiagnosis of extrapulmonary tuberculosis was reported by Wilkins and Ivanyi, who evaluated 64 patients with involvement of lymph nodes in 31, pleura and/or pericardium in 14, bones and joints in 10, meninges in 4, genitourinary tract in 3, soft tissue in 3, gastrointestinal tract in 2, and skin disease in 2.[22] Ten patients had disease in multiple extrapulmonary sites. Antibodies were detected in 73% of these patients and in 5% of uninfected controls. Mathai and coworkers studied the cerebrospinal fluid of patients having suspected tuberculous meningitis using a dot immunoassay to detect antibody to antigen 5 among 40 such patients.[23] The specificity of this assay was 100% and this technology is simpler than ELISA.

The value of ELISA serodiagnosis for tuberculosis patients who also have AIDS has not been studied extensively. Theuer et al., as well as Eriki and coworkers in a separate report, have observed that similar levels of IgG antibody to purified protein derivative were present in tuberculosis patients with and without AIDS.[24,25] Subsequently, Daniel reviewed more complete studies from his laboratory and found that approximately 10% of patients with AIDS and tuberculosis in Uganda demonstrated antibody detectable by the ELISA method.[26]

Thus, there is a large body of literature regarding ELISA serodiagnosis of tuberculosis and a comprehensive review has been published by Daniel and Debonne.[16] ELISA is well suited for use in developing countries where tuberculosis is common, and it gives information comparable to that of a direct sputum smear, and may be very useful for those patients from whom a sputum sample cannot be obtained and for patients with extrapulmonary tuberculosis. A major drawback has been the instability of antigen 5; thus, more stable antigens are being evaluated. It is not clear which of the many variations of the serodiagnostic tests will prove to be the best.

B. Immunoassays for Mycobacterial Antigens

The detection of mycobacterial antigens in clinical specimens to provide a laboratory diagnosis of tuberculosis has been reported by several groups of investigators, many of whom concentrated on its value in tuberculous meningitis. Sada et al. were the first to use ELISA for the detection of *M. tuberculosis* antigen in cerebrospinal fluid. Since this report, a number of assay techniques for this purpose have been reported using competitive inhibition ELISA, latex agglutination, hemagglutination, and double-antibody sandwich ELISA.[27,28] Radhakrishnan and Mathai studied cerebrospinal fluid from 40 patients with a clinical diagnosis of tuberculous meningitis using an inhibition ELISA technique to detect the presence of antigen 5.[29] Antigen 5 was detected in all 10 culture-positive specimens; it was detected in 21 of 30 culture-negative specimens; it was detected in none of the 40 control specimens. Krambovitis and coworkers assayed sera from patients with pulmonary and extrapulmonary tuberculosis for plasma membrane antigens and reported 45% sensitivity.[30] Wadee et al. detected *M. tuberculosis* antigens by a sandwich assay using two purified *M. tuberculosis* antibodies.[31] They studied 63 cerebrospinal fluid specimens from patients with tuberculous meningitis. A total of 253 cerebrospinal fluids specimens were studied and there were 4.3% false-positives, but no false-negatives. Radhakrishnan and Mathai developed an assay for detection of antigen 5 using an inhibition ELISA and found 85% sensitivity and 100% specificity.[32] A preliminary report by Sada et al. described the measure of LAM in the serum of patients who had tuberculosis with and without AIDS.[33] The test in persons with tuberculosis alone was 90% sensitive, with both diseases was it 85% sensitive, and overall, the test was 93% specific.

Thus, the detection of mycobacterial antigens in cerebrospinal fluid may prove to be a significant laboratory advance for the diagnosis of tuberculous meningitis, especially in countries where this diagnosis is relatively common. Its value for the study of chronic meningitis in countries where tuberculous meningitis is rare has not been sufficiently studied.

More recently several purified antigens have been prepared, which have improved the ELISA test characteristics, giving 95% specificity and 83 to 95% sensitivity in smear-positive pulmonary tuberculosis.[34] However, ELISA testing sensitivity remains below clinical usefulness for smear-negative pulmonary tuberculosis and this is especially true among patients infected by HIV.[35,36]

III. NUCLEIC ACID PROBES

DNA is composed of four repeating nucleotides: adenine, guanine, cytosine, and thymine that are joined together in a coiled, double helix, i.e., double-stranded DNA (dsDNA). The two strands are held together by hydrogen bonds that can be broken by heat or high pH. Single strands of DNA (ssDNA) are very stable and upon removal of the heat source or correction of the pH, the DNA molecule will reform (reanneal) into the double-stranded configuration. When the ssDNA molecules are from different sources, the reannealing is called hybridization. Reannealing comes about because the hydrogen bonds reform only with specific complementary bases; adenine pairs only with thymine and cytosine only with guanine. It is the same for RNA except uracil replaces thymine and pairs only with adenine. The stability of hybridization depends on the nucleotide sequence of both strands; a perfect match in the sequence of nucleotides produces a very stable dsDNA, but if there are mismatches there will be increasing instability of the molecule that leads to progressive weakening of the hybridization.

A nucleic acid probe usually is a short sequence of nucleotide bases that will bind or hybridize to highly specific regions of a target sequence of nucleotides. To develop a specific probe, a sequence of nucleotides must be found that is highly specific for the organism in question, then the probe must be reproduced in large quantity and tagged with a label that can be detected. An ideal probe usually consists of a short piece of single stranded nucleic acid composed of 15 to 30 nucleotides. It can be composed of either DNA or RNA, but DNA probes are more common. For statistical uniqueness, a minimum of 20 nucleotides are needed for a probe. Short probes hybridize at very high rates (in minutes), whereas long probes may require hours to achieve stable hybridization. Longer probes are more specific and hybridize at higher temperatures. The base sequence of the probe, and the conditions under which the probe is used, determine its specificity. It is not necessary to know the function of the target nucleic acid before a probe can be used. The only requirements are that the probe hybridize specifically to the target nucleic acids and that the target nucleic acids be unique to the cell or organism in question.

Most probes are labeled so that they can be detected after they hybridize. Isotopes such as ^{32}P, ^{35}S, and ^{125}I can be incorporated into the structure of the molecule. Enzymes such as alkaline phosphatase can be covalently linked to the probe or biotin can be incorporated into the probe and then the biotin can be detected by enzyme-labeled avidin molecules. Probes can be designed to detect genera, species, or even strains of various organisms. Targets in RNA are used because there are so many more copies per cell of RNA than DNA; this increases sensitivity of detection. Ribosomal RNA is the most useful target in a screening assay. The 16S and 23S ribosomal units are very useful for detecting taxonomic groups because these genes are highly conserved. There may be 10,000 ribosomes per cell compared with only a few or one copy of a DNA target per cell. Plasmid DNA (i.e., extrachromosomal circular DNA) may serve as a target for some organisms, but plasmids may not be present in many strains and for *M. tuberculosis,* naturally occurring plasmids have never been described.

DNA and RNA probes have proved very useful in detecting mycobacteria in a specimen if the number of organisms present is large. Two probe systems are available commercially. The Gen-Probe system (Gen-Probe, San Diego, CA) uses a labeled DNA probe complementary to the ribosomal RNA in *M. tuberculosis.* Another available probe is designated SNAP (Syngene, San Diego, CA) and it utilizes a probe labeled with alkaline phosphatase that is directed against ribosomal RNA. These probes are used after the specimen to be tested has been processed and cultured long enough for the organism to have multiplied to a large number, perhaps 10^5 organisms per sample. The probe can be used to identify organisms in a liquid or solid medium and are 99 to 100% specific.[37-40]

Another probe developed by Gen-Probe is labeled with an acridinium ester and this allows target detection using chemiluminescence. Experience indicates that this probe also is highly specific.[41] This assay is nonradioactive, rapid, and simple. Probes are also available for *M. avium, M. intracellulare, M. avium* complex, *M. gordonae,* and *M. kansasii.*[42] When probes are combined with the BACTEC system, two thirds of clinical specimens can be processed and the mycobacteria can be detected and identified as species within 2 weeks of inoculation. With this system, if the number of organisms present in the initial test sample is small, sensitivity may suffer if the probe is used after only 2 weeks incubation. This deficiency can be overcome by allowing the broth culture to reach a higher growth index before probe testing.[43]

Thus, probes are used widely in the clinical mycobacteriology laboratory to speciate mycobacteria that have been grown in large number, either in broth or on a solid medium. These probes are highly specific, but are not sensitive. The probes do not help in detecting drug resistance, but this may be possible in the future. The probes serve as a substitute for biochemical testing to identify mycobacterial species and are more accurate than biochemical methods.

IV. PHAGE TYPING FOR *M. TUBERCULOSIS*

The first phages lytic for mycobacteria were reported by Gardner and Weiser in 1947, and their report was followed by studies done by Hratko, who used a number of phages isolated from soil to type a variety of strains of rapidly growing mycobacteria.[44,45] These phages failed to infect *M. tuberculosis* or *M. bovis* and it was not until Froman et al. reported the isolation of phages D28, D29, D32, and D34 in 1954 that there were any known phages that were lytic for virulent mycobacteria.[46] They tested a large number of strains of tubercle bacilli with various phages and no clear pattern of phage susceptibility was found. Although their work suggested that some phages might be useful for identifying mycobacterial species, their technique of spotting large concentrations of phage particles onto the bacterial lawn resulted in nonspecific lysis or lysis from without. This form of lysis is highly nonspecific since the disruption of the bacterial cell wall is a result of many phages attaching to the cell wall causing cell lysis without any phage DNA penetrating the cell wall and inserting into the bacterial chromosome. Thus, there would be no phage replication. It was only after the adoption of a "routine test dilution," as proposed by Ward and Redmond, that true phage infection of *M. tuberculosis* could be detected using a spotting technique on a bacterial lawn.[47] With this technique, reproducible results were obtained and low concentrations of phage particles were shown to infect and lyse certain highly susceptible strains.

Redmond and Cater were the first to use phages isolated from soil to differeniate strains of *M. tuberculosis* and *M. bovis* from other virulent and avirulent mycobacteria with great accuracy.[48] Very significant results were obtained with phages designated DS6A and GS4E. Phage DS6A, isolated from soil, was specific for *M. tuberculosis* and *M. bovis* and would lyse no other species. Phage GS4E would lyse *M. tuberculosis* but not *M. bovis.* This work was confirmed by Murohashi et al., who studied 163 strains of *M. tuberculosis* and found all to be sensitive to phage DS6A, but noted some differences in sensitivity to phage GS4E.[49]

The first report of subdividing the species *M. tuberculosis* by phage typing was published by Bates and Fitzhugh in 1967.[50] Using 14 phages, 92 strains of *M. tuberculosis* were subdivided into three types on the basis of sensitivity to phages DS6A, BG1, GS4E, and D34. Type A strains (76%) were sensitive to DS6A only; type B strains (14%) were sensitive to DS6A, BG1, and GS4E; and type C strains (10%) were sensitive to all four phages. This nomenclature was the first system adopted for phage typing mycobacteria. No correlation was found between phage type and either the geographic location of the patient or the drug sensitivity of the strains.

Later additional studies of tubercle bacilli isolated from Europe, Africa, and Asia were reported by Bates and Mitchison.[51] A study of 255 pretreatment isolates showed that a number of strains did not give uniform results and could not be classified as type A or B, and striking differences in geographic distribution by phage type were noted. In Hong Kong, type A predominated, while in Great Britain many of the strains were type B. The strains that could not be uniformly designated type A or B were all from southern India. A number of patients were observed to relapse after treatment and the pretreatment phage type was the same as the posttreatment phage type and there was no correlation between phage type and drug sensitivity.

These studies and others laid the groundwork for the development of a reliable phage typing scheme for *M. tuberculosis.* An international working group was formed by the World Health Organization (WHO) to standardize procedures and nomenclature. This formed the foundation for the methods in general use today.[52] The phages were designated mycobacterial typing phage human (MTPH) and numbered 1 to 14. With this system most strains of *M. tuberculosis* can be reliably subdivided into phage types, although there is some variability inherent in the system. It is clear that phage type is a constant feature of the strain and does not change while the strain replicates in the host or after extensive subculturing in the laboratory. A detailed description of the technique for phage typing of *M. tuberculosis* has been published by Crawford and Bates.[53]

After the standard methods were confirmed, phage typing was carried out by the Centers for Disease Control and Prevention, U.S. Public Health Service as a service to individuals and organizations, and for its own use to study the epidemiology of selected tuberculosis outbreaks. Phage typing was used to evaluate whether or not clusters of cases of tuberculosis were epidemiologically related and it was used as an aid to study the transmission of tubercle bacilli within a closed population unit such as a hospital or prison. The data obtained by phage typing are useful, but there are marked limitations. Since such a large percentage of all strains are included within a few phage types, the sensitivity of the test is markedly limited. Thus, when two or more subjects are infected with the same phage type, it could be explained by chance alone or by direct transmission of the same phage type from subject A to subject B. The phage typing data are of greater use when the phage types of isolates from a small epidemic are not all the same. Such information will indicate that the outbreak is not due to a single source nor due to a single strain passing progressively through a susceptible population group.

Phage typing has not been adopted for routine use in service laboratories because of its expense and technical difficulty. It has never been used for laboratory identification of unknown mycobacterial species, although this is a theoretical possibility. Again, the expense and technical difficulty preclude such use. In recent years phage typing for epidemiological purposes has been replaced in many laboratories by a much more sensitive technique: restriction fragment length polymorphism.

V. MYCOBACTERIOPHAGES FOR DIAGNOSTIC STUDIES

Since mycobacteriophages may be highly specific and infect only a single species, such as *M. tuberculosis,* this specificity has been used to diagnose mycobacterial infections. Through the development of luciferace reporter phages (LRP), an inexpensive and rapid test is being evaluated in research settings.[54,55] The firefly luciferace gene is introduced into the genome of a mycobacteriophage specific for *M. tuberculosis.* When this altered phage comes into contact with *M. tuberculosis,* infection of the bacterium results and then the infected bacterium begins to produce luciferace. The product of this enzyme is a photon, which can be detected using a luminometer or photographic film. Thus, light production indicates the presence of the tubercle bacillus, confirming the diagnosis. The same technology also should be useful for rapid determination of drug sensitivity. This methodology is not yet ready for routine use, but may well be in the next few years.

VI. GENOTYPING OF *M. TUBERCULOSIS*

The use of laboratory techniques to support studies of the epidemiology of tuberculosis have been few because of the limited ability of the laboratory to differentiate among specific strains of *M. tuberculosis.* In times past, investigators were forced to depend upon comparisons of drug resistance patterns and later upon phage typing data. These methods provided only limited assistance since most strains have shown identical drug susceptibility patterns and only a few phage types were known — thus, most strains showed the same phage type. This meant that there were no highly specific laboratory tools available to aid the epidemiologist to study the movement of strains of *M. tuberculosis* through a community or other defined host group.

This deficiency was solved with the advent of a more sophisticated technique employing restriction fragment-length polymorphism (RFLP) that detects genotypic variations among members of the species *M. tuberculosis.* These studies have shown that genotyping can be used to obtain a "fingerprint" for each isolate of *M. tuberculosis.* Thus far, it appears that most tubercle bacilli show a unique fingerprint clearly different from other isolates. The exception to this rule is most commonly found when isolates are obtained from persons infected by a common source or where persons are evaluated who have experienced the spread of a particular strain from person to person in a small epidemic. However, some patients harbor isolates having the same genotype where no epidemiological links can be found. The explanation for this finding remains undetermined. Thus, the epidemiologist now has a sensitive laboratory test to aid in the study of the epidemiology of tuberculosis.

The most common fingerprinting process depends on the insertion sequence IS6110, present in the genome of all *M. tuberculosis* and *M. bovis* strains. As a general rule, strains of *M. tuberculosis* contain multiple copies of IS6110, while strains of *M. bovis* contain only a few, although there are a few exceptions.[56,57] This DNA fragment moves about within the chromosome in an almost random manner, but movement is an infrequent event. For each unrelated wild isolate, copies of IS6110 vary in number and location within the chromosome. A restriction enzyme is used which cleaves multiple areas of the chromosome, but cleaves IS6110 at a single site only. Thus, it is possible to obtain DNA fragments of varying length with which a specific probe, representing a partial sequence of IS6110, will hybridize. The number of fragments produced that will react with the probe will depend upon the number of copies of IS6110 in the chromosome. The fingerprint is produced by gel electrophoresis of the digested DNA which is then transferred to a nylon membrane where the fragments are hybridized with an IS6110-labeled probe. The banding pattern of the DNA fragments of specific sizes constitutes a "fingerprint" unique to each strain.

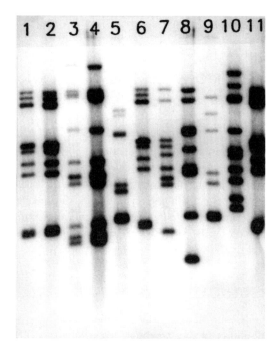

FIGURE 5.1 Shown above are 11 DNA fingerprints of *M. tuberculosis* isolated from 10 different HIV-positive patients. Note that the fingerprints in lanes 1, 2, 6, and 11 are identical although each of these strains was isolated from a different patient. The identity of the fingerprint suggests epidemiologic relatedness. The isolates in lanes 3 and 4 came from the same patient, and are identical as expected. The fingerprints in the other lanes are unique, each representing an isolate from a different patient, each with a distinct fingerprint pattern. (From Friedman, L. N., Ed., *Tuberculosis: Current Concepts and Treatment,* 1st ed., CRC Press LLC, Boca Raton, FL, 1994. With permission.)

The IS6110 fingerprinting method has been a very useful tool to study tuberculosis outbreaks. It has been used to study transmission within households, communities, and hospitals.[58-63] Data from these outbreaks (Figure 5.1) have shown that epidemiologically related groups share organisms having identical or nearly identical fingerprints, while unrelated isolates have totally different patterns. These outbreaks have demonstrated person-to-person spread that would never have been suspected based on the epidemiological data alone. In some cases the fingerprinting demonstrated that the outbreak had spread to adjacent communities even though the traditional methods of outbreak analysis had failed to reveal any links between the two communities.

Both animal models and *in vitro* studies demonstrate that the fingerprint pattern is very stable; remaining unchanged after passage of *M. tuberculosis* strains through a guinea pig for 2 months and after passage in cultured macrophages for 4 weeks.[59-64] The fingerprint of BCG strains grown in broth cultures for 6 months remain unchanged. Differences in the fingerprint may be limited to only a few bands. That is, the majority of the bands are identical except for one or two, which differ in size. The fingerprint of two different cultures of the standard laboratory strain of *M. tuberculosis* designated H37Rv differ in the size of a single band.

Genotypes from around the world can be compared as a result of the use of a standardized protocol for genotyping.[65] Additonal markers for gentotyping have been made available since the analysis of the genome sequence of *M. tuberculosis* was published. This work reveals a panel of 32 different insertion sequences, which will be candidates for genetic analysis. Another approach for genetic analysis is the use of DNA microarrays, consisting of thousands of individual gene sequences arranged on a glass microscope slide. *M. tuberculosis* is predicted to have 3924 genes and all could be arrayed on a single slide and comparisons made among different isolates.

M. tuberculosis strains having five or fewer copies of IS6110 cannot be separated with accuracy using this marker alone; thus, secondary genotyping methods are being developed. These methods are able to subdivide strains that appear to be clonal when grouped according to their IS6110 fingerprint.[66]

Currently, fingerprinting *M. tuberculosis* strains require a pure culture of the organism for DNA extraction. This delays the laboratory work and reporting of fingerprints for up to 6 months. For epidemiological use in tuberculosis control, a rapid determination of genotype is highly desirable since contact evaluation should begin very soon after a source case is diagnosed. If suspected secondary cases are discovered, knowledge of the genotype of each isolate in question will markedly strengthen the understanding of the epidemiological links. Thus a more rapid and accurate method for determining the genotype is needed and a promising method termed "spoligotyping" is being evaluated.[67] This technique enables the presence or absence of 43 segments of DNA, each having an identical nucleic acid sequence, to be detected by polymerase chain reaction technology. The results separate out isolates of *M. tuberculosis* having few copies of IS6110 that appear to be clonal. This methodology has great promise, but is not ready for routine use.

VII. POLYMERASE CHAIN REACTION

Since its introduction in 1985, the polymerase chain reaction (PCR) has transformed the way DNA analysis is performed.[68] This process involves the *in vitro* synthesis of millions of copies of a specific DNA segment and is based on the annealing and extension of two oligonucleotide primers that flank the target area in the DNA. First, the DNA is denatured and then each primer hybridizes to one of the two separated strands so that extension from each 3′ hydroxyl end is directed toward the other. The annealed primers are extended on the template strand with a DNA polymerase. These three steps (denaturation, primer binding, and DNA synthesis) represent a single PCR cycle. Repeated cycles of denaturation, primer annealing, and extension produce an exponential accumulation of a discrete fragment (target). PCR can amplify single or double-stranded DNA, and RNA can serve as a target if reverse transcription is used to make a DNA copy. This technology permits amplification of a highly specific DNA segment into millions or billions of copies in only a few hours. Thus, when once it would have been almost impossible to find a single DNA segment in a sample, PCR permits the amplification of this DNA to such a quantity that it can be detected by simple laboratory means. This technology has made possible new methods for the diagnosis of many infectious diseases, including tuberculosis.

In order to use PCR for detecting *M. tuberculosis* in clinical samples, it first was necessary to identify and characterize a DNA segment within the *M. tuberculosis* chromosome specific and unique for this organism. Hance et al. reported the detection of mycobacteria by PCR using a segment of DNA that codes for the 65-kDa antigen (the gro EL heat shock protein) as the target. However this DNA segment is present in all mycobacterial species and is not specific for *M. tuberculosis*.[69] Also, PCR using this target technique has not been shown to be sensitive enough for use in clinical samples and it is unlikely to be adopted for widespread clinical use. Manjunath identified a target segment of DNA specific for *M. tuberculosis,* and additional PCR methods for the diagnosis of tuberculosis have been reported by Pao et al., by Shanker et al., by Sjobring et al., and by Plikaytis et al.[70-74] Boddinghaus and colleagues have used the 16S ribosomal gene as a PCR target, a segment that is conserved in all mycobacterial species. This target offers the advantage of a high copy number of rRNA sequences, but despite this apparent advantage, the reported sensitivity is no higher than that obtained with single-target DNA sequences.[75]

The most attractive target specific for *M. tuberculosis* and *M. bovis* is that described by Eisenach et al.[76] The target sequence is repeated within the *M. tuberculosis* chromosome up to 20 or more times and each individual copy can be amplified using the same primers. This duplication increases the sensitivity by a factor of up to 20 or more compared to those methods that utilize a chromosomal target that occurs only once per chromosome. The target sequence is part of a larger repeated

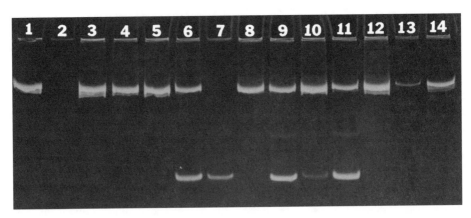

FIGURE 5.2   Shown above are examples of electrophoretic separation of mycobacterial DNA (amplified by PCR) from clinical sputum samples. Control DNA that produces a 600-base pair PCR product with the same set of primers is included in each test as an internal control. Lanes 1, 3, 4, 5, 8, 12, 13, and 14 show samples from patients without tuberculosis. Lanes 6, 7, 9, 10, and 11 show samples from patients with tuberculosis. The sample fragment migrating more rapidly is the specific amplified target (123 base pairs). The larger fragment, migrating more slowly, is the internal control. Note that lane 2 shows no amplification of control DNA, meaning that the reaction was inhibited and the test on this sample must be repeated. Note that in lane 7 the control DNA did not amplify, but the tuberculosis specific fragment is amplified. This is because the specific tuberculosis segment combined with all of the available primers so that no primer was available for annealing with the control DNA. (From Friedman, L. N., Ed., *Tuberculosis: Current Concepts and Treatment,* 1st ed., CRC Press LLC, Boca Raton, FL, 1994. With permission.)

segment that most probably is an insertion sequence that has been designated IS6110.[77] An example of a PCR analysis of several clinical sputum samples is shown in Figure 5.2.

In a clinical trial of 314 sputum samples, 93% of the patients with tuberculosis were PCR positive.[78] Among the 104 PCR positive patients, 83 were smear and culture positive, 2 were smear negative and culture positive, 16 were smear positive and culture negative, and 4 were smear and culture negative. Four patients who had completed or partially completed chemotherapy had PCR positive specimens. Of the 136 specimens obtained from patients who did not have tuberculosis (72 had nontuberculous mycobacterial infection and 64 had no known mycobacterial infection), there were 4 specimens found to be PCR positive. This study demonstrated the utility of the IS6110 PCR assay and it is expected that this assay will be adapted for use to detect *M. tuberculosis* in clinical samples of cerebrospinal fluid, pleural fluid, blood, and tissue. This test will detect low numbers of organisms in a sample, perhaps as few as 10 under ideal circumstances, and it will detect nonviable organisms as well.

Both RNA and DNA amplification systems are commercially available.[79,80] The PCR technique can be performed on sputum, spinal fluid, urine, blood, pleural fluid, and on formalin-fixed paraffin-embedded tissues. Using a clinical diagnosis as the gold standard for tuberculosis diagnosis, the sensitivity of the PCR test is approximately 81% compared to AFB smear analysis (28%) and culture (63%). When a clinical specimen is AFB-smear positive, the sensitivity of the amplification method is approximately 95% with a sensitivity of 98%.[81-83] When smear-negative specimens are examined, the sensitivity falls to approximately 50%, but the specificity remains greater than 95%. For this reason, these tests are recommended for smear-positive specimens only, but their use in this regard is changing rapidly and varies from site to site. Clearly, these methods have not replaced routine smear and culture.

Automated strand displacement amplification (SDA) is a new technology that replicates DNA at a constant temperature and, therefore, does not require a thermostable polymerase as is required for PCR replication.[84] Since each step of the reaction occurs at a single temperature, the SDA process is fast and inexpensive because temperature control blocks are not needed. This technique can detect as few as 10 organisms in a specimen and can give a 10^{10}-fold amplification of the target nucleic acid in 15 min. This methodology should be commercially available this year.

The problems with nucleic amplification methods for the diagnosis of tuberculosis include the risk of obtaining false-positive results due to contamination of clinical specimens with *M. tuberculosis* DNA product from the laboratory, the inability of the method to detect a difference between viable and nonviable organisms, and the inability of the PCR method to determine drug susceptibility. In the future it should be possible to use nucleic amplification methodology to detect drug susceptibility as the genes responsible for drug resistance are described.

VIII. HIGH PERFORMANCE LIQUID CHROMOTOGRAPHY

High performance liquid chromatography (HPLC) can detect unique mycolic acids, which are components of the cell wall of all mycobacteria.[85] Instead of using a large number of biochemical tests to reliably identify the many different species of mycobacteria, HPLC can detect unique mycolic acid patterns which are characteristic for each species. This test can be performed in only a few hours. Disadvantages include the fact that the organism to be tested must be in pure culture and the initial cost for purchase of the equipment is high. HPLC cannot separate *M. tuberculosis* from *M. bovis*.

IX. TUBERCULOSTEARIC ACID

Tuberculostearic acid (TBSA) is a structural component found in all mycobacterial species and in other members of the Actinomycetales such as diptheroids, actinomyces, and nocardia, but not in normal human tissues.[86] It is reasoned that detection of TBSA in body fluids such as sputum, gastric aspirates, urine, cerebrospinal fluid, pleural fluid, ascitic fluid, and tissue extracts indicates the likely presence of *M. tuberculosis*. A number of studies to evaluate the value of TBSA detection in clinical samples have been reported with mixed results. The expensive technology required and the highly developed skills required of the laboratory worker have limited the availability of testing to a few research laboratories only.

Frequency-pulsed electron-capture gas-liquid chromatography has been used to detect femtomole quantities of TBSA in samples.[87,88] In some situations it would seem possible to diagnose tuberculous meningitis within 3 h. In a study of 40 patients suspected of having active pulmonary tuberculosis, who could not produce sputum or whose sputum smears were negative for acid-fast bacilli, 29 were found to have tuberculosis and 23 of these showed positive TBSA tests; there were 2 false positives.[89] Brooks et al. studied clinical cases of tuberculous meningitis with gas-liquid chromatography and reported the specificity to be 91% and the sensitivity to be 95%.[90]

At present this technology should be used to evaluate the cerebrospinal fluid of patients who are suspected of having tuberculous meningitis. The fluid can be sent to the Centers for Disease Control where this test is available. Its use to diagnose tuberculosis at other sites is of less value, particularly for pulmonary disease where other mycobacteria may be found as saprophytes or as pathogens and where other actinomycetes may be present as part of the "normal flora." In all these instances one would encounter false positives.

X. ADENOSINE DEAMINASE

Adenosine deaminase (ADA) catalyzes the conversion of adenosine to inosine and is released by lymphocytes and macrophages during the cellular immune response. Increased ADA levels have been used to aid in the diagnosis of tuberculous pleural effusions, but this enzyme also is found in inflammatory fluids associated with rheumatoid arthritis, lymphoma, empyema, parapneumonic effusions, and mesothelioma.[91-94] Banales et al. studied 218 consecutive patients with exudative pleural effusions hospitalized in Mexico City.[95] In this population with a relatively high prevalence of tuberculosis, the ADA analysis was a very useful marker for tuberculosis since the determination can be made quickly and at low cost. There were 2.7% false-positive reports for patients who had cancer with pleural effusions and there was one patient with tuberculosis that had a false-negative ADA value. They reviewed results from 10 other studies, combined these reports with their own, and found a sensitivity of 99% and a specificity of 89% for the diagnosis of tuberculosis.

Additional studies have evaluated ADA levels in tuberculous peritonitis and tuberculous meningitis. In those areas where tuberculosis is very prevalent, the test may be useful. Voigt et al., working in Cape Town, South Africa, studied 41 patients with microbiologically confirmed tuberculous peritonitis together with 41 control patients having ascites from other causes such as cirrhosis, tumor, and pancreatitis.[96] They found a sensitivity of 95% and a specificity of 98% in distinguishing between the two groups. However, in geographic regions where exudative reactions of serosal surfaces often are not due to tuberculosis, the false-positive rate of elevated ADA levels in these fluids is too frequent for the test to be applied broadly.[97]

REFERENCES

1. Arloing, S., Agglutination de becille de la tuberculose vraie, *Comptes Rendues de L'Academic de Sciences*, 136, 1398, 1898.
2. Engvall, E. and Perlmann, P., Enzyme-linked immunsorbent assay, ELISA III. Quantation of specific antibodies by enzyme-labeled anti-immunoglobulin in antigen-coated tubes, *J. Immunol.*, 109, 129, 1972.
3. Young, D. B., Kaufmann, S. H. E., Hermans, P. W. M., and Thole, J. E. R., Mycobacterial protein antigens: a compilation, *Mol. Microbiol.*, 6, 133, 1992.
4. Daniel, T. M. and Janicki, B. W., Mycobacterial antigens: a review of their isolation, chemistry and immunological properties, *Microbiol. Rev.*, 42, 84, 1978.
5. Nassau, E., Parsons, E. R., and Johnson, G. D., The detection of antibodies to *Mycobacterium tuberculosis* by microplate enzyme-linked immunosorbent assay (ELISA). *Tubercle*, 57, 67, 1976.
6. Grange, J. M. and Kardijito, T., Serological tests for tuberculosis: can the problem of low specificity be overcome? *Indian J. Chest Dis.*, 24, 108, 1982.
7. Kalish, S. B., Radin, R. C., Phair, J.P ., Levitz, D., Zeiss, C. R., and Metzger, E., Use of an enzyme-linked immunosorbent assay technique in the differential diagnosis of active pulmonary tuberculosis in humans, *J. Infect. Dis.*, 147, 523, 1983.
8. Daniel, T. M., Debanne, S. M., and van der Kuyp, F., Enzyme-linked immunosorbent assay using *Mycobacterium tuberculosis* antigen 5 and PPD for the serodiagnosis of tuberculosis, *Chest*, 88, 388, 1985.
9. Benjamin, R. G., Debanne, S. M., Ma, Y., and Daniel, T. M., Evaluation of mycobacterial antigens in an enzyme-linked immunosorbent assay (ELISA) for the serodiagnosis of tuberculosis, *J. Med. Microbiol.*, 18, 309, 1984.
10. Balestrino, E. A., Daniel, T. M., de Latini, M. D. S., Latini, O. A., Ma, Y., and Scocozza, J. B., Serodiagnosis of pulmonary tuberculosis in Argentina by enzyme-linked immunosorbent assay (ELISA) of IgG antibody to *Mycobacterium tuberculosis* antigen 5 and tuberculin purified protein derivative, *Bull. WHO*, 62, 755, 1984.
11. Daniel, T. M. and Anderson, P. A., The isolation by immunosorbent affinity chromatography and physiochemical characterization of *Mycobacterium tuberculosis* antigen 5, *Am. Rev. Resp. Dis.*, 117, 533, 1978.
12. Benjamin, R. G. and Daniel, T. M., Serodiagnosis of tuberculosis using the enzyme-linked immunosorbent assay (ELISA) of antibody to *Mycobacterium tuberculosis* antigen 5, *Am. Rev. Resp. Dis.*, 126, 1013, 1982.
13. Lau, J. H. K., Long, J. C. Y., and Stroebel, A. B., A longitudinal study of antibody titers to antigen 6 in patients with bone and joint tuberculosis, *Int. Orthoped.*, 7, 205, 1983.
14. Kiran, U., Shriniwas, K. R., and Sharma, A., Efficacy of three mycobacterial antigens in the serodiagnosis of tuberculosis, *Eur. J. Resp. Dis.*, 66, 187, 1985.

15. Reggiardo, Z. and Vazquez, E., Comparison of enzyme-linked immunosorbent assay and hemogglu-tination test using mycobacterial glycolipids, *J. Clin. Microbiol.*, 13, 1007, 1981.

16. Daniel, T. M. and Debanne, S. M., The serodiagnosis of tuberculosis and other mycobacterial diseases by enzyme-linked in immunosorbent assay (ELISA), *Am. Rev. Resp. Dis.*, 135, 1137, 1987.

17. Hunter, S. W., Gaylord, H., and Brennan, P. J., Structure and antigenicity of the phosphorylated lipopolysaccharide antigens from the leprosy and tubercle bacilli, *J. Biol. Chem.*, 261, 12345, 1986.

18. Sada, E., Brennan, P. J., Herrera, T., and Torres, M., Evaluation of lipoarabinommana for the serological diagnosis of tuberculosis, *J. Clin. Microbiol.*, 28, 2587, 1990.

19. Sada, E., Aguilar, D., Torres, M., and Herrera, T., Detection of lipoarabinomannan as a diagnostic test for tuberculosis, *J. Clin. Microbiol.*, 30, 2415, 1992.

20. Charpin, D., Herbault, H., Gevaudan, M. J., Saadjian, M., De Micco, P., Arnaud, A., Vervloet, D., and Charpin, J., Value of ELISA using A60 antigen in the diagnosis of active pulmonary tuberculosis, *Am. Rev. Resp. Dis.*, 142, 380, 1990.

21. McDonough, J. A., Sada, E., Sippola, A. A., Ferguson, L. E., and Daniel, T. M., Microplate and dot immunoassays for the serodiagnosis of tuberculosis, *J. Lab. Clin. Med.*, 120, 318, 1992.

22. Wilkins, E. G. L. and Ivanyi, J., Potential value of serology for diagnosis of extrapulmonary tuber-culosis, *Lancet*, 336, 641, 1990.

23. Mathai, A., Radhakrishnan, V. V., and Thomas, M., Rapid diagnosis of tuberculous meningitis with a dot enzyme immunoassay to detect antibody in cerebrospinal fluid, *Eur. J. Clin. Microbiol. Infect. Dis.*, 10, 440, 1992.

24. Theuer, C. P., Chaisson, R. E., Elias, D., Schecter, G. L., Glassroth, J., Zeiss, C. R., Phair, J. P., and Hopewell, P. C., Detection of circulating antibodies to purified protein derivative in tuberculous patients with and without human immunodeficiency virus infection, *Am. Rev. Resp. Dis.*, 139 (Part 2), A395, 1987.

25. Eriki, P. P., Kataaha, P. K., and Daniel, T. M., The detection of IgG antibody to a 30,000 dalton antigen of *Mycobacterium tuberculosis* in the serum of HIV-positive and HIV-negative patients in Uganda, 4th Int. Conf. on AIDS and Associated Cancers in Africa, Marseilles, France, 1989.

26. Daniel, T. M., The rapid diagnosis of tuberculosis: a selective review, *J. Clin. Lab. Med.*, 116, 277, 1990.

27. Sada, E., Ruiz-Palacios, G. M., Lopez-Vidal, Y., and Ponce de Leon, S., Detection of mycobacterial antigens in the cerebrospinal fluid of patients with tuberculous meningitis by enzyme-linked immu-nosorbent assay (ELISA), *Lancet*, 2, 651, 1983.

28. Jacobs, R. F. and Eisenach, K. D., Childhood tuberculosis, *Ad. Ped. Infect. Dis.*, 8, 23, 1993.

29. Radhakrishnan, V. V. and Mathai, A., Detection of *Mycobacterium tuberculosis* antigen 5 in cere-brospinal fluid by inhibition ELISA and its diagnostic potential in tuberculous meningitis, *J. Inf. Dis.*, 163, 650, 1991.

30. Krambovitis, E., Harris, M., and Hughes, D. T. D., Improved serodiagnosis of tuberculosis using two assay test, *J. Clin. Pathol.*, 39, 779, 1986.

31. Wadee, A. A., Boting, L., and Reedy, S. G., Antigen capture assay for detection of a 43-kilodalton *Mycobacterium tuberculosis* antigen, *J. Clin. Microbiol.*, 28, 2786, 1990.

32. Radhakrishnan, V. V. and Mathai, A., Enzyme-linked immunosorbent assay to detect *Mycobacterium tuberculosis* antigen 5 and antimycobacterial antibody in cerebrospinal fluid of patients with tuber-culous meningitis, *J. Clin. Lab. Anal.*, 5, 233, 1991.

33. Sada, E., Anguilar, D., and Torres, M., Lipoarabinomannan antigenemia in patients with AIDS and tuberculosis. Presented at the 31st Interscience Conference on Antimicrobial Agents and Chemother-apy, Chicago, September 1991.

34. Schluger, M. W. and Ron, W. N., Current approaches to the dianosis of active pulmonary tuberculosis, *Am. J. Respir. Crit. Care Med.,* 149, 204, 1994.

35. Papa, F., Cruaud, P., Luquin, M., Thorel, M. F., Goh, K. S., and David, H. L., Isolation and charac-terization of serologically reactive lipooligosaccharides from *Mycobacterium tuberculosis*, *Res. Micro-biol.,* 144, 91, 1993.

36. Cavalcante, S., Kritski, A. L., Ferreira, A. S., Souza, M. A., Laszlo, A., Werneck-Barroso, E. B., and Fonseca, L. S., Associaton between an early humoral response to *Mycobacterium tuberculosis* antigens and later development of tuberculosis in human immunoldeficiency virus-infected individuals, *Int. J. Tuberc. Lung Dis.*, 1, 170, 1997.

37. Lim, S. D., Todd, J., Lopez, J., Ford, E., and Janda, J. M., Genotypic identification of pathogenic mycobacterium species by using a nonradioactive oligonucleotide probe, *J. Clin. Microbiol.*, 29, 1276, 1991.

38. Gonalez, R. and Hanna, B. A., Evaluation of Gen-Probe DNA hybridization systems for the identification of *Mycobacterium tuberculosis* and *Mycobacterium avium-intracellulare*, *Diagn. Microbiol. Infect. Dis.*, 8, 69, 1980.

39. Musial, C. E., Tice, L. S., Stockman, L., and Roberts, G. D., Identification of mycobacteria from culture by using the Gen-Probe rapid diagnostic system for *Mycobacterium avium* complex and *Mycobacterium tuberculosis* complex, *J. Clin. Microbiol.*, 26, 2120, 1988.

40. Sherman, I., Harrington, N., Rothrock, A., and George, H., Use of a cutoff range in identifying mycobacteria by the Gen-Probe rapid diagnostic system, *J. Clin. Microbiol.*, 27, 241, 1989.

41. Goto, M., Oka, S., Okuzumi, K., Kimura, S., and Shimada, K., Evaluation of acridinium-ester labeled DNA probes for identification of *Mycobacterium tuberculosis* and *Mycobacterium avium — Mycobacterium intracellulare* complex in culture, *J. Clin. Microbiol.*, 29, 2473, 1991.

42. Jacobs, R. E. and Eisenach, K. D., Childhood tuberculosis, *Ad. Ped. Infect. Dis.*, 8, 23, 1993.

43. Body, B., Warren, N. G., Spicer, A., Henderson, D., and Chery, M., Use of Gen-Probe and BACTEC for rapid isolation and identification of mycobacteria correlation of probe results with growth index, *Am. J. Clin. Pathol.*, 93, 415, 1990.

44. Gardner, G. M. and Weiser, R. S., A bacteriophage for Mycobacterium smegmates, *Proc. Soc. Exper. Biol. Med.*, 66, 205, 1947.

45. Hnatko, S. I., The isolation of bacteriophages for mycobacteria with reference to phage typing of the genus, *Can. J. Med. Sci.*, 31, 462, 1953.

46. Froman, S., Will, D. W., and Bogen, E., Bacteriophage active against virulent *Mycobacterium tuberculosis*, *Am. J. Public Health*, 44, 1326, 1954.

47. Ward, D. M. and Redmond, W. B., Spotting method of phage typing of mycobacteria, *Am. Rev. Resp. Dis.*, 85, 883, 1962.

48. Redmond, W. B. and Cater, J. D., A bacteriophage specific for *Mycobacterium tuberculosis*, varieties *hominis* and *bovis*, *Am. Rev. Resp. Dis.*, 82, 781, 1960.

49. Murohashi, T., Tokunago, T., Mizuguchi, Y., and Maruyama, Y., Phage typing of slow-growing mycobacteria, *Am. Rev. Resp. Dis.*, 88, 664, 1963.

50. Bates, J. H. and Fitzhugh, J. K., Subdivision of the species *M. tuberculosis* by mycobacteriophage typing, *Am. Rev. Resp. Dis.*, 96, 7, 1967.

51. Bates, J. H. and Mitchison, D. A., Geographic distribution of bacteriophage types of *Mycobacterium tuberculosis*, *Am. Rev. Resp. Dis.*, 100, 189, 1969.

52. Rado, T. A., Bates, J. H., Engel, H. W. B., Mankiewicz, E., Murohashi, T., Mizuguchi, Y., and Sula, L., World Health Organization studies on bacteriophage typing of mycobacteria. Subdivision of the species *Mycobacterium tuberculosis*, *Am. Rev. Resp. Dis.*, 111, 459, 1975.

53. Crawford, J. and Bates, J. H., Phage typing of mycobacteria, in *The Mycobacteria*, Part A, Kubica, G. and Wayne, L. G., Eds., Marcel Dekker Inc., New York, 1984, 123.

54. Jacobs, W. R., Barletta, R., Udani, R., Chan, J., Kalkut, G., Sarkis, G., Hatful, G. F., and Bloom, B. R., Rapid assessment of drug susceptibilities of *Mycobacterium tuberculosis* by means of luciferace reporter phages, *Science*, 260, 819, 1993.

55. Carriere, C., Riska, P. F., Zimhony, O., Kriakov, J., Bardarov, S., Bevins, J., Chan, J., and Jacobs, W. R., Conditionally replication luciferace reporter phages: improved sensitivity for rapid detection and assessment of drug susceptibility of *Mycobacterium tuberculosis*, *J. Clin. Microbiol.*, 35, 3232, 1997.

56. Cave, M. D., Eisenach, K. D., McDermott, P. F., Bates, J. H., and Crawford, J. T., IS6110: Conservation of sequence in the *Mycobacterium tuberculosis* complex and its utilization in DNA fingerprinting, *Mol. Cell Probes*, 5, 73, 1991.

57. van Soolingen, D., Hermans, P. W. M., Haas, P. E., Soll, D. R., and van Embden, J. D. A., Occurrence and stability of insertion sequences in *Mycobacterium tuberculosis* complex strains: evaluation of an insertion sequence-dependent DNA polymorphism as a tool in the epidemiology of tuberculosis, *J. Clin. Microbiol.*, 4, 2578, 1991.

58. Mazurek, G. H., Cave, M. D., Eisenach, K. D., Wallace, R. J., Bates, J. H., and Crawford, J. T., Chromosomal DNA fingerprint patterns produced with IS6110 as strain-specific markers for epidemiologic study of tuberculosis, *J. Clin. Microbiol.*, 29, 2030, 1991.

59. van Soolingen, D., Herman, P. W. M., Haas, P. E., Soll, D. R., and van Embden, J. D. A., Occurrence and stability of insertion sequence-dependent DNA polymorphism as a tool in the epidemiology of tuberculosis, *J. Clin. Microbiol.*, 4, 2578, 1991.

60. Daley, C. L., Small, P. M., Schechter, G. S., Schoolnik, G. K., McAdam, R. A., Jacobs, W. R., and Hopewell, P. C., An outbreak of tuberculosis with accelerated progression among persons infected with human immunodeficiency virus, *N. Eng. J. Med.*, 326, 231, 1992.

61. Pearson, M., Jereb, J. A., Frieden, T. R., Crawford, J. T., Davis, B. J., Dooley, S. W., and Jarvis, W. R., Nosocomial transmission of multidrug-resistant *Mycobacterium tuberculosis, Ann. Int. Med.*, 117, 191, 1992.

62. Edlin, B. R., Tokars, J. I., Grieco, M. H., Crawford, J. T., Williams, J., Sordillo, E. M., Ong, K. R., Kilburn, J. O., Dooley, S. W., Castro, K. G., Jarvis, W. R., and Holmberg, S. D., An outbreak of multidrug-resistant tuberculosis among hospitalized patients with acquired immunodeficiency syndrome, *N. Eng. J. Med.*, 326, 1514, 1992.

63. Beck-Sague, C., Dooley, S. W., Hutton, M. D., Otten, J., Bruden, A., Crawford, J. T., Pitchenik, A. E., Woodley, C., Cauthen, G., and Jarvis, W., Hospital outbreak of multidrug-resistant *Mycobacterium tuberculosis* infections, *JAMA*, 268, 1280, 1992.

64. Hermans, P. W. M., van Soolingen, D., Dale, J. W., Schuikema, A. R. J., McAdams, R. A., Catty, D., and van Embden, J. D. A., Insertion element IS986 from *Mycobacterium tuberculosis:* a useful tool for diagnosis and epidemiology of tuberculosis, *J. Clin. Microbiol.*, 28, 2051, 1990.

65. van Embden J., Cave M. D., Crawford, J. T., Dale, J. W., Eisenach, K. D., Gicquel, B., Herman, P., Martin, C., McAdam, R., Shinnick, T. M., and Small, P. M., Strain identification of *Mycobacterium tuberculosis* by DNA fingerprinting: recommendations for a standardization methodology, *J. Clin. Microbiol.*, 31, 406, 1993.

66. Chaves, F., Yang, Z. H., and El Hajj, H., Usefulness of secondary probe pTBN12 in DNA fingerprinting of *Mycobacterium tuberculosis, J. Clin. Microbiol.*, 34, 1118, 1996.

67. Kamerbeek, J. L., Schouls, M., Kolk, A., van Agterveld, M., and van Soolingen, D. L., Simultaneous detection and strain differentiation of *Mycobacterium tuberculosis* for diagnosis and epidemiology, *J. Clin. Microbiol.*, 35, 907, 1997.

68. Mullis, K. B. and Faloona, F., Specific synthesis of DNA *in vitro* via a polymerase catalyzed chain reaction, *Meth. Enzymol.*, 155, 335, 1987.

69. Hance, A. J., Grandchamp, B., Lavy-Frebault, V., Lecossier, D., Rauzier, J., Bocart, D., and Gicqual, B., Detection of mycobacteria by amplification of mycobacterial DNA, *Mol. Microbiol.*, 3, 843, 1989.

70. Manjunath, N., Evaluation of a polymerase chain reaction for the diagnosis of tuberculosis, *Tubercle*, 72, 21, 1991.

71. Pao, C. C., Yen, T. S. B., You, J. B., Maa, J. S., Fiss, E. H., and Chang, C. H., Detection and identification of *Mycobacterium tuberculosis* by DNA amplification, *J. Clin. Microbiol.*, 28, 1877, 1990.

72. Shankar, P., Manjunath, N., Lakshmi, R., Aditi, B., Seth, P., and Shriniwas, K., Identification of *Mycobacterium tuberculosis* by polymerase chain reaction, *Lancet*, 355, 423, 1990.

73. Sjobring, U., Mecklenburg, M., Anderson, A. B., and Miorner, M., Polymerase chain reaction for detection of *Mycobacterium tuberculosis*, *J. Clin. Microbiol.*, 28, 2200, 1990.

74. Plikaytis, B. B., Eisenach, K. D., Crawford, J. T., and Shinnick, T. M., Differentiation of *Mycobacterium tuberculosis* and *Mycobacterium bovis* by a polymerase chain reaction assay, *Mol. Cell Probes*, 5, 215, 1991.

75. Boddinghaus, B., Rogall, T., Flohr, T., Blocker, H., and Bottger, E. C., Detection and identification of mycobacteria by amplification of rRNA, *J. Clin. Microbiol.*, 28, 1751, 1990.

76. Eisenach, K. D., Cave, M. D., Bates, J. H., and Crawford, J. T., Polymerase chain reaction amplification of a repetitive DNA sequence specific for *Mycobacterium tuberculosis*, *J. Infect. Dis.*, 161, 977, 1990.

77. Thierry, D., Cave, M. D., Eisenach, K. D., Crawford, J. T., Bates, J. H., Gicqual, B., and Guesdon, T. L., IS6110 and IS-like element of *Mycobacterium tuberculosis* complex, *Nucl. Acids Res.*, 18, 188, 1990.

78. Eisenach, K. D., Sifford, M. D., Cave, M. D., Bates, J. H., and Crawford, J. T., Detection of *Mycobacterium tuberculosis* in sputum samples using a polymerase chain reaction, *Am. Rev. Resp. Dis.*, 144, 1160, 1991.

79. Centers for Disease Control and Prevention, Nucleic acid amplification tests for tuberculosis, *MMWR*, 45, 950, 1996.

80. Cohen, R., Muzaffar, S., Schwartz, D., Bashir, S., Luke, S., McGartland, L., and Kaul, K., Diagnosis of pulmonary tuberculosis using PCR assays on sputum collected within 24 hours of hospital admission, *Am. J. Respir. Crit. Care Med.,* 157, 156, 1998.

81. Catazaro, A., Davidson B. L., Fujiwara, P. I., Goldberger, M. J., Gordin, F., Salfinger, M., Sbabaro, J., Schluger, N. W., Sierro, M. F., and Woods, G. L., Rapid diagnosis tests for tuberculosis. What is the appropriate use? *Am. J. Respir. Crit. Care Med.,* 155, 1804, 1997.

82. Pfyffer, G. E., Diagnostic performance of amplified *Mycobacterium tuberculosis* direct test with cerebrospinal fluid, other nonrespiratory and respiratory specimens, *J. Clin. Microbiol.,* 34, 834, 1996.

83. Hellyer, T. J., Desjardin, L. E., Assaf, M. K., Eisenach, K., Cave, M. D., and Bates, J. H., Specificity of IS6110-based amplification assays for *Mycobacterium tuberculosis* complex, *J. Clin. Microbiol.,* 35, 799, 1997.

84. Spargo, C. A., Fraser, M. S., Van Cleve, M., Wright, D. J., Nycz, C. M., Spears, P. A., and Walker, G. T., Detection of *M. tuberculosis* DNA using thermophilic strand displacement amplification, *Mol. Cell Probes,* 10, 247, 1996.

85. Butler, W. R. and Kilburn, J. O., Identification of major slowly growing pathogenic mycobacteria and *Mycobacterium gordonae* by high performance liquid chromatography of their mycolic acids, *J. Clin. Microbiol.,* 26, 50, 1988.

86. Anderson, R. J. and Chargaff, E., The chemistry of the lipids of tubercle bacilli. VI. Concerning tuberculosteraric acid and phthioic acid from the acetone-soluble fat, *J. Biol. Chem.,* 85, 77, 1929.

87. Brooks, J. B., Craven, R. B., Schlossberg, D., Alley, C. C., and Pritts, F. M., Possible use of frequency-pulse-modulated electron capture gas-liquid etromalography to identify septic and aseptic causes of pleural effusions, *J. Clin. Microbiol.,* 8, 203, 1978.

88. Brooks, J. B., Daneshvar, M. I., Fast, D. M., and Good, R. C., Selective procedures for detecting femtomole quantities of tuberculostearic acid in serum and cerebrospinal fluid by frequency-pulsed electron-capture gas-liquid chromatography, *J. Clin. Microbiol.,* 25, 1201, 1987.

89. Pang, J. A., Chan, H. S., Chan, C. Y., Cheung, S. W., and French, G. L., A tuberculostearic acid assay in the diagnosis of sputum smear-negative pulmonary tuberculosis, *Ann. Int. Med.,* 111, 650, 1989.

90. Brooks, J. B., Daneshvar, M. I., Haberberger, R. L., and Mikhail, I. A., Rapid diagnosis of tuberculous meningitis by frequency-pulsed electron-capture gas-liquid chromatography detection of carboxylic acids in cerebrospinal fluid, *J. Clin. Microbiol.,* 28, 989, 1990.

91. Petterson, T., Osala, K., and Weber, T. H., Adenosine deaminase in the diagnosis of pleural effusions, *Acta. Med. Scand.,* 215, 299, 1984.

92. Ocana, I., Martinez-Vazquez, J. M., Segura, R. M., Fernandez de Sevilla, T., and Capdevila, J. A., Adenosine deaminase in pleural fluid: test for diagnosis of tuberculous pleural effusion, *Chest,* 84, 51, 1983.

93. Maritz, F. J., Malan, C., and le Roux, I., ADA estimations in the differentiation of pleural effusions, *S. Afr. Med. J.,* 62, 556, 1982.

94. Strankinga, W. F., Navta, J. J., Straub, J. P., and Stam, J., Adenosine deaminase activity in tuberculous pleural effusions: a diagnostic test, *Tubercle,* 68, 137, 1987.

95. Banales, J. L., Pineda, P. R., Fitzgerald, J. M., Rubio, H., Selman, M., and Salazar-Legama, M., Adenosine deaminase in the diagnosis of tuberculous pleural effusions, *Chest,* 99, 355, 1991.

96. Voigt, M. D., Kalvaria, I., Trey, C., Berman, P., Lombard, C., and Kirsch, R. E., Diagnostic value of ascites adenosine deaminase in tuberculous peritonitis, *Lancet,* 1, 751, 1989.

97. Van Keimpema, A. R., Sloats, E. H., and Wagenaar, J. P., Adenosine deaminase activity, not diagnostic for tuberculous pleurisy, *Eur. J. Respir. Dis.,* 71, 15, 1987.

6 Pulmonary Tuberculosis: Presentation, Diagnosis, and Treatment

Lloyd N. Friedman, M.D. and Peter A. Selwyn, M.D., M.P.H.

CONTENTS

I. PRIMARY PULMONARY TUBERCULOSIS

Historically, primary pulmonary tuberculosis has been a childhood infection (see Chapter 8). However, the frequency of infection has declined markedly, and many uninfected persons now are susceptible to infection. Myers et al. showed the prevalence of tuberculous infection in Minnesota schoolchildren to be 47.3% in 1926, 18.9% in 1936, and only 3.9% in 1954.[1] Although rates may be higher in other parts of the country, it would not be unusual today for an elderly person to be newly exposed to tuberculosis and to develop primary disease.

Although the majority of air is drawn into the lower lobes, it has been shown in autopsy studies by Ghon that the primary focus of tuberculosis is distributed equally between the upper and lower lobes, with a slight predilection for the right lung.[2] Palmer has stated that primary pulmonary tuberculosis is more common in the upper lobes.[3] On chest radiographic readings, Poulsen showed a predilection for disease in the mid-lung fields with an equal distribution of the remainder between upper and lower zones.[4] Segmental atelectasis was much more common in the upper lobes in studies by Frostad[5] and Weber et al.,[6] and similar but less pronounced differences were found by Daly.[7] In most studies, even the anterior segment of the upper lobes have a substantial number of primary complexes and atelectatic segments. Thus, an upper lobe infiltrate may represent either primary or reactivated disease.

Lymphadenopathy is common in primary tuberculosis and may exceed by far the size of the original parenchymal focus.[8] Lymphadenopathy plays a major role in the pathogenesis of atelectasis, sometimes referred to as epituberculosis,[2] and also plays a major role in the obstructive emphysema seen in children in as much as 34% of cases of primary tuberculosis.[5-7,9] The long-term sequelae of lymphadenopathy with airway involvement may be bronchostenosis, bronchiectasis, or both.

In an important study by Poulsen[4,10] of 517 Faroe Islanders, an attempt was made to document the initial time and subsequent sequelae of tuberculous infection. The Pirquet test, a scarification procedure utilizing old tuberculin, was used to document conversion. Although it is a less sensitive test than the Mantoux test, it is not clear whether this biased the findings once the group of convertors was assembled.

Initial fever was reported in 430 (83%) of the 517 known convertors. The temperature was as high as 40.5°C with more than 30% of persons having temperatures above 39.5°C. In many cases, the patients were completely unaware of the presence of fever. Although today, most patients with primary infection are thought to be asymptomatic, 117 (27%) of 430 persons in Poulsen's study with initial fever had subjective symptoms which most commonly included retrosternal and side pain, and rarely, cough, fatigue, sore throat, and joint pain. The retrosternal pain began with the onset of fever, lasted a week or two, and usually was exacerbated by swallowing. The duration of fever most commonly was 2 weeks, and was less than 6 weeks in more than 90% of persons.

Erythema nodosum occurred in 78 (15%) cases, predominantly on the shins of women and children, and appeared to coincide with the onset of delayed hypersensitivity. In five instances it involved the arms.

There were 139 (27%) of 517 convertors with parenchymal infiltrates consistent with primary tuberculosis, 44% of which were demonstrated in the first month after conversion. Hilar adenitis, more often right sided and often bilateral, occurred with or without infiltrates in 333 (64%) cases and was more common in children. The incidence of radiographic abnormalities was even higher, i.e., 86%, in persons studied during the initial fever.

Much of this study was similar to the work of Gedde-Dahl, who studied 272 tuberculin convertors (Pirquet test) and found that 41% had a primary lesion on chest radiograph and 35% had hilar adenitis. He also found erythema nodosum to be more common in women and children, and stated that its presence indicated a less favorable prognosis.[11]

Lincoln and Sewell have stated that the primary presentation of tuberculosis may mimic a typical bacterial pneumonia with fever, chills, and a lobar infiltrate.[12] Any process that causes air space consolidation cannot be distinguished from primary pulmonary tuberculosis. In addition, diseases that cause lymph node enlargement such as sarcoidosis and lymphoma may mimic primary disease.

Often the only residua of a primary tuberculous infection are a positive skin test and the Ranke complex. The Ranke complex comprises the small fibrotic parenchymal Ghon focus with an associated calcified lymph node.[13] Although the complex often is called the Ghon complex, the association of the parenchymal infiltrate and lymph node originally was made by Parrot in 1876, the significance of the association first was made clear by Kuss.[14] and the term "primary complex" was coined by Ranke.[15]

Progressive primary pulmonary tuberculosis is a condition where the primary parenchymal disease progresses either at the site of the Ghon focus, or elsewhere, usually in the upper lobes.[13] It had been reported up to 10 years after the onset of primary disease in untreated individuals,[4,11] but many of these individuals initially had normal chest radiographs and today probably would have been classified as having had reactivation tuberculosis. In Gedde-Dahl's study of tuberculin convertors, 33 (12.1%) of 272 convertors developed "progressive primary tuberculosis," with 20 (7.4%) progressing in the first year, although these were not separated by initial radiographic findings. In Poulsen's study, 20 (3.9%) of 517 infected persons with an initial parenchymal infiltrate developed progressive primary pulmonary disease with 3 (0.6%) progressing in the first year. However, today, with modern screening and therapy, it would be very unusual to see progressive primary tuberculosis ensue after initial presentation and treatment, unless the disease was unresponsive to therapy.

Cavitation was described as a sequela of this process in 8 (11%) of 78 persons with primary parenchymal infiltrates in Gedde-Dahl's group and 4 (3%) of 139 persons with primary parenchymal infiltrates in Poulsen's group.

Lincoln and Sewell have stated that calcifications may occur within 6 months in infants, require at least 1 year in children, and may take longer to appear in adults. In 964 children who survived primary pulmonary tuberculosis, 90% had calcifications on chest radiograph.[12]

Patients with primary tuberculosis often have a cough, but rarely produce adequate sputum. Gastric aspiration sometimes is successful in obtaining organisms, but as a rule, the diagnosis is based most often on the clinical findings, exposure history, radiographic findings, and skin test status. Bronchoscopy may be useful because of the high incidence of endobronchial lesions, i.e., 28% in Weber's study.[6]

A. LOWER LOBE TUBERCULOSIS IN ADULTS

Lower lobe tuberculosis has been noted in as much as 7% of pulmonary tuberculosis cases in adults.[16] It has been described in several studies and is thought to be more prevalent in patients with AIDS, diabetes, pregnancy, the elderly, and persons on steroid therapy.[16-19] It may partially reflect an increasing incidence of primary disease in older persons.

II. REACTIVATION PULMONARY TUBERCULOSIS

Reactivation, or postprimary, pulmonary tuberculosis, refers to tuberculous disease that occurs after the primary infection has resolved (see Chapter 10). When an apical calcified focus (Simon focus) or a granuloma or caseous node with dormant tuberculous organisms reactivates, the delayed hypersensitivity response may lead to massive inflammation, necrosis, liquefaction, and cavitation. The infection may involve the airways and spread to other parts of the lung, and uncommonly involves the lymph nodes. The reactivation focus usually was seeded in the well-oxygenated upper lobes during the primary lymphohematogenous dissemination, and reactivation occurs most often within 10 years after the primary infection.

There are numerous radiographic findings in tuberculosis. Fraser et al.[13] have defined "local exudative tuberculosis" as a patchy or confluent air-space consolidation, sometimes with cavitation, and "chronic fibrocaseous tuberculosis" as a finding where "the relatively poor definition of the exudative lesion is replaced by a more sharply defined shadow, usually somewhat irregular and angular in contour." Bronchogenic spread refers to a picture of bronchopneumonia where the contents of a cavity have spilled into the airways and have been aspirated into an entire segment, lobe, or lung. It has the features of a typical bacterial pneumonia, with lower lobe involvement in 19% of cases,[20] and a toxic appearing patient.

Adler found that 85% of the dominant tuberculous lesions in adults were in the apical or posterior segment of an upper lobe, and that an additional 9.5% were in the superior segment of a lower lobe.[21] Although it has been stated that reactivation tuberculosis almost never occurs solely in the anterior segment of an upper lobe, Spencer et al. have described nine adult patients with predominantly or solely anterior segment tuberculosis,[22] and Adler has shown that 3% of dominant lesions occurred in the anterior segment with an additional 36% of secondary lesions in that segment. Tuberculosis of the basilar segments was described as a dominant lesion in 1.9% of patients, and as a secondary lesion in 23.2% of patients in Adler's study.

The presence of intrathoracic lymphadenopathy does not rule out reactivation tuberculosis. Woodring et al. have found that 5% of definite cases of reactivation tuberculosis were associated with lymphadenopathy.[23]

A. CAVITATION

Vascular involvement is common in the area of active infection, and vessels may show both vasculitis and thrombosis. Endarteritis obliterans may occur and lead to necrosis and cavitation, frequent findings in advanced reactivation tuberculosis.[24] Hadlock et al.[20] have found cavitation in 51% of cases of reactivation disease, Woodring et al.[25] have found cavitation in 45% of cases, and Choyke et al.[26] have found cavitation in 7.7% of cases. The cavitation may be solitary or multiple, may vary in size and shape, may have a variable thick or thin wall, and may be internally nodular.[13,27] An air fluid level may be present and, in one study, was demonstrated in 20% of cases.[25] Changes in the cavity size or tension in the cavity may develop due to impaired drainage.[27] The cavity may rupture into the pleural space and cause an empyema. Cavities also may be a source of bleeding. A locally dilated artery in the wall of a cavity (Rasmussen's aneurysm) may cause exsanguination or, more commonly, asphyxia.[28,29] Such hemoptysis may require management with angiographic embolization.[30] As the process resolves, the natural course of the cavity is to diminish gradually in size. However, it may persist and lead to further complications such as the development of an aspergilloma.

III. ASPERGILLOMA

The Research Committee of the British Thoracic and Tuberculosis Association have studied 544 treated tuberculous patients with cavities greater than 2.5 cm in diameter who had been culture-negative for at least 1 year and found 61 (12%) to have an aspergilloma.[31] The most likely time for development of the aspergilloma in that study was within 7 to 11 years after the diagnosis of cavitary tuberculosis.[32] Another study found the average latency period to be 8.5 years.[33] Hemoptysis is common and may be massive, but rarely leads to exsanguination. Asphyxia is the major risk. Most of the patients in a study by Tomlinson and Sahn presented with varying degrees of hemoptysis, and 10 patients underwent surgical resection for massive or recurrent hemoptysis. Recommendations for management varied from watchful waiting to intracavitary instillation of amphotericin B[34] to arterial embolization to surgical resection.[33]

IV. ENDOBRONCHIAL TUBERCULOSIS

Endobronchial involvement has been described previously as a complication of advanced cavitary tuberculosis where the airway becomes infected and tracheobronchitis ensues.[35] However, it has been described with and without parenchymal involvement in adults and the elderly,[36] and may be due to lymph node erosion.[37] There often is peripheral collapse of the involved segment or lobe, and bronchostenosis is a common sequela.[37,38] The sputum is not necessarily smear positive, and in one study, 85% of cases with demonstrated endobronchial involvement were sputum smear negative.[39] In three patients with endobronchial tuberculosis and AIDS, tumor-like masses were seen, and even so, spontaneously induced sputum smears were negative.[40]

Bronchostenosis may occur due to inflammation and scarring of the bronchus, and bronchiectasis may result from bronchostenosis and obstructive pneumonitis with distal bronchiectasis, or it may occur from chronic scarring of the parenchyma with traction on the bronchus. Broncholithiasis also has been reported, usually as a complication of old inactive disease.[13]

V. TUBERCULOMA

A tuberculoma may occur during primary or reactivation tuberculosis. It is a smooth, round or ovoid lesion ranging in size from 0.5 to 4.0 cm in diameter.[41,42] Satellite lesions may be identified nearby in 80% of cases.[42] Tuberculomas may be multiple and are easily mistaken for coin lesions or metastatic disease.[18] The lesions may or may not be active, and may or may not be calcified, but activity has been reported to correlate directly with size. Cavitation may occur in 10 to 50% of tuberculomas but lymphadenopathy is a very rare association.[3]

VI. PNEUMOTHORAX AND BRONCHOPLEURAL FISTULA

A pneumothorax or pneumomediastinum may occur at any time during the disease process, even with miliary tuberculosis,[43] and probably is due to subpleural disease with formation of a cyst and subsequent rupture.

A bronchopleural fistula usually is due to rupture of a tuberculous cavity. It is a feared complication, for if the cavity is active, an empyema will result. The tear may be 1 mm to 4 cm in size,[44] and cure often requires a definitive surgical procedure.[45]

VII. RADIOLOGIC DIFFERENTIAL

Radiographic findings of other diseases may mimic tuberculosis (see Chapter 10). Upper lobe infiltrates and cavitation with or without fibrosis may be seen with atypical mycobacteria, sarcoidosis, ankylosing spondylitis, aspiration pneumonia, silicosis, Wegener's granulomatosis and other collagen vascular diseases, adenosquamous cancer, lymphomas (especially Hodgkins), infarcts, and actinomycosis.[46] Upper lobe bullous disease may be seen in emphysema and neurofibromatosis and may mimic cavitary disease, especially where there is a periemphysematous infection.[47] Thin-section computed tomography may be useful in distinguishing active pulmonary tuberculosis from other processes.[48]

In the setting of HIV infection, pulmonary tuberculosis often must be distinguished radiographically from bacterial pneumonia, upper lobe *Pneumocystis carinii* pneumonia,[49] and less commonly, nocardia and rhodococcus infections.[50,51]

VIII. ENDOCRINOLOGIC MANIFESTATIONS

Hyponatremia commonly is associated with tuberculosis and was present in 56 (10.7%) of 522 new consecutively diagnosed cases in one study.[52] The mechanism has been shown to involve the inappropriate secretion of antidiuretic hormone.[53] The syndrome resolves after several weeks of antituberculous therapy.

Hypercalcemia also is commonly associated with tuberculosis, and was present in a study by Abbasi et al. in 22 (28%) of 79 patients with tuberculosis.[54] However, 95% of the patients were receiving supplemental vitamin D. Interestingly, all patients were normocalcemic on admission, and the onset of hypercalcemia occurred within 4 to 16 weeks after therapy was started. Calcium levels returned to normal over a period of 1 to 7 months, despite the continuation of vitamin D supplementation. Resolution of the hypercalcemia appeared to correlate with the conversion to a negative sputum. Liam et al. have described hypercalcemia, after adjusting for albumin, in 27.5%

of 120 patients with tuberculosis in Malaysia.[55] Candranel et al. have confirmed the participation of the pulmonary macrophage by showing that conversion of 25 hydroxyvitamin D to 1,25 dihydroxyvitamin D was performed *in vitro* by pulmonary macrophages from a patient with pulmonary tuberculosis,[56] and in a larger study, have shown that these cells are major contributors to calcium metabolism in tuberculosis patients.[57]

Hypoadrenalism is thought to be uncommon and was not found in an extensive study of 50 patients.[58]

IX. DIAGNOSIS OF TUBERCULOSIS

A. History and Physical Examination

In pursuit of the diagnosis of tuberculosis, the history and physical examination are notoriously misleading. Reactivation tuberculosis develops insidiously and may exist for months with few symptoms. The classic symptoms of cough, hemoptysis, fever, night sweats, and weight loss rarely are seen concurrently except in advanced disease. The patient may present acutely during an upper respiratory viral infection or a superinfecting bacterial pneumonia, and it may appear that the tuberculous condition is causing the acute presentation, but often the tuberculous process has been present for months. In a study of preemployment screening where 9 (0.9%) of 970 adults had active tuberculosis, the only sensitive indicator was the presence of a cough. Other symptoms were present variably, and none of the subjects felt ill enough to seek medical attention independently, despite the presence, in some, of far advanced disease.[59]

Even when symptoms and signs are present, they are not specific for tuberculosis. Weight loss may be seen in many diseases. Night sweats have been reported in persons with nontuberculous infections, cancer, and even heavy alcohol or drug use. The physical examination sometimes adds little to the evaluation, and the classic posttussive rales often are absent in the area of involvement. Although choroidal tubercles have been shown in one study to be present in 30% of patients with pulmonary tuberculosis and were thought to be a specific finding,[60] this has not been tested widely. Therefore, the appropriate use of the history and physical examination is to prompt the physician to order a chest radiograph, sputum analysis, or both where the suspicion of tuberculosis is present.

The PPD has little use in the evaluation of reactivation tuberculosis. A positive test does not indicate that an infiltrate is tubercular in nature, and a negative test (<5 mm of induration) has been reported in 17.4 to 21.0% of cases of active tuberculosis with no known cause of anergy[61-63] (see Chapter 13).

B. Smear, Culture, and Bronchoscopy

The diagnosis of tuberculosis hinges on the procurement of several adequate sputum samples for analysis and culture (see Chapter 4). Sputum acid-fast bacilli (AFB) smears are estimated to be positive in 65 to 75% of patients who have had multiple specimens, and 30 to 40% of those with a single specimen.[64] In 1997 there were 16,285 cases reported where pulmonary tuberculosis was a major or additional site of disease. Of these, 11,481 (71%) were sputum culture-positive, and of these 6627 (58%) were smear positive (Centers for Disease Control, unpublished data).

An early morning sputum is the best specimen for the diagnosis of pulmonary tuberculosis. Pooled specimens are not advised because of problems with contamination.[65] It is recommended that if AFB are present in 2 of 3 morning specimens, it is unnecessary to continue collections. However, if no AFB are seen and if tuberculosis is strongly suspected, it is recommended that sputum collection continue, although there is little advantage to collecting more than five sputa per patient.[65] If the patient is unable to produce sputum, then sputum induction with normal or hypertonic saline should be attempted. The specimen should be labeled clearly as an induced specimen because its watery nature may cause the laboratory to mistake the sample for saliva and discard it. Another effective technique is the early morning gastric aspiration of 50 ml of fluid after an 8 to 10 h fast. This modality is especially useful in children or patients who do not produce sputum. Gastric aspirates should be processed within 4 h or they should be neutralized to a pH of 7.0 and refrigerated. Gastric smears are not thought to be reliable due to the possibility of atypical mycobacterial contaminants in food. However, in a small study in Louisiana, Klotz and Penn showed that where AFBs were identified on smear, they always were associated with true typical or atypical mycobacterial disease.[66] Also, in a study from Canada, Bahammam et al. identified smear-positive gastric aspirates in 13 (1.1%) of 1150 specimens; all 13 were culture positive for *M. tuberculosis*.[67] Positive cultures were noted in 109 (9.5%) specimens, 67 (61.5%) of which were positive for *M. tuberculosis*, and the remainder of which were atypical mycobacteria. Most of these specimens were obtained from adults. Urine also may be collected and, in one study, was reported positive in 4.7% of cases of pulmonary tuberculosis without evidence of renal disease by history, physical, or urinalysis.[68] The author stated that asymptomatic tubercle bacilluria, even without pyuria or IVP abnormalities always represents genitourinary tuberculosis. This assumption has not been proved. It certainly is possible that bacilluria can occur during bacteremia without infecting the kidneys. If the patient is very sick and the process is thought to be disseminated, blood cultures also may be drawn. They are very useful in HIV-related tuberculosis and have been shown to be positive in as much as 38% of such cases,[69] and 49% of patients where the CD4 count was 100 or fewer.[70]

If sputum cannot be obtained, or if it is imperative to make an immediate diagnosis, bronchoscopy is the next best course of action.[71] Bronchoscopy has been shown clearly to aid in the immediate diagnosis of tuberculosis. Danek and Bower have obtained 34% positive smear and 95% positive culture results with brushings, washings, and biopsies in 41 sputum smear-negative patients.[72] De Gracia et al. have obtained 18% positive smear and 88% positive culture results with lavage in 17 patients with smear-negative tuberculosis.[73] Wallace et al. have analyzed 22 patients with documented smear-negative pulmonary tuberculosis and found that, for a single procedure, the best yield for an immediate diagnosis was 30% with a transbronchial biopsy procedure that included histology and AFB stains.[74] The biopsy was exclusively positive in 26% of patients and had a far better yield than brushings or washings. Postbronchoscopy smears were considered part of the bronchoscopy procedure and added an additional 9% to the total yield. However, the prebronchoscopy sputa proved to be more sensitive for culture diagnosis than were bronchoscopic cultures, i.e., 67% vs. 44%, although the bronchoscopy cultures occasionally were positive where the sputum culture was negative. Stenson et al. also obtained their highest yield, i.e., 75%, with prebronchoscopy sputa.[75] The lower yield on bronchoscopy has been thought to be due in part to the mycobacterial inhibitory effects of the lidocaine employed as an anesthetic during the bronchoscopic procedure.[76,77] Based on these studies, one may conclude that it is important to perform a complete bronchoscopic procedure where indicated, including biopsy and lavage, and that all specimens should be stained and cultured. It also is important to collect postbronchoscopy sputa. For information on diagnostic modalities in HIV-related tuberculosis, see Section X.

Careful cleaning of the bronchoscope is essential to reduce the risk of cross-contamination of specimens,[78] and the risk of actual transmission of tuberculosis to the next patient in whom bronchoscopy is performed.[79] Various cleaning regimens and solutions have been recommended, and glutaraldehyde, phenol, or ethylene oxide are effective agents.[80-82] Guidelines for decontamination have been published,[83,84] and include careful cleaning followed by at least 20 min of immersion in 2% glutaraldehyde (see Chapter 3). Rapid diagnostic methods are discussed in Chapter 5.

X. HIV INFECTION AND PULMONARY TUBERCULOSIS

The presentation of pulmonary tuberculosis in patients early in the course of HIV disease may not be different from the presentation in the normal host, tending to occur at a CD4 count of 300 cells per mm^3 or less.[50,51,85,86] The skin test may be less reactive, but otherwise the body still is capable of responding to and controlling tuberculosis in the usual way.[50,87] Since 1993, HIV-positive individuals who develop tuberculosis have been considered to have AIDS and, thus, the spectrum of AIDS-related tuberculosis may range from mild to severe disease, depending on the CD4 count. The development of tuberculosis early in the course of HIV disease often indicates that other more severe manifestations of AIDS will follow soon.[88-90] Where tuberculosis develops in persons with advanced AIDS, the T helper cell count usually is less than 200 cells per mm^3,[85,86,91] and both cell-mediated immunity and delayed-type hypersensitivity are depressed. The body is less able to fight the infection, but also is less able to respond with destructive processes such as caseation, lique-faction, and cavitation.[19,92,93] Tuberculous pneumonia may present typically, and has been associated with cavitation, or it may present atypically with a diffuse or miliary pattern, a mid or lower lung field infiltrate and, frequently, hilar adenopathy.[19,50,92,94] In fact, AIDS patients occasionally may present with pulmonary tuberculosis and a normal chest radiograph.

Pulmonary tuberculosis in HIV-positive patients often coexists with extrapulmonary disease. Extrapulmonary disease occurs commonly in as much as 20% of most series of tuberculosis cases without HIV infection, but may occur in over 50% of cases of HIV-related tuberculosis at advanced stages of immunosuppression.[85,86,95,96] De Cock et al., in a review of tuberculosis and AIDS, have determined that the median CD4 count at the time of diagnosis of localized extrapulmonary tuberculosis was approximately 240 cells per mm^3, compared to 140 cells per mm^3 for meningeal tuberculosis, and less than 100 cells per mm^3 for disseminated tuberculosis.[85] Jones et al. have found extrapulmonary tuberculosis to be present in 30 (70%) of 43 patients with CD4 counts of 100 cells/mm^3 or less, and mycobacteremia was present in 18 (49%) of 37 patients in whom blood cultures were obtained.[70] Small et al. showed that 42 (32%) of 132 patients with HIV-related tuberculosis had coexistent pulmonary and extrapulmonary disease.[97] Therefore, in addition to the lungs, other sites such as urine, stool, blood, lymph nodes, bone marrow, and cerebrospinal fluid may yield a diagnosis. Further discussion on this matter may be found in Chapter 7.

It is not clear what proportion of tuberculosis in AIDS patients represents primary vs. reacti-vation tuberculosis, and indeed, there is evidence for both mechanisms. Data from early in the AIDS epidemic, especially among HIV-infected patients who did not have AIDS at the time they were diagnosed with tuberculosis, suggest that reactivation of latent infection was the primary mechanism to explain the increased risk of tuberculosis in AIDS.[50,51,98-100] Numerous studies have shown that the highest risk for tuberculosis is in HIV-infected drug users with positive skin tests[101-104] (see Chapter 13), although others have shown that in the right setting, PPD-negative drug users at risk for HIV in the inner city have the same risk for tuberculosis as PPD-positive drug users.[105] Studies now show that as much as 40% of new tuberculosis cases in urban centers may be due to recent infection.[106-108] Also, data obtained through investigations of nosocomial outbreaks of tuber-culosis among HIV-infected patients, have indicated that primary infection with *Mycobacterium tuberculosis* and rapid disease progression may be an important mechanism for the increased risk of tuberculosis in this population, especially in late-stage AIDS patients.[109-113] Studies by Di Perri et al. and Daley et al. have documented high tuberculosis attack rates and rapid disease progression within weeks to months in HIV-infected patients exposed to an active tuberculosis index case in a residential or hospital setting.[110,111] Some of these investigations have been carried out through the use of restriction fragment length polymorphisms and other molecular genetic techniques which enable investigators to link cases epidemiologically and to document person-to-person transmis-sion.[109,110,113] These data strongly suggest that highly immunosuppressed patients may be at risk not only for acquiring tuberculosis but also for developing symptomatic disease in the short term.

Several studies have examined the yield and sensitivity of sputum examination in diagnosing tuberculosis in HIV-infected patients. Although some have found sputum analysis to be extremely sensitive, i.e., 61 to 83% smear positive and 88 to 100% culture positive, in four studies of HIV-positive patients,[94,97,99,114] others have postulated that the lower incidence of cavitary disease and necrosis makes it less likely that sputum examination will yield positive results. Klein et al. showed that only 11 (29%) of 38 AIDS/ARC patients had an initial positive smear compared with 35 (61%) of 57 controls.[115] Five smears increased the yield to 40% as opposed to 87.1% of the control group.

Another study found that the failure to diagnose tuberculosis promptly in HIV-infected patients was not due to decreased sensitivity of sputum smear examination, but rather to a failure to obtain the recommended minimum number of sputum smears.[69] Long et al.[116] addressed this issue more definitively in 289 Haitian patients with culture-proven pulmonary mycobacterial disease (tuberculous and nontuberculous). He found the sensitivity of AFB smears in culture-positive pulmonary tuberculosis in 55 HIV-positive patients and 181 HIV-negative patients to be 67.3% vs. 79.0%, respectively. In an analysis of the entire cohort of 289 patients, the positive predictive accuracy of a positive smear in diagnosing pulmonary tuberculosis in HIV-positive vs. HIV-negative patients was 80% vs. 90%, respectively. The authors concluded that although tuberculous smear positivity was slightly reduced in HIV-positive disease, it was still a sensitive and accurate means of diagnosis in the right epidemiologic setting.

Bronchoscopy data also vary widely. Smear positivity in three studies ranged from 10 to 47%, while culture-positivity ranged from 43 to 89%.[69,97,114] Granulomas were present in 19% of biopsies in one study[69] and, thus, support the use of biopsy. Salzman et al.[117] also have shown the utility of transbronchial biopsy in HIV-related pulmonary tuberculosis. Their study has shown that an immediate diagnosis by smear or histology was made in 12 (39%) of 31 patients; in 7 it was the sole means of an immediate diagnosis. Data from Miro et al.[118] did not support the use of the transbronchial biopsy, although their data did show an increase in yield with brushings and biopsy. The lack of significance in their study may be due to a relatively small sample size.

The acuity of the process and the atypical presentations often lead the practitioner to pursue other diagnoses, and unsuspected tuberculosis is found on autopsy in a substantial number of AIDS cases.[69,119] Also, HIV-infected patients are more likely to be colonized with atypical mycobacteria and may be more susceptible to symptomatic disease with organisms such as *M. kansasii* and *M. avium-intracellulare*.[120,121] Thus, in individuals who harbor both tuberculous and nontuberculous mycobacteria, overgrowth with atypical organisms may, in some cases, obscure the tuberculous disease.[122] Thus, when tuberculosis is suspected in an HIV-positive person, it is important to pursue the diagnosis aggressively at multiple sites, since a delay in treatment has been strongly associated with mortality.[123]

XI. DIAGNOSTIC CLASSIFICATION OF TUBERCULOSIS

All tuberculosis cases must be categorized and reported to the Centers for Disease Control and Prevention according to the "Diagnostic Standards and Classification of Tuberculosis in Adults and Children,"[124] a joint statement of the American Thoracic Society (ATS) and the Centers for Disease Control and Prevention (CDC). The classifications are found in Table 6.1.

XII. TREATMENT OF DISEASE

The goal of therapy is to eradicate the tuberculous organisms in the various environments within the host, and to prevent the emergence of drug-resistant strains. Accordingly, Mitchison has described four basic environments, three of which are targeted for attack.[125,126] First are the extracellular organisms which grow most rapidly along cavity walls and in a liquid necrotic medium, and represent the largest load of bacilli. These are killed most effectively by isoniazid. Second are the slower growing semidormant extracellular organisms sometimes found in caseous material that may have only spurts of activity. These are killed most effectively by rifampin because it has the fastest onset of action (15 to 20 min) and is the drug most capable of killing the organism during one of the growth spurts. Third are the slowly growing or semidormant bacilli found intracellularly in the acidic environment (pH 5.5) of macrophages. These are attacked most effectively by pyrazinamide which works best at an acid pH, although some believe that the pH of the macrophage actually is neutral.[127] The fourth environment contains the dormant organisms which cannot be

TABLE 6.1
Diagnostic Classification of Tuberculosis

Class	Diagnosis
0	No tuberculosis exposure, not infected.
1	Tuberculosis exposure, no evidence of infection, i.e., a negative skin test.
2	Latent tuberculosis infection, no disease, i.e., a positive skin test and no evidence of disease (indicate mm of induration).
3	Tuberculosis, clinically active. The location of the disease should be listed as pulmonary, pleural, lymphatic, bone and/or joint, genitourinary, disseminated (miliary), meningeal, peritoneal, and/or other. The predominant site should be listed and the bacteriologic status, chemotherapy status, chest radiograph findings, and tuberculosis skin test reaction should be recorded.
4	Tuberculosis, not clinically active. The diagnosis is made either by history or by a positive skin test with a stable radiograph consistent with tuberculosis. The past or present chemotherapy status should be recorded.
5	Tuberculosis suspect (diagnosis pending). Persons may only remain in this category for 3 months. When diagnostic procedures have been completed, they should be placed in one of the other categories. The chemotherapy status should be recorded.

Source: Adapted from American Thoracic Society/Centers for Disease Control and Prevention, *Am. J. Respir. Crit. Care Med.,* 161, 1376, 2000.

killed until they begin to grow. Although isoniazid and rifampin work best in the environments described, they are each effective in all but the fourth environment.

These mechanisms, in part, explain the philosophy of utilizing three of the currently prescribed drugs, i.e., isoniazid, rifampin, and pyrazinamide, in the initial phase of short-course therapy. Other reasons for using multidrug chemotherapy include the rapid decrease of the burden of organisms and a decreased chance for the emergence of resistant strains. According to David, the highest proportions of resistant organisms that were found in unselected populations in 1970 were: 3.5×10^{-6} for isoniazid, 3.1×10^{-8} for rifampin, 3.8×10^{-6} for streptomycin, and 5×10^{-5} for ethambutol.[128] These *in vitro* studies have indicated that there may be a significant number of resistant organisms found in cavities, which may harbor as many as 10^9 organisms, and explain why more than one drug must be used to treat active tuberculosis. The chance occurrence of an organism that is resistant to more than one drug is equal to the product of the resistance rates for each drug. Therefore, the use of three bactericidal drugs makes it very unlikely that a resistant organism will emerge. Furthermore, the actual mutation rate per generation is approximately 100 times less frequent than the above rates, and explains why two-drug maintenance therapy is adequate once the initial burden of organisms is reduced and the initially resistant strains largely are eliminated. The low burden of organisms in tuberculous infection without disease explains why isoniazid may be used alone in chemoprophylaxis without leading to the development of resistance, and why less rigorous therapy may be used in smear-negative disease.

Because of the slow replication time, as long as the bacillus is exposed to adequate antimicrobial levels at some period of time over several divisions (i.e., several days), therapy will be effective. This allows for daily, thrice-weekly, or twice-weekly therapy even if blood levels are inadequate for a portion of the day or week.

A. CURRENT THERAPY

Since 1970, therapy has been shortened from 18 months of isoniazid and ethambutol to 9 months of isoniazid and rifampin, and then to the current 6-month regimen. This was due largely to the introduction of rifampin, and then to the addition of pyrazinamide. The basis for adopting any new short-course regimen may be found in the statement by the Centers for Disease Control that "an acceptable short course chemotherapy regimen should allow reduction in the duration of therapy while resulting in a rate of relapse not greater than 5%."[129] Pyrazinamide seems to be the key

TABLE 6.2
Current Recommendations for Therapy of Actual or Probable Drug Sensitive Tuberculosis in HIV-Negative Individuals

6-Month Therapy

Option 1:

Eight weeks of daily isoniazid, rifampin, and pyrazinamide, followed by 16 weeks of isoniazid and rifampin, daily or 2 to 3 times per week. In areas where the isoniazid resistance rate is not documented to be less than 4%, ethambutol or streptomycin should be added to the initial regimen until susceptibility to isoniazid and rifampin is demonstrated. If the results of susceptibility studies are not available at 8 weeks and the rate of isoniazid resistance is not documented to be less than 4%, then pyrazinamide may be discontinued, but the fourth drug (i.e., either ethambutol or streptomycin) must be continued until the isolate is shown to be drug susceptible. The treatment duration should total at least 6 months, and 3 months beyond culture conversion. All regimens administered twice or thrice weekly should by monitored by directly observed therapy. A tuberculosis medical expert should be consulted if the patient is symptomatic or smear or culture positive after 3 months.

Option 2:

Two weeks of daily isoniazid, rifampin, pyrazinamide, and streptomycin or ethambutol followed by 6 weeks of the same drugs, twice weekly, administered by directly observed therapy, followed by 16 weeks of isoniazid and rifampin administered twice weekly by directly observed therapy in cases where the organism is shown to be drug susceptible. A tuberculosis medical expert should be consulted if the patient is symptomatic or smear or culture positive after 3 months.

Option 3:

Thrice weekly isoniazid, rifampin, pyrazinamide, and ethambutol or streptomycin for 6 months, administered by directly observed therapy. (The strongest evidence from clinical trials shows the effectiveness of all 4 drugs administered for the full 6 months. There is weaker evidence that streptomycin can be discontinued after 4 months if the isolate is susceptible to all drugs. The evidence for stopping pyrazinamide before the end of 6 months is equivocal for the thrice-weekly regimen, and there is no evidence for the effectiveness of this regimen with ethambutol for less than the full 6 months.) A tuberculosis medical expert should be consulted if the patient is symptomatic or smear or culture positive after 3 months.

9-Month Therapy

Nine months of daily isoniazid and rifampin, or 1 to 2 months of daily isoniazid and rifampin followed by 7 to 8 months of daily or twice weekly isoniazid and rifampin for a total of 9 months of therapy. Directly observed therapy should be used for twice-weekly administration. Ethambutol or streptomycin should be added for the first 2 months in areas where the isoniazid resistance rate is not documented to be less than 4%.

4-Month Therapy

Treat as per Options 1, 2, or 3 under 6-Month Therapy, truncated after 4 months in patients who are not at high risk and have smear-negative, culture-negative pulmonary tuberculosis.

Note: For cases where isoniazid, rifampin, or pyrizinamide cannot be used, please see the text for therapy modifications.

Source: Adapted from The American Thoracic Society/Centers for Disease Control and Prevention, *Am. Rev. Respir. Dis.*, 149, 1359, 1994, and Centers for Disease Control and Prevention, *MMWR*, 47(No. RR-20), 1, 1998.

additional drug in 6-month regimens.[130] At least one other drug must be used where isoniazid resistance is possible. Twice-weekly or thrice-weekly therapy allows for easier monitoring by public health officers.

Current therapy recommendations for new cases of tuberculosis in HIV-negative individuals are displayed in Table 6.2 and are based on statements from the American Thoracic Society and the Centers for Disease Control and Prevention.[130,131] New recommendations for HIV-related tuberculosis based on recent CDC recommendations[132] may be found in Table 6.3 and will be discussed later. The dosages of the first- and second-line drugs are displayed in Tables 6.4 and 6.5, respectively. Further descriptions of these agents may be found in Chapter 11.

TABLE 6.3
HIV-Related Tuberculosis

Rating	Drugs	Induction Phase — Interval and Duration	Drugs	Continuation Phase — Interval and Duration	Considerations for HIV Therapy	Comments
6-Month RFB-Based Therapy (May be Prolonged[a] to 9 Months)						
A.II	• INH • RFB • PZA[b] • EMB[b]	Daily for 2 months (8 weeks) or	• INH • RFB	Daily or 2 times/week for 4 months (18 weeks) or	RFB should not be used concurrently with hard-gel saquinavir (Invirase™) or delavirdine. A 20%–25% increase in the dose of protease inhibitors or NNRTIs might be necessary.	If the patient also is taking indinavir, nelfinavir, or amprenavir, the daily dose of RFB is decreased from 300 mg to 150 mg. The twice-weekly dose of RFB (300 mg) remains unchanged if the patient is also taking these protease inhibitors.
	• INH • RFB • PZA[b] • EMB[b]	Daily for 2 weeks and then 2 times/week for 6 weeks	• INH • RFB	2 times/week for 4 months (18 weeks)	The patient should be monitored carefully for RFB drug toxicity (arthalgia, uveitis, leukopenia) if RFB is used concurrently with protease inhibitors or NNRTIs. Evidence of decreased antiretroviral drug activity should be assessed periodically with HIV RNA levels. No contraindication exists for the use of RFB with NRTIs.	If the patient also is taking efavirenz, the daily or twice weekly dose of RFB is increased from 300 mg to 450 mg. Three-times-a-week administration of RFB used in combination with antiretroviral therapy has not been studied.
9-Month SM-Based Therapy (May be Prolonged[a] to 12 Months)						
B.II	• INH • SM • PZA • EMB	Daily for 2 months (8 weeks) or	• INH • SM • PZA	2–3 times/week for 7 months (30 weeks) or	Can be used concurrently with antiretroviral regimens that include protease inhibitors, NRTIs, and NNRTIs.	SM is contraindicated for pregnant women. Every effort should be made to continue administering SM for the total duration of treatment. When SM is not used for the recommended 9 months, EMB should be added to the regimen and the treatment duration should be prolonged from 9 months (38 weeks) to 12 months (52 weeks).
	• INH • SM • PZA • EMB	Daily for 2 weeks and then 2–3 times/week for 6 weeks	• INH • SM • PZA	2–3 times/week for 7 months (30 weeks)		

6-Month RIF-Based Therapy (May be Prolonged[a] to 9 Months)

A.I	• INH • RIF • PZA[c] • EMB[c] (or SM)	Daily for 2 months (8 weeks)	• INH • RIF	Daily or 2–3 times/week for 4 months (18 weeks)	Protease inhibitors or NNRTIs should not be administered concurrently with RIF. NRTIs can be administered concurrently with RIF. If appropriate, patients should be assessed every 3 months to evaluate the decision to initiate antiretroviral therapy. A 2-week "P-450 induction washout" period may be necessary between the last dose of RIF and the first dose of protease inhibitors or NNRTIs.	SM is contraindicated for pregnant women.
		or				
	• INH • RIF • PZA[c] • EMB[c] (or SM)	Daily for 2 weeks and then 2–3 times/week for 6 weeks	• INH • RIF	2–3 times/week for 4 months (18 weeks)		
		or				
	• INH • RIF • PZA • EMB (or SM)	3 times/week for 2 months (8 weeks)	• INH • RIF • PZA • EMB (or SM)	3 times/week for 4 months (18 weeks)		

Note: EMB = ethambutol; INH = isoniazid; PZA = pyrazinamide; RFB = rifabutin; RIF = rifampin; SM = streptomycin; NNRTI = nonnucleoside reverse transcriptase inhibitor; NRTI = nucleoside reverse transcriptase inhibitor. If PIs or NNRTIs are administered, an expert in these drug interactions must be consulted.

[a] Duration of therapy should be prolonged for patients with delayed response to therapy. Criteria for delayed response should be assessed at the end of the 2-month induction phase and include (a) lack of conversion of the *Mycobacterium tuberculosis* culture from positive to negative or (b) lack of resolution or progression of signs or symptoms of TB.

[b] Continue PZA and EMB for the total duration of the induction phase (8 weeks).

[c] Continue PZA for the total duration of the induction phase (8 weeks). EMB can be stopped after susceptibility test results indicate *Mycobacterium tuberculosis* susceptibility to INH and RIF.

Source: Adapted from Centers for Disease Control and Prevention, *MMWR*, 47(No. RR-20), 1, 1998.

It is recommended that drug susceptibility studies be performed on all initial isolates from patients with newly diagnosed tuberculosis.[130] Furthermore, as noted in Table 6.2, it is essential to begin therapy with four drugs in areas where the prevalence of isoniazid resistance has not been demonstrated to be less than 4%.

There have been numerous studies in HIV-negative individuals to document the effectiveness of the 6-month regimen defined in Table 6.2, Options 1 and 2.[133-137] Although most of these regimens were effective in smear-positive disease, a study from Hong Kong has suggested that the initial addition of a fourth drug, i.e., streptomycin, in smear-positive disease is superior to the three-drug regimen.[138]

Pyrazinamide is the best third drug to add to isoniazid and rifampin for short-course therapy[130] and, for patients receiving the regimen outlined in Table 6.2, Options 1 or 2, there is no advantage to the use of pyrazinamide after the first 2 months of therapy for drug-susceptible tuberculosis.[139] However, if the organism is resistant to isoniazid, it may be discontinued, but pyrazinamide should be continued for the entire 6-month duration of treatment, as noted below.

The course of therapy outlined in Table 6.2, Option 3, i.e., thrice-weekly, four-drug therapy for 6 months, is based on a study performed in Hong Kong where five different 6-month regimens were compared, two of which were four-drug, thrice-weekly regimens using isoniazid, rifampin, pyrazinamide, and either ethambutol or streptomycin.[140] In drug-susceptible patients who were followed over a 5-year period, there were 2 (1.3%) relapses in 151 patients who were taking the regimen containing streptomycin, and there were 7 (4.4%) relapses in 160 patients who were taking the regimen containing ethambutol. Overall, the rate of relapse in the regimens containing pyrazinamide vs. the regimen that did not contain pyrazinamide was 3.4% vs. 10.3%, respectively. Therefore, it was suggested that for thrice-weekly therapy, pyrazinamide was beneficial where used for the entire 6-month period,[130] although the Hong Kong study did not address this issue specifically because there was no comparison with a 6-month regimen that used initial pyrazinamide for 2 months only. Analysis of a small group of 131 patients who were resistant to isoniazid, streptomycin, or both, showed that those who took pyrazinamide fared much better than those who did not; there were 4 (3.8%) relapses in 104 patients in the pyrazinamide series vs. 6 (22.2%) in 27 patients in the nonpyrazinamide series. Therefore, in all treatment options in Table 6.2 where isoniazid cannot be used due to resistance or toxicity, pyrazinamide should be continued for the entire 6 month duration of therapy.[130]

Two other studies have shown success with intermittent therapy started immediately without a daily induction phase. One was a 6-month supervised intermittent trial in Haiti where isoniazid, rifampin, pyrazinamide, and ethambutol were administered thrice weekly for 8 weeks followed by 18 weeks of isoniazid and rifampin.[141] The relapse rate in HIV-negative individuals was 2.8%, and in HIV-positive individuals, 5.4%. A similar study also has shown good results, i.e., a relapse rate of 3.3% for a regimen of isoniazid, rifampin, pyrazinamide, and streptomycin every other day for 2 months followed by isoniazid and rifampin for 4 months.[142] Initial intermittent therapy may help to ease the burden on public health workers who administer directly observed therapy to patients who are diagnosed and treated as outpatients.

In cases where both isoniazid and pyrazinamide cannot be used, it has been recommended that ethambutol and rifampin be administered for a minimum of 12 months.[130] This is based largely on a study by the National Research Institute for Tuberculosis, Poland, where a regimen of 12 weeks of daily therapy (rifampin, 600 mg, and ethambutol, 25 mg/kg) followed by twice-weekly rifampin (600 mg) and ethambutol (50 mg/kg) for a total of 12 months of therapy, was used in the treatment of 40 patients with isoniazid-resistant pulmonary tuberculosis.[143,144] There was a 10% overall failure rate (5% treatment failures plus 5% relapses). The results from a similar Hong Kong study were even less favorable.[145] Better results were obtained with a similar regimen used by Lees et al. and Nitti et al.[146,147] These overall failure rates are not acceptable and we recommend that a third drug be added to this regimen.

TABLE 6.4
Antituberculosis Medications: Doses, Toxicities, and Monitoring Requirements

Drug	Dose in mg/kg (maximum dose) Route of Administration						Adverse Reactions	Monitoring	Comments
	Daily		Two times/week[a]		Three times/week[a]				
	Children[b]	Adults	Children[b]	Adults	Children[b]	Adults			
INH	10–20 (300 mg) PO or IM	5 (300 mg) PO or IM	20–40 (900 mg) PO or IM	15 (900 mg) PO or IM	20–40 (900 mg) PO or IM	15 (900 mg) PO or IM	• Rash • Hepatic enzyme elevation • Hepatitis • Peripheral neuropathy • Mild central nervous system effects • Drug interactions resulting in increased phenytoin (Dilantin) or disulfiram (Antabuse) levels	Liver function tests Repeat measurements if • Baseline results are abnormal • Patient is pregnant or at high risk for adverse reactions • Patient has symptoms of adverse reactions	Hepatitis risk increased with age and alcohol consumption. Pyridoxine (Vitamin B_6) might prevent peripheral neuropathy and central nervous system effects.
RIF	10–20 (600 mg) PO or IV	10 (600 mg) PO or IV	10–20 (600 mg) PO or IV	10 (600 mg) PO or IV	10–20 (600 mg) PO or IV	10 (600 mg) PO or IV	• Rash • Hepatitis • Fever • Thrombocytopenia • Flu-like symptoms associated with intermittent dosing • Orange-colored body fluids (secretions, urine, tears)	Complete blood count, platelets, and liver function tests Repeat measurements if • Baseline results are abnormal • Patient has symptoms of adverse reactions	RIF use contraindicated for patients taking PIs or NNRTIs. Decreases levels of many drugs (e.g., methadone, dapsone, ketoconazole, hormonal contraceptives). Might permanently discolor soft contact lenses.

TABLE 6.4 *(continued)*
Antituberculosis Medications: Doses, Toxicities, and Monitoring Requirements

| | Dose in mg/kg *(maximum dose)* Route of Administration | | | | | | | | |
| | Daily | | Two times/week[a] | | Three times/week[a] | | | | |
Drug	Children[b]	Adults	Children[b]	Adults	Children[b]	Adults	Adverse Reactions	Monitoring	Comments
RFB[c]	10–20 (*300 mg*) PO or IV	5 (*300 mg*) PO or IV	10–20 (*300 mg*) PO or IV	5 (*300 mg*) PO or IV	Not Known	Not Known	• Rash • Hepatitis • Fever • Thrombocytopenia • Orange-colored body fluids (secretions, urine, tears)	Complete blood count, platelets, and liver function tests	RFB is contraindicated for patients taking saquinavir (Invirase™) or delavirdine. Reduces levels of many drugs (e.g., PIs, NNRTIs, methadone, dapsone, ketoconazole, hormonal contraceptives). Might permanently discolor soft contact lenses.
	or	or	or	or				Repeat measurements if • Baseline results are abnormal • Patient has symptoms of adverse reactions	
	NA[d] (*150 mg*) PO or IV	NA[d] (*150 mg*) PO or IV	10–20[d] (*300 mg*) PO or IV	5 (*300 mg*) PO or IV	Not Known	Not Known	With increased levels of RFB: • Severe arthralgias • Uveitis • Leukopenia	Use adjusted daily dose of RFB[d], and monitor for decreased antiretroviral activity and for RFB toxicity if RFB is taken concurrently with PIs or NNRTIs.	
	or	or	or	or					
	NA[e] (*450 mg*) PO or IV	NA[e] (*450 mg*) PO or IV	NA[e] (*450 mg*) PO or IV	NA[e] (*450 mg*) PO or IV	Not Known	Not Known			
PZA	15–30 (*2.0 g*) PO	15–30 (*2.0 g*) PO	50–70 (*3.5 g*) PO	50–70 (*3.5 g*) PO	50–70 (*2.5 g*) PO	50–70 (*2.5 g*) PO	• Gastrointestinal upset • Hepatitis • Rash • Arthralgias • Hyperuricemia • Gout (rare)	Liver function tests and uric acid; Repeat measurements if • Baseline results are abnormal • Patient has symptoms of adverse reactions	Treat hyperuricemia only if patient has symptoms. Might make glucose control more difficult in persons with diabetes.

Drug						Adverse reactions	Monitoring	Comments
EMB[f]	15–25 (1600 mg) PO	50 (4000 mg) PO	50 (4000 mg) PO	25–30 (2000 mg) PO	25–30 (2000 mg) PO	• Optic neuritis (decreased red-green color discrimination), decreased visual acuity • Rash	Baseline and monthly tests of visual acuity and color vision	Optic neuritis might be unilateral; check each eye separately.
SM	20–40 (1 g) IM or IV	15 (1 g) IM or IV	25–30 (1.5 g) IM or IV	25–30 (1.5 g) IM or IV	25–30 (1.5 g) IM or IV	• Ototoxicity (hearing loss or vestibular dysfunction) • Nephrotoxicity	Baseline and repeat as needed audiometry and renal function tests	Ultrasound and warm compresses to injection site might reduce pain. Maximum dose for patients ≥60 years is 1.0 g.

Note: EMB = ethambutol; INH = isoniazid; PZA = pyrazinamide; RFB = rifabutin; RIF = rifampin; SM = streptomycin. NNRTIs = nonnucleoside reverse transcriptase inhibitors; PI = protease inhibitor. IM = intramuscular; IV = intravenous; PO = by mouth. If PIs or NNRTIs are administered, an expert in these drug interactions must be consulted. Please refer to the text for information update.

[a] All intermittent dosing should be administered with directly observed therapy.

[b] Children are ≤ 12 years old.

[c] The concurrent use of RFB is contraindicated with saquinavir (Invirase™) and delavirdine. Information regarding the use of rifabutin with saquinavir (Fortovase™), amprenavir, efavirenz, and nevirapine is limited. If rifabutin is used in a patient receiving antiretroviral agents, an expert in the use of antiretroviral agents should be consulted on proper dosing since the information in this field is changing rapidly.

[d] Not applicable. If nelfinavir, indinavir, or amprenavir is administered with RFB, blood concentrations of these protease inhibitors decrease. Thus, when RFB is used concurrently with any of these three drugs, the daily dose of RFB is reduced from 300 mg to 150 mg (the twice-weekly dose of RFB is unchanged, however).

[e] NA = not applicable. If efavirenz is administered with RFB, blood concentrations of RFB decrease. Thus, when RFB is used concurrently with efavirenz, the dose of RFB for both daily and twice weekly administration should be increased from 300 mg to 450 mg.

[f] Ethambutol generally is not recommended for children whose visual acuity cannot be monitored (< 8 years) unless they are HIV-positive or unless the organism is resistant to other drugs and susceptibility to ethambutol has been demonstrated or is likely.

Source: From the American Thoracic Society/Centers for Disease Control and Prevention, *Am. Rev. Respir. Dis.,* 149, 1359, 1994, and Centers for Disease Control and Prevention, *MMWR,* 47(No. RR-20), 1, 1998.

TABLE 6.5
Second Line Antituberculosis Drugs[a]

Drug	Dosage Forms	Daily Dose in Children and Adults[b] (mg/kg)	Maximal Daily Dose in Children and Adults (g)	Major Adverse Reactions	Recommended Regular Monitoring
Capreomycin	Vials: 1 g	15 to 30 IM	1	Auditory, vestibular, and renal toxicity	Vestibular function, audiometry, blood urea nitrogen, and creatinine
Kanamycin	Vials: 75 mg, 500 mg, 1 g	15 to 30 IM	1	Auditory and renal toxicity, rare vestibular toxicity	Vestibular function, audiometry, blood urea nitrogen, and creatinine
Ethionamide	Tablets: 250 mg	15 to 20 PO	1	Gastrointestinal disturbance, hepatotoxicity, hypersensitivity	Hepatic enzymes
ρ-Aminosalicylic acid	Tablets: 500 mg, 1 g; delayed release granules; bulk powder	150 PO	12	Gastrointestinal disturbance, hypersensitivity, hepatotoxicity, sodium load	Hepatic enzymes
Cycloserine	Capsules: 250 mg	15 to 20 PO	1	Psychosis, convulsions, rash	Assessment of mental status

[a] These drugs are more difficult to use than drugs listed in Table 6.4. They should be used only when necessary and should be given and monitored by health providers experienced in their use.
[b] Doses based on weight should be adjusted as weight changes.

Source: Adapted from the American Thoracic Society/Centers for Disease Control and Prevention, *Am. Rev. Respir. Dis.,* 149, 1359, 1994.

In cases where rifampin cannot be used, isoniazid, pyrazinamide, and streptomycin may be used daily for 9 months,[148] or isoniazid and ethambutol may be used daily or twice weekly for 18 months.[149,150] Ethambutol always should be started at a daily dose of 25 mg/kg during the induction phase.

In cases where rifampin and pyrazinamide cannot be used, isoniazid and ethambutol may be used as noted above.

In cases where both isoniazid and rifampin cannot be used because of toxicity, it would be wise to apply the principles of treatment for multidrug-resistant tuberculosis (see Chapter 12). In these instances, it is preferable to use at least three new drugs, one of which is an injectable drug, and continue until culture conversion is documented, followed by at least 12 months of two-drug therapy. Often, a total of 24 months is administered empirically.[130]

In the treatment regimens noted above, where the sensitivities are not known, consideration should be given to adding an additional drug during the induction phase, until the drug susceptibilities are known.

The previous standard of 9-month therapy was established in 1980[129] and has been shown to be very effective in most forms of tuberculosis.[134,151-156] In fact, there are still those who prefer to use this regimen. In view of the rising problems with isoniazid resistance, it is prudent in most cases to add ethambutol during the initial phase until culture sensitivity reports are available, and recommended strongly where the incidence of isoniazid resistance is not documented to be less than 4%.

Although the quinolones, e.g., levofloxocin, ofloxacin, ciprofloxacin, and others, have antimycobacterial activity, they should not be considered adequate substitutions for first line drugs.[157-160]

In general, it appears that the smaller the bacillary load in pulmonary tuberculosis, the less vigorous the therapy. Dutt et al. have shown success in smear-negative, culture-positive pulmonary tuberculosis with 6 months of isoniazid and rifampin,[161] and have shown further success in smear-negative, culture-negative pulmonary tuberculosis with 4 months of isoniazid and rifampin.[162] Furthermore, there is evidence that smear-negative pulmonary tuberculosis, with or without positive cultures, responds well to 4 months of either daily or thrice-weekly, four-drug therapy.[163] Therefore, in smear-negative, culture-negative tuberculosis, the ATS and CDC have recommended that it is acceptable to reduce the basic 6-month regimen to 4 months.[130] Recommendations for the treatment of tuberculosis in pregnant women, children, and neonates may be found in Chapter 8.

1. HIV-Related Treatment

The principles of treatment of HIV-related tuberculosis are similar to those of normal hosts. The primary differences relate to the need for increased vigilance when assessing the response to therapy, and to drug dosage adjustments during the concurrent use of antiretroviral agents. The Advisory Committee for the Elimination of Tuberculosis has recommended that antituberculous therapy be started as soon as AFB are seen in a specimen from the respiratory tract of a person with known or suspected HIV infection.[164] The basic recommendations for therapy, which now may include rifabutin, are shown in Table 6.3.[132]

The available data show that a 6-month regimen is acceptable in some patients who are HIV-infected,[141,165,166] but not in all such patients.[167] Experts have concluded that a 6-month regimen may be used in HIV-positive persons with pansensitive tuberculosis who are receiving directly observed therapy (usually in the U.S.) if there is a good clinical response and rapid sputum conversion, i.e., within 2 months.[132] Otherwise, a 9-month or longer regimen might be indicated. This duration has been shown to be very effective.[165,168] Four-drug therapy should be continued throughout the 2-month induction phase for rifabutin-based regimens.[132]

Persons with HIV-related tuberculosis often respond well to antituberculous chemotherapy and, once effectively treated, usually do not die from tuberculosis. Even with advanced HIV infection, Small et al. have shown good results in 125 persons with pulmonary and/or extrapulmonary tuberculosis who received either 6 or 9 months of short-course therapy.[97] There were 52 deaths during therapy, but only 8 (6.4%) were due to tuberculosis. In general, sputa were cleared of acid-fast organisms after a median of 10 weeks of therapy, and there were only 3 (5%) relapses in 58 patients who completed therapy, all due to poor compliance.

Patients who are receiving antiretroviral agents and develop tuberculosis are given special consideration. Unfortunately the protease inhibitors (PI) and the nonnucleoside reverse transcriptase inhibitors (NNRTI) generally cannot be administered with rifampin because of problems with drug metabolism, although the nucleoside reverse transcriptase inhibitors (NRTI) may be given with rifampin. In the past, patients were taken off their antiretroviral agents while they were treated for tuberculosis, and could not restart these agents until 2 weeks after the last dose of rifampin. Now it is recommended that therapy be administered concurrently by substituting rifabutin for rifampin and making appropriate dosage adjustments with very close clinical monitoring (see Tables 6.3, 6.4, and below). Rifabutin has been shown to be effective in 6-month regimens in HIV-positive individuals.[169-171]

Rifabutin is not as potent a P450 enzyme inducer as rifampin, and can be used, with dosage adjustments (150 mg for daily regimens; no change for intermittent regimens), with the PIs nelfinavir, indinavir, and amprenavir.[132,172] It is not known whether rifabutin dose modifications are needed where soft-gel saquinavir (Fortavase™) is used, and it may be best to avoid the use of this drug with rifabutin. Information about efavirenz also is limited, but because it reduces the concentration of rifabutin, it has been recommended that the daily and twice-weekly dose of rifabutin be increased to 450 mg.[132] Rifabutin is contraindicated with hard-gel saquinavir (Invirase™) and delavirdine.[132] For information on the use of ritonavir, refer to Chapter 13. Information about the interactions of these drugs with rifabutin is controversial and is changing rapidly. Therefore, it is strongly recommended that an expert in the use of antiretroviral agents be consulted for dosage adjustments when a patient receiving these medications also must receive antituberculosis medications. (See Chapter 13.)

Rifapentine is not recommended as a rifampin substitute because its safety and effectiveness have not been established in patients with HIV-related tuberculosis.[132]

The clinician should be familiar with other drug interactions with the rifamycins that might cause the need for dosage adjustments. Such drugs include methadone, barbiturates, hormonal contraceptives, dapsone, ketoconazole, fluconazole, itraconazole, narcotics, anticoagulants, corticosteroids, cardiac glycosides, hypoglycemics (sulfonylureas), diazepam, beta-blockers, anticonvulsants, and theophylline.

In low-income countries, fixed-dose combination pills are recommended to prevent the development of drug resistance.[173] Also, there are data from Africa indicating an unacceptably high relapse rate in HIV-infected patients treated with regimens that include thiacetazone.[174,175] This, along with the unacceptably high rate of adverse reactions, make HIV-positivity a contraindication for the use of thiacetazone.[173]

B. Monitoring Response to Therapy

Patients should be seen every month to monitor the response to treatment and encourage adherence. Directly observed therapy is recommended unless there is evidence that the patient will adhere to therapy. In sputum smear-positive patients, monthly sputum analysis is mandatory, and weekly sputum smears with quantification is encouraged strongly.[130] Otherwise, sputum should be obtained each month until culture conversion is documented. After 2 months of therapy with a standard regimen containing both isoniazid and rifampin, more than 85% of positive sputum cultures should have converted to negative.[130] If the sputum has not converted by that time, the patient should be evaluated carefully and drug susceptibility tests should be repeated. The patient also should be started on directly observed therapy. Treatment should be continued with an emphasis on adherence and, where necessary, supervised therapy.

Fever may be present for prolonged periods. In one study, 34% of patients treated with isoniazid and PAS with or without streptomycin were still febrile at 2 weeks.[176] In another study with more effective therapy (i.e., isoniazid, rifampin, and ethambutol) only 10% were still febrile at 2 weeks.[177] The duration of fever was longer than 100 days in rare cases and correlated with the extent of disease. The presence of fever during the first few weeks should not be of great concern if the patient is improving clinically. A chest radiograph should be performed 2 or 3 months into therapy to assess the radiographic resolution of the disease. If the sputum culture converts within 2 months, the chest radiograph improves, and the patient improves clinically, then a final sputum and chest radiograph should be performed at the completion of therapy. Further follow-up is not necessary. Monitoring and follow-up of high-risk patients should be more intensive and individualized. Patients who have been slow to respond, have significant residual radiographic findings upon completion of treatment, or who are immunosuppressed should be reevaluated 6 months after the completion of treatment, or earlier if symptoms occur.[130] For patients with negative pretreatment sputa, the course of therapy should be followed clinically and by chest radiograph.

If a nonimmunosuppressed compliant patient with a pansensitive organism is failing therapy, antibiotic drug levels should be considered. In one study on non-HIV-infected patients with a slow clinical response, treatment failure or a relapse, 68 and 64% had low levels of isoniazid and rifampin, respectively.[178]

Patients whose sputum cultures do not convert after 5 or 6 months are considered treatment failures. Therapy may be continued pending drug susceptibility tests, or the patient may be started immediately on at least two new drugs while continuing the previous regimen, pending the susceptibility report. Direct supervision of therapy should be implemented. In one study, 10 (2.2%) of 453 patients had a positive smear at the end of therapy: 8 were culture negative and 2 grew atypical organisms.[179] It is important to note that smears may contain acid-fast organisms, even at the end of therapy, without representing worsening disease. If the patient has improved clinically, the organism most likely is nonviable or atypical, and the clinician can wait for the culture report.

Patients who relapse after completing a regimen containing both isoniazid and rifampin may be restarted on their original therapy as the organisms usually still are susceptible to the original drugs.[130,180] Patients who relapse after a regimen that did not contain both isoniazid and rifampin should be treated as if they are resistant to all previous drugs (see Chapter 12).

1. HIV-Related Issues

Directly observed therapy should be used in all patients who are HIV positive.[132] If the patient is adherent, the lack of sputum conversion at 2 months is strongly suggestive of a delayed response to treatment.[132] This also is true even if the patient has converted his sputum but continues to have persistent fever or progressive weight loss, and an increase in the size of lymph nodes, abscesses, or other tuberculous lesions, none of which can be accounted for by other processes, such as a paradoxical reaction (see below). If a delayed response is diagnosed, rifamycin-based regimens should be prolonged from 6 months to 9 months (or to 4 months after culture conversion is documented). If it is a nonrifamycin streptomycin-based regimen, therapy should be prolonged from 9 months to 12 months (or to 6 months after culture conversion is documented).[132]

Another reason for the lack of an appropriate response to therapy is the malabsorption of antituberculous drugs. This seems to be especially common in HIV-positive individuals,[181-184] although in one study, there was no difference in absorption between HIV-positive and HIV-negative individuals.[185] Therapeutic drug monitoring is not recommended in the routine management of HIV-positive individuals,[132] but there are circumstances such as treatment failures or the management of multidrug-resistant tuberculosis where it might be appropriate.

The response of patients receiving rifabutin with antiretroviral agents must be monitored very closely because of the alterations in the metabolism of the drugs.

Completion of therapy is based more on the total number of doses received than on the actual duration of therapy. Usually, if an interruption of therapy is brief, the patient may restart his original medications. However, if the interruption lasts 2 months or more, sputum samples should be obtained for smear, culture, and drug-susceptibility studies.[132]

When antiretroviral agents are administered during tuberculous chemotherapy, the immune system may become partially reconstituted and the patient may experience a paradoxical reaction.[132,186,187] This reaction has been reported in as much as 36% of patients studied.[186] The reaction may consist of worsening symptoms and signs including a worsening chest radiograph, uncontrollable fever, airway compromise from enlarging lymph nodes, enlarging effusions in the pleura, pericardium, or peritoneum, or a sepsis-like syndrome. Such patients also may recover from their anergic states and develop a positive tuberculin skin test.[186] When the reaction is mild, the patient should be seen every 2 weeks with no change in therapy, but when it is severe, hospitalization may be required with the administration of steroids, 60 to 80 mg/day for 1 to 2 weeks with gradual reduction over 4 to 6 weeks.

C. MONITORING FOR ADVERSE REACTIONS

Baseline evaluation for one of the standard regimens should include a complete blood count with platelets, liver function tests, blood urea nitrogen, creatinine, and calcium. If pyrazinamide is used, uric acid should be obtained; if ethambutol is used, uric acid, visual acuity, and red/green color perception should be assessed; and if streptomycin is used, renal and auditory tests should be performed. Isoniazid toxicity should be monitored as described in Table 6.4 and Chapter 13. Patients should be instructed about the complications of therapy and the natural course of the disease. If symptoms develop that suggest drug toxicity, a full evaluation should ensue.[130] For techniques on reintroducing drugs after an adverse reaction, refer to Chapter 12.

1. HIV-Related Adverse Reactions

Adverse reactions to antituberculous medications have been found to be more prevalent in HIV-positive individuals by some authors,[97,165,167] but not others.[141] One report has shown that HIV-infected patients have a higher incidence than expected of allergic reactions to rifampin, which occurred in approximately 20% of patients.[97] The incidence of adverse reactions necessitating a change in therapy was 18%, and was due to rashes, hepatitis, gastrointestinal distress, and anaphylaxis. Pyridoxine (25 to 50 mg daily or 50 to 100 mg twice weekly) should be administered to all HIV-infected patients receiving isoniazid to reduced the incidence of nervous system side effects. Patients on rifabutin and clarithromycin should be monitored closely for the development of uveitis (see Chapter 11).

The incidence of allergic reactions to thiacetazone is so troublesome that the International Union Against Tuberculosis and Lung Disease states that thiacetazone is contraindicated in HIV-infected patients.[132]

D. IMMUNOCOMPROMISED HOSTS WITHOUT HIV

Non-HIV immunocompromised patients respond well to chemotherapy unless they have extensive tuberculous disease. In one study, tuberculosis in patients immunocompromised by cancer, cancer chemotherapy, transplant therapy, hemopathy, or steroid therapy responded well to a regimen of isoniazid, rifampin, and ethambutol for 3 months followed by isoniazid and rifampin for 9 to 12 months.[188] However 2 of 30 patients died, 1 before therapy and 1 just after it began. All others did well. In addition, both Bobrowitz et al.[190] and Fulkerson et al.[189] noted that persons with coexistent tuberculosis and lung cancer could be irradiated successfully with full doses as long as adequate antituberculous chemotherapy was administered. Therefore, it would seem reasonable for all significantly immunocompromised hosts to follow the same guidelines set forth for the treatment of tuberculosis in HIV infection, but it might be wise to administer at least 9 months of therapy since the rapid response to treatment has not been documented as well as it has in HIV-related tuberculosis.

E. SILICOTUBERCULOSIS

As noted earlier, tuberculosis is particularly difficult to treat in the setting of silicosis and relapses are common, presumably due to the cytotoxicity of silica for alveolar macrophages.[191] Some have recommended continuous therapy once silicotuberculosis has been diagnosed.[192]

Dubois et al.[193] had success with initial therapy of tuberculosis in 27 silicotic individuals with a regimen of three to four drugs (including rifampin and ethambutol) given until sputum conversion occurred, followed by two drugs for 6 months, and then by isoniazid for 1 year. Sputum conversion occurred in all persons by 5 months, and there was one relapse during a 2- to 6-year period. Escreet et al. have claimed success in 36 patients with a 9-month regimen that included thiacetazone.[194] However, their relapse rate was 9%. Lin et al. studied a regimen of 2 months of isoniazid, rifampin, pyrazinamide, and streptomycin, followed by 7 months of isoniazid and rifampin.[195] They had 5% treatment failures and 5% relapses. Cowie et al. treated 1085 cases with 4.5 months of a weekday regimen of isoniazid, rifampin, pyrazinamide, and streptomycin with no treatment failures and a gross relapse rate of 3.8% after 36 months of follow-up;[196] it was estimated that 14% of the assembled group had atypical mycobacteria. Neither the atypical mycobacteria nor the initial resistance patterns appeared to affect the rate of relapse. Other regimens in the same study with a less intensive initial phase and without rifampin during the maintenance phase were much less successful. The Hong Kong Chest Service compared 6 months vs. 8 months of a thrice-weekly, four-drug regimen of isoniazid, rifampin, pyrazinamide, and streptomycin, supplemented by ethambutol if the patient had been treated previously. Sputum conversion occurred in 98% of patients at 3 months, but the relapse rate was 7% in the 8-month group, and 22% in the 6-month group.[197]

The recommendation of the ATS and the CDC is that in cases of culture positive silicotuberculosis, the usual therapy must be extended by at least 2 months.[130] As noted above, 8 months of a thrice-weekly, four-drug regimen might be effective.

F. SURGERY

Surgery for pulmonary tuberculosis rarely is performed today. Before the chemotherapy era, it was an important adjunct for "resting" the lung, for resection of cavities and progressive local disease, and for managing empyemas and fibrothoraces. Operations such as the artificial pneumothorax, artificial pneumoperitoneum, artificial phrenic nerve paralysis, plombage, thoracoplasty, pulmonary resection, cavity drainage, Eloesser flap, and decortication had been performed.[198,199] Currently, the indications for surgery are few. They include active localized disease unresponsive to adequate chemotherapy (e.g., a multidrug-resistant strain), empyema or bronchopleural fistula unresponsive to closed pleural space evacuation, and life-threatening hemoptysis unresponsive to arteriographic embolization.[200] In one study of 206 patients, the major indications were cavitary sequelae, bronchiectasis, and hemoptysis.[201] The overall mortality rate was 3% and the morbidity rate was 29%. The complication rate was lower in patients who where smear negative and had had an adequate course of chemotherapy before surgery was undertaken. Video-assisted thoracoscopic surgery has been used for pleural biopsies, wedge resections, empyema drainage, and lobectomies in 37 tuberculosis patients with no morbidity or mortality.[202]

Iseman et al. have studied surgical resection as adjunctive therapy for multidrug-resistance in 29 patients. Of 27 survivors (there were 2 unrelated deaths), 25 (93%) remained sputum culture-negative at 36 months postresection.[203]

If drug resistance continues to be a major problem, surgery may again become important in the management of tuberculosis (see Chapter 12).

G. CORTICOSTEROIDS

Notwithstanding their beneficial use in tuberculous meningitis and pericarditis (see Chapter 7), corticosteroids do not play a role in the management of typical pulmonary tuberculosis, unless it is associated with fulminant miliary disease and/or the adult respiratory distress syndrome,[204-207] or severe obstructive intrathoracic lymphadenopathy in primary disease.[208] They may be useful in severe HIV-related tuberculosis,[209] or where there is a paradoxical response (see Section XII.B.1.). Signs and symptoms may resolve sooner in typical pulmonary[210] and pleural disease,[211,212] but a long-term benefit has not been demonstrated. If a patient does require corticosteroids while receiving antituberculous medications, there is no diminishment in the clinical response to the infection.[213]

REFERENCES

1. Myers, J. A., Gunlaugson, F. G., Meyerding, E. A., et al., Importance of tuberculin testing of school children — a twenty-eight year study, *JAMA*, 159, 185, 1955.
2. Caffey, J., Ed., *Caffey's Pediatric X-Ray Diagnosis*, 7th ed., Year Book Medical Publishers, Chicago, 1985.
3. Palmer, P. E. S., Pulmonary tuberculosis — usual and unusual radiographic presentations, *Semin. Roentgenol.*, 14, 204, 1979.
4. Poulsen, A., Some clinical features of tuberculosis. II. Initial fever. III. Erythema nodosum. IV. Tuberculosis of lungs and pleura in primary infection. V. Extrapulmonary tuberculosis. VI. Spread of infection. VII. Sequelae of primary tuberculous infection, *Acta Tuberc. Scand.*, 33, 37, 1951.
5. Frostad, S., Segmental atelectasis in children with primary tuberculosis, *Am. Rev. Tuberc.*, 79, 597, 1959.
6. Weber, A. L., Bird, K. T., and Janower, M. L., Primary tuberculosis in childhood with particular emphasis on changes affecting the tracheobronchial tree, *Am. J. Roentgenol.*, 103, 123, 1968.
7. Daly, J. F., Endoscopic aspects of primary tuberculosis in children, *Ann. Otol. Rhinol. Laryngol.*, 67, 1089, 1958.
8. Smith, M. H. D. and Marquis, J. R., Tuberculosis and other mycobacterial infections, in Feigin, R. D. and Cherry, J. D., Eds., *Textbook of Pediatric Infectious Diseases*, Saunders, Philadelphia, 1987.
9. Singh, D. and Richards, W. F., Obstructive emphysema in primary pulmonary tuberculosis, *Tubercle*, 38, 397, 1957.
10. Poulsen, A., Some clinical features of tuberculosis: I. Incubation period, *Acta Tuberc. Scand.*, 24, 311, 1950.
11. Gedde-Dahl, T., Tuberculous infection in the light of tuberculin matriculation, *Am. J. Hyg.*, 56, 139, 1952.
12. Lincoln, E. M. and Sewell, E. M., Tuberculosis in children, McGraw Hill, New York, 1963.
13. Fraser, R. S., Pare, J. A. P., Fraser, R. G., and Pare, P. D., Eds., *Synopsis of Diseases of the Chest*, 2nd ed., Saunders, Philadelphia, 1994.
14. Fried, B. M., The primary complex (initial anatomic lesion in childhood type of tuberculosis), *Arch. Pathol.*, 22, 829, 1936.
15. Pinner, M., Pulmonary tuberculosis in the adult: its fundamental aspects, Charles C. Thomas, Springfield, IL, 1945.
16. Chang, S. C., Lee, P. Y., and Perng, R. P., Lower lung field tuberculosis, *Chest*, 91, 230, 1987.
17. Berger, H. W. and Granada M. G., Lower lung field tuberculosis, *Chest*, 65, 522, 1974.
18. Khan, M. A., Kovnat, D. M., Bachus B., et al., Clinical and roentgenographic spectrum of pulmonary tuberculosis in the adult, *Am. J. Med.*, 62, 31, 1977.
19. Pitchenik, A. E. and Rubinson H. A., The radiographic appearance of tuberculosis in patients with the acquired immune deficiency syndrome and pre-AIDS, *Am. Rev. Respir. Dis.*, 131, 393, 1985.
20. Hadlock, F. P., Park, S. K., Awe, R. J., et al., Unusual radiographic findings in adult pulmonary tuberculosis, *Am. J. Radiol.*, 134, 1015, 1980.
21. Adler, H., Phthisiogenetic studies by means of tomography in cases of localized pulmonary tuberculosis in adults, *Acta Tuberc. Scand.*, 47, 13, 1959.

22. Spencer, D., Yagan, R., Blinkhorn, R., et al., Anterior segment upper lobe tuberculosis in the adult: occurrence in primary and reactivation disease, *Chest*, 97, 384, 1990.
23. Woodring, J. H., Vandiviere, H. M., and Lee, C., Intrathoracic lymphadenopathy in postprimary tuberculosis, *South. Med. J.*, 81, 992, 1988.
24. Cudkowicz, L., The blood supply of the lung in pulmonary tuberculosis, *Thorax*, 7, 270, 1952.
25. Woodring, J. H., Vandiviere, H. M., Fried, A. M., et al., Update: the radiographic features of pulmonary tuberculosis, *Am. J. Radiol.*, 146, 497, 1986.
26. Choyke, P. L., Sostman, H. D., Curtis, A. M., et al., Adult-onset pulmonary tuberculosis, *Radiology*, 148, 357, 1983.
27. Jacobson, H. G. and Shapiro, J. H., Pulmonary tuberculosis, *Radiol. Clin. North Am.*, 1, 411, 1963.
28. Auerbach, O., Pathology and pathogenesis of pulmonary arterial aneurysm in tuberculous cavities, *Am. Rev. Tuberc.*, 39, 99, 1939.
29. Plessinger, V. A. and Jolly, P. N., Rasmussen's aneurysms and fatal hemorrhage in pulmonary tuberculosis, *Am. Rev. Tuberc.*, 60, 589, 1949.
30. Muthuswamy, P. P., Akbik, F., Franklin, C., et al., Management of major or massive hemoptysis in active pulmonary tuberculosis by bronchial arterial embolization, *Chest*, 92, 77, 1987.
31. British Thoracic Association, Aspergilloma and residual tuberculous cavities — the results of a resurvey, *Tubercle*, 51, 227, 1970.
32. British Thoracic Association, Aspergillus in persistent lung cavities after tuberculosis, *Tubercle*, 49, 1, 1968.
33. Tomlinson, J. R. and Sahn, S. A., Aspergilloma in sarcoid and tuberculosis, *Chest*, 92, 505, 1987.
34. Munk, P. L., Vellet, A. D., Rankin, R. N., Muller, N. L., and Ahmad, D., Intracavitary aspergilloma: transthoracic percutaneous injection of amphotericin gelatin solution, *Radiology*, 181, 821, 1993.
35. Auerbach, O., Tuberculosis of the trachea and major bronchi, *Am. Rev. Tuberc.*, 60, 604, 1949.
36. Van den Brande, P. M., Van de Mierop F., Verbeken, E. K., et al., Clinical spectrum of endobronchial tuberculosis in elderly patients, *Arch. Intern. Med.*, 150, 2105, 1990.
37. Chang, S. C., Lee, P. Y., and Perng R. P., Clinical role of bronchoscopy in adults with intrathoracic tuberculous lymphadenopathy, *Chest*, 93, 314, 1988.
38. Hoheisel, G., Chan, B. K. M., Chan, C. H. S., Chan, K. S., Teschler, H., and Costabel, U., Endobronchial tuberculosis: diagnostic features and therapeutic outcome, *Resp. Med.*, 88, 593, 1994.
39. Ip, M. S. M. and Lam, W. K., Endobronchial tuberculosis revisited, *Chest*, 89, 727, 1986.
40. Wasser, L. S., Shaw, G. W., and Talavera, W., Endobronchial tuberculosis in the acquired immunodeficiency syndrome, *Chest*, 94, 1240, 1988.
41. Bleyer, J. M. and Marks J. H., Tuberculomas and hamartomas of the lung: comparative study of 66 proved cases. *Am. J. Radiol.*, 77, 1013, 1957.
42. Sochocky, S., Tuberculoma of the lung, *Am. Rev. Tuberc.*, 78, 403, 1958.
43. Narang, R. K., Kumar, S., and Gupta, A., Pneumothorax and pneumomediastinum complicating acute miliary tuberculosis, *Tubercle*, 58, 79, 1977.
44. Johnson, T. M., McCann, W., and Davey, W. N., Tuberculous bronchpleural fistula, *Am. Rev. Respir. Dis.*, 107, 30, 1973.
45. Light, R. W., *Pleural Diseases*, 2nd ed., Lea and Febiger, Philadelphia, 1990.
46. Laforet, E. G. and Laforet, M. T., Nontuberculous cavitary disease of the lungs, *Dis. Chest*, 31, 665, 1957.
47. Mahler, D. A. and D'Esopo, N. D., Peri-emphysematous lung infection, *Clin. Chest Med.*, 2, 51, 1981.
48. Lee, K. S., Hwang, J. W., Chung, M. P., Hojoong, K., and Kwon, O. J., Utility of CT in the evaluation of pulmonary tuberculosis in patients without AIDS, *Chest*, 110, 977, 1996.
49. Sarkar, S., Dube, M. P., Jones, B. E., and Sattler, F. R., *Pneumocystis carnii* pneumonia masquerading as tuberculosis, *Arch. Intern. Med.*, 157, 351, 1997.
50. Barnes, P. F., Bloch, A. B., Davidson, P. T., and Snider, D. E., Tuberculosis in patients with human immunodeficiency virus infection, *N. Engl. J. Med.*, 324, 1644, 1991.
51. Hopewell, P. C., Impact of human immunodeficiency virus infection on the epidemiology, clinical features, management, and control of tuberculosis, *Clin. Infect. Dis.*, 15, 540, 1992.
52. Chung, D. K. and Hubbard, W. W., Hyponatremia in untreated active pulmonary tuberculosis, *Am. Rev. Respir. Dis.*, 99, 595, 1969.

53. Hill, A. R., Uribarri, J., Mann, J., et al., Altered water metabolism in tuberculosis: role of vasopressin, *Am. J. Med.*, 88, 357, 1990.

54. Abbasi, A. A., Chemplavil, J. K., Farah, S., et al., Hypercalcemia in active pulmonary tuberculosis, *Ann. Intern. Med.*, 90, 324, 1979.

55. Liam, C. K., Lim, K. H., Srivivas, P., and Poi, P. J. H., Hypercalcaemia in patients with newly diagnosed tuberculosis in Malaysia, *Int. J. Tuberc. Lung Dis.*, 2, 818, 1998.

56. Cadranel, J., Hance, A. J., Milleron, B., et al., Vitamin D metabolism in tuberculosis: production of $1,25(OH)_2D_3$ by cells recovered by bronchoalveolar lavage and the role of this metabolite in calcium homeostasis, *Am. Rev. Respir. Dis.*, 138, 984, 1988.

57. Cadranel, J. L., Garabedian, M., Milleron, B., Guillozzo, H., Valeyre, D., Paillard, F., Akoun, G., and Hance, A. J., Vitamin D metabolism by alveolar immune cells in tuberculosis: correlation with calcium metabolism and clinical manifestations, *Eur. Respir. J.*, 7, 1103, 1994.

58. Post, F. A., Soule, S. G., Willcox, P. A., and Levitt, N. S., The spectrum of endocrine dysfunction in active pulmonary tuberculosis, *Clin. Endocrinol.*, 40, 367, 1994.

59. Friedman, L. N., Sullivan, G. M., Bevilaqua, R. P., et al., Tuberculosis screening in alcoholics and drug addicts, *Am. Rev. Respir. Dis.*, 136, 1188, 1987.

60. Massaro D., Katz S., and Sachs, M., Choroidal tubercles: a clue to hematogenous tuberculosis, *Ann. Intern. Med.*, 60, 231, 1964.

61. Holden M., Dubin, M. R., and Diamond P. H., Frequency of negative intermediate-strength tuberculin sensitivity in patients with active tuberculosis, *N. Engl. J. Med.*, 285, 1507, 1971.

62. McMurray, D. N. and Echeverri, A., Cell-mediated immunity in anergic patients with pulmonary tuberculosis, *Am. Rev. Respir. Dis.*, 118, 827, 1978.

63. Rooney, J. J., Crocco, J. A., Kramer, S., and Lyons, H. A., Further observations on tuberculin reactions in active tuberculosis, *Am. J. Med.*, 60, 517, 1976.

64. Daniel, T. M., Rapid diagnosis of tuberculosis: laboratory techniques applicable in developing countries, *Rev. Infect. Dis.*, 11(Suppl. 2), S471, 1989.

65. Kubica, G. P., Gross, W. M., Hawkins, J. E., et al., Laboratory services for mycobacterial diseases, *Am. Rev. Respir. Dis.*, 112, 773, 1975.

66. Klotz, S. A. and Penn, R. L., Acid-fast staining of urine and gastric contents is an excellent indicator of mycobacterial disease, *Am. Rev. Respir. Dis.*, 136, 1197, 1987.

67. Bahammam, A., Choudhri, S., and Long, R., The validity of acid-fast smears of gastric aspirates as an indicator of pulmonary tuberculosis, *Int. J. Tuberc. Lung Dis.*, 3, 62, 1999.

68. Bentz, R. R., Dimcheff, D. G., Neimiroff, M. J., et al., The incidence of urine cultures positive for mycobacterium tuberculosis in a general tuberculosis patient population, *Am. Rev. Respir. Dis.*, 111, 647, 1975.

69. Kramer, F., Modilevsky, T., Waliany, A. R., Leedom, J. M., and Barnes, P. F., Delayed diagnosis of tuberculosis in patients with human immunodeficiency virus infection, *Am. J. Med.*, 89, 451, 1990.

70. Jones, B. E., Young, S. M. M., Antoniskis, D., Davidson, P. T., Kramer, F., and Barnes, P. F., Relationship of the manifestations of tuberculosis to CD4 cell counts in patients with human immunodeficiency virus infection, *Am. Rev. Respir. Dis.*, 148, 1292, 1993.

71. Fulkerson, W. J., Fiberoptic bronchoscopy, *N. Engl. J. Med.*, 311, 511, 1984.

72. Danek, S. J. and Bower, J. S., Diagnosis of pulmonary tuberculosis by flexible fiberoptic bronchoscopy, *Am. Rev. Respir. Dis.*, 119, 677, 1979.

73. De Gracia, J., Curull, V., Vidal, R., et al., Diagnostic value of bronchoalveolar lavage in suspected pulmonary tuberculosis, *Chest*, 93, 329, 1988.

74. Wallace, J. M., Deutsch, A. L., Harrall, J. H., et al., Bronchoscopy and transbronchial biopsy in evaluation of patients with suspected active tuberculosis, *Am. J. Med.*, 78, 1189, 1981.

75. Stenson, W., Aranda, C., and Bevelaqua, F. A., Transbronchial biopsy culture in pulmonary tuberculosis, *Chest*, 83, 883, 1983.

76. Conte, B. A. and Laforet, E. G., The role of the topical anesthetic agent in modifying bacteriologic data obtained by bronchoscopy, *N. Engl. J. Med.*, 267, 957, 1962.

77. Schmidt, R. M. and Rosenkranz, H. S., Antimicrobial activity of local anesthetics: lidocaine and procaine, *J. Infect. Dis.*, 121, 597, 1970.

78. Dawson, D. J., Armstrong, J. G., and Blacklock, Z. M., Mycobacterial cross-contamination of bronchoscopy specimens, *Am. Rev. Respir. Dis.*, 126, 1095, 1982.

79. Nelson, K. E., Larson, P. A., Schraufnagel, D. E., et al., Transmission of tuberculosis by flexible fiberbronchoscopes, *Am. Rev. Respir. Dis.*, 127, 97, 1983.
80. Best M., Sattar A., Springthorpe, V. S., et al., Efficacies of selected disinfectants against *Mycobacterium tuberculosis, J. Clin. Microbiol.*, 28, 2234, 1990.
81. Davis, D., Bonekat, H. W., Andrews, D., et al., Disinfection of the flexible fibreoptic bronchoscope against *Mycobacterium tuberculosis* and *M. gordonae, Thorax*, 39, 785, 1984.
82. Leers, W. D., Disinfecting endoscopes: how not to transmit *Mycobacterium tuberculosis* by bronchoscopy, *Can. Med. Assoc. J.*, 123, 275, 1980.
83. Rutala, W. A. and Weber, D. J., FDA labeling requirements for disinfection of endoscopes: a counterpoint, *Infect. Cont. Hosp. Epidemiol.*, 16, 231, 1995.
84. Rutala, W. A., APIC guideline for selection and use of disinfectants, *Am. J. Infect. Cont.*, 18, 99, 1990.
85. De Cock, K. M., Soro, B., Lucas, S. B., and Coulibaly, I. M., Tuberculosis and HIV infection in sub-Saharan Africa, *JAMA*, 268, 1581, 1992.
86. Shafer, R. W., Chirgwin, K. D., Glatt, A. E., Dahdouh, M. A., Landesman, S. H., and Suster, B., HIV prevalence, immunosuppression, and drug resistance in patients with tuberculosis in an area endemic for AIDS, *AIDS*, 5, 399, 1991.
87. Chaisson, R. E. and Slutkin, G., Tuberculosis and human immunodeficiency virus infection, *J. Infect. Dis.*, 159, 96, 1989.
88. Centers for Disease Control, Tuberculosis and AIDS — Connecticut, *MMWR*, 36, 133, 1987.
89. Centers for Disease Control, Tuberculosis and acquired immunodeficiency syndrome — Florida, *MMWR*, 35, 587, 1986.
90. Centers for Disease Control, Tuberculosis and acquired immunodeficiency syndrome — New York City, *MMWR*, 36, 785, 1987.
91. Theuer, C. P., Hopewell, P. C., Elias, D., et al., Human immunodeficiency virus infection in tuberculosis patients, *J. Infect. Dis.*, 162, 8, 1990.
92. Pozniak, A. L., MacLeod, G. A., Ndlovu, D., Ross, E., Mahari, M., and Weinberg, J., Clinical and chest radiographic features of tuberculosis associated with human immunodeficiency virus in Zimbabwe, *Am. J. Respir. Crit. Care Med.*, 152, 1558, 1995.
93. Fournier, A. M., Dickinson, G. M., Erdfrocht, I. R., et al., Tuberculosis and nontuberculous mycobacteriosis in patients with AIDS, *Chest*, 93, 772, 1988.
94. Long, R., Maycher, B., Scalcini, M., et al., The chest roentgenogram in pulmonary tuberculosis patients seropositive for human immunodeficiency virus type 1, *Chest*, 99, 123, 1991.
95. Elder, N. C., Extrapulmonary tuberculosis, *Arch. Fam. Med.*, 1, 91, 1992.
96. Braun, M. M., Byers, R. H., Heyward, W. L., Ciesielski, C. A., Bloch, A. B., et al., Acquired immunodeficiency syndrome and extrapulmonary tuberculosis in the United States, *Arch. Intern. Med.*, 150, 1913, 1990.
97. Small, P. M., Schecter, G. F., Goodman, P. C., et al. Treatment of tuberculosis in patients with advanced human immunodeficiency virus infection, *N. Engl. J. Med.*, 324, 289, 1991.
98. Centers for Disease Control, Tuberculosis — United States, 1985 — and the possible impact of human T-lymphotropic virus type III/lymphadenopathy-associated virus infection, *MMWR*, 35, 74, 1986.
99. Chaisson, R. E. and Slutkin, G., Tuberculosis and human immunodeficiency virus infection, *J. Infect. Dis.*, 159, 96, 1989.
100. Centers for Disease Control, Tuberculosis and HIV infection: recommendations of the advisory committee for the elimination of tuberculosis (ACET), *MMWR*, 38, 236, 1989.
101. Selwyn, P. A., Hartel, D., Lewis, V. A., Schoenbaum, E. E., Vermund, S. H., Klein, R. S., Walker, A. T., and Friedland, G. H., A prospective study of the risk of tuberculosis among intravenous drug users with human immunodeficiency virus infection, *N. Engl. J. Med.*, 320, 545, 1989.
102. Pape, J. W., Jean, S. S., Ho, J. L., Hafner, A., and Johnson, W. D., Effect of isoniazid prophylaxis on incidence of active tuberculosis and progression of HIV infection, *Lancet*, 342, 268, 1993.
103. Moreno, S., Miralles, P., Diaz, M. D., Baraia, J., Padilla, B., Berenguer, J., and Alberdi, J. C., Isoniazid preventive therapy in human immunodeficiency virus-infected persons: long-term effect on development of tuberculosis and survival, *Arch. Intern. Med.*, 157, 1729, 1997.
104. Whalen, C. C., Johnson, J. L., Okwera, A., Hom, D. L., Huebner, R., Mugyenyi, P., Mugwera, R. D., and Ellner, J. J., A trial of three regimens to prevent tuberculosis in Ugandan adults infected with the human immunodeficiency virus, *N. Engl. J. Med.*, 337, 801, 1997.

105. Friedman, L. N., Williams, M. T., Singh, T. P., and Frieden, T. R., Tuberculosis, AIDS, and death among substance abusers on welfare in New York City, *N. Engl. J. Med.,* 334, 828, 1996.

106. Alland, D., Kalkut, G. E., Moss, A. R., McAdam, R. A., Hahn, J. A., Bosworth, W., Drucker, E., and Bloom, B. R., Transmission of tuberculosis in New York City: an analysis by DNA fingerprinting and conventional epidemiologic methods, *N. Engl. J. Med.,* 330, 1710, 1994.

107. Small, P. M., Hopewell, P. C., Singh, S. P., Paz, A., Parsonnet, J., Ruston, D. C., Schecter, G. F., Daley, C. L., and Schoolnik, G. K., The epidemiology of tuberculosis in San Francisco: a population-based study using conventional and molecular methods, *N. Engl. J. Med.,* 330, 1703, 1994.

108. Bishai, W. R., Graham, N. M. H., Harrington, S., Pope, D. S., Hooper, N., Astemborski, J., Sheely, L., Vlahov, D., Glass, G. E., and Chaisson, R. E., Molecular and geographic patterns of tuberculosis transmission after 15 years of directly observed therapy, *JAMA,* 280, 1679, 1998.

109. Beck-Sague, C., Dooley, S. W., Hutton, M. D., et al., Hospital outbreak of multidrug-resistant *Mycobacterium tuberculosis* infections, *JAMA,* 268, 1280, 1992.

110. Di Perri, G., Cruciani, M., Danzi, M. C., et al., Nosocomial epidemic of active tuberculosis among HIV-infected patients, *Lancet,* 2, 1502, 1989.

111. Daley, C. L., Small, P. M., Schecter, G. F., et al., An outbreak of tuberculosis with accelerated progression among persons infected with the human immunodeficiency virus: an analysis using restriction-fragment-length-polymorphisms, *N. Engl. J. Med.,* 26, 231, 1992.

112. Fischl, M. A., Uttamchandani, R. B., Daikos, G. L., et al., An outbreak of tuberculosis caused by multiple-drug-resistant tubercle bacilli among patients with HIV infection, *Ann. Intern. Med.,* 117, 177, 1992.

113. Pearson, M. L., Jereb, J. A., Frieden, T. R., et al., Nosocomial transmission of multidrug-resistant *Mycobacterium tuberculosis, Ann. Intern. Med.,* 117, 191, 1992.

114. Modilevsky, T., Sattler, F. R., and Barnes, P. F., Mycobacterial disease in patients with human immunodeficiency virus infection, *Arch. Intern. Med.,* 149, 2201, 1989.

115. Klein, N. C., Duncanson, F. P., Lenox, T. H., et al., Use of mycobacterial smears in the diagnosis of pulmonary tuberculosis in AIDS/ARC patients, *Chest,* 95, 1190, 1989.

116. Long R., Scalcini S., Manfreda J., Jean-Baptiste M., and Hershfield E., The impact of HIV on the usefulness of sputum smears for the diagnosis of tuberculosis, *Am. J. Publ. Health,* 81, 1326, 1991.

117. Salzman, S. H., Schindel, M. L., Aranda, C. P., Smith, R. L., and Lewis M. L., The role of bronchoscopy in the diagnosis of pulmonary tuberculosis in patients at risk for HIV infection, *Chest,* 102, 143, 1992.

118. Miro, A. M., Gibilara, E., Powell, S., and Kamholz, S. L., The role of fiberoptic bronchoscopy for diagnosis of pulmonary tuberculosis in patients at risk for AIDS, *Chest,* 101, 1211, 1992.

119. Flora, G. S., Modilevsky T., Antoniskis D., et al., Undiagnosed tuberculosis in patients with human immunodeficiency virus infection, *Chest,* 98, 1056, 1990.

120. Levine, B. and Chaisson, R. E., *Mycobacterium kansasii:* a cause of treatable pulmonary disease associated with advanced human immunodeficiency virus (HIV) infection, *Ann. Intern. Med.,* 114, 861, 1991.

121. Horsburgh, C. R., *Mycobacterium avium* complex infection in the acquired immunodeficiency syndrome, *N. Engl. J. Med.,* 19, 132, 1991.

122. Burnens, A. P. and Vurma-Rapp, U., Mixed mycobacterial cultures — occurrence in the clinical laboratory, *Zentralbl. Bacteriol. Mikrobiol.,* 271, 85, 1989.

123. Pablos-Mendez, A., Sterling, T. R., and Frieden, T. R., The relationship between delayed or incomplete treatment and all-cause mortality in patients with tuberculosis, *JAMA,* 276, 1223, 1996.

124. American Thoracic Society/Centers for Disease Control and Prevention, Diagnostic standards and classification of tuberculosis in adults and children, *Am. J. Respir. Crit. Care Med.,* 161, 1376, 2000.

125. Mitchison D. A., The action of antituberculosis drugs in short-course chemotherapy, *Tubercle,* 66, 219, 1985.

126. Mitchison D. A., Basic mechanisms of chemotherapy, *Chest,* 76(Suppl.), 771, 1979.

127. Crowle, A. J., Dahl, R., Ross, E., et al., Evidence that vesicles containing living, virulent *Mycobacterium tuberculosis* or *Mycobacterium avium* in cultured human macrophages are not acidic, *Infect. Immun.,* 59, 1823, 1991.

128. David H. L., Probability distribution of drug-resistant mutants in unselected population of *Mycobacterium tuberculosis, Appl. Microbiol.,* 20, 810, 1970.

129. Centers for Disease Control, Guidelines for short-course tuberculosis chemotherapy, *MMWR,* 29, 97, 1980.

130. American Thoracic Society/Centers for Disease Control and Prevention, Treatment of tuberculosis and tuberculosis infection in adults and children, *Am. Rev. Respir. Dis.*, 149, 1359, 1994.

131. Centers for Disease Control, Initial therapy for tuberculosis in the era of multidrug resistance: recommendations of the advisory council for the elimination of tuberculosis, *MMWR*, 42(No. RR-7), 1, 1992.

132. Centers for Disease Control and Prevention, Prevention and treatment of tuberculosis among patients infected with human immunodeficiency virus: principles of therapy and revised recommendations, *MMWR*, 47(No. RR-20), 1, 1998.

133. Snider, D. E., Graczyk J., Bek E., et al., Supervised six-months treatment of newly diagnosed pulmonary tuberculosis using isoniazid, rifampin, and pyrazinamide with and without streptomycin, *Am. Rev. Respir. Dis.*, 130, 1091, 1984.

134. Combs, D. L., O'Brien, J., and Geiter, L. J., USPHS tuberculosis short-course chemotherapy trial 21: effectiveness, toxicity, and acceptability: the report of final results, *Ann. Intern. Med.*, 112, 397, 1990.

135. Cohn, D. L., Catlin, B. J., Peterson, K. L., et al., A 62-dose, 6-month therapy for pulmonary and extrapulmonary tuberculosis: a twice-weekly, directly observed, and cost-effective regimen, *Ann. Intern. Med.*, 112, 407, 1990.

136. Singapore Tuberculosis Service/British Medical Research Council, Five-year follow-up of a clinical trial of three 6-months regimens of chemotherapy given intermittently in the continuation phase in the treatment of pulmonary tuberculosis, *Am. Rev. Respir. Dis.*, 137, 1147, 1988.

137. Singapore Tuberculosis Service/British Medical Research Council, Assessment of a daily combined preparation of isoniazid, rifampin, and pyrazinamide in a controlled trial of three 6-month regimens for smear-positive pulmonary tuberculosis, *Am. Rev. Respir. Dis.*, 143, 707, 1991.

138. Hong Kong Chest Service/British Medical Research Council, Controlled trial of 2, 4, and 6 months of pyrazinamide in 6-month, three-times-weekly regimens for smear-positive pulmonary tuberculosis, including an assessment of a combined preparation of isoniazid, rifampin, and pyrazinamide: results at 30 months, *Am. Rev. Respir. Dis.*, 143, 700, 1991.

139. Singapore Tuberculosis Service/British Medical Research Council, Long-term follow-up of a clinical trial of six-month and four-month regimens of chemotherapy in the treatment of pulmonary tuberculosis, *Am. Rev. Respir. Dis.*, 133, 779, 1986.

140. Hong Kong Chest Service/British Medical Research Council, Five-year follow-up of a controlled trial of five 6-month regimens of chemotherapy for pulmonary tuberculosis, *Am. Rev. Respir. Dis.*, 136, 1339, 1987.

141. Chaisson, R. E., Clermont, H. C., Holt, E. A., Cantave, M., Johnson, M. P., Atkinson, J., Davis, H., Boulos, R., Quinn, T. C., and Halsey, N. A., (the JHU-CDS research team), Six-month supervised intermittent tuberculosis therapy in Haitian patients with and without HIV infection, *Am. J. Respir. Crit. Care Med.*, 154, 1034, 1996.

142. Cao, J. P., Zhang, L. Y., Zhu, J. Q., and Chin, D. P., Two-year follow-up of directly-observed intermittent regimens for smear-positive pulmonary tuberculosis in China, *Int. J. Tuberc. Lung Dis.*, 2, 360, 1998.

143. National Research Institute for Tuberculosis, Poland, A comparative study of daily, followed by twice- or once-weekly, regimens of ethambutol and rifampicin in the retreatment of patients with pulmonary tuberculosis: 2nd report, *Tubercle*, 57, 105, 1976.

144. Zierski, M., Prospects of retreatment of chronic resistant pulmonary tuberculosis patients: a critical review, *Lung*, 154, 91, 1977.

145. Hong Kong Tuberculosis Treatment Services/Brompton Hospital/British Medical Research Council, A controlled trial of daily and intermittent rifampicin plus ethambutol in the retreatment of patients with pulmonary tuberculosis: results up to 30 months, *Tubercle*, 56, 179, 1972.

146. Lees, A. W., Allan, G. W., Smith, J., et al., Rifampin in association with isoniazid in initial therapy of pulmonary tuberculosis and rifampin and ethambutol in retreatment cases, *Chest*, 61, 579, 1972.

147. Nitti, V., Catena, E., Veneri, F. D., et. al., Rifampin in association with isoniazid, streptomycin, and ethambutol, respectively, in the initial treatment of pulmonary tuberculosis, *Am. Rev. Respir. Dis.*, 103, 329, 1971.

148. Hong Kong Chest Service/British Medical Research Council, Controlled trial of 6-month and 9-month regimens of daily and intermittent streptomycin plus isoniazid plus pyrazinamide for pulmonary tuberculosis in Hong Kong: results up to 30 months, *Am. Rev. Respir. Dis.*, 115, 727, 1977.

149. American Thoracic Society, Treatment of mycobacterial disease, *Am. Rev. Respir. Dis.*, 115, 185, 1977.

150. American Thoracic Society, Intermittent chemotherapy for adults with tuberculosis, *Am. Rev. Respir. Dis.,* 110, 374, 1974.

151. British Thoracic Association, A controlled trial of six months chemotherapy in pulmonary tuberculosis, 1st report: results during chemotherapy, *Br. J. Dis. Chest,* 75, 141, 1981.

152. Dutt, A. K., Moers D., and Stead W. W., Short-course chemotherapy for tuberculosis with mainly twice-weekly isoniazid and rifampin: community physicians' seven-year experience with mainly outpatients, *Am. J. Med.,* 77, 233, 1984.

153. Dutt, A. K., Jones L., and Stead W. W., Short-course chemotherapy for tuberculosis with largely twice-weekly isoniazid-rifampin, *Chest,* 75, 441, 1979.

154. Dutt, A. K. and Stead, W. W., Chemotherapy of tuberculosis for the 1980s, *Clin. Chest Med.,* 1, 243, 1980.

155. Dutt, A. K., Moers, D., and Stead, W. W., Short-course chemotherapy for extrapulmonary tuberculosis: nine year's experience, *Ann. Intern. Med.,* 104, 7, 1986.

156. Slutkin G., Schecter, G. F., and Hopewell, P. C., The results of 9-month isoniazid-rifampin therapy for pulmonary tuberculosis under program conditions in San Francisco, *Am. Rev. Respir. Dis.,* 138, 1622, 1988.

157. Mohanty, K. C. and Dhamgate, T. M., Controlled trial of ciprofloxacin in short-term chemotherapy for pulmonary tuberculosis, *Chest,* 104, 1194, 1993.

158. Kennedy, N., Berger, L., Curram, J., Fox, R., Gutmann, J., Kisyombe, G. M., Ngowi, F. I., Ramsay, A. R. C., Saruni, A. O. S., Sam, N., Tillotson, G., Uiso, L. O., Yates, M., and Gillespie, S. H., Randomized controlled trial of a drug regimen that includes ciprofloxacin for the treatment of pulmonary tuberculosis, *Clin. Infect. Dis.,* 22, 827, 1996.

159. Kennedy, N., Fox, R., Kisyombe, G. M., Saruni, A. O. S., Uiso, L. O., Ramsay, A. R. C., Ngowi, F. I., and Gillespie, S. H., Early bactericidal and sterilizing activities of ciprofloxacin in pulmonary tuberculosis, *Am. Rev. Respir. Dis.,* 148, 1547, 1993.

160. Alangaden, G. J. and Lerner, S. A. The clinical use of fluoroquinolones for the treatment of myco-bacterial diseases, *Clin. Infect. Dis.,* 25, 1213, 1997.

161. Dutt, A. K. and Stead, W. W., Smear-negative, culture-positive pulmonary tuberculosis: six-month chemotherapy with isoniazid and rifampin, *Am. Rev. Respir Dis.,* 141, 1232, 1990.

162. Dutt, A. K. and Stead, W. W., Smear- and culture-negative pulmonary tuberculosis: four-month short-course chemotherapy, *Am. Rev. Respir. Dis.,* 139, 867, 1989.

163. Hong Kong Chest Service/Tuberculosis Research Centre, Madras/British Medical Research Council, A controlled trial of 3-month, 4-month, and 6-month regimens of chemotherapy for sputum-smear-negative pulmonary tuberculosis: results at 5 years, *Am. Rev. Respir. Dis.,* 139, 871, 1989.

164. Centers for Disease Control, Tuberculosis and human immunodeficiency virus infection: recommendations of the Advisory Committee for the Elimination of Tuberculosis, *MMWR,* 38, 236, 1989.

165. El-Sadr, W. M., Perlman, D. C., Matts, J. P., Nelson, E. T., Cohn, D. L., Salomon, N., Olibrice, M., Medard, F., Chirgwin, K. D., Mildvan, D., Jones, B. E., Telzak, E. E., Klein, O., Heifets, L., and Hafner, R., Evaluation of an intensive intermittent-induction regimen and duration of short-course treatment for human immunodeficiency virus-related pulmonary tuberculosis, *Clin. Infect. Dis.,* 26, 1148, 1998.

166. Kassim, S., Sassan-Morokro, M., Ackah, A., Abouya, L. Y., Digbeu, H., Yesso, G., Coulibaly, I. M., Coulibaly, D., Whitaker, P. J., Doorly, R., Vetter, K. M., Brattegaard, K., Gnaore, E., Greenberg, A. E., Wiktor, S. Z., and De Cock, K. M., Two-year follow-up of persons with HIV-1- and HIV-2-associated pulmonary tuberculosis treated with short-course chemotherapy in West Africa, *AIDS,* 9, 1185, 1995.

167. Perriens, J. H., St. Louis, M. E., Mukadi, Y. B., Brown, C., Prignot, J., Pouthier, F., Portaels, F., Willame, J. C., Mandala, J. K., Kaboto, M., Ryder, R. W., Roscigno, G., and Piot, P., Pulmonary tuberculosis in HIV-infected patients in Zaire: a controlled trial of treatment for either 6 or 12 months, *N. Engl. J. Med.,* 332, 779, 1995.

168. Jones, B. E., Otaya, M., Antoniskis, D., Sian, S., Wang, F., Mercado, A., Davidson, P. T., and Barnes, P. F., A prospective evaluation of antituberculosis therapy in patients with human immunodeficiency virus infection, *Am. J. Respir. Crit. Care Med.,* 150, 1499, 1994.

169. Schwander, S., Rusch-Gerdes, S., Mateega, A., Lutalo, T., Tugume, S., Kityo, C., Rubaramira, R., Mugyenyi, P., Okwera, A., Mugerwa, R., Aisu, R., Moser, R., Ochen, K., M'Bonye, B., and Dietrich, M., A pilot study of antituberculosis combinations comparing rifabutin with rifampicin in the treatment of HIV-1 associated tuberculosis, *Tuberc. Lung Dis.,* 76, 210, 1995.

170. Gonzalez-Montaner, L. J., Natal, S., Yongchaiyud, P., and Olliaro, P., (the Rifabutin Study Group), Rifabutin for the treatment of newly-diagnosed pulmonary tuberculosis: a multinational randomized, comparative study versus rifampicin, *Tuberc. Lung Dis.*, 75, 341, 1994.

171. McGregor, M. M., Olliaro, P., Wolmarans, L., Mabuza, B., Bredell, M., Felten, M. K., and Fourie, P. B., Efficacy and safety of rifabutin in the treatment of patients with newly diagnosed pulmonary tuberculosis, *Am. J. Respir. Crit. Care Med.*, 154, 1462, 1996.

172. Havlir, D. V. and Barnes, P. F., Tuberculosis in patients with human immunodeficiency virus infection, *N. Engl. J. Med.*, 340, 367, 1999.

173. International Union Against Tuberculosis and Lung Disease, Treatment regimens in HIV-infected tuberculosis patients, *Int. J. Tuberc. Lung Dis.*, 2, 175, 1998.

174. Perriens, J. H., Colebunders, R. L., Karahunga, C., et al., Increased mortality and tuberculosis treatment failure rate among human immunodeficiency virus (HIV) seropositive compared with HIV seronegative patients with pulmonary tuberculosis treated with "standard" chemotherapy in Kinshasa, Zaire, *Am. Rev. Respir. Dis.*, 144, 750, 1991.

175. Hawken, M., Nunn, P., Gathua, S., Brindle, R., Godfrey-Faussett, P., Githui, W., Odhiambo, J., Batchelor, B., Gilks, C., Morris, J., and McAdam, K., Increased recurrence of tuberculosis in HIV-1-infected patients in Kenya, *Lancet,* 342, 332, 1993.

176. Berger, H. W., Prolonged fever in patients treated for tuberculosis, *Am. Rev. Respir. Dis.*, 97, 140, 1968.

177. Kiblawi, S. S. O., Jay, S. J., Stonehill, R. B., and Norton, J., Fever response of patients on therapy for pulmonary tuberculosis, *Am. Rev. Respir. Dis.*, 123, 20, 1981.

178. Kimerling, M. E., Phillips, P., Patterson, P., Hall, M., Robinson, A., and Dunlap, N. E., Low serum antimycobacterial drug levels in non-HIV-infected tuberculosis patients, *Chest,* 113, 1178, 1998.

179. Vidal, R., Martin-Casabona, N., Juan, A., Falgueras, T., and Miravitlles, M., Incidence and significance of acid-fast bacilli in sputum smears at the end of antituberculous treatment, *Chest,* 109, 1562, 1996.

180. Costello, H. D., Caras, G. J., and Snider D. E., Drug resistance among previously treated tuberculosis patients, a brief report, *Am. Rev. Respir. Dis.*, 121, 313, 1980.

181. Sahai, J., Gallicano, K., Swick, L., Tailor, S., Garber, G., Seguin, I., Oliveras, L., Walker, S., Rachlis, A., and Cameron, D. W., Reduced plasma concentrations of antituberculosis drugs in patients with HIV infection, *Ann. Intern. Med.*, 127, 289, 1997.

182. Patel, K. B., Belmonte, R., and Crowe, H. M., Drug malabsorption and resistant tuberculosis in HIV-infected patients, *N. Engl. J. Med.*, 332, 336, 1995.

183. Gordon, S. M., Horsburgh, C. R., Peloquin, C. A., et al., Low serum levels of oral antimycobacterial agents in patients with disseminated *Mycobacterium avium* complex disease, *J. Infect. Dis.*, 168, 1559, 1993.

184. Peloquin, C. A., MacPhee, A. A., and Berning, S. E., Malabsorption of antimycobacterial medications, *N. Engl. J. Med.*, 329, 1122, 1993.

185. Taylor, B. and Smith, P. J., Does AIDS impair the absorption of antituberculosis agents? *Int. J. Tuberc. Lung Dis.*, 2, 670, 1998.

186. Narita, M., Ashkin, D., Hollender, E. S., and Pitchenik, A. E., Paradoxical worsening of tuberculosis following antiretroviral therapy in patients with AIDS, *Am. J. Respir. Crit. Care Med.*, 158, 157, 1998.

187. Chien, J. W. and Johnson, J. L., Paradoxical reactions in HIV and pulmonary TB, *Chest,* 114, 933, 1998.

188. Dautzenberg, B., Grosset, J., Fechner, J., et al., The management of thirty immunocompromised patients with tuberculosis, *Am. Rev. Respir. Dis.*, 129, 494, 1984.

189. Bobrowitz, I. D., Elkin, M., Evans, J. C., et al., Effect of direct irradiation on the course of pulmonary tuberculosis (using cancerocidal doses), *Dis. Chest*, 40, 397, 1961.

190. Fulkerson, L. L., Perlmutter, G. S., Zack, M. B., et al., Radiotherapy in chest malignant tumors associated with pulmonary tuberculosis, *Radiology,* 106, 645, 1973.

191. Allison, A. C. and Hart, P. D., Potentiation by silica of the growth of *Mycobacterium tuberculosis* in macrophage cultures, *Br. J. Exp. Path.*, 49, 465, 1968.

192. Morgan, E. J., Silicosis and tuberculosis, *Chest*, 75, 202, 1979.

193. Dubois, P., Gyselen, G., and Prignot, J., Rifampin-combined chemotherapy in coal worker's pneumoconio-tuberculosis, *Am. Rev. Respir. Dis.*, 115, 221, 1977.

194. Escreet, B. C., Langton, M. E., and Cowie R. L., Short-course chemotherapy for silicotuberculosis, *S. Afr. Med. J.*, 66, 327, 1984.

195. Lin, T. P., Suo, J., Lee, J. J., et al., Short-course chemotherapy of pulmonary tuberculosis in pneumoconiotic patients, *Am. Rev. Respir. Dis.*, 136, 808, 1987.

196. Cowie, R. L., Langton, M. E., and Becklake, M. R., Pulmonary tuberculosis in South African gold miners, *Am. Rev. Respir. Dis.*, 139, 1086, 1989.

197. Hong Kong Chest Service/British Medical Research Council, A controlled clinical comparison of 6 and 8 months of antituberculous chemotherapy in the treatment of patients with silicotuberculosis in Hong Kong, *Am. Rev. Respir. Dis.*, 143, 262, 1991.

198. Gaensler, E. A., The surgery for pulmonary tuberculosis, *Am. Rev. Respir. Dis.*, 125 (3, Part 2), 73, 1982.

199. Newman, M. M., The olden days of surgery for tuberculosis, *Ann. Thorac. Surg.*, 48, 161, 1989.

200. Harrison, L. H., Current aspects of the surgical management of tuberculosis, *Surg. Clin. North Am.*, 60, 883, 1980.

201. Rizzi, A., Rocco, G., Robustellini, M., Rossi, G., Della Pona, C., and Massera, F., Results of surgical mangagement of tuberculosis: experience in 206 patients undergoing operation, *Ann. Thorac. Surg.*, 59, 896, 1995.

202. Yim, A. P. C., The role of video-assisted thoracoscopic surgery in the management of pulmonary tuberculosis, *Chest*, 110, 829, 1996.

203. Iseman, M. D., Madsen, L., Goble, M., et al., Surgical intervention in the treatment of pulmonary disease caused by drug-resistant *Mycobacterium tuberculosis, Am. Rev. Respir. Dis.*, 141, 623, 1990.

204. Johnson, J. R., Turk, T. L., and Macdonald, F. M., Corticosteroids in pulmonary tuberculosis. III. Indications, *Am. Rev. Respir. Dis.*, 96, 62, 1967.

205. Huseby, J. S. and Hudson, L. D., Miliary tuberculosis and adult respiratory distress syndrome, *Ann. Intern. Med.*, 85, 609, 1976.

206. Dyer, R. A., Chappell, W. A., and Potgieter, P. D., Adult respiratory distress syndrome associated with miliary tuberculosis, *Crit. Care Med.*, 13, 12, 1985.

207. Murray, H. W., Tuazon, C. U., Kirmani, N., and Sheagren, J. N., The adult respiratory distress syndrome associated with miliary tuberculosis, *Chest*, 73, 37, 1978.

208. Nemir, R. L., Cardona, J., Vaziri, F., et al., Prednisone as an adjunct in the chemotherapy of lymph node-bronchial tuberculosis in childhood: a double-blind study. II. Further term observation, *Am. Rev. Respir. Dis.*, 95, 402, 1967.

209. Masud, T. and Kemp, E., Corticosteroids in treatment of disseminated tuberculosis in patient with HIV infection, *Br. Med. J.*, 296, 464, 1988.

210. Muthuswamy, P., Hu, T. C., Carasso, B., Antonio, M., and Dandamudi, N., Prednisone as adjunctive therapy in the management of pulmonary tuberculosis: report of 12 cases and review of the literature, *Chest,* 107, 1621, 1995.

211. Wyser, C., Walzl, G., Smedema, J. P., Swart, F., van Schalkwyk, E. M., and van de Wal, B. W., Corticosteroids in the treatment of tuberculous pleurisy: a double-blind, placebo-controlled, randomized study, *Chest*, 110, 333, 1996.

212. Lee, C. H., Wang, W. J., Lan, R. S., Tsai, Y. H., and Chiang, Y. C., Corticosteroids in the treatment of tuberculous pleurisy: a double-blind, placebo-controlled, randomized study, *Chest*, 94, 1256, 1988.

213. Dooley, D. P., Carpenter, J. L., and Rademacher, S., Adjunctive corticosteroid therapy for tuberculosis: a critical reappraisal of the literature, *Clin. Infect. Dis.*, 25, 872, 1997.

7 Extrapulmonary Tuberculosis

Wilfredo Talavera, M.D., Rodolfo Miranda, M.D.,
Klaus-Dieter K. L. Lessnau, M.D., and Ari Klapholz, M.D.

CONTENTS

I. INTRODUCTION

Tuberculosis (TB) in organs other than the lung had been observed for many centuries but was not recognized as such. Skeletal TB was present in Egypt in 3500 B.C.[1] Ancient physicians divided

TABLE 7.1
Historical Terminology

Bouchut's tubercles	Choroidal tubercles in miliary MTB
Eales' disease	Retinal periphlebitis, retinal vasculitis, retinal hemorrhage with possible retinal detachment and neovascularization
Empyema necessitatis	Empyema with invasion of chest wall or lung
Ghon complex	Calcified area in the chest radiograph due to healed primary tuberculosis
Gibbus	Anterior erosion of vertebral bone leads to collapse and sharp kyphosis (Victor Hugo's Quasimodo; latin for hump, convex, protuberant, humpbacked)
Lupus vulgaris	Cutaneous tuberculosis
Phthisis	Wasting syndrome, "consumption"
Poncet's disease	Polyarthritis, hypersensitivity induced
Pott's disease	Vertebral tuberculosis, tuberculous spondylitis, spinal caries
Scrofula	Cervical lymph nodes (king's evil); latin for "glandular swelling"
Spina ventosa	Tuberculous osteitis of the phalanges in children; "ballooned-out" appearance (ventosa)
Tabes mesenterica	Mesenteric tuberculous lymphadenitis

Source: Adapted from Friedman, L. N., *Tuberculosis: Current Concepts and Treatment,* 1st ed., CRC Press LLC, Boca Raton, FL, 1994. With permission.

phthisis (consumption) into many supposedly distinct diseases. Throughout history, extrapulmonary tuberculosis was referred to by many names (Table 7.1), such as Pott's disease of the spine, lupus vulgaris of the skin, and scrofula of the cervical lymph nodes. It was described as an "evil omen" and a disease that "carried men off after their candle had flickered but a short time." The discovery of the tubercle bacillus in 1882 by Robert Koch advanced the understanding of TB as a systemic infection with varying clinical manifestations.

The classic definition of extrapulmonary TB is the tuberculous involvement of an organ outside of the lung. It includes disseminated disease and bacteremia, pleural disease, and intrathoracic lymphatic disease. It may occur in the presence or absence of pulmonary involvement. The course of extrapulmonary TB may be acute and overwhelming, or chronic and slowly progressive over many years, and any organ may be involved. The spectrum of clinical presentations may mimic other systemic diseases and is partly responsible for misdiagnosis and diagnostic delay.

Approximately 10 million of the 250 million people who live in the U.S. are infected with the tubercle bacillus.[2] Each year from 1964 to 1989 there were approximately 20,000 reported new cases of TB of which approximately 20% resulted in extrapulmonary involvement.[3-5] In 1997, there were 19,851 cases of TB reported in the U.S., of which 3554 (17.9%) cases were exclusively extrapulmonary.[6] Of those cases, 41.3% were lymphatic, 20.7% were pleural, 11.2% involved bones or joints, 6.6% were urogenital, 5.2% were meningeal, 4.3% were peritoneal, and 10.7% involved other sites.[6] In developing countries, the annual incidence of tuberculosis was approximately 7 million cases, of which 5 to 10% were extrapulmonary.[7] This apparent underestimation may be due to the difficulty in diagnosis, particularly with the unavailability of advanced technology in some third world countries.[8,9] Between 20 and 50% of cases of extrapulmonary TB are diagnosed at autopsy only.[3,9,10]

Historically, extrapulmonary TB has afflicted children, has decreased in incidence with age, and then has peaked in the elderly.[3] In the post-AIDS era in this country, 1008 patients (22%) with extrapulmonary tuberculosis were older than 65 years old.[11] However, meningitis, lymphadenopathy (scrofula), and miliary disease are more common among children less than 5 years old.[12] Extrapulmonary disease is more common in Hispanics (4-fold), Blacks (6-fold), Asians (11-fold), foreign born, and Native Americans.[3,9]

Specific medical risk factors for extrapulmonary TB include HIV infection with low CD4+ cell counts, immunosuppression, chronic renal disease and hemodialysis,[13,14] bone marrow transplantation,[15] and jejunoileal bypass.[16,17] A questionable risk factor is pregnancy.[18]

Low CD4+ cell counts are associated with a greater probability of extrapulmonary disease in patients with AIDS. For example, mean CD4+ cell counts of 350 have been reported with pulmonary disease, 250 with localized extrapulmonary TB (lymph nodes or effusion), 140 with meningitis, and 70 with bacteremia.[19,20]

It has been estimated that more than 4 million persons worldwide have been infected with both HIV and TB. Two thirds of these patients potentially have extrapulmonary involvement.[21] In the U.S., between 6000 and 9000 new cases of tuberculosis are estimated to occur annually in patients with HIV infection.[22] Extrapulmonary disease appears to be common among patients infected with HIV in this country. Of 292 HIV-positive patients with TB compiled from several retrospective studies, 181 patients (62%) had extrapulmonary TB (with or without pulmonary disease), 216 patients (74%) had pulmonary TB (with or without extrapulmonary disease), and 36% had both.[23] In a retrospective study undertaken at our institution,[24] of 178 cases of TB in HIV-infected patients, 55(31%) had extrapulmonary involvement. In the U.S., during the period of October 1987 through March 1989, 48,712 persons with AIDS were reported to the Centers for Disease Control and Prevention (CDC). Of these, 1239 patients (2.5%) were diagnosed with extrapulmonary tuberculosis.[25]

In patients with AIDS, multiple sites of infection are common. The bacilli may be found in lymph nodes, blood, bone marrow, urinary tract, liver, gastrointestinal tract, central nervous system, cardiovascular system, skin, and soft tissues.[26,27,28] Thus, in HIV-infected patients with persistent undiagnosed fever, a search for extrapulmonary tuberculosis should be undertaken.[29]

In a study of 44 patients with AIDS or ARC and tuberculosis, published by Handwerger et al., 13 patients (29.5%) had extrapulmonary disease alone.[30] In another study of 35 patients with both AIDS and TB, 9 patients (26%) had extrapulmonary disease alone.[31] Both reports were published before the AIDS case definition included extrapulmonary tuberculosis. In 1991, Shafer et al. reported 199 patients with AIDS and extrapulmonary TB at a major New York City hospital; 76 patients (38%) had extrapulmonary involvement alone.[32] More unusual presentations have been seen in HIV-positive patients,[33] such as skeletal disease, scrotal disease, and bacteremia.[34] Miliary and lymphatic disease often are observed, and unusual presentations such as spinal and breast abscesses, and esophagobronchial fistulas have been described.[35] Extrapulmonary TB has become a significant cause of morbidity and mortality in HIV-infected patients in the 1990s.

The diagnosis of extrapulmonary TB often is difficult. The shortest delay in diagnosis is in pleural disease, and the longest is in skeletal disease, probably because tissue is less accessible and symptoms are more subtle.[36] Twenty to fifty percent of extrapulmonary TB is discovered at autopsy, in contrast to 5% of pulmonary TB. Those numbers may be increased in the elderly and in HIV patients.[3,37] Unfortunately there is no inexpensive, rapid, and noninvasive screening test, and a high degree of clinical suspicion is a prerequisite for a timely diagnosis.

Although short-course therapy for pulmonary tuberculosis has been well established, there are few data available on the use of short-course chemotherapy in extrapulmonary tuberculosis. The extrapulmonary site of disease probably is less consequential since the mycobacterial population is smaller in extrapulmonary vs. cavitary pulmonary disease. Dutt et al.[38] reported their experience with short-course chemotherapy in 350 patients with extrapulmonary tuberculosis. Nine-month therapy with isoniazid and rifampin was successful in 95% of patients.[38,39] Cohn et al.[40] reported success with a 62-dose, largely twice-weekly, 6-month tuberculosis treatment regimen in 7 patients with both pulmonary and extrapulmonary disease and 17 patients with extrapulmonary tuberculosis alone who had directly observed therapy. Although it appears that a 6-month short course of therapy may be adequate in selected patients with extrapulmonary tuberculosis, caution must be taken when extrapolating small series of patients. Specific treatment for each extrapulmonary site will be considered below.

II. LYMPH NODES

A. EXTRATHORACIC

1. Epidemiology

Tuberculous lymphadenitis was the most common type of extrapulmonary tuberculosis in the U.S. in 1997. It accounted for 41.3% (1469 patients) of cases of exclusively extrapulmonary disease and 7.4% of all cases of tuberculosis.[6] Historically, tuberculous lymphadenitis has comprised 31% of extrapulmonary disease and 2 to 5% of all cases of TB, of which approximately 70% has been cervical in location.[41-43]

Mycobacterial tuberculous lymphadenitis has been described as a disease of children and often occurs within the first 6 months of infection.[44] Recent studies suggest that the peak incidence now occurs in young adults between the ages of 20 to 40 years.[45-48] This probably reflects the decreasing rate of childhood tuberculosis in developed countries, and in this age group, atypical mycobacteria now predominate.[47,49]

Both sex and ethnicity play a major role in the development of tuberculous lymphadenitis. Most studies show a female to male predominance of greater than 2:1,[42,49,50] and in the developed world, Indian, Asian, and Blacks, especially women, appear to be predisposed.[43,45,49,51] Considering that pulmonary tuberculosis is more common in males, this female preponderance is paradoxical.[3]

An additional risk factor for the development of tuberculous lymphadenitis is HIV infection. In fact, lymphadenopathy is a prominent feature in patients with AIDS and tuberculosis. Peripheral tuberculous lymphadenopathy occurs in 22 to 31% of patients with AIDS.[31,32,52,53]

2. Clinical

The cervical form of this disease, or scrofula, was well recognized by the 17th century in Europe, where it was called the "King's evil," because of the belief that it could be cured by the hands of a sovereign. Charles II of England is reputed to have applied the "royal touch" to the scrofulous over 90,000 times.[54]

Tuberculous lymphadenitis may represent a localized process or an expression of disseminated disease. In adults, most cases are due to reactivation of the initial lymphatic spread of primary pulmonary infection.[55,56] Seventy percent of patients with tuberculous lymphadenitis have cervical lymph node involvement. Sixty percent of reported cases are unilateral.[41] This may include both the anterior and posterior cervical chains.[42,57] Bilateral cervical lymphadenitis is uncommon, accounting for less than 10% of cases.[42] Enlarged lymph nodes also may affect the submandibular region, the supraclavicular space, the superior portion of the neck, and the submental and preauricular areas.[45,46] Cervical lymph nodes may be isolated, may extend from an adjacent focus, such as intrathoracic or paratracheal lymph nodes, may develop from subclinical pulmonary disease, or hematogenously from an unrecognized site.[41,51] Infected tonsils or adenoids may be a focus.[41]

Typically, there is slow, painless enlargement in the neck.[46] The nodes are usually discrete and "rubbery-soft" to palpation. As the disease progresses there may be significant induration, fluctuance, and necrosis, and a sinus tract may form.[43,45,49,58] Progression to draining sinus tracts occurs in less than 10% of patients.[42,49,59] In a study by Malik and others, the average size of lymph nodes on biopsy was 5 × 5 cm (range, 2 to 8 cm), and the average number of nodes found was four.[58]

Tuberculous lymphadenitis may be bilateral, but diffuse lymphadenopathy is distinctly uncommon,[49] unless associated with childhood miliary tuberculosis.[60] Systemic symptoms such as fever, weight loss, anorexia, and fatigue occur in less than 20% of patients,[45] but in a recent study of 47 patients (including 10 patients with HIV disease), 43% had systemic symptoms.[59] Constitutional symptoms seem to be more common in HIV patients.[32] When isolated peripheral lymphadenopathy is seen, such as in the epitrochlear, axillary, or inguinal regions, a more distal focus must be identified.[61]

Other less common presentations of tuberculous lymphadenopathy may occur. These include chronic abdominal pain from retroperitoneal lymph node involvement, jaundice from biliary tract obstruction, and generalized lymphadenopathy mimicking neoplasia.[62]

In a study by Shafer et al. of 199 HIV-positive patients with extrapulmonary tuberculosis, 44 patients (22%) had peripheral lymphadenopathy. Of this group 37 patients (84%) had cervical disease, 8 patients (18%) had axillary disease, and 1 patient (2.3%) had inguinal disease. In the majority of these patients, the clinical presentation was dominated by systemic symptoms. Only 20 of these patients (45%) had symptoms referable to enlarged lymph nodes. This suggests that the lymphadenopathy is only one facet of a more generalized process. An additional 24 patients (12%) had intraabdominal lymphadenopathy which was present invariably with disseminated tuberculosis.[32]

3. Diagnosis

Since the differential diagnosis of tuberculous lymphadenopathy is vast, many other conditions including infections and neoplasia must be considered before rendering empiric therapy. A careful history, chest radiograph, and tuberculin skin test are important in the evaluation of the patient with suspected tuberculous lymphadenitis. Less than 20% of adults have a history of exposure to tuberculosis,[45] and 24 to 46% of patients have chest radiographic abnormalities consistent with tuberculosis.[42,45,59] Tuberculin skin testing may be positive in 90% of patients unless the patient is HIV positive.[41,42,45,46,51,59] If the diagnosis of tuberculous lymphadenitis remains in doubt, a lymph node biopsy with AFB smear, culture, and histological evaluation is required.

Total excisional biopsy has been long recommended since incomplete excision may result in chronic fistulous tract formation.[43,51] With the chemotherapeutic armamentarium presently available, needle biopsy or aspiration may be safe[63-65] in most cases of cervical tuberculous lymphadenitis. Cervical abscess formation may require total excisional surgery. In a study of 40 patients with tuberculous cervical abscesses, 17 (77%) of the 22 patients who had a simple drainage procedure required a second operation because of sinus tract formation. Of those having a complete excisional procedure, 17 (94%) of 18 patients required no further surgical intervention.[66]

In a study by Dandapat et al. of 80 cases of peripheral tuberculous lymphadenitis, fine-needle aspiration (FNA) provided a positive diagnosis in 66 patients (83%) including a positive culture in 52 patients (65%). Biopsy of the largest affected lymph node gave histological confirmation in 100%.[57] In another study, FNA or biopsy of cervical lymph nodes showed caseous material and/or granulomas in 80% of patients and culture positivity in 60% of patients.[67] The yield of AFB smear positivity of tuberculous lymph nodes varied from 35 to 56%.[42,57,59]

FNA of lymph nodes usually is diagnostic in the HIV-positive population and should be used as the initial diagnostic procedure.[26] In a study by Shriner et al., all FNAs performed were diagnostic for tuberculosis.[41] In HIV-positive patients the smear is positive in 70 to 90% of patients,[32,53,41,68] and culture positivity reaches 90 to 100%.[32,53,41] This undoubtedly reflects a higher burden of organisms in patients with low CD4+ cell counts.[53] Lymph node biopsies are diagnostic in approximately 90% of patients,[32] and offer little advantage over FNA in this group. Lymph node aspiration is a simple, rapid, and inexpensive diagnostic procedure in HIV-positive patients with peripheral nodes equal to or larger than 1.5 cm.[68] Note that although FNA is a practical, cost-effective alternative to excisional biopsy and may also lead to a rapid diagnosis, it has not been shown to be superior to excisional biopsy. Excisional biopsy remains the diagnostic procedure of choice in HIV-negative patients, since FNA appears to result in a low diagnostic yield in this population of patients.[69]

Thoracic and abdominal sonography, computed tomography (CT) of the chest and abdomen, and whole-body gallium scanning are useful adjuncts in detecting mediastinal, hilar, and intraabdominal lymph nodes and helpful in directing biopsies or aspiration.[70-73]

4. Treatment

Treatment of tuberculous lymphadenopathy includes antimicrobial therapy and the judicious use of surgical excision in selected patients. Nine months of isoniazid (INH) and rifampin (RIF), supplemented initially by 2 months of ethambutol, has been shown to be effective therapy with excellent response rates in most studies.[57,63,74,75] Another study showed that 6 months of INH, RIF, pyrazinamide (PZA), and streptomycin was similar to a 9-month, 3-drug regimen.[76] However, the incidence of residual enlarged lymph nodes varied from 5% to 14.5%.[41,63,76] In some patients, extension of therapy up to 18 months was required before most lymph nodes regressed.[58]

5. Complications

Complete surgical excision can relieve discomfort caused by enlarging lymph nodes and may be helpful with scars or fistulas that do not improve with 6 months of therapy.[59,75] Incision and drainage may be required with cervical abscesses.[66] A second procedure may be necessary when there is persistent discharge, recurrent abscesses, or increasing lymphadenopathy.[64] Excision alone without antituberculous therapy has a relapse rate of 83%.[75,77] During therapy, lymph nodes may enlarge or new nodes may develop. These often are transient and do not necessarily indicate relapse or treatment failure.[49]

B. Intrathoracic

Intrathoracic lymphadenopathy is an uncommon manifestation of adult tuberculosis, although it is quite common in children.[49] In a study by Silver and Steel, intrathoracic tuberculous lymphadenopathy has been found to be more common in Asians and Blacks.[78] Although mediastinal nodes are the most common primary regional draining sites, they account for only 5% of lymph node tuberculosis.[54]

In adults, enlarging lymph nodes rarely lead to luminal obstruction with respiratory symptoms such as cough, sputum production, localized wheezing, and dyspnea. Usually, fever, weight loss, anorexia, night sweats, and fatigue prevail. The patient may be asymptomatic with an abnormal chest radiograph.[79,80] Two thirds of mediastinal nodes involve the right paratracheal region.[81]

HIV-positive patients with suspected intrathoracic tuberculous lymphadenopathy frequently have palpable extrathoracic lymph nodes.[69] Hilar lymphadenopathy occurred in 33 to 40% of patients in several studies.[52,53,82,83] In a study of 199 patients with AIDS and extrapulmonary tuberculosis by Shafer et al., 28 patients (14%) had mediastinal tuberculosis diagnosed at mediastinoscopy or at autopsy. CT scanning was very useful in assessing the various groups of lymph nodes involved, and in finding low central density areas consistent with necrosis.[32] Endobronchial obstruction from mediastinal lymphadenopathy, mimicking lung cancer, can occur in patients with AIDS.[84]

In intrathoracic lymphadenopathy due to tuberculosis, mediastinoscopy and fiberoptic bronchoscopy may be useful. The latter, when coupled with brush and bronchial biopsy, has a diagnostic yield of 75%.[85] This high yield has been explained by the presence of endobronchial disease. Mediastinoscopy or exploratory thoracotomy rarely is required for diagnosis.

Treatment comprises standard antituberculous chemotherapy including isoniazid, rifampin, and ethambutol or pyrazinamide.[75,86]

Severe complications such as rupture of a lymph node into adjacent tissue including the esophagus, bronchus, superior vena cava, aorta, and pericardium may occur. Local nerve compression may cause Horner syndrome[76] or unilateral laryngeal palsy with hoarseness.[49]

III. PLEURA

A. Epidemiology

Worldwide, tuberculosis still is a significant cause of pleural effusions. In some parts of the world (e.g., Spain, Rwanda), tuberculosis remains the most frequent cause of pleural effusions in the absence of an obvious pulmonary lesion.[87,88] In the U.S., tuberculosis is responsible for only a small percentage of all pleural effusions, the incidence varying from less than 1 to 13% of all exudative

TABLE 7.2
Pleural Tuberculosis

Characteristic	Percentage and References
Clinical	
Weight loss (>5 kg)	28–35[93,105]
Night sweats	46[105]
Dyspnea	38–52[93,105]
Cough	55–80[92,93,105]
Chest pain	50–75[92,105]
Leukocytosis (>10,000/mm³)	5–15[92,102]
Insidious onset	33[92,102]
Acute onset and pain	67[92,102]
Symptoms <1 week	31–62[92,102]
Symptoms <1 month	62[102]
Fever	65–85[92,93,105]
More than 50% lymphocytes in effusion	62–90[92,93]
Radiography	
Unilateral effusion	90[92,93,105]
Hemorrhagic effusion	2–9[92]
Radiographic pulmonary lesion	
CXR	22–35[92,105]
CT	80[104]
Stain	
Sputum	7–8[92,107]
Pleural fluid	0–9[93,107]
Pleural biopsy	21–39[92,107]
Pathology	
Pleural biopsy	57–97[92,93,107]
Culture	
Sputum (without infiltrate)	4–11[91,93]
Sputum (with infiltrate)	18–89[91,97,105]
Thoracentesis	23–60[91-93,105,107]
Pleural biopsy (only culture)	39–65[92,93,107]
Pleural biopsy (culture and pathology)	90[114]

Source: Adapted from Friedman, L. N., Ed., *Tuberculosis: Current Concepts and Treatment,* 1st ed., CRC Press LLC, Boca Raton, FL, 1994. With permission.

effusions.[89,90] In a study of 1738 cases of pulmonary tuberculosis, 70 patients (4.9%) with tuberculous effusions were identified.[91] In 1997, of all cases that were exclusively extrapulmonary, 20.7% were pleural.[6] Pleural TB may affect any age group, although there are peaks at 20 to 40 years and in the elderly population.[92,93]

B. CLINICAL

The clinical and laboratory characteristics of pleural tuberculosis are included in Table 7.2. Tuberculous pleurisy frequently is associated with primary disease and, in those instances, results from the rupture of a subpleural caseous focus, which may not be evident radiographically.[94,95] It also may result secondarily from intrapulmonary cavitary disease or lymphohematogenous dissemination, or spread from an adjacent source, e.g., lymph node or spine.[94] Tuberculous pleuritis traditionally has been regarded as a manifestation of primary tuberculosis. However, a study in Edinburgh[96] has shown that tuberculous pleural effusions are more common in reactivation (64%) than in primary disease. In a study by Antoniskis et al.,[97] tuberculous pleurisy was a manifestation of reactivation in 27 of 59 patients (46%), altering the classic view of the pathogenesis of tuberculous effusions. This study also suggests that these patients are less capable of mounting an effective immunologic response to the tubercle bacillus.

Delayed hypersensitivity appears to play a pivotal role in the pathogenesis of tuberculous pleuritis. When tuberculin protein is injected into the pleural space of previously immunized laboratory animals, a large exudative effusion results within 2 days. It is likely that delayed hypersensitivity also plays a major role in the development of tuberculous pleuritis in humans, and explains the small bacterial load seen. Thus, the yield of smears and cultures of the pleural fluid is expected to be low. The intense inflammatory reaction obstructs the lymphatic pores of the parietal pleura and explains the high biopsy yield.[95]

Typically, a tuberculous pleural effusion occurs 3 to 6 months after the primary infection,[98] but it may occur with postprimary (i.e., reactivated) disease. In HIV-positive patients, it may appear as early as 4 to 12 weeks after the initial infection.[99]

The natural history of an untreated isolated tuberculous effusion is spontaneous resolution, only to recur as active parenchymal disease at a later date.[95] In a Finnish Armed Forces study of 2816 men with undiagnosed pleural effusions, 43% developed tuberculosis during a 7-year follow-up period.[100] In another study by Roper and Waring[101] of 141 military personnel with a positive purified protein derivative (PPD) and a pleural effusion, most patients completely reabsorbed their effusions and became asymptomatic within 2 to 4 months. This response required prolonged bed rest and most recuperated with minimal chest radiographic changes and minimal pleural thickening. Ninety-two of these 141 individuals (65%) developed active tuberculosis within 5 years, 88% of these within 3 years. This proclivity for the development of subsequent active tuberculosis makes it imperative to treat those with documented or presumed tuberculous pleuritis.

The onset of pleurisy is typically abrupt and may resemble bacterial pneumonia with fever and a dry cough. The onset of effusion is acute in approximately two thirds of patients.[92,102] Effusions usually are small or moderate in size, but may involve the entire hemithorax. Massive effusions occur in 14 to 29% of patients with primary disease.[92] More than 90% of effusions are unilateral, and bilateral effusions usually are associated with miliary spread.[92,93] Effusions more commonly were present on the left side in 57% of patients in a study by Berger and Mejia,[92] but more commonly on the right side in 65% of patients in a study by Epstein et al.[93] The primary pulmonary focus often is undetectable on chest radiograph, but in a study of 70 patients with pleural tuberculosis, 50% had an accompanying infiltrate.[91] Chest radiographs also may aid in classifying the disease as primary or reactivation. Lower lung infiltrates with hilar adenopathy suggest primary infection, whereas upper lobe involvement suggests reactivation. Upper lobe infiltrates may be seen in as much as 20% of those with primary disease.[103] The chest CT scan is especially useful in those patients with no obvious parenchymal disease on conventional chest radiograph. In one study of 14 such patients, 11 patients (78.5%) had additional cavities or parenchymal infiltrates on CT scan. Sites of communication between the parenchyma and pleural space also were demonstrated.[104]

Tuberculous pleuritis has been reported in 9 to 20% of patients with HIV infection and tuberculosis.[32,52,53] In one study, tuberculous effusions in patients with AIDS often were a manifestation of a disseminated process.[105] In a study of 199 HIV-positive patients with extrapulmonary TB, 32 patients (16%) had pleural effusions; 75% of whom had respiratory symptoms including cough, pleuritic chest pain, and dyspnea. Most effusions were present on admission, but, in nine patients (28%), the effusions developed during the hospital stay. The effusions invariably were exudative, were bilateral in six patients (15.6%), and were more likely to be culture positive (91%).[32]

Extrapulmonary tuberculosis is more common in HIV patients, and as many as 37% of such patients develop pleural reactions.[53] In one study, pleural reactions were seen more frequently in the HIV population with tuberculosis, i.e., 11% vs. 6%.[106]

C. DIAGNOSIS

An unexplained exudative pleural effusion in the presence of a positive PPD skin test may suggest that more aggressive measures are needed to diagnose tuberculous pleurisy, but a negative skin test does not eliminate its possibility. Tuberculin skin test positivity in tuberculous pleurisy, as reflected in several studies, ranges from 47 to 93%.[91-93,97,105,107] In a study of tuberculous pleurisy by Berger and Mejia,[92] 11 of 36 patients (30.5%) had a negative intermediate tuberculin skin test. Upon retesting, all patients converted their skin test to positive. This skin test negativity has been attributed to sequestration of specific T-lymphocytes in the pleural space.[108] In some patients the negative skin test may represent true anergy. We recommend retesting patients with a suspected tuberculous effusion and a negative tuberculin skin test in 4 to 8 weeks.

The diagnosis is made definitively by a positive culture from pleural tissue or pleural fluid, and presumptively by a positive sputum culture along with appropriate radiographic findings. The effusion almost always is exudative, may be serosanguinous on occasion, and rarely is grossly bloody. The protein content invariably is greater than 3 g/dl and in 77% of patients is greater than 5 g/dl. The lactate dehydrogenase (LDH) levels are elevated.[92] Although in the past, pleural fluid glucose levels were thought to be low, more recent studies[92,93] demonstrate that most effusions have glucose levels greater than 60 mg/dl; levels less than 30 mg/dl occur rarely. The pleural pH may range from 7.00 to 7.50, paralleling the pleural glucose levels, but often is nonspecific.[95] Pleural fluid that is exudative by LDH criteria alone, that is bloody (RBC > 100,000/mm^3), that has more than 10% eosinophils, or that has more than 1% mesothelial cells is unlikely to be tuberculous.[90,92,109-113]

During an early tuberculous effusion, neutrophils (PMNs) predominate. Monocytes increase between days 2 and 5. After 6 days, the classic finding of small lymphocytes, which constitute less than 50% of cells, are present in 90% of effusions.[91,93,95,114] Subsequent thoracenteses show a greater proportion of smaller lymphocytes as the disease becomes chronic.[92] The CD4+ lymphocytes are elevated[108] and eosinophils rarely are seen. Mesothelial cells typically are absent in tuberculous pleurisy. They usually are decreased with extensive pleural inflammation and increased with neoplasia; therefore, their presence or absence is nondiagnostic.[95]

Proposed rapid methods for diagnosing tuberculous pleurisy involve assaying products of T-lymphocyte activation or mycobacterial markers. Measurement of adenosine deaminase (ADA) levels in pleural effusions are useful in ascertaining the diagnosis of tuberculous pleuritis, although not readily used in this country. This enzyme is a product of activated T-lymphocytes and, therefore, is elevated where cellular immunity is stimulated. ADA levels in tuberculous effusions have a sensitivity and specificity of 80%. Levels above 70 U/l are 90% specific and levels below 40 U/l have not been observed in TB.[115,116] Similar results have been reported by Fontan-Bueso[87] in 138 patients with tuberculous and malignant effusions. In the same study, a ratio of pleural fluid to serum lysozyme above 1.2 was found to be 80% sensitive and specific, and was especially helpful when used in conjunction with ADA. Measurement of pleural fluid lysozyme may be useful in differentiating tuberculous from malignant effusions. False-positive ADA tests have been observed in rheumatoid disease, undifferentiated lymphoma, and chronic lymphatic leukemia.[117,118] ADA activity will have a high positive predictive value in circumstances where the incidence of tuberculosis exceeds any other cause of a lymphocytic pleural effusion.[119] One day, γ-interferon levels and SC5b-9, generated by the activation of complement and measured by a simple and rapid enzyme immunoassay, may be useful diagnostic tools.[120,121] γ-interferon levels are as sensitive and specific as ADA activity but are more expensive.[120] Amplification of mycobacterial DNA by the use of the polymerase chain reaction (PCR) is a rapid and sensitive diagnostic test for TB. In a study evaluating 84 patients with pleural effusions, including 53 patients with TB, the sensitivity of PCR for tuberculous pleural fluid was 81%. The sensitivity of pleural fluid culture, pleural biopsy culture, and histology of the biopsy was 52.8%, 69.8%, and 77.3%, respectively.[122] The advantage of PCR is that it does not require an intact immune system and it is very specific.[123]

Since a definitive diagnosis of tuberculous pleurisy requires demonstration of the tubercle bacilli in the sputum, pleural fluid, or pleural biopsy, these specimens should be cultured for mycobacteria whenever this condition is suspected. Chan et al.[107] reported 83 patients with tuberculous effusions, 7 (8%) of whom were sputum smear-positive and 18 (22%) were culture positive. The percentage of positive sputum cultures is dependent on the presence or absence of concomitant parenchymal infiltration. Cultures were more likely to be positive if there was underlying parenchymal disease (see Table 7.2).

The recovery of the tubercle bacilli from smear and culture of pleural fluid varies substantially depending on the study (see Table 7.2). They are demonstrable on smear in less than 10% of cases.[93] In most series, pleural fluid cultures show *Mycobacterium tuberculous* in approximately 25% of cases, but some studies show yields as much as 66%.[91-93,105,107] The diagnostic yield improves with large fluid samples and centrifugation.[124]

Parietal pleural biopsy is diagnostic, i.e., positive smear, culture, or granuloma formation, in 70 to 95% of cases, depending on the technique employed.[91,107] The smear of the biopsy specimen has been shown to be positive in 21 to 39% of cases,[92,107] the culture in 39 to 65% of cases,[92,93,107] and granulomas have been identified in 57 to 97% of cases.[92,93,107] When the microscopic examination of the biopsy specimen is combined with biopsy culture, the diagnosis can be made in 90% of patients,[114] especially with the use of multiple biopsies.[95,125,126] We recommend that a thoracentesis and a minimum of three pleural biopsy specimens for culture and histology be obtained when tuberculous pleuritis is suspected.

Pleuroscopy, or thoracoscopy, is a safe, rapid, and useful adjunct to the diagnosis of tuberculous pleurisy due to direct visualization of affected tissue. It may obviate the need for open pleural biopsy and, as a result, may decrease complications.[127,128] In a study by Sarkar et al. of 40 patients with undiagnosed pleural effusions, a diagnosis of tuberculosis was made by pleuroscopic biopsy in 17 patients (42.5%). The yield for tuberculosis was 100% and the overall specific diagnostic yield in this study was 92.5%.[127] The pleuroscopic findings included hyperemia, shiny opalescent pleural thickening and small white-gray tubercular nodules.[127,129] In another study, thoracoscopic pleural biopsy had a yield of 90%.[129] Open thoracotomy for pleural biopsy rarely is necessary today.

D. Treatment

The goals of therapy of tuberculous effusions are to prevent the subsequent development of active pulmonary disease, to relieve the patient's symptoms and to prevent associated complications.[95]

Nine-month therapy with INH (300 mg) and RIF (600 mg) daily is a highly efficacious regimen with no relapses.[130] Standard 6-month therapy is equally efficacious,[40] with extension to 9 months in patients with AIDS.[131]

Even shorter durations of therapy may be effective in the management of tuberculous effusions. In a study by Dutt et al., 198 patients with tuberculous effusions were treated with INH (300 mg) and RIF (600 mg) daily for 1 month followed by INH (900 mg) plus RIF (600 mg) twice weekly for an additional 5 months. There were no relapses in the 161 patients who completed therapy, and side effects occurred in only 6.6% of patients. The therapy was efficacious even in the presence of a parenchymal infiltrate.[132]

With appropriate treatment, symptoms and signs of the disease slowly subside. Most patients are afebrile by the second week of therapy, but fever persists for as much as 2 months in some patients. Radiologic resolution occurs at approximately 6 weeks but may take as long as 12 weeks in some patients.[133] Tuberculous effusions have been treated with a combination of antimicrobials and corticosteroids, with more rapid improvement in signs and symptoms. Lee et al.,[134] in a double-blind, prospective, randomized study showed that resolution of clinical symptoms and pleural fluid was greater in the group receiving corticosteroids. The effusions were not drained and the development of residual pleural thickening was not influenced by the use of corticosteroids. However, in a study by Wyser et al., after complete drainage of the effusions, corticosteroids did not appear to influence symptoms, resolution of the pleural effusion, residual pleural thickening, or pulmonary function.[135] Once a definitive diagnosis is established and therapy is prescribed, corticosteroid therapy may be beneficial if symptoms are severe or if the pleural effusion is particularly large, but cannot be recommended routinely.

E. COMPLICATIONS

The most common sequelum of tuberculous pleuritis is residual pleural thickening, which usually is present upon diagnosis and may be seen in as much as 50% of patients after treatment. Repeated thoracenteses are indicated only for the relief of symptomatic effusions since they do not diminish the amount of residual pleural thickening.[136] Chest tube drainage is useful primarily for the treatment of empyemas and bronchopleural fistulas. Pleurectomy or decortication rarely may be required for a "trapped lung" resulting from a thick fibrin peel.[107,137]

Tuberculous empyema is characterized by a purulent exudate and numerous organisms on smear. Although historically, it is a consequence of previous pleurisy, collapse pneumothorax therapy or thoracoplasty, tuberculous empyema may result from the rupture of an underlying cavity.[95] Tuberculous empyema may occur alone or as a "mixed" empyema with superinfection by anaerobic bacteria such as bacteroides species. Repeated thoracenteses or chest tube insertion have been used, but may lead to a mixed infection.[138] Surgical intervention with decortication, thoracoplasty, extrapleural pneumonectomy, or an Eloesser flap may be required.[95,139] Repeated thoracentesis and 24 months of triple drug therapy without tube drainage or surgery has been succesful in nonsurgical candidates.[140] In patients with AIDS, tuberculous empyema may be the result of lymphohematogenous dissemination; a subpleural caseous focus or bronchopleural fistula may not be present.[141] More serious complications include empyema necessitatis, which may burrow through the parietal pleura, esophagus, retroperitoneum, flank, groin, pericardium, or vertebral column.[142] A chylothorax, due to obstruction of the thoracic duct, also may be seen with *Mycobacterium tuberculosis*.[143]

Tuberculous bronchopleural fistulas are uncommon today and usually can be managed with antituberculous therapy. Like tuberculous empyemas, they occur primarily in those who were treated prior to effective chemotherapy.[95,139] Shafer et al. reported 32 HIV-infected patients with pleural tuberculosis, of whom 3 (9.4%) developed a bronchopleural fistula.[32] A bronchopleural fistula with pneumothorax usually requires closed chest tube drainage but definitive surgical management may be necessary.[139]

Non-Hodgkin's lymphoma and pleural sarcoma have been reported after complicated tuberculous pleurisy or therapeutic pneumothorax.[144-146] They occur 15 to 50 years after the development of tuberculous pleurisy and are attributed to chronic inflammation.[147]

IV. SKELETAL

A. VERTEBRAL

1. Epidemiology

Skeletal tuberculous was the third most common type of extrapulmonary tuberculosis in the U.S. in 1997.[6] It accounted for 11.2% (399 patients) of all cases of exclusively extrapulmonary disease and 2% of all cases of tuberculosis.[6] Previously, bone and joint tuberculosis occurred primarily in children afflicted with pulmonary tuberculosis.[44] Today it is a disease of the elderly in America and Europe, but still is a disease of children in developing countries.[148] The incidence of skeletal tuberculosis in patients with HIV infection largely is unknown. In several series of HIV-related tuberculosis, 0 to 9% of patients had bone or joint involvement.[20,31,32,52] Skeletal TB remains an important crippling disease worldwide.

Skeletal tuberculosis typically involves the vertebrae as well as the weight-bearing bones and joints. Farer et al. in a retrospective study published in 1979 noted 676 cases of bone and joint tuberculosis. The spine was involved in 40.7% of cases, the hips in 13.3% of cases, the knees in 10.3% of cases, and other areas such as ankles, long bones, wrist, elbow, shoulder, ribs, sacroiliac joint, foot, and hand in 35.7% of cases. This disease process may involve any bone or joint.[54,149] Recent statistics have shown spinal involvement in 50% of patients (50% thoracic, 25% cervical, 25% lumbar); pelvic involvement in 12%; hip and femur involvement in 10%; rib involvement in 7%; ankle, shoulder, elbow, or wrist involvement in 2%; and multiple site involvement in 3% of cases.[150]

2. Clinical

Vertebral TB or Pott's disease usually results from lymphohematogenous dissemination from a primary focus such as lung. It also may result from direct invasion of a paravertebral focus, or lymphangitic spread from paravertebral lymph nodes or the pleural space.[149] Mechanical factors seem to play a role in the pathogenesis, and it has been suggested that trauma is responsible for this increased susceptibility of weight-bearing joints.[149]

The basic lesion in skeletal tuberculosis is a combination of osteomyelitis and arthritis. Involvement of the joint space may occur from an adjacent epiphyseal bone or through hematogenous dissemination. Early synovitis, granulation tissue, and effusion ensues. Destruction of cartilage, bone demineralization, and caseation necrosis eventually occur. The cartilage is destroyed peripherally first, preserving the integrity of the joint space. The proteolytic enzymes that usually destroy cartilage, as in pyogenic processes, are not produced in tuberculous infections. Focal osteolysis and marginal sclerosis are other features which differentiate it from nontuberculous infections.[151] At this early stage, intermittent pain and tenderness over the affected area are seen.[149,152]

Later, as paraosseous abscesses form and gibbus formation occurs due to the collapse of adjacent vertebrae and narrowing of the disk space, an increase in pain is noted.[149,152] Paravertebral abscesses are "cold" (i.e., without erythema or warmth), may be fluctuant, and either nontender or slightly painful on palpation. They may descend and involve caudal areas, may extend along fascial planes to the retroperitoneal, inguinal, gluteal, or pelvic regions, or rarely as far as the popliteal space. They may form a psoas abscess, and even pleural, cervical, and supraclavicular soft tissue masses have been described.[148] Regardless of location, abscesses may calcify after 1 to 2 years. In the late stage the lesions may disseminate or heal spontaneously with fibrosis and ankylosis.[149,152] Complete destruction with collapse of the vertebral body, kyphosis and adjacent arthritis eventually ensues.[152]

The midthoracic spine is the area most frequently involved. In the child there is a tendency toward upper or cervical spine involvement, while in the adult, infection of the lower thoracic and lumbar spine predominates.[148,152,153] In nonwhites, tuberculous spondylitis has a more atypical presentation involving multiple singular vertebral bodies, primarily on the posterior part of the vertebrae.[154]

Pain is the most common complaint noted, but sinus drainage, joint swelling, and limitation of motion also may be seen. Systemic symptoms such as fever, chills, weight loss, and fatigue are present in only 20% of patients with skeletal tuberculosis.[148] Characteristically, the onset is insidious, developing 2 to 3 years after primary infection.[98] Extensive destruction of the spine may lead to various neurologic syndromes, including paralysis.

Skeletal tuberculosis as a manifestation of AIDS has not been well described. Despite frequent bone marrow involvement in patients with AIDS, tuberculous bone and joint infections are uncommon.[32] One case report described a patient with multifocal osteitis,[155] and another study described two patients with psoas abscess formation.[30]

3. Diagnostic

Early diagnosis is critical to the preservation of the cartilage and joint space. Prompt diagnosis and treatment allows for maintenance of good joint function. The chronicity of the complaints attributable to tuberculous spondylitis may lead to a delay in diagnosis from 4 months to 2 years.[156]

Although skin test results are reported variably in the literature, available data suggests that positivity occurs in 76 to 100% of patients.[148,153] As many as 58% of patients have normal chest radiographs.[157]

Radiographic techniques are of benefit in the diagnosis and treatment of tuberculous spondylitis (see Chapter 10). A paravertebral mass can be seen on chest or abdominal roentgenogram, although there is a greater likelihood of detection with CT scanning.[152] Lesions are evaluated better by CT scanning or magnetic resonance imaging (MRI) techniques.[157,158] CT findings in 11 patients with tuberculosis of the spine have included vertebral body destruction (10 patients), psoas or paraspinous abscesses (10 patients), and intervertebral disk space narrowing (6 patients).[157] Atypical cases may be seen.[159] Bone scintigraphy with technetium is more sensitive than radiographs and useful in early stages,[152] but may be negative in 35% of patients with spinal tuberculosis.[153] Scanning with gallium occasionally may show unsuspected sites not detected by bone scanning and clinical evaluation,[160] but in one study was negative in 70% of patients with tuberculous spondylitis.[153]

Confirmation of tuberculous spondylitis requires microbiological confirmation as early as possible to avoid an unnecessary delay in treatment. Although, historically, it is a disease requiring surgical intervention for diagnosis, tuberculosis of the spine occasionally may be diagnosed by fine-needle aspiration.[161]

Tuberculous spondylitis is characterized by an uncommonly small mycobacterial population.[162] In some cases, even with extensive surgery and large amounts of abscess fluid, cultures are positive in only 40%,[148,162] although if infected bone is obtained, the yield has been shown to be 80 to 95%.[148] In one study, a positive smear was obtained in 30% of cases, and granulomas were present in 90% of specimens obtained.[36] A percutaneous needle biopsy may supplant surgery for diagnosis in early cases.[36]

4. Treatment

In general, response to medical therapy usually is complete although large lesions may require drainage. The British Medical Research Council has undertaken several clinical trials in the treatment of tuberculous spondylitis. Chemotherapy with isoniazid, PAS, and streptomycin plus a radical procedure (Hong Kong operation) with extensive debridement and autologous bone grafting achieved a favorable response at 18 months (89%) and was essentially the same during the 5-year follow-up period. Eighteen months of chemotherapy alone led to a favorable response at 18 months (67%), at 3 years (85%), and at 5 years (88%). On the basis of these results, it has been recommended that tuberculous spondylitis is best treated by a combination of chemotherapy and the Hong Kong procedure.[162]

The chemotherapy used today clearly is superior to the regimens used in the British Medical Research Council trials. Although tuberculosis authorities have recommended treatment of all forms of extrapulmonary tuberculosis with a shorter course regimen employing INH, RIF, and PZA for a period of 6 to 9 months, its efficacy in skeletal tuberculosis has yet to be proved.[163] Dutt et al. found that when short-course therapy with INH and RIF was employed in 21 patients with Pott's disease, 4 patients (19%) failed therapy. Six additional patients required radical surgery early in the course of therapy.[38] In another study by Omari et al. of 19 patients with Pott's disease treated with INH, RIF, and ethambutol (EMB), 8 patients (42%) still required surgery for progressive neurologic deficits, spinal deformities, progressive enlargement of psoas abscesses, and poor response to medical therapy.[157]

Most patients with Pott's disease will respond to conventional antituberculous chemotherapy. Standard treatment with INH, RIF, and PZA in the first 2 months and INH and RIF over 6 to 9 months is sufficient for those without neurologic deficit.[152] Whether therapy should be continued for 2 years for some patients remains to be determined.[152] If medical therapy alone is employed, careful medical and radiologic assessment must be undertaken if treatment failure and progressive neurologic deterioration is to be identified.[148] With acute or progressive neurologic deficits, immediate surgery for decompression is required.[152] Restoration, especially of the vertebral spine, can be astonishing; however, destruction of the joints often is permanent.[152] A trial of empiric therapy is reasonable if a biopsy or surgery otherwise is contraindicated.

5. Complications

Complications include kyphosis with typical gibbus formation, fistulas, superinfection, myelopathy, cold abscess, and spinal cord compression with radiculopathy or even paraplegia.[148,152]

The paralysis of Pott's disease remains the most serious complication of tuberculous spondylitis and may occur early or late in the course of the disease. Early paralysis during active disease may respond to medical therapy alone. Paralysis associated with healed disease is problematic and almost always is associated with kyphosis. Surgical success is neither uniform nor complete.[162]

B. Foot and Ankle

Tuberculosis of the foot and ankle is much less common than disease of the spine, hip, and knee.[164] It accounts for less than 10% of all skeletal TB, and between 0.1% and 0.3% of all extrapulmonary cases.[165] The spectrum of clinical presentations of tuberculosis of the bones and joints of the foot and ankle includes soft tissue infections, arthritis, synovitis, and osteomyelitis.[164,166] Not uncommonly, bone disease spreads to the neighboring joint space.[166] Tuberculous synovitis, especially of the ankle, also may result. In a review of 200 cases of adult skeletal tuberculosis diagnosed between 1930 and 1970,[166] there were 13 patients with disease of the foot distal to the tarsus. Of these 13 cases, 3 had soft tissue involvement, 6 had metatarsal joint involvement, and 4 had metatarsal-phalangeal joint involvement. Additionally, Dhillon et al.,[165] have reported 22 cases of TB of the bones and joints of the foot evaluated between 1989 and 1992. The site of involvement included the calcaneus in 5 cases alone, and 2 additional cases with involvement of the talus and metatarsus. There were 4 cases of metatarsal TB and one case of cuboidal TB. The ankle joint was involved in 8 cases, and there was one case each of talonavicular joint and tarsometatarsal joint involvement. In a review by Martini et al,.[167] of 125 patients with tuberculous osteomyelitis, 20 cases were found to have involvement of the foot. Of these 20 cases, 10 involved the calcaneus, 2 involved the talus, 6 involved the metatarsals, and 2 involved the phalanges (toes).

Tuberculosis of the foot and ankle normally occurs as a result of hematogenous dissemination at the time of the initial pulmonary infection, but it also may be caused by intracanalicular extension, lymphatic drainage, or direct invasion.[168a] Its presentation is that of a chronic monoarticular arthritis, especially when there has been involvement of a single bone or joint for several years. It also may complicate long-standing arthritis.[149] The clinical presentation of TB of the foot and ankle is nonspecific. Symptoms may include one or more of the following: pain, soft tissue swelling, chronic inflammation, constitutional symptoms, fevers, draining sinus tract, and lymphadenopathy.[165] Tuberculosis is considered only after a routine workup has failed to provide a diagnosis. Specific diagnosis requires a biopsy (with stains and culture), along with a detailed history and physical examination, a tuberculin skin test, and radiographic studies.

Radiographic evidence of active pulmonary disease has been described in 19 to 57% of cases.[149,168a] However, a comprehensive study by Mann[168b] found that abnormal chest radiographs were found more in the younger population, especially children, than adults. In the older population, by the time the bone manifestation occurred, the pulmonary lesion had healed. Therefore, a negative chest radiograph in an adult should not deter the physician from considering TB. The presence of a positive tuberculin skin test in an immunocompetent patient should add to the consideration of TB.

The radiographic findings of tuberculous infection of the foot and ankle are nonspecific, and there are no pathognomonic lesions. The radiographic presentation may vary from purely or diffusely destructive to well-delineated cystic lesions. Early in the disease, soft tissue swelling, periosteitis, and osteopenia are present. These may progress to bone destruction and joint surface irregularities, ending in cavitation and cystic lesions, marginal osteosclerosis, sequestra, and spina ventosa.[165,166] In a study of 22 patients by Dhillon et al.,[165] osteoporosis was observed in 12 patients, soft tissue swelling in 12, hazy/irregular joint surfaces in 10, cavitary/cystic lesions in 6, marginal osteosclerosis in 5, spina ventosa in 3, and sequestrum formation in 2.

The aim of treatment is to achieve microbiologic cure of the disease and a painless, mobile foot. Patients typically respond to conventional antituberculous chemotherapy, although occasionally, surgical intervention is required. Surgery such as arthrodesis or debridement is indicated when a juxtaarticular focus threatens a joint space or there is a painful, destroyed joint. Response to therapy is marked by the disappearance of symptoms and radiologic evidence of remineralization, obliteration of cavities, restoration of trabeculae, and improvement of osteoporosis.[164,165] Early diagnosis and treatment is paramount to prevent joint involvement from periarticular bone lesions.

C. OTHER BONES

The rich vascular supply of the epiphysis and metaphysis of long bones explains the predilection of tuberculous infection for the proximal end of the femur, pelvis, rib, shoulder, elbow, and wrist. Disease of the fingers or the skull is rare.[169] "Spina ventosa" describes the periosteal thickening of finger bones in children.[170] Tuberculosis develops slowly, often without pain, and may be confused with a metastatic carcinoma, especially if osteolytic lesions are present. Adjacent monoarticular arthritis may be present, presumably due to lymphatic communication.[152] The roentgenographic findings include cartilage destruction, a widened joint space, erosions, and cysts. Most lesions are osteolytic; osteoblastic lesions are seen rarely. Aspiration of the bone usually yields the diagnosis.[36] Antituberculous chemotherapy is appropriate before resorting to surgical debridement.[36] Abscesses and sinuses are observed frequently.[152]

D. JOINTS

Tuberculous arthritis is a local manifestation of a more systemic disorder which, if left untreated, may eventuate in the complete destruction of the joint.[171]

Weight bearing joints are most frequently involved. In a study of 25 patients with tuberculous arthritis, the knees were involved in 6 patients (24%), the hip in 5 patients (20%), the wrist in 5 patients (20%), the ankle in 3 patients (12%), the elbow in 2 patients (8%), and 1 each for the tarsal-metatarsal, shoulder, carpal-metacarpal, and proximal interphalangeal joint.[171] Although polyarticular involvement has been reported, monoarticular infection is the rule.[171]

The most common early symptom of disease is the insidious onset of joint pain and swelling. Twenty percent of patients denied constitutional symptoms and 13 of 25 patients (52%) had local or systemic predisposing factors. These included trauma, narcotic addiction, intraarticular corticosteroid injections, systemic lupus erythematosus (SLE), and diabetes mellitus. Tuberculin skin testing was positive in all patients tested.[171]

Five of 25 patients (20%) had active pulmonary or pleural tuberculosis and an additional 9 patients (36%) had chest radiographic changes of previous pulmonary TB. Nonarticular extrapulmonary foci were seen in 13 patients (52%) and only 4 patients (16%) had joint disease alone.[171] Roentgenograms of the joints reveal metaphyseal and subchondral erosions; however, films may be normal in 12% of patients.[171] Narrow joint spaces signal an advanced stage.[152]

Tuberculous arthritis requires aspiration and possible synovial biopsy. Aspiration of the joint space often shows an exudative effusion with high protein, low glucose, and a leukocyte count of 10,000 to 20,000 cell/mm^3 (predominantly neutrophils). A positive smear is seen in 25% of patients and a positive fluid culture is seen in 94% of patients. Synovial biopsy with histology produces a yield of 95%.[171]

The treatment of tuberculous arthritis is similar to that of other forms of skeletal tuberculosis, but relapses may occur.[130] Surgery should be reserved for failure of medical therapy, or the need for decompression, as in the hip joint. Destroyed joints cannot be restored. Ankylosis is an option, but insertion of a prosthetic device should be attempted only after significant chemotherapy is given.[152] In patients with no prior history of TB, joint arthroplasty complicated by TB is uncommon. Spinner et al., noted that of 18 cases of periprosthetic tuberculous infections occurring in patients without prior evidence or history of TB, 13 were in the hip.[172]

E. PONCET'S DISEASE

Poncet's disease is otherwise known as "tuberculous rheumatism." It originally was described as a rare polyarthritis associated with abdominal TB without evident bacterial joint involvement.[173-175] This differs from monoarticular tuberculous arthritis where the synovial fluid cultures and histology are positive. Since TB may regress and arthritis progress, there is some controversy as to whether this disease represents a coincidental arthritis. Treatment of TB is required for resolution of the syndrome. If no improvement occurs, other diagnoses such as rheumatoid arthritis, osteoarthrosis, acute rheumatic fever, and ankylosing spondylitis should be considered.[176]

V. GENITOURINARY

A. UROLOGICAL TB

1. Epidemiology

Genitourinary tuberculous was the fourth most common type of extrapulmonary tuberculosis in the U.S. in 1997 and accounted for 6.6% (233 patients) of all cases of exclusively extrapulmonary disease and 1.2% of all cases of tuberculosis.[6] In Western European countries, it was the second most common form of extrapulmonary tuberculosis, with a frequency of 30 to 40%.[177] Tuberculosis of the genitourinary tract may affect the kidney, ureter, bladder, prostate, and genitalia. The most commonly affected organs of the genitourinary tract are the kidneys and prostate.[191]

The clinical manifestations of renal tuberculosis are rare in childhood and there is a peak incidence at 20 to 45 years.[178] There is a long latent period between the initial pulmonary infection and the subsequent clinical disease. The mean interval varies from 8 to 22 years after the primary infection.[179,180] As a result there is a reservoir of disease in the elderly population as well.[180]

The exact incidence of renal tuberculosis is not known in HIV-positive patients with tuberculosis. Several series of patients with HIV infection and tuberculosis, with or without bacteremia, have reported positive urine cultures in 0 to 44% of patients.[26,31,34,52,53,83,181,182] In one study of 79 patients with HIV infection and disseminated tuberculosis, 18 patients (22.7%) had at least one urine culture positive for *Mycobacterium tuberculosis* (MTB).[82]

2. Clinical

Renal tuberculosis originates from a primary lung focus with subsequent lymphohematogenous dissemination leading to bilateral cortical seeding. The subsequent tubercles in the renal cortex may remain silent for years before spreading toward the papillae. Granulomas may eventually rupture into the collecting and calyceal system. Infection descends via the ureter and may involve the contralateral organ or the genitalia. Without therapy, the course may be protracted and eventually fatal. Cavitation, abscess formation, fibrosis, and calcification are typical features. Untreated infection may lead ultimately to ureteral strictures, hydronephrosis, and endstage renal disease. Progressive destruction may be limited to one kidney.[178]

There is no characteristic clinical presentation; symptoms generally are related to local organ involvement. In a study by Simon et al. of 78 patients with genitourinary tuberculosis, 41 patients were identified with active urinary tract disease.[183] The presenting urinary tract signs and symptoms in these 41 patients were dysuria in 34%, hematuria in 27%, flank pain in 10%, and pyuria in 5%. Other presenting signs and symptoms such as a flank mass, recurrent UTIs, and gross hematuria also have been noted.[180] Constitutional symptoms such as fever and weight loss occurred in 14% of patients. No symptoms attributable to tuberculosis were noted in 20% of patients.

Although some patients had physical signs attributable to active or old tuberculous disease, 78% had no findings related to active urinary tract tuberculosis. Of these 41 patients, 66% had an abnormal chest radiograph, representing inactive disease in 58% and active disease in 7%. Tuberculin skin testing was positive in 20 of 21 patients (95%) on whom it was performed.[183]

In a study by Shafer et al. of 199 HIV-infected patients with extrapulmonary tuberculosis, the genitourinary tract was a site of disease in 73 patients (37%).[32] Sixty-one patients (83.5%) had positive urine cultures for MTB, 11 patients (15%) had kidney or bladder involvement at autopsy, and the remaining patients had genital disease. Only three patients had genitourinary TB without involvement of other sites, indicating that the GU tract was seldom the sole site of infection. Overall, 77% of those patients who had urine specimens cultured grew MTB, suggesting that most had subclinical genitourinary tuberculosis. Presenting localized signs or symptoms rarely indicated genitourinary involvement. Two patients had symptoms referable to involvement of the epididymis and prostate and no patient had gross hematuria or flank pain. Pyuria occurred in 40% of the patients with genitourinary disease.[32]

3. Diagnosis

The diagnosis of renal tuberculosis requires the isolation of the organism from the urinary tract. This can be done by collection of three to six consecutive morning clean-catch urine specimens for culture. The direct AFB smear may be misleading since nonpathogenic mycobacteria in the smegma may be confused with MTB. Consecutive morning urine cultures are as reliable as culture of a 24-hour urine collection specimen.[178] When the urine specimen is collected and processed properly the yield is very high. In 38 patients with urinary tract tuberculosis who had urine cultures sent, 90% were positive. The few negative results were attributed to inadequate cultures. The urine sediment by microscopic analysis was abnormal in 93% of patients, i.e., pyuria, hematuria, or both.[183] Percutaneous kidney biopsy may yield the diagnosis.[184]

A plain abdominal film may show punctate calcifications in the renal parenchyma or calyceal system.[185] The intravenous pyelogram (IVP), performed in 30 of 41 patients with urinary tuberculosis, showed an abnormality in 93% of cases.[183] Intravenous pyelography may show calcification, cavitation, parenchymal scarring, calyceal dilatation or deformity, calculi, or stricture formation.[183,185] Retrograde pyelography may be performed safely in patients with renal dysfunction. Ultrasonography also may show the spectrum of morphologic abnormalities of genitourinary tuberculosis.[186] Gallium scanning may show persistent renal uptake after 48 to 120 hours.[160]

4. Treatment

Nine-month chemotherapy has been shown to be effective for the treatment of renal tuberculosis.[38] Other studies have shown 4- to 6-month short-course therapy to be effective in conjunction with adjunctive surgery.[187,188] If concerns remain about persistent bacilli at the end of treatment, cavities may be sampled and cultured by needle aspiration.[189] With persistent infection, isotope renography may show persistent enhancement.[189] At least 1 year of follow-up is required posttreatment; even longer in the presence of strictures or renal calcifications. The latter may involve the intramural ureters and eventually obliterate the urinary system.[185] Urinalysis should be performed monthly or bimonthly, and excretory urograms or renal scans should be obtained after 6 and 12 months if structural aberrations are present,[189] although ultrasonography is less invasive. With modern treatment regimens, the majority of patients do not require follow-up for more than 2 years after the completion of therapy.

5. Complications

Complications may include secondary amyloidosis, fistulas, parenchymal destruction, and uremia. Nephrectomy is indicated for relief of intractable pain, unresponsive hypertension due to parenchymal destruction,[190] uncontrollable fever from obstruction, life-threatening hematuria, or resistant disease not amenable to conventional medical treatment.[188] Some advocate nephrectomy as an adjunct to a 4-month course of chemotherapy.[188] Ureteral strictures can be relieved by retrograde dilation or by the use of Double-J ureteral catheters. If strictures progress after 1 month of chemotherapy, steroids may be of benefit.[187] Infundibular stenosis, nondraining calyces, and pelvic obstructions all can be manipulated endoscopically.[189] Surgical augmentation can be performed for a shrunken and contracted bladder.[189]

B. Genital TB

1. Males

The male genital organs may be affected by urinary, contiguous, or hematogenous spread. There is no evidence to support the concept that infected urine and upward transmission through the urethra are causes of prostatic or renal spread.[191,192] The most common sites of involvement are the prostate followed by the seminal vesicles, epididymis, and testes.[193,194] The most common presentation of male genital tuberculosis is epididymitis.[195] Abscess formation may lead to a palpable mass and a chronic draining sinus. Orchitis and prostatitis may occur. Other manifestations include painful inflammation of the vas deferens and seminal vesicles; infections of the urethra and penis are rare. Except for one case of *M. celatum* affecting the penis, penile mycobacterial infections have only been described with *M. tuberculosis*.[196] Penile tuberculous infections usually present as ulcerating lesions, although subcutaneous nodules have been described.[197] Involvement of the epididymis and prostate has been described in patients with HIV infection.[26,32] Constitutional symptoms are seen rarely.[178] Prostatic tuberculosis becomes symptomatic when the epididymis is involved or when perianal abscesses develop.[191] The prostate usually is normal in size with painless, palpable, well-localized indurated areas likely representing fibrosis. Focal necrosis with caseation and calcification may occur.[198] The urinalysis usually is normal and the PSA may be normal or increased. The urine culture usually is negative, although the prostatic fluid usually contains mycobacteria.[199]

A sonogram is helpful for the evaluation of this condition.[200] The diagnosis of genital tuberculosis may be made by biopsy and culture of the genital mass.[183] Culture of semen may lead to a diagnosis in 11% of patients.[193] Some recommend 9-month short-course therapy, but others recommend 18 months of INH and RIF because potential prostatic involvement may require longer therapy.[193] Chemotherapy may be supplemented with surgery if there is abscess formation, stricture formation, or failure to respond to medical therapy. Sterility develops in 50% of patients and all patients with clinical lesions have abnormal semen.[178]

2. Females

Tuberculous infection of the genital tract in women usually is due to lymphohematogenous spread from a pulmonary or abdominal focus or, rarely, directly by coitus.[178,201] Disease can occur at any age from puberty to menopause. The distal end of the salpinges are affected in approximately 85%, the endometrium in 70 to 75%, and the ovary in 30 to 35% of patients. Involvement of the vagina and vulva is rare.[178,201]

Symptoms usually are few or absent. Presenting symptoms are pelvic-abdominal pain (20%), leukorrhea, metrorrhagia, dysmenorrhoea (30%), amenorrhea, and dyspareunia (10%). Abdominal and pelvic examination are normal in 60% of women.[202] Useful diagnostic tests include first-voided, early-morning urine; premenstrual endometrial culture and biopsy; hysterosalpingography; and laparoscopy.[178,202] The culture of menstrual blood is extremely sensitive and can be used as a screening test.[203,204]

Treatment with isoniazid and rifampin for 15 months supplemented with an initial 3 months of streptomycin led to a 93% response rate in 38 patients.[205] Surgery for large tuboovarian abscesses may be necessary. Fibrotic fallopian tubes may cause sterility. Tuberculosis is the cause of sterility in 10% of women worldwide and 1% in industrialized countries.[186] Other complications include pelvic inflammatory disease with salpingo-oophoritis, endometritis, peritubal abscess, peritonitis, and ascites. Pyometria may develop with an occluded cervical canal.[178]

VI. DISSEMINATED TB

A. EPIDEMIOLOGY

Historically, miliary tuberculosis has been a disease of children, with more than a third of cases occurring in those younger than 3 years old. Today, most cases occur in adults, especially those older than 65 years.[206] Prior to effective antituberculous chemotherapy, dissemination was invariably due to a pulmonary focus. Since the advent of effective antituberculous therapy, an extrapulmonary focus can account for dissemination in approximately 75% of cases.[207] Men and Blacks are more likely to be affected than women and Caucasians.[207]

Medical risk factors for acute dissemination include immunosuppression (especially cancer and chemotherapy),[208] alcoholism, starvation, chronic hemodialysis,[209] and viral infections (measles, influenza).[203,206] Surgical procedures such as incision and drainage of an abscess, partial resection of a lymph node, tubal surgery,[210] transurethral prostatectomy, urinary instrumentation,[211] lithotripsy treatment,[212] and prosthetic valve replacement[213] on occasion may activate a focus and precipitate dissemination. In the prechemotherapy era, miliary disease was observed after surgery for skeletal tuberculosis.[152] Predictors of mortality from dissemination are age greater than 60 years, lymphopenia, thrombocytopenia, hypoalbuminemia, elevated transaminases, and delay in appropriate therapy.[214] Mortality also has been shown to increase with overwhelming disease, an altered mental status,[215] and HIV infection.[24] One of the most common forms of extrapulmonary tuberculosis in patients with HIV infection is disseminated disease.

B. CLINICAL

Historically, miliary tuberculosis has been defined as disseminated TB, with multiple nodular lesions on chest radiograph that are 1 to 2 mm in diameter. It was described first by Manget, who compared the tiny disseminated lesions to millet seeds, hence the term "miliae." The term miliary often has mistakenly been used to characterize dissemination.[215-217] Disseminated lesions can range from miliae to larger nodules to tuberculomas. They originate from a specific focus and spread via the hematogenous route. The lesion may spread from a newly acquired infection or a long-standing focus. Indolent forms of disease, e.g., bone, renal, and lymphatic, result only rarely in dissemination.[206]

Disseminated TB is defined by the involvement of two or more noncontiguous tuberculous sites or the presence of bacteremia. It may mimic a variety of diseases and requires a high index of suspicion to diagnose. Of all cases of disseminated TB found at autopsy, 33 to 80%[218,219] were missed antemortem. In the prechemotherapy era, disseminated TB was rare and invariably fatal.[215]

Miliary tuberculosis may occur in three separate distinct forms:[220] (1) acute (acute primary and late generalized),[207,221] (2) chronic (chronic hematogenous or cryptic),[220,222,223] and (3) nonreactive (typhobacillosis of Landouzy).[224]

The acute form is a rapidly progressive process which is uniformly fatal if not treated. It may occur at the time of primary infection or later as a manifestation of a distant reactivated focus.[207] Several autopsy studies showed that the lungs, liver, and spleen are involved 75 to 95% of the time. Next most commonly involved are the kidneys, bone marrow, central nervous system (CNS), adrenal glands, and peritoneum. Less commonly involved are the thyroid, heart, skeleton, genitalia, and the gastrointestinal tract.[207,225,226]

Signs and symptoms are nonspecific and frequently include fever, weight loss, malaise, anorexia, and fatigue. The average duration of symptoms before diagnosis varied significantly depending on the series.[207,214,215,221,225,227] Less common symptoms are headache, dyspnea, and abdominal pain. Headache is an ominous sign and signifies meningeal involvement,[221,225] abdominal pain indicates intraabdominal disease,[226] and dyspnea suggests significant pulmonary disease or impairment of lung diffusing capacity.[228] Physical signs include hepatomegaly, and less commonly, splenomegaly and lymphadenopathy.[214,215,227] Choroidal tubercles have been reported in disseminated disease from "rare" to "almost all cases,"[229] but also may be seen in pulmonary tuberculosis without dissemination.[227,229]

Chronic or cryptic miliary tuberculosis, as defined by Proudfoot,[222] is miliary tuberculosis where the classical and radiological features of miliary TB are not present. The disease is insidious before it becomes acute, typically affects the elderly, presents as a fever of unknown origin, and the diagnosis often is delayed. As a result the diagnosis frequently is made postmortem. The overall mortality is approximately 80%.[222,223,230] This syndrome rarely is associated with the typical miliary pattern on chest radiograph, and frequently is associated with an underlying malignancy or blood dyscrasia.[222,223]

Nonreactive miliary tuberculosis is a fatal form of the disease where many organs show areas of caseous necrosis surrounded by normal or near normal parenchyma. The clinical spectrum ranges from an acute and overwhelming illness to a chronic persistent condition. It is associated with an abnormal blood picture.[224]

Bacteremia is not an uncommon occurrence among patients who are HIV-infected with tuberculosis, but is not necessarily synonymous with miliary tuberculosis.[34,82,83,181,182,231] In a study by Shafer et al. of 199 HIV-infected patients with extrapulmonary tuberculosis, 76 patients (38%) had disseminated disease including the bone marrow in 32 patients, the blood in 28 patients, the liver in 25 patients, and more than 2 noncontiguous extrapulmonary sites in 56 patients.[32] Fever and respiratory symptoms predominated in 67% of patients. Twenty-four patients (32%) had miliary infiltrates on chest radiographs and 9 of these developed the infiltrates during hospitalization. In HIV-positive patients, disseminated TB is seen more commonly, may be rapidly progressive and overwhelming, requiring an aggressive diagnostic approach and early therapy.[232] The majority (90%) of patients are anergic.[32,82]

C. Diagnosis

The chest radiograph is the single most important screen for detecting miliary tuberculosis, although it may be normal in 25 to 50% of patients,[214,233] and may remain that way for several weeks. It may also exhibit a vast array of abnormalities including pleural effusions, hilar adenopathy, interstitial infiltrates, and extensive parenchymal consolidation (ARDS). The retrocardiac space on the lateral view is a very sensitive area for assessment of miliae.[206] This miliary pattern may be confused with congestive heart failure, sarcoidosis, fungal infections, bacterial pneumonia, and even *Pneumocystis carinii* pneumonia in patients with AIDS.[217,234] In one series of patients with HIV infection and tuberculosis, a miliary pattern was seen in 30% of patients.[131] The high resolution CT is a more sensitive indicator of disease.[233] The gallium scan frequently is positive.[235]

The sputum smear is positive in approximately 30% of patients with miliary TB, and increases with additional lesions, e.g., cavitation, in as much as 70% of patients. Sputum cultures are positive in almost two thirds of patients.[214,215,221]

Histologic confirmation of disseminated tuberculosis is best achieved by biopsy of the lung, bone marrow, liver, lymph node, skin, or any other tissue that is clinically involved. Fiberoptic bronchoscopy with bronchoalveolar lavage (BAL) and transbronchial biopsy (TBB) remains an invaluable tool in the immediate diagnosis of miliary TB. Three studies show an immediate (histology and/or +AFB smear) diagnostic rate of 64 to 79% with cultures providing an additional 4 to 10% yield. The definitive diagnostic yield from transbronchial biopsy and bronchial washings or lavage is 73 to 86%.[214,236,237] This procedure is quite useful, provides a high diagnostic yield and has supplanted the liver biopsy as the initial diagnostic procedure. In a study including 76 patients with disseminated tuberculosis and HIV infection, only 26% had histologic evidence of TB on fiberoptic bronchoscopy with transbronchial biopsy.[32] Therefore, this procedure cannot be relied upon to exclude disseminated disease in HIV-infected patients.

Percutaneous liver biopsies have been used frequently and reveal granulomata in 50 to 100% of patients.[214,225,226] Organisms were more likely to be seen when caseation was present, and caseation was seen in 20 to 45% of cases. In one study of 199 patients with extrapulmonary tuberculosis and HIV infection, 76 patients (38%) had disseminated disease. In those with dissemination, liver biopsy revealed histologic evidence of TB in 14 of 18 (78%) patients where it was performed.[32]

Because of its rich blood supply, bone marrow involvement occurs and may lead to aplastic anemia, granulocytopenia, leukemoid reaction, a "left shift," and pancytopenia.[238] Bone marrow examination has been reported to be positive in as much as 83% of HIV-negative patients with miliary tuberculosis.[214,221,226,239] The marrow is more likely to be positive if a biopsy, rather than an aspirate, is performed and yields are improved by culture of the marrow. The yield of a bone marrow biopsy is even higher where there are hematologic abnormalities such as anemia, leukopenia, or thrombocytopenia.[214,238]

Bone marrow aspiration and biopsy also are helpful but less so in HIV-positive patients.[240] AFB stains of the bone marrow are positive in 22% of patients and culture is positive in 29% of patients with disseminated TB.[241] Histologic evidence of tuberculosis is seen in 25 to 52% of patients having a bone marrow biopsy.[32,241]

Blood cultures are useful in tuberculous bacteremia especially in patients who are HIV-infected, where blood cultures may be positive in as much as 38% of cases.[83,181,231] Specimens of gastric washings,[173,174,184] urine,[214,215,225,242] and cerebrospinal fluid[214] should always be cultured.

Bronchoscopy with BAL and TBB, bone marrow biopsy and liver biopsy have a relatively high yield and, if the diagnosis is suspected, should be performed early to prevent therapeutic delay.[243]

D. TREATMENT

With acute and overwhelming disease, it is reasonable to start early empiric therapy with the standard four-drug regimen. A delay of even 1 to 8 days contributes to a high mortality rate.[217,244] The decision to embark upon empirical therapy without having obtained appropriate tissue can be a difficult one. The effects of early therapy on culture results and the potentially serious adverse effects of antituberculous agents must be weighed against the risk of treatment delay.

Even with appropriate therapy, the mortality rate may reach 16 to 24%.[214,215,221,225] In one study, most deaths occurred within the first 2 weeks of admission.[214] This reinforces the fact that patients frequently present late in the natural course of this illness and emphasizes the importance of early diagnosis and treatment. Most cases respond to conventional short course chemotherapy.[30,214] The practice of the addition of corticosteroids to patients who are severely ill in an attempt to accelerate the clinical response remains controversial.[206]

In a study by Shafer et al. of 76 patients with disseminated tuberculosis, most of the patients treated with antituberculous therapy survived. Thirty-four patients (45%) died during hospitalization and 21 of these died without a definitive diagnosis or specific therapy.[32]

E. COMPLICATIONS

The complications of miliary tuberculosis are numerous and may potentially involve any organ. "Sepsis tuberculosis gravissima" is acute overwhelming septic shock with multiple complications such as respiratory failure,[217] ARDS,[216,245,246] cholestatic jaundice, acute pancreatitis,[247] hepatic and renal failure, and disseminated intravascular coagulation.[214] Multisystem organ failure has a mortality of as much as 90%.[248] Autopsy studies in these patients may show extensive necrosis with no granuloma formation and few inflammatory cells,[249] granulomatous inflammation of the interstitial space, exudative alveolitis, or obliterative arteritis.[217]

VII. NEUROLOGIC

A. MENINGES

1. Epidemiology

Neurotuberculosis is a life threatening complication which can affect all regions of the CNS, although there is a predilection for the basilar meninges. Tuberculosis of the nervous system can affect the meninges, brain, spinal cord, cranial and peripheral nerves, ears, and eyes.

Tuberculous meningitis was the fifth most common form of extrapulmonary tuberculosis in the U.S. in 1997.[6] It accounted for 5.2% (186) of all cases of exclusively extrapulmonary disease and 0.7% of all cases of tuberculosis reported.[6]

Tuberculous meningitis may occur at any age, but historically is a disease of children in the first 5 years of life. It is uncommon in children less than 6 months of age and rare under the age of 3 months.[250] Auerbach found that, in a series of 97 cases of fatal tuberculosis in children under 13 years old, 42.2% had tuberculous meningitis.[251] In the same study, only 2.7% of 2236 adult deaths due to tuberculosis resulted from meningitis. Riggs et al. found meningeal involvement at postmortem in 19.3% of patients with tuberculosis who were less than 20 years old and in 5.9% of patients who were older than 20.[252] The incidence of tuberculous meningitis in adults has been increasing in recent years, probably due to a later age of acquisition of tuberculous infection.[253]

Predisposing medical conditions for tuberculous meningitis include alcoholism, substance abuse, corticosteroid use, head trauma, and HIV infection.[254,255]

2. Clinical

Meningitis may develop either from a local activated dormant focus or from a distant site, e.g., lung or paravertebral abscess, through hematogenous spread, or as the result of miliary tuberculosis. Regardless of the site of origin, there must be rupture of a caseous focus into the arachnoid space. This focus usually lies adjacent to the meninges.[251]

Pathologically, only a small number of living bacilli may be seen in the parenchyma, and serous meningitis may result without evident organisms. Hyperemia, capillary damage, scars, and edema are observed. A thick gelatinous exudate may collect at the base of the brain, interfering with cranial nerve function, and hydrocephalus may occur. Basal meningeal inflammation may spread focally to adjacent tissues. Granulomas are seen within the choroid plexus in 75% of cases and the ependyma in 90% of cases. Small discrete gray white tubercles may be visible over the entire surface of the brain.[256]

The onset of tuberculous meningitis is insidious with a 2-week prodromal period before meningeal symptoms occur.[257] The clinical features include fever, anorexia, malaise, nausea, vomiting, headache, apathy, and mental alterations. Physical findings include nuchal rigidity, basilar cranial nerve involvement, focal neurologic deficits, pupillary changes, funduscopic changes, papilledema, and peripheral adenopathy.[254,256] A waxing and waning course with sudden acceleration may occur, especially in children.[256] Nonneurologic tuberculosis is associated with 37% of patients.[258]

Most cases of tuberculous meningitis progress through three stages. The first stage occurs with low grade fever, personality changes, and irritability, and lasts 1 to 2 weeks. Confusion may be an early sign in the elderly. The cerebrospinal fluid (CSF) shows few neutrophils and a borderline normal glucose and protein. During the second stage there is an increase in the intracranial pressure with nausea, vomiting, nuchal rigidity, photophobia, seizures, and cranial nerve palsies (3rd, 6th, and 7th) are seen. The CSF shows lymphocytes, an increased protein and a decreased glucose content. The last stage is associated with high fever, confusion, stupor, and coma. Decortication and herniation eventually may ensue. Prechemotherapy mortality was 45% in stage 1, 70% in stage 2, and 90% in stage 3.[257,259]

HIV infection may be complicated by tuberculous infection of the nervous system. Bishburg et al. reported tuberculous meningitis in 10 of 52 patients (19.2%) with HIV infection and tuberculosis.[255] In a study of 199 patients with extrapulmonary tuberculosis and HIV infection, 27 patients (14%) had disease of the central nervous system.[32] Of these 21 had meningitis and 6 had tuberculomas. Ninety-six percent of patients had neurologic signs or symptoms and were not dissimilar from the HIV-negative controls, a finding confirmed by two other studies of HIV-related tuberculous meningitis.[20,258] The presence of peripheral, intrathoracic, and intraabdominal lymphadenopathy was more common in patients with HIV infection. Patients with a lower CD4+ count had a poorer prognosis.[258]

3. Diagnosis

The tuberculin skin test can be negative in as much as 50% of cases,[254,257,260] but usually becomes positive during chemotherapy.[261] Tuberculin skin testing was positive (greater than 10 mm in induration) in 22.5%, and 29% of patients with HIV infection in two studies.[20,258] Hyponatremia is common and usually is secondary to inappropriate secretion of antidiuretic hormone.[257]

Chest radiographs are abnormal and suggestive of tuberculosis in 31 to 74% of patients.[20,254,262] In a study by Dubé et al. of 31 patients with tuberculous meningitis, chest radiographs were abnormal in 81% of HIV-negative patients and 67% of HIV-positive patients.[20] A miliary pattern was predominant in both (44% vs. 33%). Abnormal chest radiographs were seen in 54% of patients in another study.[258]

The widespread use of CT and MRI scanning has been useful in the management of tuberculous meningitis. Hydrocephalus; meningeal enhancement (with contrast CT or gadolinium MRI);[263] thickened basilar meninges; and nonenhancing, enhancing, hyperdense, or isodense lesions, sometimes with surrounding edema, may be seen.[264-267] Abnormalities on CT scan of the head were seen in 60 to 69% of patients in several studies and they included hydrocephalus, mass lesions, and meningeal enhancement. This yield appears to be increased by the use of MRI scanning.[20,32,258] CT and MRI scanning may be useful in the follow-up process.

Examination of the CSF is the most valuable procedure in the diagnosis of meningeal tuberculosis. The opening pressure during lumbar puncture usually is elevated. The CSF protein is elevated and ranges from 100 to 500 mg/dl, and may rise considerably higher if there is a spinal block with xanthochromia.[20,257] An increasing protein concentration is common during therapy and does not necessarily portend treatment failure.[258] The CSF glucose concentration usually is below 40 mg/dl. The CSF/blood glucose ratio is below 0.5 in 50 to 85% of patients,[257,258] although it is often normal in diabetics.[151] The glucose concentration declines in untreated cases. Intravenously administered glucose should be avoided 2 hours before the lumbar puncture.[250] In two studies of HIV-related tuberculous meningitis, the HIV-positive patients had CSF abnormalities which were comparable to those found in patients without HIV infection. A normal CSF protein concentration was found with higher frequency in patients with HIV infection than in those without.[20,258]

The cellular changes in the CSF reflect a tuberculin reaction provoked by the presence of tuberculoproteins.[257] There may be a moderate degree of pleocytosis, usually with less than 500 cells/mm^3 and rarely greater than 1200 cells/mm^3. More than 80 to 95% are lymphocytes, but a predominance of polymorphonuclear cells may be seen early.[257]

The AFB smear of the CSF has been reported to be positive in 10 to 40% of specimens,[253,260] but the yield may increase to 85 to 87% with repeated or centrifuged specimens.[268-270] Serial lumbar punctures, even after the onset of therapy, may contain the organism.[271] The AFB smear was reported to be positive in 0 to 27% of patients with HIV infection.[19,28,217] Tubercle bacilli may be isolated by culture in 50 to 80% of cases.[152,257,260,262,268]

Achieving the diagnosis at an early stage is critical but often onerous because cerebrospinal fluid may be normal in as much as 20% of HIV-positive patients.[258] If the CSF remains normal within 2 weeks of presentation, the diagnosis of tuberculous meningitis is unlikely. It may be reasonable to withdraw treatment and follow the patient over the next few months with repeat lumbar punctures.[151]

More elaborate tests have been utilized in an attempt to establish the diagnosis of tuberculous meningitis. Adenosine deaminase (ADA) is elevated in the CSF and 60% of patients have levels greater than 10 IU/ml. Unfortunately ADA also may be increased in bacterial meningitis and, therefore, is nondiagnostic.[272] In one study in HIV-infected patients, the sensitivity of ADA was 63%, better than the AFB smear.[258] Enzyme-linked immunoabsorbent assay (ELISA) to detect soluble mycobacterial antigen (e.g., antigen 5) may be useful, with a sensitivity of 80% and a specificity nearing 100%.[273-275] An immunoblot technique using mycobacterial antigen 60 (A60) has been developed. The early appearance of antimycobacterial immunoglobulins to this complex may be seen in the CSF of patients with tuberculous meningitis.[276] Detection of tuberculostearic acid, a fatty acid present only in mycobacteria, provides a diagnostic test with a high degree of accuracy. This may represent the best approach to the rapid diagnosis of tuberculous meningitis.[277]

The bromide (^{82}Br) partition test[151] and lactate levels[278] are less useful, but the polymerase chain reaction (PCR) technique can yield a sensitivity above 75%; specificity is lower.[279] PCR performed on stored CSF increases specificity by decreasing possible laboratory contamination.[279] Multicenter trials would be most helpful in establishing the clinical usefulness of these various tests.[280] A meningeal biopsy or brain biopsy may be necessary, on occasion, but carries significant risk, including postoperative epidural hematoma and hydrocephalus.[281]

4. Treatment

Early and immediate treatment is critical for improving outcome. With appropriate chemotherapy, complete recovery is increased to 95%, 80%, and 20% in stages 1, 2 and 3, respectively.[259] The best agents in tuberculous meningitis are INH, RIF, PZA, and streptomycin, all of which enter the CSF well in the presence of meningeal inflammation.[256] Ethambutol is less effective in meningeal disease unless used at higher doses.[282] Ethionamide (15 mg/kg/day),[259] cycloserine, and ofloxacin also may be effective.[283] Intrathecal drugs usually are not necessary.

Dutt et al. showed that a 9-month, short-course chemotherapy regimen was effective in 18 patients with tuberculous meningitis.[38] Another study showed similar results but emphasized the need for corticosteroids or surgery to treat complications such as hydrocephalus or arachnoiditis.[284] The duration of conventional therapy is 6 to 9 months, although some authors still recommend up to 24 months of therapy.[259,285] Children must be treated for 12 months along with adjunctive corticosteroids (see Chapter 8). Patients who have had meningitis should be kept under medical supervision for a minimum of 2 years.[151] The use of corticosteroids in adults is controversial, and may be indicated in the presence of elevated intracranial pressure, altered consciousness, focal neurologic findings, or spinal block.[257] The overall mortality is 20%,[258] and probably is higher in the elderly. The overall mortality rate for patients with HIV infection and tuberculous meningitis receiving conventional antituberculous therapy was 20% and 33% in two studies.[20,258] Even with appropriate medical therapy and rapid clinical response, patients should be monitored for any complication requiring adjunctive therapy, e.g., anticonvulsants or surgical intervention.

Surgical intervention for hydrocephalus, tuberculoma, or abscess formation rarely is required. Hydrocephalus, which develops in 20% of patients, or opening pressures greater than 50 cm H$_2$O, may be improved by diuretics,[151] but most physicians would resort to a ventriculoatrial or ventriculoperitoneal shunt.[203,250] Early shunt placement may improve outcome. External ventricular drainage may be indicated in more severe cases.[286] Hyaluronidase has been used in spinal arachnoiditis with excellent results in more than 15 patients.[287]

Opticochiasmatic arachnoiditis is due to an inflammatory reaction in the area of the optic chiasm leading to loss of visual acuity. It may be associated with hydrocephalus and responds well to surgery and corticosteroids.[288]

5. Complications

Complications include hydrocephalus, cranial nerve palsies and nerve compression (e.g., bilateral 6th nerve palsy), cerebral infarction, and blockage of CSF flow. A steep rise in CSF protein appears before a spinal block develops.[151] Obstruction of capillaries from multiple small tuberculous emboli leads to microinfarcts (tuberculids). They may persist, enlarge or caseate, and large tuberculomas may lead to focal neurological deficits. An abscess or spinal leptomeningitis may develop, and endarteritis may account for focal areas of cerebral infarction.[257] "Paradoxical" tuberculomas may develop during the course of treatment of drug-sensitive TB.[267,289] Continuation of the same therapy and the addition of corticosteroids have helped these patients.[266,289]

Some degree of neurologic deficit remains in 50% of patients, and a decreased IQ is the rule in infantile meningitis.[257] Severe late sequelae such as paralysis or aphasia may persist. Thirty-five percent of survivors have serious disabilities such as memory loss, mental retardation, involuntary movements, paralysis, panhypopituitarism, and epilepsy. Late events are arachnoiditis ossificans and arachnoid cysts.[256] Meningeomyeloradiculitis can be life threatening with advancing paraplegia and rising CSF protein levels.[290]

B. Brain/Nerve Lesions

Hematogenous dissemination leads to perivascular microscopic foci that form tubercles with central caseation, epithelioid, and giant cells. Gradually they enlarge to form numerous small macroscopic tuberculomas which then may coalesce. Tuberculomas, which are rare, may be asymptomatic, or present with symptoms and signs of a focal lesion, or elevated intracranial pressure.[266] They may mimic almost any disease of the brain including glioma, glioblastoma, metastasis, hemorrhage, or abscess.[265] Tuberculomas constitute 33% of intracranial space-occupying lesions in patients in developing countries. Although characteristically solitary, 15 to 34% are multiple.[291] Calcification may be present within the contrast enhanced ring, creating a "target sign," and probably is a sign of reactivation.[265] The CSF may be normal in the presence of parenchymal disease.[256] Tuberculomas may be visualized by CT and MRI scanning techniques in as much as 45% of patients with meningitis,[263] and may be more common in patients with HIV infection.[20,32,258]

Surgical intervention is controversial and generally not required because of the use of corticosteroids and antituberculous drugs, but debulking may be necessary if vital structures such as the optic pathway are compromised. Tuberculomas respond slowly to medical therapy and require several months to 1 year for resolution, although partial improvement may be seen within 6 to 8 weeks.[289] Thirty-four cases of paradoxical progression of tuberculomas despite adequate tuberculostatic chemotherapy have been reported worldwide.[291] Complications include clinical meningitis, spinal cord compression, radiculomyelitis, and seizures.[257]

Brain abscesses are tuberculomas that develop into pus-filled cavities and indicate poor defense mechanisms.[63] They are rare and may require surgical excision.[264] A paravertebral cold abscess may cause local deficits. Rarely, the abscess may flow through the intervertebral foramen into the epidural space and cause paraplegia.[266]

Epidural tuberculosis compresses the spine, does not involve bones, and can be confused with carcinomas (spinal tumor syndrome).[151,250] Spinal cord TB can be focal (with root pain, paraplegia, or loss of bladder control), ascending, or multifocal.[151] Corticosteroids are useful therapy if worsening neurologic deficits occur secondary to edema (e.g., dexamethasone 0.2 mg/kg/day for the first 2 weeks).

Peripheral polyneuropathy has not been attributed to TB. When described, it has been seen with pyridoxine (vitamin B_6) deficiency in malnourished patients on INH therapy or with supranormal supplementation of pyridoxine (greater than 200 mg/day).[292]

C. Ocular

Ocular manifestations occur in approximately 1% of patients with tuberculosis.[293] Although usually the result of hematogenous dissemination, ocular tuberculosis may extend from surrounding tissues or from direct inoculation with the patient's own sputum.[293] In some developing countries, it accounts for 30% of all uveitis diagnosed.[294]

The cornea and choroidae are most frequently affected, but every segment of the eye and its adnexae (except the lens) including the uvea, retina, sclera, iris, and optic nerve may be involved. External structures, such as the lid, orbit, and lacrimal gland, rarely are affected.[293] The clinical presentation is variable. A primary "tuberculous chancre" may occur on the lid and the conjunctiva and may appear as an ulcerated lesion with regional lymphadenopathy.[295] Chronic keratoconjunctivitis, anterior and posterior uveitis, iris nodules, retinal vasculitis, and panophthalmitis have been described.[295]

Phlyctenular (Greek for "blister") keratoconjunctivitis was a major cause of visual loss in the U.S. at the beginning of the century among Eskimos and Native Americans. It probably is a hypersensitivity reaction to the presence of tuberculoproteins, but may be due to local implantation.[296,297] Careful examination may reveal elevated limbal lesions migrating toward the central cornea carrying a "leash" of vessels and leaving a triangular scar. Phlyctenular lesions may cause intense pain, lacrimation, and photophobia.[298]

Superficial scleritis also is a hypersensitivity reaction, while deep scleritis usually results from direct inoculation. Tuberculous scleritis characteristically is painless.[295]

A classic finding in miliary tuberculosis is multiple bilateral choroidal tubercles (Bouchut's tubercles) or many small discrete yellowish nodules in the posterior pole of the eye.[229] These are normally visible on funduscopic examination.

Intraocular involvement may include retinal neovascularization and ischemic retinal vasculitis.[294,299] Vitreous hemorrhage may occur from neovascularization and is referred to as Eales' disease. As a result, sudden loss of vision in one eye or visual impairment with scotoma or floating spots may occur.[293,300] Optic neuropathy may lead to blindness.[293]

A complete evaluation includes funduscopy and a slit-lamp examination. Fluorescein angiography is useful in the follow-up assessment of choroidal lesions.[301] In the absence of a positive ocular culture, the diagnosis of ocular TB may be established by the characteristic findings of ocular TB plus a positive culture from another source and/or the response of lesions to chemotherapy. The bacillus may be recovered directly from the cornea or sclera. Chorioretinal endobiopsy or vitreous aspiration with culture are helpful, but rarely necessary.[294]

Antituberculous therapy is effective, but local instillation or systemic use of corticosteroids may be required as adjuvant therapy (e.g., in phlyctenular keratoconjunctivitis). The use of topical corticosteroids may prevent focal corneal scarring.[294] For anterior uveitis, topical mydriatic agents are used.[293] Direct or panretinal[302] photocoagulation is indicated for neovascularization and retinal capillary closure.[293]

Complications of ocular TB usually are reversible, although retinal detachment, glaucoma, and cataract formation have been described. Rarely exophthalmus may develop secondary to an optochiasmatic tuberculoma. A tuberculoma of the orbit can produce proptosis and, therefore, may mimic other diseases.[298]

D. OTOLOGIC

Historically, tuberculous involvement of the ear has been observed in approximately 2% of all patients with active pulmonary TB.[303] Now there are almost none. However, at the beginning of the century, TB was responsible for up to 20% of all otitis media.[303]

The mucosa of the middle ear thickens and produces a discharge and effusion, which may appear in the nasopharynx. The tympanic membrane may thicken and reveal yellow spots, representing caseating granulomata.[304] The breakdown of a previous tympanoplasty or developing granulation tissue should suggest TB. Large or multiple perforations of the tympanic membrane may develop and produce the characteristic otorrhea. Painless perforation with chronic discharge is characteristic and may linger for many years. Hearing impairment occurs early and may antedate other symptoms. The hearing loss may be conductive (due to ossicle destruction), sensorineural, or both. Mastoiditis also may develop.[303]

The diagnosis is evident by obtaining positive mycobacterial cultures, but the diagnosis may be masked by the presence of bacterial superinfection. The yield of smear and culture from secretions is low, although the yield is higher from granulation tissue. Histology frequently is unrevealing and granuloma formation may be lacking. The most sensitive tests are the AFB smear and culture of a biopsy specimen.[303] The possibility of permanent hearing loss makes early diagnosis critical.

Treatment of otologic tuberculosis requires at least INH and RIF for as long as 18 to 24 months.[305] Surgical intervention after a failed medical regimen may be necessary for facial nerve palsy, subperiosteal abscess, or persistent fistulas.

Typical complications are postauricular fistula development, preauricular lymphadenopathy, and facial nerve palsy. The most serious complication is arterial invasion and bleeding from the spread of a contiguous focus. These complications are rare, occur late, and usually differentiate TB from bacterial otitis.[305] Other rare complications include periosteal abscess formation, labyrinthitis, fistulas, and extension of infection into the CSF.[303]

VIII. ABDOMINAL

A. Peritoneal TB

1. Epidemiology

Tuberculosis of the abdomen includes disease of the peritoneum, gastrointestinal tract, liver and biliary tract, pancreas, tonsils, tongue, and mouth. At the turn of the century, intraabdominal involvement was present in 25% of patients with far advanced pulmonary disease, it now accounts for approximately 4.2% of all cases of extrapulmonary TB.[306] The peritoneum is the major site of intraabdominal involvement and, in a study by Farer from 1969 to 1973, was five times as common as all other forms of abdominal tuberculosis combined.[54] Peritoneal tuberculosis was the sixth most common form of extrapulmonary tuberculosis in the U.S. in 1997.[6] It accounted for 4.2% (151 patients) of all cases of exclusively extrapulmonary disease and 0.8% of all cases of tuberculosis reported.[6]

Historically, tuberculous peritonitis occurred most commonly in young adults but was observed at any age. Although it may occur in both men and women, recent studies suggest a male predominance.[307,308] It has been described among Blacks, North American Indians, and Asian and West Indian immigrants. Alcoholism, and its associated malnutrition, appears to be a major risk factor.[306,308] Tuberculous peritonitis has been described in long-term peritoneal dialysis patients.[309] Half of all ascites in developing countries are due to tuberculosis.[308]

2. Clinical

Peritoneal tuberculosis occurs from rupture of a latent caseous peritoneal focus that results from hematogenous dissemination of a primary infection. It may result from rupture of a caseous abdominal lymph node or extend from an intestinal source or genitalia.[310-312]

The symptoms of peritonitis are insidious over several months, although occasionally may be abrupt if bowel perforation occurs. Symptoms include abdominal pain and swelling, and generalized symptoms of fever, chills, anorexia, and malaise.[313] The physical examination reveals diffuse or local abdominal tenderness, ascites, omental masses, and, on rare occasions, a "doughy abdomen."[308]

There are two forms of tuberculous peritonitis frequently encountered: wet (ascitic) and dry (associated with a scant or localized effusion).[306] Ascites almost always is present, although the effusion is large only when complicated by hepatic cirrhosis. A pleural effusion, either unilateral or bilateral, is seen in 22 to 32% of patients.[307,308,310] As much as 50% of cases of tuberculous peritonitis are associated with active pulmonary tuberculosis.[307,310,311,314]

Tuberculin skin testing generally is not helpful and the range of positivity varies significantly depending on age. Nonreactors tend to be older and have coexistent liver disease; younger patients tend to be reactors.[308,310,313]

In a study by Shafer et al., 27 of 199 HIV-positive patients (13.5%) with extrapulmonary tuberculosis had intraabdominal involvement.[32] Of these, 24 had lymphadenopathy and 6 had peritoneal involvement. Intraabdominal lymphadenopathy was a universal finding in patients with disseminated tuberculosis. Six patients had pancreatic abscesses originating from peripancreatic lymph nodes and two patients had liver abscesses from portahepatic nodes. Five patients had intestinal perforation from contiguous lymphadenitis. Twenty-one patients (78%) had symptoms of abdominal pain, tenderness, or ascites. Gastrointestinal fistulous tracts from other organs, such as stomach, esophagus, ileum, and rectum, also were observed.

3. Diagnosis

There is leukocytosis in less than 30% of patients and anemia in less than 20% of patients. Liver function tests usually are normal unless there is underlying liver disease.[308,315]

Gallium scanning, ultrasonography, and CT scanning are of considerable diagnostic value. Gallium scanning with prolonged uptake is nonspecific and may merely reflect peritoneal inflammation.[316] Computed tomography is nonspecific except for lymphadenopathy with low-density centers suggesting tuberculosis, especially in patients with HIV infection.[32,317] Ultrasonography facilitates aspiration of localized effusions.[306]

Tuberculous peritonitis may be diagnosed by culture of the peritoneal fluid and possibly by biopsy of the peritoneum. The ascitic fluid is exudative and the protein concentration usually is above 2.5 to 3.0 g/l, although it may be lower with supervening cirrhosis.[315] The ascitic fluid/blood glucose ratio is below 1.0 in 80% of cases.[318] The ascitic fluid shows a lymphocytic predominance, although neutrophils also may be present.[314]

In tuberculous peritonitis, the AFB smear is positive in less than 5% of cases,[310,315] while the culture is positive in as much as 68% of cases.[308,314] Examining a large amount (1 l) of centrifuged fluid has a sensitivity of 83%.[310]

Adenosine deaminase (ADA) is increased fivefold when compared to control groups, but decreased with low-protein ascites (false-negative). The ADA ratio of ascitic fluid to serum also is increased.[308,319]

Blind peritoneal needle biopsy has a diagnostic yield of approximately 65%, but rarely is recommended since bleeding or perforation may occur, especially if fibroadhesions are present.[306] Sonogram or CT scan-guided fine-needle aspiration of an intraabdominal mass or lymph node may be helpful.[320] Peritoneoscopy or laparoscopy are useful and in one study, peritoneoscopy with biopsy led to a diagnosis of tuberculosis in 77% of cases.[321] Biopsy may show a thickened or inflamed peritoneum, miliary yellow-white tubercles of the peritoneum, serosa, and omentum, or fibroadhesions between the liver and parietal peritoneum. Procedural complications include a postparacentesis ascitic fluid leakage in 3% of cases, fecal fistulas in 2% of cases, and gastrointestinal hemorrhage.[308]

4. Treatment

Medical therapy usually is adequate and early diagnosis usually averts surgical intervention. In a study by Dutt et al., 17 patients with tuberculous peritonitis were successfully treated with 9-month short-course therapy.[38]

5. Complications

Late complications of TB peritonitis include retroperitoneal fibrosis with ureteral obstruction,[308] and adhesions between visceral and parietal peritoneum. These adhesions may, on occasion, obstruct the bowel and require surgical resection. Partial obstruction may respond to antituberculous medication. Intestinal obstruction may transpire during or following therapy.[308] The mortality of tuberculous peritonitis has decreased from 50% to 10% with appropriate therapy. Mortality is higher with delayed or missed diagnosis, concomitant liver disease, and age above 60 years.[308]

B. Enteric Tuberculosis

1. Epidemiology

Tuberculosis can effect any portion of the gastrointestinal tract. The ileocecal region most commonly is affected but the large colon, esophagus, stomach, duodenum, jejunum, appendix, and anorectal areas also may be involved.[307,322,323] In a study of 341 cases of abdominal tuberculosis, 21% of patients had ileocecal disease, 20% had anorectal disease, and 1% had involvement of the sigmoid colon.[307] This disease remains more common among immigrants from India, the Middle East, Africa, and Asia, especially in women.[307,308]

2. Clinical

Tuberculous enteritis may occur as a result of direct invasion by ingested organisms, lymphohematogenous dissemination, extension from a contiguous site, or biliary secretions.[308] Gastrointestinal involvement due to ingestion of organisms may occur in as much as 46% of patients with smear-positive pulmonary TB.[312] With reduced gastric acid production (e.g., postgastrectomy state or achlorhydria, and cavitary lung disease), there is an increased risk of tuberculous enteritis with swallowed organisms reaching the ileum and cecum.[312]

The clinical features of tuberculous enteritis are relatively nonspecific. Symptoms may be acute, associated with obstruction or perforation, chronic for many years, or asymptomatic and found on autopsy.[308,323] There may be crampy abdominal pain, weight loss, fever, anorexia, and diarrhea. On occasion there may be severe gastrointestinal hemorrhage.[323]

Esophageal involvement resulting in dysphagia may occur due to compression by paratracheal and subcarinal nodes. Subcarinal lymph nodes may erode into the esophagus and cause hematemesis, hemorrhage, or fistulous tracts.[324] A fistula to the trachea or the bronchial system or esophageal perforation has been reported in a patient with HIV infection.[325] An intraluminal mass can mimic a tumor and an ulceration may cause hemorrhage.[324]

TB of the stomach and duodenum may exhibit symptoms of chronic peptic ulceration or may resemble a carcinoma. Gastric outlet or duodenal obstruction may occur.[326]

Jejunal involvement produces malabsorption and may cause severe diarrhea and weight loss. Small bowel disease, especially in the ileocecal region, may lead to chronic weight loss, abdominal cramps, colicky pain, diarrhea, hematochezia, and mimic Crohn's disease.[308] Intestinal involvement may cause a mass effect, obstruction, perforation, strictures, ileus, bleeding, or diarrhea. Perforation proximal to stricture formation may occur. As much as 2% of appendicitis in India is due to tuberculosis,[327] but is a rare finding in this country. Anorectal disease usually presents as an ulceration but may present as a verrucous or lupoid lesion, mass, perirectal abscess especially in males, or fistulous formation.[328]

Tuberculous enteritis may present as an acute abdomen, mimic carcinoma, or complicate hepatic cirrhosis.[329] Thirty percent present as surgical emergencies, another 10% are diagnosed at surgery, and as much as 40% are diagnosed postmortem.[308,330]

Stool smears and cultures for *M. tuberculosis* have been described in 16 and 29%, respectively, of patients with HIV infection.[53,83] This may represent swallowed organisms rather than true tuberculous enteritis in these patients.[131] Further workup, including barium studies, CT scan, and endoscopy with biopsy, may be required.

3. Diagnosis

The diagnosis of tuberculous enteritis requires positive cultures from secretions or biopsy material. Tuberculin skin testing may be negative and represent malnutrition or may be positive in 80% of patients.[307]

The barium enema remains relatively nonspecific and may show an irregular coarse mucosal lining said to be suggestive of TB [331] Computed tomography of the abdomen also is nonspecific but may be suggestive of ileocecal tuberculosis.[308,332]

Upper endoscopy and colonoscopy may show nodular areas, ulcerations, fistulas, scarring, mucosal hypertrophy, ileocecal and ascending colon involvement, or pancolitis.[333] Granulomas are submucosal in location, may be missed by the biopsy forceps, and grow mycobacteria in less than 50% of specimens. The yield increases with colonoscopic fine-needle aspiration.[334] Arteriograms usually are not required, although they may reveal hypervascularity (with ulcerations), occlusion of arteries (with strictures), stretching, crowding, or encasement.[335] With smear-positive pulmonary TB there is gastrointestinal disease by colonoscopy in as much as 45% of cases, mostly in the ileocecal region.[312] Laparoscopy and laparotomy occasionally are useful in diagnosis.

4. Treatment

Antituberculous therapy is highly effective, and adjunctive surgery is indicated only for perforation, abscess formation, or complete obstruction.[335] Nine-month short-course chemotherapy has been successful in a small number of patients.[30] Despite conventional antituberculous chemotherapy, 50% of patients in one study required surgery for diagnosis or treatment.[336] Narrowing and adhesions generally respond to antituberculous medication, although they may develop even on therapy.[310]

5. Complications

Adhesions and subacute obstruction in acute tuberculous disease may require medical therapy only. Obstruction due to cicatricial healing may occur. Bypass procedures are useful primarily for the treatment of stricture formation and intestinal obstruction. Resection or stricture-plasty usually is preferable.[337]

C. Hepatic TB

The liver may be involved in all forms of tuberculosis, including pulmonary, extrapulmonary, and miliary or disseminated disease. Noncaseating hepatic granulomas have been described in 25% of patients with pulmonary tuberculosis without evidence of clinical hepatitis.[338] Percutaneous liver biopsies may show granulomata in 50 to 100% of patients with miliary tuberculosis.[62,214,226] Liver involvement usually occurs with dissemination, but can be an isolated process in 5% of patients.[62] Hepatic tuberculosis may be seen with granulomatous disease, isolated or multiple abscesses, fibrosis, cirrhosis, or chronic hepatitis.[62]

Histologically there is miliary-micronodular, pseudotumoral-macronodular, or pericanalicular involvement with cholestasis. Nonspecific reactive hepatitis may be present with fatty infiltration, inflammatory cell infiltrates, portal inflammation and fibrosis, Kupffer cell hyperplasia, and fatty metamorphosis. The spectrum of hepatic disease extends from granulomas, tuberculids, tuberculomas (coalescing granulomas), abscesses,[339] peliosis hepatis (blood filled lakes), cirrhosis, and hepatic failure.[62]

Hepatic tuberculosis may be asymptomatic, or manifest with fever, right upper quadrant pain, or jaundice and may mimic a variety of conditions from infections to neoplasms.[62] Often there are no localizing symptoms. In one study, 10% of patients with clinically unexplained hepatomegaly had tuberculosis.[312] The alkaline phosphatase is elevated with space-occupying granulomas in 30% of patients, transaminases often are normal, and hyperbilirubinemia is minimal or absent.[62] Hepatomegaly is present in 50% of patients and splenomegaly in 30% of patients with hepatic granulomas.[340]

The diagnosis can be established by sonogram-guided percutaneous biopsy in 70% of patients or laparoscopy in 90% of patients, although stains are negative in 50 to 90% of cases.[340] The sonogram may show periportal lymph nodes that potentially may obstruct the biliary system.[341] Computed tomography of the abdomen may show hepatomegaly or a mass lesion.[382]

Surgery is indicated for diagnosis and possibly for abscess drainage.[342] Mortality due to hepatic tuberculosis is related to respiratory insufficiency, peritonitis, portal vein thrombosis, and portal hypertension with variceal hemorrhage.[62]

D. OTHER DISEASE

TB can involve all sites from the mouth to the anus and atypical presentations such as mouth ulcers, tongue lesions, and tonsillitis have been described.[323,343]

Tuberculosis of the spleen is a rare clinical entity in non-AIDS patients.[344] It may result from lymphohematogenous dissemination or may be an isolated process. Sonography and CT scan of the abdomen may show densities, which often are multiple and 4 to 20 mm in size. These abscesses may be isolated findings without pulmonary tuberculosis in patients with AIDS.[345] Splenic tuberculosis has been diagnosed by needle aspiration, although we would not recommend this in view of bleeding complications.[344] It may take 2 to 4 months for these lesions to resolve on therapy. Splenectomy is indicated only if no improvement with medical therapy occurs.[344] Calcifications represent healed disease and occur in approximately half of the patients.[203]

The biliary tract rarely is involved in tuberculosis. Jaundice most commonly is associated with fulminant intrahepatic disease and only rarely from biliary obstruction.[341] However, on occasion, enlarged periportal lymph nodes may obstruct the biliary tract and lead to jaundice.[341] Intrahepatic tubercles may rupture into the ductules.[62] Biliary involvement occurs in as much as 7% of patients with abdominal TB and usually is accompanied by multiple small cavities. It is associated with other organs drained by the portal circulation, including mesenteric lymph nodes in 89% of patients, gastrointestinal ulcerations in 73% of patients, and peritonitis in 27% of patients.[62] It may be seen only at autopsy, especially in patients with miliary TB. Abdominal symptoms are present in 15% of patients and hepatomegaly in 30% of patients.[62] Primary tuberculosis of the gallbladder is seen rarely. It usually occurs in women over the age of 30 years and presents as cholecystitis. Treatment includes chemotherapy in conjunction with cholecystectomy, or ERCP if there is common bile duct obstruction.[62]

Pancreatic involvement is uncommon, found in only 2.7% of autopsies in miliary disease.[346] Although abdominal tuberculosis is frequent in patients with AIDS, few cases of pancreatic tuberculosis have been reported as their AIDS-defining illness.[346] In the absence of any other intraabdominal disease, tuberculous pancreatitis is rare.[347] It may present as obstructive jaundice[348,349] gastrointestinal (GI) bleeding,[350] acute pancreatitis, or a pancreatic mass.[348,351-353] Constitutional symptoms include low grade fever, weight loss, malaise, and nausea. A tuberculous mass in the pancreatic head may mimic carcinoma.[354] Peripancreatic tuberculous lymphadenitis may occur and may be found by sonography or CT scan.[355]

In HIV-positive patients, atypical abscess formation has been observed in the pancreatic, retroperitoneal, and subhepatic areas, and even within the abdominal wall.[342] Twenty percent of AIDS patients with TB have abdominal disease. Enlarged lymph nodes (10%), hepatic (10%), ileal and peritoneal involvement (5%) may be seen.[356] Splenic TB may occur even more often.[344,345]

IX. CARDIOVASCULAR

A. PERICARDIAL

1. Epidemiology

Cardiovascular tuberculosis in industrialized countries is rare and accounts for 1% of all cases of extrapulmonary TB.[357] It is a manifestation of disseminated disease in more than 50% of patients.[358] Cardiovascular tuberculosis includes disease of the pericardium, myocardium, and major arteries such as the aorta. The pericardium is the area most frequently involved. In a study of 136 patients with extrapulmonary tuberculosis at Boston City Hospital, four patients (3%) had pericardial disease.[359] Tuberculosis accounts for as much as 4% of all acute pericarditis and 7% of all cardiac tamponade.[360] In some third-world countries and in a study of patients with AIDS, it was the leading cause of pericarditis.[203,361] It generally occurs in the middle aged,[362] and there appears to be a predilection for Black males.[363] Pericardial effusions have been reported in patients with HIV infection,[32,364-366] and in one study, the incidence was approximately 8%.[367]

2. Clinical

Pericardial tuberculosis frequently arises from hematogenous dissemination from a distant focus. It also may arise from other sources such as a contiguous mediastinal or peribronchial lymph node, contiguous pleuritis, or a primary pericardial focus.[203] It is likely that hypersensitivity to a tuberculoprotein plays a role in the pathogenesis, as with pleuritis and meningitis. The natural course of untreated tuberculous pericarditis includes death during the acute phase, seen in as much as 31% of patients, spontaneous reabsorption of the effusion, or progression to constriction.[363] The disease usually is insidious but may present in an acute manner with cardiac tamponade.[368]

The most common symptoms are weight loss, cough, dyspnea, orthopnea, chest pain, peripheral edema, and night sweats. Tachycardia, increased venous pressure, hepatomegaly, pulsus paradoxicus, and friction rubs also may be observed.[363,369,370] A pulmonary infiltrate or a pleural effusion may appear on chest radiograph in 32% and 36% of patients, respectively.[363,371] Cardiomegaly is found with a subacute or chronic effusion, and a small heart size is seen with fibrosis or a rapidly evolving effusion. An acute effusion, with as little as 200 ml, can cause tamponade and be life threatening, while late and chronic effusions may lead to restrictive disease.[203,363,369,370] Constrictive pericarditis occurs in approximately 20% of patients and calcification in 50%.[203,363] Cardiomegaly is common and, in one study, 190 of 193 patients had cardiomegaly on chest radiograph.[372]

The tuberculin skin test is positive in most patients with tuberculous pericarditis,[363,372] but yields as low as 54% have been reported.[373]

Tuberculous pericarditis has been described as the first manifestation of AIDS.[374] Kinney et al. have reported five patients who presented with tuberculous pericarditis as the initial infectious manifestation of AIDS.[367] All patients had cardiac tamponade and all required a pericardiectomy. The smears and cultures were positive for TB in all cases. In another series, three patients had tuberculous pericarditis with tamponade and all required pericardial windows.[32]

3. Diagnosis

The diagnosis of tuberculous pericarditis is based on finding the tubercle bacilli in the pericardial fluid, on pericardial histology, or proof of TB elsewhere with unexplained pericarditis.

The presence of a thickened pericardium with effusion is characteristic of this disease and the echocardiography is 100% sensitive for this finding.[360,362] In the absence of pericardial fluid or if there is only pericardial thickening, the search for disease elsewhere must ensue to obtain a definitive diagnosis. Calcification of the pericardium may be detected by echocardiography, chest radiography, fluoroscopy, or CT scan,[375] and usually is associated with chronic or inactive disease. Gallium scanning may be useful in diagnosing tuberculous pericarditis.[376]

The pericardial fluid usually is serosanguinous but may be grossly hemorrhagic or even purulent.[360,377] The fluid is exudative with an increased protein concentration. There is an increased leukocyte count, with lymphocytes and monocytes predominating but neutrophils may be prevalent in the first 2 weeks.[360]

AFB smears of the pericardial fluid in HIV-negative patients almost invariably are negative.[373,378] However, in patients with HIV infection, one study reported 14.3% smear positivity,[361] and another study reported a yield of 100%.[367] The pericardial fluid may show culture positivity in as much as 86% of patients.[360,363,373,378] Pericardial biopsy is a sensitive procedure yielding positive histology in 83% and 100% of patients in two studies.[363,378] Adenosine deaminase levels in tuberculous pericardial fluid are above 60 U/l and have a sensitivity and specificity of approximately 80%.[379]

4. Treatment

The treatment of tuberculous pericarditis includes both the eradication of the tubercle bacilli and control of the pericardial inflammation. Standard therapy, identical to that for pulmonary tuberculosis, has been recommended.[380] A 9-month course of chemotherapy appeared to be adequate in a study of 12 patients with pericardial tuberculosis.[38] However, in two studies by Strang et al., 6 months of chemotherapy alone was associated with significant morbidity and mortality.[372,381]

The more difficult task is minimizing the risk of significant pericardial inflammation. Corticosteroid therapy may be useful when the effusion persists or recurs despite adequate chemotherapy, but its use still is controversial. Several studies failed to show its long-term benefit.[363,373,378,382] Two controlled prospective studies, using 11 weeks of corticosteroids in addition to a modern 6-month short-course chemotherapy regimen, were undertaken in effusive and constrictive pericarditis.[372,381] Both studies demonstrated a decline in mortality rate and a decrease in the need for pericardiectomy. A significant number still required pericardiectomy. A study by Strang et al., found that antituberculous drugs plus steroids did not reduce the likelihood of constriction, although improvement in the acute stage of tuberculous pericarditis was significantly more rapid.[383] Pericardiocentesis provides prompt symptomatic relief from accumulation of pericardial fluid and cardiac tamponade but a pericardial window is recommended for a large effusion. If pericardial thickening is found during the window procedure, early pericardiectomy is recommended.[373] Surgical resection of the pericardium is indicated in life-threatening tamponade, persistent elevation of central venous pressure unrelieved by pericardiocentesis, and a nonresolving effusion.[357] As much as 30% of patients will require pericardiectomy despite adequate drug therapy.[381] Since surgical mortality is higher during the late calcific or chronic phase of constrictive pericarditis, early pericardiectomy is recommended.[360] Although some authors recommend pericardiectomy for all patients,[384] most do not.

Both specific antituberculous therapy and adjunctive surgical procedures are required for good therapeutic results.[367,374] The incidence of chronic constrictive pericarditis in patients with HIV infection is largely unknown.

5. Complications

The mortality from tuberculous pericarditis has declined from 80 to 85% prior to the introduction of chemotherapy to below 50%, and as low as 3% in some studies.[359,360,372] The mortality in treated patients is due to cardiac tamponade, congestive heart failure, and advanced TB.[203]

B. CARDITIS

Tuberculosis also can involve the endocardium or the myocardium, and in most patients is found in association with disseminated TB.[385] Nodular tuberculomas, miliary nodules, diffuse infiltrations, and focal lymphocytic lesions have been described pathologically.[358,386] In an autopsy study of 243 patients with disseminated tuberculosis, Rose reported myocardial involvement in 8% of patients.[358] It has been described as a tumor mass of the tricuspid valve and even as congestive heart failure.[385] Carditis may cause arrhythmias, impaired contractility, and even ventricular aneurysm and rupture.[358,387] Endocardial tuberculomas associated with ventricular tachycardia have been described.[388] Involvement of coronary vessels is very rare and may be due to arteritis, intimal lesions, or adjacent mediastinal or pericardial lymph node enlargement.[385]

Although most cases are diagnosed postmortem, diagnostic tests such as CT scan, MRI, and echocardiogram can be useful.[386] Treatment must be individualized and surgery occasionally may be necessary.[386]

C. AORTITIS

Tuberculous aortitis is a very rare condition and may lead to infectious ("mycotic") aneurysms, rupture, and fatal hemorrhage.[357,389,390] Although usually thought to arise from hematogenous dissemination, extension from a lymph node or another contiguous focus is possible.[391] A tuberculous aortic aneurysm is rare but fatal if the diagnosis is delayed. In a patient with active or miliary TB, a tuberculous aortic aneurysm should be suspected in the setting of persistent chest, abdominal, or back pain, hypovolemic shock, or a paraaortic mass (palpable or radiographically visible).[392] Aneurysmal dilatation of the thoracic or abdominal aorta occurs in 50% of patients[357,390] and esophagoaortic fistulas[393] also have been described. Transesophageal echocardiogram and abdominal sonogram or CT scan are potentially helpful in suspected aortitis. Surgical intervention is recommended if the patient is symptomatic and combined medical and surgical therapy is preferred since together they are superior to either individual therapy for curing the lesion.[394] Medical treatment includes antituberculous chemotherapy and mindful attention to potential complications. Complications such as aortic valve insufficiency and aneurysm formation and rupture may occur. Surgery usually is indicated. The thoracic aorta can be repaired or replaced by prosthetic grafts.[390]

X. UPPER AIRWAYS

Upper airway structures such as the nose, epiglottis, larynx, and pharynx can be infected with *M. tuberculosis*. These structure are bathed continuously by organisms in the expectorated sputum of active cavitary lung disease.[343] Upper airway involvement is associated primarily with severe cavitary pulmonary disease and rarely with miliary tuberculosis.[395] In one North American study of a large number of patients with active tuberculosis, laryngeal lesions were found in 1.5% of patients.[396]

Laryngitis is highly infectious, with a tremendous load of live bacilli, and usually is accompanied by severe cavitary pulmonary disease or endobronchial disease.[395] The chest radiograph is abnormal in 95% of cases.[395] Hoarseness, cough, and throat pain are common symptoms. The anterior two thirds of the vocal cords are involved in 70% of patients.[395] There is hypertrophy with a pale or pink appearance, odynophagia, ulceration, edema, and stridor.[395] Pathology may show a superficial lesion, an ulceration, or granuloma. It may mimic a laryngeal cancer or papilloma, although concomitant carcinoma is possible.[395] Unusual presentations mimicking a salivary gland tumor, sebaceous cyst, or carotid body tumor have been reported.[397] Occasionally the epiglottis, the false cords, the aryepiglottic folds, or the hypopharynx are involved.[343] Paralysis of the vocal cords, especially the left, is secondary to lymphatic or pleural disease.[343] There is a dramatic therapeutic response with chemotherapy and pain will usually subside within 1 to 2 weeks.[395] Stenosis secondary to fibrosis or cricoarytenoid fixation is rare.

XI. DERMAL

Tuberculosis of the dermal system includes the skin, subcutaneous tissue and the breast. A high index of suspicion is necessary to diagnose cutaneous TB. Histology may show only acute and chronic inflammation, and staining and culture of the biopsy is required.[398] The course usually is benign, but at times may be serious.

There are three distinct categories of disease,[399] based on the source, including exogenous, endogenous, and hematogenous. Exogenous infection of the intact skin occurs by inoculation in less than 2% of patients with cutaneous TB.[400] It may appear as a verrucous lesion (prosector's wart, "anatomical tubercle") or a hyperkeratotic papule with hyperplasia and dense inflammation.[399,400] There usually is no lymph node involvement, and it has been previously referred to as "tuberculosis verrucosa cutis" and "tuberculosis cutis verruca et necrogenica."[400] It is acquired primarily in the autopsy room or by touching contaminated specimens.[401] Lesions can be treated with chemotherapy and in some cases by excision alone. Spontaneous resolution in immunocompetent patients may conceivably occur. Primary inoculation also may resemble an ulcer (tuberculous chancre) and is referred to as a cutaneous primary complex or a cutaneous Ghon complex. Lymph nodes may enlarge 3 to 6 weeks after inoculation. The primary cutaneous infection occurs mostly in children and is associated with regional adenopathy.[400]

Tuberculosis of the skin may occur through contiguous spread, e.g., from cervical lymph nodes, osteomyelitis, or epididymitis. This is called scrofuloderma or tuberculosis colliquativa cutis, and is "the fistulous opening of sinuses originated in glands or bones previously infected with tuberculosis."[402] Disease also may occur secondary to excretion of organisms and autoinoculation and is called orificial tuberculosis. Painful ulcers of the anal, oral, labial openings, and the surrounding skin can be seen. This is referred to as "tuberculosis ulcerosa cutis et mucosae" or "tuberculosis cutis orificialis."[398]

There is a form of cutaneous TB from hematogenous spread which is divided into three subsets: lupus vulgaris, acute dissemination, and nodules or abscesses. Lupus vulgaris is seen primarily in women. It presents with "apple-jelly" plaques or nodules upon diascopy, scarring ulcers, and severe deformities of the nose, neck, ear lobe, or face.[399] Its hallmark is chronicity and it may be indolent and missed clinically for years.[398] With long-standing chronic ulcers, carcinoma may develop in as much as 8% of patients.[403] Antituberculous chemotherapy usually is necessary.

Acute disseminated TB may cause multiple skin lesions (tuberculosis cutis miliaris disseminata),[404] which appear as blue-red to brown papules the size of a pinhead and may be mistaken for folliculitis.[404] It is rare and primarily a disease of infants and children.[400] Cutaneous vasculitis is rare.

Subcutaneous cold abscesses may be isolated to the breast, chest wall, axilla, buttocks, and extremities.[400] Mastitis or a breast abscess may appear in younger women and usually is accompanied by axillary lymphadenopathy.[406] It occurs as the result of retrograde lymphatic extension from adjacent lymph nodes. It may be difficult to diagnose and often is confused with carcinoma.[400] The yield on stain and culture is only 15% and histologic diagnosis is crucial.[406] Pathologically, it may be confused with ductal ectasia, foreign body, or idiopathic reactions. Surgical excision is the treatment of choice but chemotherapy also may be required.[406] Complications include discharge, ulcer with inflammation, recurring abscess, fistula, and sclerosis with nipple retraction. Open abscesses treated with irrigation may aerosolize organisms and cause infection.[407]

TB may manifest in HIV-positive patients as acneiform papules that mimic folliculitis, indurated crusted plaques, multiple tender skin nodules, abscesses, or swollen lymph nodes with overlying erythema. Sometimes ill-defined macules or ecthymatous lesions have been noted.[408] Chronic recurrent perirectal abscesses have been observed. Tuberculosis cutis miliaris disseminata with numerous 2 to 3 mm follicular papules has been described.[405] Lesions with purulent discharge may be infectious.[409] Localized cutaneous disease may respond to excision and drainage.[408] PCR has been used to detect mycobacterial DNA in the skin; however, it is susceptible to technical error, has resulted in false-positive as well as false-negative results, and is unable to differentiate viable from nonviable mycobacteria.[410]

Tuberculids are a heterogenous group of cutaneous lesions with caseation necrosis and perivascular infiltrates (hypersensitivity reaction secondary to dissemination), which include erythema induratum, papulonecrotic tuberculid, lichen scrofulosorum, and papular lesions of tuberculid hypersensitivity.[400]

XII. ENDOCRINE

A. Adrenal

In Addison's original description of adrenal insufficiency, 7 of 11 patients had tuberculosis. At least 80 to 90% of the glands must be destroyed for significant insufficiency to occur.[411] As much as 30% of cases of chronic adrenal insufficiency were considered to be due to TB.[359] The adrenals have been involved in approximately 53% of patients with disseminated TB, but adrenal insufficiency has been present in less than 1% of patients, even with severe or chronic disease.[207,412] Nine patients with tuberculosis of the adrenal gland diagnosed at autopsy were reported in one study of extrapulmonary tuberculosis.[32]

Histopathology may show massive caseation and enlargement of both glands in acute disease.[413] Calcification is a sign of chronicity, develops within 6 to 24 months, and is 95% specific for TB.[414] With TB of less than 2 years duration, enlarged glands are typical; at more than 2 years, they are normal or small. Therefore, adrenal size can be a clinical clue to the duration of disease. Sonography or CT scan-guided, fine-needle aspiration/biopsy may be helpful in achieving the diagnosis.[415]

HIV-positive patients with miliary TB may develop acute adrenal insufficiency. Rifampin may increase the catabolism of corticosteroids and unmask subclinical adrenal insufficiency.[416] With suspected adrenal insufficiency, it is prudent first to perform an ACTH stimulation test, administer dexamethasone therapy (to avoid interference with testing), and then change to hydrocortisone, 100 mg every 6 hours.[417]

B. THYROID

For unknown reasons, TB of the thyroid is very unusual despite the relatively high organ perfusion. There were only two patients with TB among 75,000 thyroid biopsies.[418] Tuberculosis of the thyroid may present as an abscess, or a cold or warm nodule. The patient may have pain, tenderness, hoarseness, dysphagia, or accompanying dyspnea.[413] Only one case of hypothyroidism with myxedema due to TB has been reported, most patients are euthyroid.[418]

In a study by Shafer et al., of 199 cases of extrapulmonary tuberculosis, three patients had thyroid involvement at autopsy.[32]

C. PITUITARY

Pituitary gland involvement may cause fever, headache, visual disturbances, and usually is associated with preexisting pituitary adenomas or meningitis.[250,419] A hypophyseal tuberculoma may impair or destroy function. Diabetes insipidus, hypogonadism, growth failure, and panhypopituitarism are subjects of case reports only.[420] However, hypopituitarism was documented in 10 of 49 patients years after recovery from tuberculous meningitis in childhood.[421]

REFERENCES

1. Morse, D., Brothwell, D. R., and Ucko, P. J., Tuberculosis in ancient Egypt, *Am. Rev. Resp. Dis.*, 90, 524, 1964.
2. Centers for Disease Control/American Thoracic Society, Core curriculum on tuberculosis, American Lung Association, New York, 1990.
3. Rieder, H. L., Snider, D. E., and Cauthen, G.. M., Extrapulmonary tuberculosis in the United States, *Am. Rev. Respir. Dis.*, 141, 347, 1990.
4. Anon., Extrapulmonary tuberculosis in the United States, U.S. Department of Health, Education, and Welfare, Center for Disease Control, Atlanta, GA, 1978.
5. Anon., Cases of specified notifiable diseases, United States, *MMWR*, 38, 241, 1989.
6. Centers for Disease Control and Prevention, Reported Tuberculosis in the United States, Atlanta, GA, 1997, 1998.
7. Centers for Disease Control, Tuberculosis in developing countries, *MMWR*, 39, 561, 1990.
8. Richter, C., Ndosi, B., Mwammy, A. S., and Mbwambo, R. K., Extrapulmonary tuberculosis — a simple diagnosis, *Tropic Geograph. Med.*, 43, 375, 1991.
9. Rieder, H. L., Kelly, G. D., Bloch, A. B., Cauthen, G. M., and Snider, D. E., Jr., Tuberculosis diagnosed at death in the United States, *Chest*, 100, 678, 1991.
10. Chastonay, P. and Gardiol, D., Extensive active tuberculosis at autopsy: retrospective study of a collection of adult autopsies (1961-1985), *J. Suisse Med.*, 117, 925, 1987.

11. U.S. Department of Health and Human Services, 1990 tuberculosis statistics in the United States, Centers for Disease Control, Atlanta, GA, 1992.
12. Lester, T. W., Extrapulmonary tuberculosis, *Clin. Chest Med.*, 2, 219, 1980.
13. Cuss, F. M. C., Carmichael, D. J. S., Linington, A., and Hulme, B., Tuberculosis in renal failure: a high incidence in patients born in the third world, *Clin. Nephrol.*, 25, 129, 1986.
14. Andrew, O. T., Schoenfeld, P., Hopewell, C., and Humphries, M. H., Tuberculosis in patients with endstage renal disease, *Am. J. Med.*, 68, 59, 1980.
15. Navari, R. M., Sullivan, K. M., Springmeyer, S. C., Siegel, M. S., Meyers, J. D., Buckner, C. D., Sanders, J. E., Stewart, P. S., Clift, R. A., Fefer, A., Storb, R., and Thomas, E. D., Mycobacterial infections in marrow transplant patients, *Transplantation*, 36, 509, 1983.
16. Bruce, R. M. and Wise, L., Tuberculosis after jejunoileal bypass for obesity, *Ann. Int. Med.*, 87, 574, 1982.
17. Snider, D. E., Jejunoileal bypass for obesity: a risk factor for tuberculosis, *Chest*, 81, 531, 1982.
18. Warner, T. T., Khoo, S. H., and Wilkins, E. G., Reactivation of tuberculous lymphadenitis during pregnancy, *J. Inf.*, 24, 181, 1992.
19. De Cock, K. M., Soro, B., Coulibaly, I. M., and Lucas, S. B., Tuberculosis and HIV infection in sub-Saharan Africa, *JAMA*, 268, 1581, 1992.
20. Dubé, M. P., Holtom, P. D., and Larsen, R. A., Tuberculous meningitis in patients with and without human immunodeficiency virus infection, *AJM*, 93, 520, 1992.
21. Raviglione, M. C., Narain, J. P., and Kochi, A., HIV-associated tuberculosis in developing countries: clinical features, diagnosis, and treatment, *Bull. World Health Org.*, 70, 515, 1992.
22. Markowitz, N., Hansen, N. I., Hopewell, P. C., et al., Incidence of tuberculosis in the United States among HIV-infected persons, *Ann. Intern. Med.*, 126, 123, 1997.
23. Pitchenik, A. E. and Fertel, D., Tuberculosis and nontuberculous mycobacterial disease, *Med. Clin. N. Am.*, 76, 121, 1992.
24. Mehta, J. R., Klapholz, A., Staniloae, C., and Talavera, W., The spectrum of extrapulmonary tuberculosis in patients infected with human immunodeficiency virus, *Chest,* 110(Suppl.), A69, 1996.
25. Braun, M. M., Byers, R. H., Heyward, W. L., Ciesielski, C. A., Bloch, A. B., Berkelman, R. L., and Snider, D. E., Acquired immunodeficiency syndrome and extrapulmonary tuberculosis in the United States, *Arch. Intern. Med.*, 150, 1913, 1990.
26. Flora, G. S., Modilevsky, T., Antoniskis, D., and Barnes, P. F., Undiagnosed tuberculosis in patients with human immunodeficiency virus infection, *Chest*, 98, 1056, 1990.
27. Gilks, C. F., Brindle, R. J., Otieno, L. S., Bhatt, S. M., Newnham, R. S., Simani, P. M., Lule, G. N., Okelo, G. B. A., Watkins, W. M., Waiyaki, P. G., Were, J. O. B., and Warrell, D.,A., Extrapulmonary and disseminated tuberculosis in HIV-1-seropositive patients presenting to the acute medical services in Nairobi, *AIDS*, 4, 981, 1990.
28. Chaisson, R. E. and Slutkin, G., Tuberculosis and human immunodeficiency virus infection, *J. Infect. Dis.*, 159, 96, 1989.
29. Havlir, D. V. and Barnes, P. F., Tuberculosis in patients with human immunodeficiency virus infection, *N. Engl. J. Med.*, 340, 367, 1999.
30. Handwerger, S., Mildvan, D., Senie, R., and McKinley, F. W., Tuberculosis and the acquired immunodeficiency syndrome at a New York City hospital: 1978–1985, *Chest*, 91, 176, 1987.
31. Chaisson, R. E., Schecter, G. F., Theuer, C. P., et al., Tuberculosis in patients with the acquired immunodeficiency syndrome, *Am. Rev. Respir. Dis.*, 136, 570, 1987.
32. Shafer, R. W., Kim, D. S., Weiss, J. P., and Quale, J. M., Extrapulmonary tuberculosis in patients with human immunodeficiency virus infection, *Medicine*, 70, 384, 1991.
33. Hopewell, P. C., Impact of human immunodeficiency virus infection on the epidemiology, clinical features, management, and control of tuberculosis, *Clin. Inf. Dis.*, 15, 540, 1992.
34. Barnes, P. F. and Arevalo, C., Six cases of *Mycobacterium tuberculosis* bacteremia, *J. Inf. Dis.*, 156, 377, 1987.
35. Hartstein, M. and Leaf, H. L., Tuberculosis of the breast as a presenting manifestation of AIDS, *Clin. Inf. Dis.*, 15, 692, 1992.
36. Marini, M., Ed., *Tuberculosis of the Bone and Joints,* Springer Verlag, Berlin, 1988.
37. Edlin, G. P., Active tuberculosis unrecognised until necropsy, *Lancet*, 1, 8076, 650, 1978.
38. Dutt, A. K., Moers, D., and Stead, W. W., Short-course chemotherapy for extrapulmonary tuberculosis: nine years' experience, *Ann. Int. Med.*, 104, 7, 1986.

39. Dutt, A. K. and Stead, W. W., Treatment of extrapulmonary tuberculosis, *Sem. Resp. Inf.*, 4, 225, 1989.

40. Cohn, D. L., Catlin, B. J., Peterson, K. L., Judson, F. N., and Sbarbaro, J. A., A 62-dose, 6-month therapy for pulmonary and extrapulmonary tuberculosis, a twice-weekly, directly observed, and cost-effective regimen, *Ann. Int. Med.*, 112, 407, 1990.

41. Shriner, K. A, Mathisen, G. E., and Goetz, M. B., Comparison of mycobacterial lymphadenitis among persons infected with human immunodeficiency virus and seronegative controls, *Clin. Inf. Dis.*, 1, 601, 1992.

42. Shikhani, A. H., Hadi, U. M., Mufarrij, A. A., and Zaytoun, G. M., Mycobacterial cervical lymphadenitis, *ENT J.*, 68, 660, 1989.

43. Hooper, A. A., Tuberculous peripheral lymphadenitis, *Br. J. Surg.*, 9, 33, 1972.

44. Lincoln, E. M. and Sewell, E. M., *Tuberculosis in Children*, McGraw-Hill, New York, 1963.

45. Kent, D. C., Tuberculous lymphadenitis: not a localized disease process, *Am. J. Med. Sci*, 24, 866, 1967.

46. Ord, R. J. and Matz, G. J., Tuberculous cervical lymphadenitis, *Arch. Otolaryngol.*, 99, 327, 1974.

47. Lai, K. K., Stottmeier, K. D., Sherman, I. H., and McCabe, W. R., Mycobacterial cervical lymphadenopathy, *JAMA*, 21, 1286, 1984.

48. Summers, G. D. and McNicol, M. W., Tuberculosis of superficial lymph nodes, *Br. J. Dis. Child.*, 74, 369, 1980.

49. Powell, D. A., Tuberculous lymphadenitis, in Schlossberg, D., Ed., *Tuberculosis*, Springer Verlag, New York, 1993, 143.

50. Huhti, E., Brander, E., Paloheimo, S., and Sutinen, S., Tuberculosis of the cervical lymph nodes: a clinical, pathological and bacteriological study, *Tubercle*, 56, 27, 1975.

51. Cantrell, R. W., Jensen, J. H., and Reid, D., Diagnosis and management of tuberculous cervical adenitis, *Arch. Otolaryngol.*, 101, 53, 1975.

52. Pitchenik, A. E., Burr, J., Suarez, M., Fertel, D., Gonzalez, G., and Moas, C., Human T-cell lymphotropic virus-III (HTLV-III) seropositivity and related disease among 71 consecutive patients in whom tuberculosis was diagnosed, *Am. Rev. Respir. Dis.*, 13, 87, 1987.

53. Modilevsky, T., Sattler, F. R., and Barnes, P. F., Mycobacterial disease in patients with human immunodeficiency virus infection, *Arch. Int. Med.*, 149, 2201, 1989.

54. Farer, L. S., Lowell, A. M., and Meador, M. P., Extrapulmonary tuberculosis in the United States, *Am. J. Epidemiol.*, 109, 20, 1979.

55. Thompson, B. C., The pathogenesis of tuberculosis of peripheral lymph nodes: a clinical study of 324 cases, *Tubercle,* 21, 217, 1940.

56. Miller, F. J. W. and Cashman, J. M., Origin of peripheral tuberculous lymphadenitis in childhood, *Lancet*, 1, 286, 1958.

57. Dandapat, M. C., Mishra, B. M., Dash, S. P., and Kar, P. K., Peripheral lymph node tuberculosis: a review of 80 cases, *Br. J. Surg.*, 77, 911, 1990.

58. Malik, S. K., Behera, D., and Gilhotra, R., Tuberculous pleural effusion and lymphadenitis treated with rifampin-containing regimen, *Chest*, 92, 902, 1992.

59. Lee, K. C., Tami, T. A., Lalwani, A. K., and Schecter, G., Contemporary management of cervical tuberculosis, *Laryngoscope*, 102, 60, 1992.

60. Schuit, K. E., Miliary tuberculosis in children: clinical and laboratory manifestation in 19 patients, *Am. J. Dis. Child.*, 133, 83, 1979.

61. Kecharvarz-Oliai, L. and Warren, W. S., Peripheral tuberculous lymphadenitis, *Am. J. Dis. Child.*, 122, 74, 1971.

62. Lewis, J. H. and Zimmerman, H. J., Tuberculosis of the liver and biliary tract, in Schlossberg, D., Ed., *Tuberculosis*, Springer Verlag, New York, 1993, 199.

63. British Thoracic Society Research Committee, Short course chemotherapy for tuberculosis of lymph nodes: a controlled trial, *BMJ*, 290, 1106, 1985.

64. Campbell, I. A. and Dyson, A. J., Lymph node tuberculosis: a comparison of various methods of treatment, *Tubercle*, 8, 171, 1977.

65. Campbell, I. A. and Dyson, A. J., Lymph node tuberculosis: a comparison of treatments 18 months after completion of chemotherapy, *Tubercle*, 60, 9, 1979.

66. Cheung, W. L., Siu, K. F., and Ng, A., Tuberculous cervical abscess: comparing the results of total excision against simple incision and drainage, *Br. J. Surg.*, 7, 63, 1988.

67. Lau, S. K., Kwan, S., Lee, J., and Wei, W. I., Source of tubercle bacilli in cervical lymph nodes: a prospective study, *J. Laryng. Otol.*, 10, 8, 1991.

68. Pithie, A. D. and Chicksen, B., Fine-needle extrathoracic lymph node aspiration in HIV-associated sputum-negative tuberculosis, *Lancet*, 340, 104, 1992.

69. Artenstein, A. W., Kim, J. H., Williams, W. J., and Chung, R. C. Y., Isolated peripheral tuberculous lymphadenitis in adults: current clinical and diagnostic issues, *Clin. Infect. Dis.,* 20, 876, 1995.

70. Ganz, W. I. and Serafini, A. N., The diagnostic role of nuclear medicine in the acquired immunodeficiency syndrome, *J. Nucl. Med.*, 30, 193, 1989.

71. Radin, D. R., Intraabdominal *Mycobacterium tuberculosis* versus *Mycobacterium avium*-intracellulare infections in patients with AIDS: distinction based on CT findings, *Am. J. Roentgenol.*, 16, 487, 1991.

72. Skarzynski, J. J., Sherman, W., Lee, H. K., and Berger, H., Patchy uptake of gallium in the lungs of AIDS patients with atypical mycobacterial infection, *Clin. Nucl. Med.*, 12, 7, 1987.

73. Shiota, Y., Kitade, M., Ueda, N., and Furuya, K., Tuberculous mediastinal lymphadenitis in an adult patient, *Jpn. J. Med.*, 28, 382, 1989.

74. Anon., Six-months versus nine-months chemotherapy for tuberculosis of lymph nodes: preliminary results, *Resp. Med.*, 86, 1, 1992.

75. Campbell, I. A., The treatment of superficial tuberculous lymphadenitis, *Tubercle*, 71, 1, 1990.

76. Cheung, W. L., Siu, K. F., and Ng, A., Six-month combination chemotherapy for cervical tuberculous lymphadenitis, *J. R. Coll. Edinb.*, 3, 293, 1990.

77. Illes, P. B. and Emerson, P. A., Tuberculous lymphadenitis, *Br. Med. J.*, 1, 143, 1974.

78. Silver, C. P. and Steel, S. J., Mediastinal lymphatic gland tuberculosis in Asian and coloured immigrants, *Lancet*, 1, 124, 1961.

79. Dhand, S., Fisher, M., and Fewell, J. W., Intrathoracic tuberculous lymphadenopathy in adults, *JAMA*, 241, 1, 1979.

80. Liu, C., Fields, W. R., and Shaw, C., Tuberculous mediastinal lymphadenopathy in adults, *Radiology*, 126, 369, 1978.

81. Im, J. G., Song, K. S., Kang, H. S., Park, J. H., Yeon, K. M., Han, M. C., and Kim, C. W., Mediastinal tuberculous lymphadenitis: CT manifestations, *Radiology*, 164, 11, 1987.

82. Hill, A. R., Premkur, S., Brustein, S., Vaidya, K., Powell, S., Li, P., and Suster, B., Disseminated tuberculosis in the acquired immunodeficiency syndrome era, *Am. Rev. Resp. Dis.*, 144, 1164, 1991.

83. Kramer, F., Modilevsky, T., Waliany, A. R., Leedom, J. M., and Barnes, P. F., Delayed diagnosis of tuberculosis in patients with human immunodeficiency virus infection, *Am. J. Med.*, 89, 41, 1990.

84. Wasser, L. S., Shaw, G. W., and Talavera, W., Endobronchial tuberculosis in the acquired immunodeficiency syndrome, *Chest*, 94, 1240, 1988.

85. Chang, S. C., Lee, P. Y., and Perng, R. P., Clinical role of bronchoscopy in adults with intrathoracic tuberculous lymphadenopathy, *Chest*, 93, 314, 1988.

86. American Thoracic Society, Treatment of tuberculosis and tuberculosis infection in adults and children, *Am. Rev. Respir. Dis.*, 134, 3, 1986.

87. Fontan-Bueso, J. F., Hernando, V., Garcia-Buela, J. P., Juncal, L. D., Egaña, M. T. M., and Martinez, M. C. M., Diagnostic value of simultaneous determination of pleural adenosine deaminase and pleural lysozyme/serum lysozyme ratio in pleural effusions, *Chest*, 93, 303, 1988.

88. Pugatch, R. D., Faling, L. J., Robbins, A. H., et al, Differentiation of pleural lesions using computed tomography, *J. Comput. Assist. Tomograph.*, 2, 601, 1978.

89. Storey, D. D., Dines, D. E., and Coles, D. T., Pleural effusion — a diagnostic dilemma, *JAMA*, 236, 2183, 1976.

90. Light, R. W., Macgregor, I. M., Luchsinger, P. C., and Ball, W. C., Pleural effusions, the diagnostic separation of transudates and exudates, *Ann. Int. Med.*, 77, 507, 1972.

91. Seibert, A. F., Haynes, J., Jr., Middleton, R., and Bass, J. B., Jr., Tuberculous pleural effusion: twenty-year experience, *Chest*, 99, 883, 1991.

92. Berger, H. W. and Mejia, E., Tuberculous pleurisy, *Chest*, 63, 88, 1973.

93. Epstein, D. M., Kline, L. R., Albelda, S. M., and Miller, W. T., Tuberculous pleural effusions, *Chest*, 91, 106, 1987.

94. Rossman, M. D. and Mayock, R. L., Pulmonary tuberculosis, in Schlossberg, D., Ed., *Tuberculosis*, Springer Verlag, New York, 1993, 95.

95. Light, R. W., Tuberculous pleural effusions, in Light, R. W., Ed., *Pleural Diseases*, 2nd ed., Lea and Febiger, Philadelphia, 1990, 11.

96. Moudgil, H., Sridhar, G., and Leitch, A., Reactivation disease: the commonest form of tuberculous pleural effusion in Edinburgh, *Respir. Med.*, 88, 301, 1994.

97. Antoniskis, D., Amin, K., and Barnes, P. F., Pleuritis as a manifestation of reactivation tuberculosis, *AJM*, 89, 447, 1990.

98. Wallgren, A., The timetable of tuberculosis, *Tubercle*, 22, 24, 1948.

99. Fischl, M. A., Uttamchandani, R. B., and Daikos, G. L., An outbreak of tuberculosis caused by multiple-drug-resistant tubercle bacilli among patients with HIV infection, *Ann. Int. Med.*, 117, 177, 1992.

100. Patiala, J., Initial tuberculous pleuritis in the Finnish Armed Forces in 1939–1944 with special reference to eventual post pleuritic tuberculosis, *Acta Tuberc. Scand.*, Suppl. 36, 1, 1948.

101. Roper, W. H. and Waring, J. J., Primary serofibrinous pleural effusion in military personnel, *Am. Rev. Resp. Dis.*, 71, 616, 1984.

102. Levine, H., Szanto, P. B., and Cugell, D. W., Tuberculous pleurisy: an acute illness, *Arch. Int. Med.*, 122, 329, 1968.

103. Gedde-Dahl, T., Tuberculous infection in the light of tuberculin matriculation, *Am. J. Hygiene*, 56, 139, 214, 1952.

104. Hulnick, D. H., Naidich, D. P., and McCauley, D. I., Pleural tuberculosis evaluated by computed tomography, *Radiology*, 149, 79, 1983.

105. Ankobiah, W. A., Finch, P., Powell, S., Heurich, A., Shivaram, I., and Kamholz, S. L., Pleural tuberculosis in patients with and without AIDS, *J. Assoc. Acad. Min. Phys.*, 1, 20, 1990.

106. Frye, M., Pozsik, C., and Sahn, S., Tuberculous pleurisy is more common in AIDS than in non-AIDS patients with tuberculosis, *Chest*, 112, 393, 1997.

107. Chan, C. H., Arnold, M., Chan, C. Y., Mak, T. W., and Hoheisel, G. B., Clinical and pathological features of tuberculous pleural effusion and its long-term consequences, *Respiration*, 8, 171, 1991.

108. Rossi, G. A., Balbi, B., and Manca, F., Tuberculous pleural effusions, *Am. Rev. Respir. Dis.*, 136, 7, 1987.

109. Light, R., Erozan, Y., and Ball, W., Jr., Cells in pleural fluid: their value in differential diagnosis, *Arch. Intern. Med.*, 132, 854, 1973.

110. Adelman, M., Albelda, S. M., Gottlieb, J., et al., Diagnostic utility of pleural fluid eosinophilia, *Am. J. Med.*, 77, 915, 1984.

111. Spriggs, A. and Boddington, M., Absence of mesothelial cells from tuberculous pleural effusions, *Thorax*, 15, 169, 1960.

112. Hurwitz, S., Leiman, G., and Shapiro, C., Mesothelial cells in pleural fluid: TB or not TB? *S. African Med. J.*, 57, 937, 1980.

113. Lau, K., Numerous mesothelial cells in tuberculous pleural effusions, *Chest*, 96, 438, 1989.

114. Levine, H., Metzger, W., Lacera, D., and Kay, L., Diagnosis of tuberculous pleurisy by culture of pleural biopsy specimen, *Arch. Int. Med.*, 126, 269, 1970.

115. Bañales, J. L., Pineda, P. R., Fitzgerald, J. M., Rubio, H., Selman, M., and Salazar-Lezama, M., Adenosine deaminase in the diagnosis of tuberculous pleural effusions, *Chest*, 99, 355, 1991.

116. Ocaña, I., Martinez-Vazquez, J. M., Segura, R. M., Fernandez de Sevilla, T., and Capdevila, J. A., Adenosine deaminase in pleural fluids, *Chest*, 84, 51, 1983.

117. Ocana, I., Ribera, E., Martinez-Vasquez, J. M., Ruiz, I., Bejarano, E., Pigrau, C., et al., Anosine deaminase activity in rheumatoid pleural effusion, *Ann. Rheum. Dis.*, 47, 394, 1988.

118. Valdes, L., San Jose, E., Alvarez, D., Sarandeses, A., Pose, A., Chomon, B., et al., Diagnosis of tuberculous pleurisy using the biologic parameters adenosine deaminase, lysozyme and interferon gamma, *Chest*, 103, 458, 1993.

119. Bothamley, G. H., Tuberculous pleurisy and adenosine deaminase, *Thorax*, 50, 593, 1995.

120. Ribera, E., Ocaña, I., Martinez-Vazquez, J. M., Rossell, M., Espanel, T., and Ruibal, A., High level of interferon gamma in tuberculous pleural effusion, *Chest*, 93, 308, 1988.

121. Hara, N., Abe, M., Inuzuka, S., Kawarada, Y., and Shigematsu, N., Pleural SCb-9 in differential diagnosis of tuberculous, malignant, and other effusions, *Chest*, 102, 1060, 1992.

122. de Wit, D., Maartens, G., and Steyn, L., A comparative study of the polymerase chain reaction and conventional procedures for the diagnosis of tuberculous pleural effusion, *Tuberc. Lung Dis.*, 73, 262, 1992.

123. de Lassence, A., Lecossier, D., Pierre, C., Cadranel, J., Stern, M., and Hance, A. J., Detection of mycobacterial DNA in pleural fluid from patients with tuberculous pleurisy by means of the polymerase chain reaction: comparison of two protocols, *Thorax*, 47, 265, 1992.

124. Maartens, G. and Bateman, E., Tuberculous pleural effusions: increased culture yield with bedside inoculation of pleural fluid and poor diagnostic value of adenosine deaminase, *Thorax*, 46, 96, 1991.

125. Sahn, S. A., The pleura, *Am. Rev. Respir. Dis.*, 138, 184, 1988.

126. Nance, K. V., Shermer, R. W., and Askin, F. B., Diagnostic efficacy of pleural biopsy as compared with that of pleural fluid examination, *Mod. Path.*, 4, 320, 1991.

127. Sarkar, S. K., Purohit, S. D., Sharma, T. N., Sharma, V. K., Ram, M., and Singh, A. P., Pleuroscopy in the diagnosis of pleural effusion using a fiberoptic bronchoscope, *Tubercle*, 66, 141, 1988.

128. Menzies, R. and Charbonneau, M., Thoracoscopy for the diagnosis of pleural disease, *Ann. Int. Med.*, 114, 271, 1991.

129. Boutin, C., Astoul, P., and Seitz, B., The role of thoracoscopy in the evaluation and management of pleural effusions, *Lung*, 168, 1113, 1990.

130. Dutt, A. K., Moers, D., and Stead, W. W., Short-course chemotherapy for pleural tuberculosis, *Chest*, 90, 112, 1986.

131. Barnes, P. F., Bloch, A. B., Davidson, P. T., and Snider, D. E., Tuberculosis in patients with human immunodeficiency virus infection, *NEJM*, 324, 1644, 1991.

132. Dutt, A. K., Moers, D., and Stead, W. W., Tuberculous pleural effusion: 6-month therapy with isoniazid and rifampin, *Am. Rev. Respir. Dis.*, 14, 1429, 1991.

133. Tani, P., Poppius, H., and Makiyaja, J., Cortisone therapy for exudative tuberculous pleurisy in the light of the follow-up study, *Acta Tuberc. Scand.*, 44, 303, 1964.

134. Lee, C. H., Wang, W. J., Lan, R. S., Tsai, Y. H., and Chiang, Y. C., Corticosteroids in the treatment of tuberculous pleurisy: a double-blind, placebo-controlled, randomized study, *Chest*, 94, 126, 1988.

135. Wyser, C., Wazl, G., Smedema, J., et al., Corticosteroids in the treatment of tuberculous pleurisy, a double blind, placebo-controlled, randomized study, *Chest*, 110, 333, 1996.

136. Large, S. E. and Levick, R. K., Aspiration in the treatment of primary tuberculous pleural effusion, *BMJ*, 1, 112, 1989.

137. Barbas, C. S., Cukier, A., de Varvalho, C. R., Barbas, F. J. V., and Light, R. W., The relationship between pleural findings and the development of pleural thickening in patients with pleural tuberculosis, *Chest*, 100, 1264, 1991.

138. Singh, P. P., Sridharan, K. B., Bhagi, R. P., and Singla, R., Anaerobic infection of the lung and pleural space in tuberculosis, *Ind. J. Chest Dis. All. Sci.*, 31, 8, 1989.

139. Johnson, T. M., McCann, W., and Davey, W. N., Tuberculous bronchopleural fistula, *Am. Rev. Resp. Dis.*, 107, 30, 1973.

140. Neihart, R. E. and Hof, D. G., Successful nonsurgical treatment of tuberculous empyema in an irreducible pleural space, *Chest*, 88, 792, 1985.

141. Cendan, I., Talavera, W., Busillo, C., Garner, G., and Mullen, M., Empyema thoracis: a complication of disseminated *Mycobacterium tuberculosis* (MTB) in AIDS, *Am. Rev. Respir. Dis.*, 143(Suppl.), A281, 1991.

142. Glicklich, M., Mendelson, D. S., Gendal, E. S., and Teirstein, A. S., Tuberculous empyema necessitatis — computed tomography findings, *Clin. Imag.*, 14, 23, 1990.

143. Vennera, M. C., Moreno, R., Cot, J., Marin, A., Sanchez-Lloret, J., Picado, C., and Agusti-Vidal, A., Chylothorax and tuberculosis, *Thorax*, 38, 694, 1983.

144. Fugiwara, T., Kashara, H., Tanohata, K., et al., Fast spin-echo MR imaging of non-Hodgkin lymphoma arising from chronic tuberculous empyema, *J. Thorac. Imag.*, 10, 82, 1995.

145. Takanami, I., Imamura, T., Morota, N., et al., Malignant fibrous histiocytoma of the chest wall developing after pleuropneumonectomy performed for tuberculous pyothorax: report of an unusal case, *J. Thorac. Cardiovasc. Surg.*, 108, 395, 1994.

146. Iuchi, K., Ichimaya, A., Akashi, A., et al., Non-Hodgkin's lymphoma of the pleural cavity developing from longstanding pyothorax, *Cancer*, 60, 1771, 1987.

147. Myouki, A., Aozasa, K., Iuchi, K., et al., Soft tissue sarcoma of the pleural cavity, *Cancer,* 68, 1550, 1991.

148. Gorse, G. J., Pais, M. J., Kusske, J. A., and Cesario, T. C., Tuberculous spondylitis, *Medicine,* 62, 178, 1983.

149. Davidson, P. T. and Horowitz, I., Skeletal tuberculosis: review with patient presentation and discussion, *Am. J. Med.,* 48, 77, 1970.

150. Watts, H. and Lifeso, R. M., Current concepts review: tuberculosis of bones and joints, *J. Bone Joint Surg.,* 78, 288, 1996.

151. Parsons, M., *Tuberculous Meningitis,* Oxford University Press, Oxford, U.K., 1988.

152. Thijn, C. J. P. and Steensma, J. T., *Tuberculosis of the Skeleton,* 1st ed., Springer, New York, 1990.

153. Lifeso, R. M., Weaver, P., and Harder, E. H., Tuberculous spondylitis in adults, *J. Bone Joint Surg.,* 67A, 1410, 1985.

154. Frankel, D. G., Daffner, R. H., and Wang, S. E., Case report 64, *Skeletal Radiol.,* 20, 130, 1991.

155. Gros, T., Soriano, V., Gabarre, E., Tor, J., and Sabria, M., Multifocal tubercular osteitis in a female patient infected with the human immunodeficiency virus (Spanish), *Rev. Clin. Esp.,* 191, 3, 1992.

156. Walker, G. F., Failure of early recognition of skeletal tuberculosis, *BMJ,* 1, 682, 1968.

157. Omari, B., Robertson, J. M., Nelson, R. J., and Chiu, L. C., Pott's disease: a resurgent challenge to the thoracic surgeon, *Chest,* 9, 14, 1989.

158. Sharif, H. S., Clark, D. C., Aabed, M. Y., Haddad, M. C., Al Deeb, S. M., Yaqub, B., and Al Moutaery, K. R., Granulomatous spinal infections: MR imaging, *Radiology,* 177, 101, 1990.

159. Babhulkar, S. S., Tayade, W. B., and Babhulkar, S. K., Atypical spinal tuberculosis, *J. Bone Joint Surg.,* 66, 239, 1984.

160. Sarkar, S. D., Ravikrishnan, K. P., Woodbury, D. H., Carson, J. J., and Daley, K., Gallium-67 citrate scanning — a new adjunct in the direction and follow-up of extrapulmonary tuberculosis: concise communication, *J. Nucl. Med.,* 20, 833, 1979.

161. Silverman, J. F., Larkin, E. W., Carney, M., Weaver, M. D., and Norris, H. T., Fine needle aspiration cytology of tuberculosis of the lumbar vertebrae (Pott's disease), *Acta Cytol.,* 30, 538, 1986.

162. Griffiths, D. L., Tuberculosis of the spine: a review, *Adv. Tuberc. Res.,* 20, 93, 1980.

163. Medical Section of the American Lung Association, Treatment of tuberculosis and tuberculosis infection in adults and children (joint statement of the American Thoracic Society and the Centers for Disease Control), *Am. Rev. Resp. Dis.,* 134, 358, 1986.

164. Talavera, W. and Cortes, J. A., Mycobacterial tuberculosis infections of the bones and joints, including the foot and ankle, *Lower Extrem.,* 3, 215, 1996.

165. Dhillon, M. S., Sharma, S., Gill, S. S., and Nagi, O. N., Tuberculosis of bones and joints of the foot: an analysis of 22 cases, *Foot Ankle,* 14, 505, 1993.

166. Feldman, F., Auerbach, R., and Johnston, A., Tuberculous dactylitis in the adult, *Am. J. Roentgenol.,* 112, 460, 1971.

167. Martini, M., Adjrad, A., and Bondjema, A., Tuberculous osteomyelitis: a review of 125 cases, *Int. Orthop.,* 10, 201, 1986.

168a. Reifler, J. F., Extrapulmonary tuberculosis, *Infect. Med.,* 9, 50, 1992.

168b. Mann, K. J., Lung lesions in skeletal tuberculosis: review of 500 cases, *Lancet,* 2, 744, 1946.

169. Jensen, C. M., Jensen, C. H., and Paerregaard, A., A diagnostic problem in tuberculous dactylitis, *J. Hand Surg.,* 16(2), 202, 1991.

170. Rigauts, H., Van Holsbeeck, M., and Lechat, A., Spina ventosa: the forgotten diagnosis. Report of one case, review of the literature, *J. Belg. Rad.,* 72, 13, 1989.

171. Berney, S., Goldstein, M., and Bishko, F., Clinical and diagnostic features of tuberculous arthritis, *Am. J. Med.,* 3, 36, 1972.

172. Spinner, R. J., Sexton, D. J., Goldner, R. D., and Levin, L. S., Periprosthetic infections due to *Mycobacterium tuberculosis* in patients with no prior history of tuberculosis, *J. Arthrop.,* 11, 217, 1996.

173. Poncet, M. A., Rhumatisme tuberculeux ou pseudo-rhumatisme d'origine bacillaire, *Bull. de l'Academie Nationale Medecine,* 46, 194, 1901, and Poncet, M. A., De la polyarthrite tuberculeuse, deformante ou pseudorheumatisme chronic tuberculeux, *Congres Francaise de Chirurgie,* 1, 732, 1897.

174. Pandy, D., Dubey, A. P., and Choudhury, P., Poncet's disease, *Ind. Pediatr.,* 26, 828, 1989.

175. Isaacs, A. J. and Sturrock, R. D., Poncet's disease — fact or fiction? *Tubercle,* 55, 135, 1974.

176. Dall, L., Long, L., and Stanford, J., Poncet's disease: tuberculous rheumatism, *Rev. Inf. Dis.*, 11, 105, 1989.

177. Carl, P. and Stark, L., Indications for surgical management of genitourinary tuberculosis, *World J. Surg.*, 21, 505, 1997.

178. Weinstein, A. J., Genitourinary tuberculosis, in Schlossberg, D., Ed., *Tuberculosis*, Springer Verlag, New York, 1993, 155.

179. Cinman, A. C., Genitourinary tuberculosis, *Urology*, 20, 33, 1982.

180. Christensen, W. I., Genitourinary tuberculosis: review of 102 cases, *Medicine*, 3, 377, 1974.

181. Shafer, R. W., Goldberg, R., Sierra, M., and Glatt, A. E., Frequency of *Mycobacterium tuberculosis* bacteremia in patients with tuberculosis in an area endemic for AIDS, *Am. Rev. Resp. Dis.*, 140, 1611, 1989.

182. Barber, T. W., Craven, D. E., and McCabe, W. R., Bacteremia due to *Mycobacterium tuberculosis* in patients with human immunodeficiency virus infection: a report of 9 cases and a review of the literature, *Medicine*, 69, 37, 1990.

183. Simon, H. B., Weinstein, A. J., Pasternak, M. S., Swartz, M. N., and Kunz, L. J., Genitourinary tuberculosis: clinical features in a general hospital population, *Am. J. Med.*, 63, 410, 1977.

184. Shariff, S. and Thomas, J. A., Fine needle aspiration cytodiagnosis of clinically suspected tuberculosis in tissue enlargement, *Acta Cytol.*, 3, 333, 1991.

185. Kollins, S. A., Hartman, G. W., Carr, D., Segura, J. W., and Hattery, R. R., Roentgenographic findings in urinary tract tuberculosis: a 10-year review, *Am. J. Roentgenol.*, 121, 487, 1974.

186. Das, K. M., Indudhara, R., and Vaidyanathan, S., Sonographic features of genitourinary tuberculosis, *Am. J. Roentgenol.*, 18, 327, 1992.

187. Gow, J. G., Genitourinary tuberculosis: a 7-year review, *BMJ*, 1, 239, 1979.

188. Gow, J. G. and Barbosa, S., Genitourinary tuberculosis: a study of 1117 cases over a period of 34 years, *Br. J. Urol.*, 6, 449, 1984.

189. Weinberg, A. C. and Boyd, S. D., Short-course chemotherapy and role of surgery in adult and pediatric genitourinary tuberculosis, *Urology*, 31, 95, 1988.

190. Ehrlich, R. M. and Lattimer, J. K., Genitourinary tuberculosis, *Surg. Ann.*, 6, 439, 1974.

191. *Smith's General Urology*, 13th ed., Appleton and Lange, CA, 1992, 240.

192. *Campbell's Urology*, 6th ed., Saunders, Philadelphia, 1993, 1037.

193. Gorse, G. J. and Belshe, R. B., Male genital tuberculosis: a review of the literature with instructive case reports, *Rev. Inf. Dis.*, 7, 511, 1985.

194. Medlar, E. M., Spain, D. M., and Holliday, R. W., Post-mortem compared with clinical diagnosis of genito-urinary tuberculosis in adult males, *J. Urol.*, 61, 1079, 1949.

195. Wechsler, H., Westfall, M., and Lattimer, J. K., The earliest signs and symptoms in 127 male patients with genitourinary tuberculosis, *J. Urol.*, 83, 801, 1960.

196. Lewis, E., Tuberculosis of the penis: a report of 5 new cases, and a complete review of the literature, *J. Urol.*, 56, 737, 1946.

197. Baskin, L. S. and Mee, S., Tuberculosis of the penis presenting as a subcutaneous nodule, *J. Urol.*, 141, 1430, 1989.

198. Auerbach, O., Pathology of urogenital tuberculosis, *New Intern. Clin.*, 3, 21, 1940.

199. Sporer, A. and Auerbach, O., Tuberculosis of prostate, *Urology*, 11, 362, 1978.

200. Chung, T. and Harris, R. D., Tuberculous epididymo-orchitis: sonographic findings, *J. Clin. Ultrasound*, 19, 367, 1991.

201. Davids, A. M., Genital tuberculosis in females, *J. Mt. Sinai Hosp.* New York, 23, 567, 1956.

202. Marana, R., Muzii, L., Lucisano, A., Ardito, F., Muscatello, P., Bilancioni, E., Maniccia, E., and Dell'Acqua, S., Incidence of genital tuberculosis in infertile patients submitted to diagnostic laparoscopy: recent experience in an Italian university hospital, *Int. J. Fertil.*, 36, 104, 1991.

203. Rao, K. N., Viswanathan, R., Deshmukh, M. D., Pamra, S. P., Sen, P. K., Bordia, N. L., and Dingley, H. B., Eds., *Textbook of Tuberculosis,* 2nd ed., Vikas Publishing, New Delhi, 1981.

204. Margolis, K., Wranz, P. A. B., Kruger, T. F., Joubert, J. J., and Odendaal, H. J., Genital tuberculosis at Tyberberg hospital — prevalence, clinical presentation and diagnosis, *S. Afr. Med. J.*, 81, 12, 1992.

205. Sutherland, A. M., Drug treatment of tuberculosis of the female genital tract, *J. Obs. Gyn.*, 6, 51, 1985.

206. Menitove, S. and Harris, H. W., Miliary tuberculosis, in Schlossberg, D., Ed., *Tuberculosis*, Springer Verlag, New York, 1993, 233.

207. Slavin, R. E., Walsh, T. J., and Pollack, A. D., Late generalized tuberculosis: a clinical pathologic analysis and comparison of 100 cases in the preantibiotic and antibiotic eras, *Medicine*, 59, 352, 1980.

208. Kaplan, M. H., Armstrong, D., and Rosen, P., Tuberculosis complicating neoplastic disease: a review of 201 cases, *Cancer*, 33, 80, 1974.

209. Pradhan, R. P., Katz, L. A., Nidus, B. D., Matalon, R., and Eisinger, R. P., Tuberculosis in dialyzed patients, *JAMA*, 229, 798, 1974.

210. Ballon, S. C., Clewell, W. H., and Lamb, E. J., Reactivation of silent pelvic tuberculosis by reconstructive tubal surgery, *Am. J. Obst. Gyn.*, 122, 991, 1975.

211. Yekanath, H., Gross, P. A., and Vitenson, J. H., Miliary tuberculosis following ureteral catheterization, *Urology*, 16, 197, 1980.

212. Federmann, M. and Kley, H. K., Miliary tuberculosis after extracorporeal shock-wave lithotripsy, *N. Engl. J. Med.*, 323, 1210, 1990.

213. Yamane, H., Fujiwara, T., Doko, S., Inada, H., Nogami, A., Masaki, H., Kanazawa, S., Hara, T., Kondo, J., and Yoshida, H., Two cases of miliary tuberculosis following prosthetic valve replacement (Japanese), *Kokyu To Junkan — Resp. Circ.*, 37, 803, 1989.

214. Maartens, G., Willcox, P. A., and Benatar, S. R., Miliary tuberculosis: rapid diagnosis, hematologic abnormalities, and outcome in 109 treated adults, *AJM*, 89, 291, 1990.

215. Kim, J. H., Langston, A. A., and Gallis, H. A., Miliary tuberculosis: epidemiology, clinical manifestations, diagnosis, and outcome, *Rev. Inf. Dis.*, 12, 583, 1990.

216. Dyer, R. A., Chappel, W. A., and Potgieter, P. D., Adult respiratory distress syndrome associated with miliary tuberculosis, *Crit. Care Med.*, 13, 12, 1985.

217. Heffner, J. E., Strange, C., and Sahn, S. A., The impact of respiratory failure on the diagnosis of tuberculosis, *Arch. Int. Med.*, 148, 1103, 1988.

218. Gee, W. M., The frequency of unsuspected tuberculosis found post-mortem in a geriatric population, *Z. Gerontol.*, 22, 311, 1989.

219. Rossi, S., Reale, D., and Grandi, E., Rilievo di patologia tuberculare in una casistica autoptica. Correlazione tra diagnosi clinica e anatomopatologica, *Pathologica*, 80, 449, 1988.

220. Cameron, S. J., Tuberculosis and the blood — a special relationship? *Tubercle*, 55, 55, 1974.

221. Munt, P. W., Miliary tuberculosis in the chemotherapy era: with a clinical review in 69 American adults, *Medicine*, 1, 139, 1971.

222. Proudfoot, A. T., Akhtar, A. J., Douglas, A. C., and Horne, N. W., Miliary tuberculosis in adults, *BMJ*, 2, 273, 1969.

223. Yu, Y. L., Chow, W. H., Humphries, M. J., Wong, R. W. S., and Gabriel, M., Cryptic miliary tuberculosis, *Q. J. Med.*, 228, 421, 1986.

224. O'Brien, J. R., Non-reactive tuberculosis, *J. Clin. Pathol.*, 7, 216, 1954.

225. Gelb, A. F., Leffler, C., Brewin, A., Mascatello, V., and Lyons, H. A., Miliary tuberculosis, *Am. Rev. Resp. Dis.*, 108, 1327, 1973.

226. Prout, S. and Benatar, S. R., Disseminated tuberculosis: a study of 62 cases, *S. Afr. Med. J.*, 8, 83, 1980.

227. Sahn, S. A. and Neff, T. A., Miliary tuberculosis, *Am. J. Med.*, 6, 49, 1974.

228. Williams, N. H., Jr., Kane, C., and Yoo, O. H., Pulmonary function in miliary tuberculosis, *Am. Rev. Resp. Dis.*, 107, 858, 1973.

229. Massaro, D., Katz, S., and Sachs, M., Choroidal tubercles, *Ann. Int. Med.*, 60, 231, 1964.

230. Bobrowitz, I. D., Active tuberculosis undiagnosed until autopsy, *Am. J. Med.*, 72, 60, 1982.

231. Saltzman, B. R., Motyl, M. R., Friedland, G. H., McKitrick, J. C., and Klein, R. S., *Mycobacterium tuberculosis* bacteremia in the acquired immunodeficiency syndrome, *JAMA*, 26, 390, 1986.

232. Gachot, B., Wolff, M., Clair, B., and Regnier, B., Severe tuberculosis in patients with human immunodeficiency virus infection, *Int. Care Med.*, 16, 491, 1990.

233. McGuinness, G., Naidich, D. P., Jagirdar, J., Leitman, B., and McCauley, D. I., High resolution CT findings in miliary lung disease, *J. Comp. Ass. Tomo.*, 16, 384, 1992.

234. Wasser, L. S., Brown, E., and Talavera, W., Miliary PCP in AIDS, *Chest*, 96, 693, 1989.

235. Grieff, M. and Lisbona, R., Detection of miliary tuberculosis by Ga-67 scintigraphy, *Clin. Nucl. Med.*, 16, 910, 1991.

236. Willcox, P. A., Potgieter, P. D., Bateman, E. D., and Benatar, S. R., Rapid diagnosis of sputum negative miliary tuberculosis using the flexible fibreoptic bronchoscope, *Thorax*, 41, 681, 1986.

237. Pant, K., Chawla, R., Mann, P. S., and Jaggi, O. P., Fiberbronchoscopy in smear-negative miliary tuberculosis, *Chest*, 9, 111, 1989.

238. Cucin, R. L., Coleman, M., Eckhardt, J. J., and Silver, R. T., The diagnosis of miliary tuberculosis: utility of peripheral blood abnormalities, bone marrow and liver needle biopsy, *J. Chronic Dis.*, 26, 355, 1973.

239. Heinle, E. W., Jensen, W. N., and Westerman, M. P., Diagnostic usefulness of marrow biopsy in disseminated tuberculosis, *Am. Rev. Resp. Dis.*, 91, 701, 1965.

240. Uribe-Botero, G., Prichard, J. G., and Kaplowitz, H. J., Bone marrow in HIV infection, *Am. J. Clin. Path.*, 91, 313, 1989.

241. Nichols, J., Florentine, B., Lewis, W., Sattler, F., Rarick, M. U., and Brynes, R. K., Bone marrow examination for the diagnosis of mycobacterial and fungal infections in the acquired immunodeficiency syndrome, *Arch. Pathol. Lab. Med.*, 115, 1125, 1991.

242. Bentz, R. R., Dimcheff, D. G., Nemiroff, M. J., Tsang, A., and Weg, J. G., The incidence of urine cultures positive for MTB in a general tuberculosis patient population, *Am. Rev. Respir. Dis.*, 111, 647, 1969.

243. Kissner, D. G., Missed opportunities, *Arch. Int. Med.*, 147, 2037, 1987.

244. Counsell, S. R., Tan, J. S., and Dittus, R. S., Unsuspected pulmonary tuberculosis in a community teaching hospital, *Arch. Int. Med.*, 149, 1274, 1989.

245. Huseby, J. S. and Hudson, L. D., Miliary tuberculosis and adult respiratory distress syndrome, *Ann. Intern. Med.*, 8, 609, 1976.

246. Murray, H. W., Tuazon, C. U., Kirmani, N., and Sheagren, J. N., The adult respiratory distress syndrome associated with miliary tuberculosis, *Chest*, 73, 37, 1978.

247. Knowles, K. F., Saltman, D., Robson, H. G., and Lalonde, R., Tuberculous pancreatitis, *Tubercle*, 71, 65, 1990.

248. Piqueras, A. R., Marruecos, L., Artigas, A., and Rodriguez, C., Miliary tuberculosis and adult respiratory distress syndrome, *Int. Care Med.*, 13, 175, 1987.

249. Ahuja, S. S., Ahuja, S. K., Phelps, K. R., Thelmo, W., and Hill, A. R., Hemodynamic confirmation of septic shock in disseminated tuberculosis, *Crit. Care Med.*, 20, 901, 1992.

250. Tandon, P. N., Tuberculous meningitis (cranial and spinal), in Vinken, P. J., Bruyn, G. W., and Klawans, H. L., Eds., *Handbook of Clinical Neurology: Infections of the Nervous System*, North Holland Publishing Company, Amsterdam, 33, 193, 1978.

251. Auerbach, O., Tuberculous meningitis: correlation of therapeutic results with the pathogenesis and pathologic changes, *Am. Rev. Tuberc.*, 64, 408, 1943.

252. Riggs, H. E., Rupp, C., and Ray, H., Clinicopathologic study of tuberculous meningitis in adults, *Am. Rev. Tuberc.*, 74, 830, 1956.

253. Hinman, A. R., Tuberculous meningitis at Cleveland Metropolitan General Hospital 1959–1963, *Am. Rev. Resp. Dis.*, 9, 670, 1967.

254. Ogawa, S. K., Smith, M. A., Brennessel, D. J., and Lowy, F. D., Tuberculous meningitis in an urban medical center, *Medicine*, 66, 317, 1987.

255. Bishburg, E., Sunderam, G., Reichman, L. B., and Kapila, R., Central nervous system tuberculosis with the acquired immunodeficiency syndrome and its related complex, *Ann. Int. Med.*, 105, 210, 1986.

256. Kasik, J. E., Central nervous system tuberculosis, in Schlossberg, D., Ed., *Tuberculosis*, Springer Verlag, New York, 1993, 129.

257. Molavi, A. and LeFrock, J. L., Tuberculous meningitis, *Med. Clin. N. Am.*, 69, 315, 1985.

258. Berenguer, J., Moreno, S., Laguna, F., Vicente, T., Adrados, M., Ortega, A., González-LaHoz, J., and Bouza, E., Tuberculous meningitis in patients infected with the human immunodeficiency virus, *NEJM*, 326, 668, 1992.

259. Humphries, M., The management of tuberculous meningitis, *Thorax*, 47, 77, 1992.

260. Haas, E. J., Madhavan, T., Quinn, E. L., Cox, F., Fisher, E., and Burch, K., Tuberculous meningitis in an urban general hospital, *Arch. Int. Med.*, 137, 1518, 1977.

261. Rooney, J. J., Jr., Crocco, J. A., Kramer, S., and Lyons, H. A., Further observations on tuberculin reactions in active tuberculosis, *Am. J. Med.*, 60, 17, 1976.

262. Klein, N. C., Damsker, B., and Hirschman, S. Z., Mycobacterial meningitis: retrospective analysis from 1970 to 1983, *Am. J. Med.*, 79, 29, 1985.

263. Offenbacher, H., Fazekas, F., Schmidt, R., Kleinert, R., Payer, F., Kleinert, G., and Lechner, H., MRI in tuberculous meningoencephalitis: report of four cases and review of the neuroimaging literature, *J. Neurol.*, 238, 340, 1991.

264. Whitener, D. R., Tuberculous brain abscess, *Arch. Neurol.*, 3, 148, 1978.

265. Jinkins, J. R., Computed tomography of intracranial tuberculosis, *Neuroradiology*, 33, 126, 1991.

266. Lees, A. J., Marshall, J., and MacLeod, A. F., Cerebral tuberculomas developing during treatment of tuberculous meningitis, *Lancet*, ii, 1208, 1970.

267. van Bommel, E. F., Stiegelis, W. F., and Schermers, H. P., Paradoxical response of intracranial tuberculomas during chemotherapy: an immunologic phenomenon? *Neth. J. Med.*, 38, 126, 1991.

268. Kennedy, D. H. and Fallon, R. J., Tuberculous meningitis, *JAMA*, 241, 264, 1979.

269. Illingworth, R. S., Miliary and meningeal tuberculosis: difficulties in diagnosis, *Lancet*, 271, 646, 1956.

270. Stewart, S. M., Technical methods: the bacteriological diagnosis of tuberculous meningitis, *J. Clin. Pathol.*, 6, 241, 1936.

271. Leonard, J. M. and Des Prez, R. M., Tuberculous meningitis, *Inf. Dis. Clin. N. Am.*, 4, 769, 1990.

272. Chawla, R. K., Seth, R. K., Raj, B., and Saini, A. S., Adenosine deaminase levels in cerebrospinal fluid in tuberculosis and bacterial meningitis, *Tubercle*, 72, 190, 1991.

273. Daniel, T. M., New approaches to the rapid diagnosis of tuberculous meningitis, *J. Inf. Dis.*, 1, 599, 1987.

274. Kadival, G. V., Mazarelo, T. B. M. S., and Chaparas, S. D., Sensitivity and specificity of enzyme-linked immunosorbent assay in the detection of antigen in tuberculous meningitis cerebrospinal fluids, *J. Clin. Microbiol.*, 23, 901, 1986.

275. Kadival, G. V., Samuel, A. M., Mazarelo, T. B. M. S., and Chaparas, S. D., Radioimmunoassay for detection of *Mycobacterium tuberculosis* antigen in cerebrospinal fluids of patients with tuberculous meningitis, *J. Inf. Dis.*, 155, 608, 1987.

276. Cocito, C. G., Properties of the mycobacterial antigen complex A60 and its applications to the diagnosis and prognosis of tuberculosis, *Chest*, 100, 1687, 1991.

277. Daniel, T. M., The rapid diagnosis of tuberculosis: a selective review, *J. Lab. Clin. Med.*, 116, 277, 1990.

278. Tang, L. M., Serial lactate determinations in tuberculous meningitis, *Scand. J. Inf. Dis.*, 20, 81, 1988.

279. Shankar, P., Manjunath, N., Mohan, K. K., Prasad, K., Behari, M., Shriniwas, and Ahuja, G. K., Rapid diagnosis of tuberculous meningitis by polymerase chain reaction, *Lancet*, 337, 5, 1991.

280. Cameron, D., Ansari, B. M., and Boyce, J. M. H., Rapid diagnosis of tuberculous meningitis, *J. Inf. Dis.*, 24, 334, 1992.

281. Bouchama, A., Al-Kawi, M. Z., Kanaan, I., Coates, R., Jallu, A., Rahm, B., and Siqueira, E. B., Brain biopsy in tuberculoma: the risks and benefits, *Neurosurgery*, 28, 405, 1991.

282. Bobrowitz, I. D., Ethambutol in tuberculous meningitis, *Chest*, 61, 629, 1972.

283. Alegre, J., Fernández de Sevilla, T., Falcó, V., and Martinez Vazquez, J. M., Ofloxacin in miliary tuberculosis, *Eur. Respir. J.*, 3, 238, 1990.

284. Parenti, F., New experimental drugs for the treatment of tuberculosis, *Rev. Inf. Dis.*, 11(Suppl.), S479, 1989.

285. Goel, A., Pandya, S. K., and Satoskar, A. R., Whither short-course chemotherapy for tuberculous meningitis? *Neurosurgery*, 27, 418, 1990.

286. Palur, R., Rashekhar, V., Chandy, M. J., Joseph, T., and Abraham, J., Shunt surgery for hydrocephalus in tuberculous meningitis: a long-term follow-up study, *J. Neurosurg.*, 74, 64, 1991.

287. Gourie-Devi, M. and Satish, P., Hyaluronidase as an adjuvant in the treatment of cranial arachnoiditis complicating meningitis, *Acta Neurol. Scand.*, 62, 368, 1980.

288. Navarro, I. M., Peralta, V. H. R., Leon, J. A. M., Varela, E. A. S., and Cabrera, J. M. S., Tuberculous optochiasmatic arachnoiditis, *Neurosurgery*, 9, 64, 1981.

289. Chambers, S. T., Hendrickse, W. A., Record, C., Rudge, P., and Smith, H., Paradoxical expansion of intracranial tuberculomas during chemotherapy, *Lancet*, 2, 181, 1984.

290. Naidoo, D. P., Desai, D., and Kranidiotis, L., Tuberculous meningomyeloradiculitis — a report of two cases, *Tubercle*, 72, 66, 1991.

291. Hejazi, N. and Hassler, W., Multiple intracranial tuberculomas with atypical response to tuberculostatic chemotherapy: literature review and a case report, *Infection*, 25, 233, 1997.

292. Marcus, R. and Coulston, A. M., Water-soluble vitamins, in Gilman, A. G., Rall, T. W., Nies, A. S., and Taylor, E., Eds., *The Pharmacological Basis of Therapeutics*, W.B. Saunders, Philadelphia, 1992, 139.

293. Albert, D. M. and Dehm, E. J., Ocular tuberculosis, in Schlossberg, D., Ed., *Tuberculosis*, Springer Verlag, New York, 1993, 119.

294. Rosen, P. H., Spalton, D. J., and Graham, E. M., Intraocular tuberculosis, *Eye*, 4, 486, 1990.

295. Duke-Elder, S., Summary of systemic ophthalmology, in Duke-Elder, S., Ed., *System of Ophthalmology*, Vol. 1, CV Mosby Company, St. Louis, 1976, 160.

296. Philip, R. N. and Comstock, G. W., Phlyctenular keratoconjunctivitis among Eskimos in southwestern Alaska: I. Epidemiologic characteristics, *Am. Rev. Resp. Dis.*, 91, 171, 1965.

297. Philip, R. N. and Comstock, G. W., Phlyctenular keratoconjunctivitis among Eskimos in southwestern Alaska: II. Isoniazid prophylaxis, *Am. Rev. Resp. Dis.*, 91, 188, 1965.

298. Friedlaender, M. H., *Allergy and Immunology of the Eye,* Raven Press, New York, 1993, 139.

299. Fountain, J. A. and Werner, R. B., Tuberculous retinal vasculitis, *Retina*, 4, 48, 1984.

300. Eales, H., Cases of retinal haemorrhage associated with epistaxis and constipation, *Birmingham Med. Rev.*, 9, 262, 1880.

301. Gur, S., Silverstone, B. Z., Sylberman, R., and Berson, D., Chorioretinitis and extrapulmonary tuberculosis, *Ann. Opthalmol.*, 19, 112, 1987.

302. Magargal, L. E., Walsh, A. W., Magargal, H. O., and Robb-Doyle, E., Treatment of Eales' disease with scatter laser photocoagulation, *Ann. Ophthalmol.*, 21, 300, 1989.

303. Skolnik, P. R., Nadol, J. B., and Baker, A. S., Tuberculosis of the middle ear: review of the literature with an instructive case report, *Rev. Inf. Dis.*, 8, 403, 1986.

304. Vomero, E. and Ratner, S. J., Diagnosis of miliary tuberculosis by examination of middle ear discharge, *Arch. Otolaryng. Head Neck Surg.*, 114, 1029, 1988.

305. Pankey, G. A., Otologic tuberculosis, in Schlossberg, D., Ed., *Tuberculosis*, Springer Verlag, New York, 1993, 115.

306. Israel, H. L., Tuberculous peritonitis, in Schlossberg, D., Ed., *Tuberculosis*, Springer Verlag, New York, 1993, 193.

307. Jakubowski, A., Elwood, R. K., and Enarson, D. A., Clinical features of abdominal tuberculosis, *J. Inf. Dis.*, 18, 687, 1988.

308. Fitzgerald, J. M., Menzies, R. I., and Elwood, R. K., Abdominal tuberculosis: a critical review, *Dig. Dis.*, 9, 269, 1991.

309. Cheng, I. K., Chan, P. C., and Chan, M. K., Tuberculous peritonitis complicating long-term peritoneal dialysis: report of 3 cases and review of the literature, *Am. J. Nephrol.*, 9, 155, 1989.

310. Singh, M. M., Bhargave, A. N., and Jain, K. P., Tuberculous peritonitis: an evaluation of pathogenetic mechanisms, diagnostic procedures and therapeutic measures, *N. Engl. J. Med.*, 281, 1091, 1969.

311. Sochocky, S., Tuberculous peritonitis: a review of 100 cases, *Am. Rev. Resp. Dis.*, 9, 398, 1967.

312. Pettengell, K. E., Larsen, C., Garb, M., Mayet, F. G. H., Simjee, A. E., and Pirie, D., Gastrointestinal tuberculosis in patients with pulmonary tuberculosis, *Q. J. Med.*, 74, 303, 1990.

313. Bastani, B., Shariatzadeh, M. R., and Dehdashti, F., Tuberculous peritonitis — report of 30 cases and review of the literature, *Q. J. Med.*, 56, 549, 1985.

314. Sherman, S., Rohwedder, J. J., Ravikrishman, K. P., and Weg, J. G., Tuberculous enteritis and peritonitis: report of 36 general hospital cases, *Arch. Int. Med.*, 140, 6, 1980.

315. Karney, W. W., O'Donoghue, J. M., Ostrow, J. H., Holmes, K. K., and Beaty, H. N., The spectrum of tuberculous peritonitis, *Chest*, 72, 310, 1977.

316. Lerer, S., Romano, T., and Denmark, L., Gallium-67-citrate scanning in tuberculous peritonitis, *Am. J. Gastroenterol.*, 71, 264, 1979.

317. Hulnick, D. H., Megibow, A. J., Naidich, D. P., Hilton, S., Cho, K. C., and Balthazar, E. J., Abdominal tuberculosis: CT evaluation, *Radiology*, 157, 199, 1985.

318. Wilkens, E. G., Tuberculous peritonitis: diagnostic value of the ascitic/blood glucose ratio, *Tubercle*, 6, 47, 1984.

319. Voigt, M. D., Trey, C., Lombard, C., Kalvaria, I., Berman, P., and Kirsch, R. E., Diagnostic value of ascites adenosine deaminase in tuberculous peritonitis, *Lancet*, 1, 71, 1989.

320. Thapa, B. R., Yachha, S. K., and Mehta, S., Abdominal tuberculosis, *Ind. Ped.*, 28, 1093, 1991.

321. Geake, T. M. S., Spitaels, J. M., Moshal, M. G., and Simjee, A. E., Peritoneoscopy in the diagnosis of tuberculous peritonitis, *Gastrointest. Endosc.*, 27, 66, 1981.

322. Bhansali, S. K., Abdominal tuberculosis: experience with 300 cases, *Am. J. Gastroenterol.*, 67, 324, 1977.
323. Paustian, F. F. and Stahl, M. G., Tuberculosis enteritis, in Schlossberg, D., Ed., *Tuberculosis*, Springer Verlag, New York, 1993, 189.
324. Eng, J. and Sabanathan, S., Tuberculosis of the esophagus (4 cases), *Dig. Dis. Sci.*, 36, 36, 1991.
325. Allen, C. M., Craze, J., and Grundy, A., Case report: tuberculous broncho-oesophageal fistula in the acquired immunodeficiency syndrome, *Clin. Rad.*, 43, 60, 1991.
326. Vijayraghavan, M., Arunabh, K., Sarda, A. K., Sharma, A. K., and Chatterjee, T. K., Duodenal tuberculosis: a review of the clinicopathologic features and management of twelve cases, *Jap. J. Surg.*, 20, 526, 1990.
327. Gupta, S. C., Gupta, A. K., Keswani, N. K., Singh, P. A., Tripathi, A. K., and Krishna, V., Pathology of tropical appendicitis, *J. Clin. Path.*, 42, 1169, 1989.
328. Sen, P., Kapila, R., Salaki, J., and Louria, D. B., The diagnostic enigma of extra-pulmonary tuberculosis, *J. Chron. Dis.*, 30, 321, 1977.
329. Gilinsky, N. H., Marks, I. N., Kottler, R. E., and Price, S. K., Abdominal tuberculosis: a 10-year review, *S. Afr. Med. J.*, 84, 849, 1983.
330. Aston, N. O. and de Costa, A. M., Abdominal tuberculosis, *Br. J. Clin. Pract.*, 44, 58, 1990.
331. Thoeni, R. F. and Margulis, A. R., Gastrointestinal tuberculosis, *Sem. Roentgenol.*, 14, 283, 1979.
332. Balthazar, E. J., Gordon, R., and Hulnick, D., Ileocecal tuberculosis: CT and radiologic evaluation, *Am. J. Roentgenol.*, 14, 499, 1990.
333. Shah, S., Thomas, V., Mathan, M., Chacko, A., Chandy, G., Ramakrishna, B. S., and Rolston, D. D. K., Colonoscopic study of 50 patients with colonic tuberculosis, *Gut*, 33, 347, 1992.
334. Kochhar, R., Rajwanshi, A., Goenka, M. K., Nijhawan, R., Sood, A., Nagi, B., Kochhar, S., and Mehta, S. K., Colonoscopic fine needle aspiration cytology in the diagnosis of ileocecal tuberculosis, *Am. J. Gastroenterol.*, 86, 102, 1991.
335. Shah, P. and Ramakantan, R., Role of vasculitis in the natural history of abdominal tuberculosis — evaluation by mesenteric angiography, *Ind. J. Gastroent.*, 10, 127, 1991.
336. Palmer, K. R., Patil, D. H., Basran, G. S., Riordan, J. F., and Silk, D. B. A., Abdominal tuberculosis in urban Britain — a common disease, *Gut*, 26, 1296, 1985.
337. Goldman, M., The surgical management of abdominal tuberculosis, *Surg. Ann.*, 21, 363, 1989.
338. Bowry, S., Chan, C. H., Weiss, H., Katz, S., and Zimmerman, H. J., Hepatic involvement in pulmonary tuberculosis: histologic and functional characteristics, *Am. Rev. Resp. Dis.*, 101, 941, 1970.
339. Weinberg, J. J., Cohen, P., and Malhotra, R., Primary tuberculous abscess associated with the human immunodeficiency virus, *Tubercle*, 69, 145, 1988.
340. Harrington, P. T., Gutiérrez, J. J., Ramírez-Ronda, C. H., Quiñones-Soto, R., Bermúdez, R. H., and Chaffey, J., Granulomatous hepatitis, *Rev. Inf. Dis.*, 4, 638, 1982.
341. Ratanarapee, S. and Pausawasdi, A., Tuberculosis of the common bile duct, *HPB Surg.*, 3, 205, 1991.
342. Lupatkin, H., Braeu, N., Flomenberg, P., and Simberkoff, M. S., Tuberculous abscesses in patients with AIDS, *Clin. Inf. Dis.*, 14, 1040, 1992.
343. Rohwedder, J. J., Upper respiratory tract tuberculosis, in Schlossberg, D., Ed., *Tuberculosis*, Springer Verlag, New York, 1993, 107.
344. Khalil, T., Uzoaru, I., Nadimpalli, V., and Wurtz, R., Splenic tuberculous abscess in patients positive for HIV: report of two cases and review, *Clin. Inf. Dis.*, 14, 1266, 1992.
345. Wolff, M. J., Bitran, J., Northland, R. G., and Levy, I. L., Splenic abscesses due to *M. tuberculosis* in patients with AIDS, *Rev. Inf. Dis.*, 13, 373, 1991.
346. Desmond, N. M., Beale, T. J., Tanner, A. G., et al., Tuberculous pancreatic abscess: an unusual manifestation of HIV infection, *J. R. Soc. Med.*, 88, 109, 1995.
347. Brusko, G., Melvin, W. S., Fromkes, J. J., and Ellison, E. C., Pancreatic tuberculosis, *Am. Surg.*, 61, 513, 1995.
348. Watanapa, P. and Vathonopas, V., Tuberculous pancreatic abscess: a rare condition mimicking carcinoma, *HPB Surg.*, 5, 209, 1992.
349. Crowson, M. C., Perry, M., and Burden, E., Tuberculosis of the pancreas: a rare cause of obstructive jaundice, *Br. J. Surg.*, 71, 239, 1984.
350. Fan, S. T., Yan, K. W., Lau, Y. W., and Wong, K. K., Tuberculosis of the pancreas: a rare cause of massive gastrointestinal bleeding, *Br. J. Surg.*, 73, 373, 1986.

351. Rushing, J. L., Hanna, C. J., and Slecky, P. A., Pancreatitis as the presenting manifestation of miliary tuberculosis, *West. J. Med.*, 129, 432, 1978.

352. Stock, K. P., Rieman, J. F., Stadler, W., and Rosh, W., Tuberculosis of the pancreas, *Endoscopy*, 13, 178, 1981.

353. Chandrasekara, K. L., Iyer, S. K., Staneck, A. E., and Herbstman, H., Pancreatic tuberculosis mimicking carcinoma, *Gastrointest. Endosc.*, 31, 386, 1985.

354. Desai, D. C., Swaroop, V. S., Mohandas, K. M., Borges, A., Dhir, V., Nagral, A., Jagannath, P., and Sharma, O. P., Tuberculosis of the pancreas: report of three cases, *Am. J. Gastrol.*, 86, 761, 1991.

355. Allen, J. R., Bauer, L. A., Evans, L., and Watson, K., Primary pancreatic tuberculosis, *Miss. Med.*, 88, 766, 1991.

356. Soriano, E., Mallolas, J., Gatell, J. M., Latorre, X., Miró, J. M., Pecchiar, M., Mensa, J., Trilla, J., and Moreno, A., Characteristics of tuberculosis in HIV-infected patients: a case-control study, *AIDS*, 2, 429, 1988.

357. Crocco, J. A., Cardiovascular tuberculosis, in Schlossberg, D., Ed., *Tuberculosis*, Springer Verlag, New York, 1993, 179.

358. Rose, A. G., Cardiac tuberculosis, *Arch. Pathol. Lab. Med.*, 111, 422, 1987.

359. Alvarez, S. and McCabe, W. R., Extrapulmonary tuberculosis revisited: a review of experience at Boston City and other hospitals, *Medicine*, 63, 2, 1984.

360. Fowler, N. O., Tuberculous pericarditis, *JAMA*, 266, 99, 1991.

361. Reynolds, M. M., Hecht, S. R, Berger, M., Kolokathis, A., and Horowitz, S. F., Large pericardial effusions in the acquired immunodeficiency syndrome, *Chest*, 102, 1746, 1992.

362. Larrieu, A. J., Tyers, F. O., Williams, E. H., and Derrick, J. R., Recent experience with tuberculous pericarditis, *Ann. Thorac. Surg.*, 29, 464, 1980.

363. Rooney, J. J., Crocco, J. A., and Lyons, H. A., Tuberculous pericarditis, *Ann. Int. Med.*, 72, 73, 1970.

364. Cegielski, J. P., Ramaiya, K., Lallinger, G. J., Mtulia, I. A., and Mbaga, I. M., Pericardial disease and human immunodeficiency virus in Dar es Salaam, Tanzania, *Lancet*, 33, 209, 1990.

365. D'Cruz, I. A., Sengupta, E. E., Abrahams, C., Reddy, H. K., and Turlapati, R. V., Cardiac involvement, including tuberculous pericardial effusion, complicating acquired immune deficiency syndrome, *Am. Heart J.*, 112, 1100, 1986.

366. de Miguel, J., Pedreira, J. D., Campos, V., Gomez, A. P., and Porto, J. A. L., Tuberculous pericarditis and AIDS, *Chest*, 97, 1273, 1990.

367. Kinney, E. L., Monsuez, J. J., Kitzis, M., and Vittecoq, D., Treatment of AIDS-associated heart disease, *Angiology*, 40, 970, 1989.

368. Guberman, B. A., Fowler, N. O., Engel, P. J., Gueron, M., and Allen, J. M., Cardiac tamponade in medical patients, *Circulation*, 3, 633, 1981.

369. Desai, H. N., Tuberculous pericarditis, *S. Afr. Med. J.*, 55, 877, 1979.

370. Hageman, J. H., D'Esopo, N. D., and Glenn, W. W. L., Tuberculosis of the pericardium, *N. Engl. J. Med.*, 270, 327, 1964.

371. Fowler, N. O. and Manitsas, G. T., Infectious pericarditis, *Prog. Cardiovasc. Dis.*, 16, 323, 1973.

372. Strang, J. I. G., Gibson, D. J., Mitchison, D. A., Girling, D. J., Kakaza, H. H. S., Allen, B. W., Evans, D. J., and Nunn, A. J., Controlled clinical trial of complete open surgical drainage and of prednisolone in treatment of tuberculous pericardial effusion in Transkei, *Lancet*, 2, 8614, 79, 1988.

373. Quale, J. M., Lipschik, G. Y., and Heurich, A. E., Management of tuberculous pericarditis, *Ann. Thorac. Surg.*, 43, 63, 1987.

374. Dalli, E., Quesada, A., Juan, G., Navarro, R., Payá, R., and Tormo, V., Tuberculous pericarditis as the first manifestation of acquired immunodeficiency syndrome, *Am. Heart J.*, 114, 905, 1987.

375. Suchet, I. B. and Horwitz, T. A., CT in tuberculous constrictive pericarditis, *J. Comp. Ass. Tomogr.*, 16, 391, 1992.

376. Haase, D., Marrie, T. J., Martin, R., and Hayne, O., Gallium scanning in tuberculous pericarditis, *Clin. Nucl. Med.*, 6, 27, 1981.

377. Schepers, G. W. H., Tuberculous pericarditis, *Am. J. Cardiol.*, 9, 248, 1962.

378. Sagristá-Sauleda, J., Permanyer-Miralda, G., and Soler-Soler, J., Tuberculous pericarditis: ten-year experience with a prospective protocol for diagnosis and treatment, *J. Am. Coll. Cardiol.*, 11, 724, 1988.

379. Telenti, M., Fdez, J., de Quiros, B., Susano, R., and Moreno, T. A., Tuberculous pericarditis: diagnostic value of adenosine deaminase, *Presse Medicale Paris*, 20, 637, 1991.

380. Bass, J. B., Farer, L. S., Hopewell, P. C., and Jacobs, R. F., Treatment of tuberculosis and tuberculous infection in adults and children, *Am. Rev. Resp. Dis.*, 134, 358, 1986.
381. Strang, J. I. G., Gibson, D. G., Nunn, A. J., Kakaza, H. H. S., Girling, D. J., and Fox, W., Controlled trial of prednisolone as adjuvant in treatment of tuberculous constrictive pericarditis in Transkei, *Lancet*, 2, 1418, 1987.
382. Gooi, H. C. and Smith, J. M., Tuberculous pericarditis in Birmingham, *Thorax*, 33, 94, 1978.
383. Volini, F. I., Olfield, R. C., Jr., Thompson, J. R., et al., Tuberculosis of the aorta, *JAMA,* 181, 98, 1962.
384. Carson, T. J., Murray, G. F., Wilcox, B. R., and Starek, P. J. K., The role of surgery in tuberculous pericarditis, *Ann. Thorac. Surg.*, 17, 163, 1974.
385. Kannangara, D. W., Salem, F. A., Rao, B. S., and Thadepalli, H., Cardiac tuberculosis: TB of the endocardium, *Am. J. Med. Sci.*, 287, 45, 1984.
386. Halim, M. A., Mercer, E. N., and Guinn, G. A., Myocardial tuberculoma with rupture and pseudoaneurysm formation — successful surgical treatment, *Br. Heart J.*, 4, 603, 1982.
387. Wallis, P. J. W., Branfoot, A. C., and Emerson, P. A., Sudden death due to myocardial tuberculosis, *Thorax*, 39, 155, 1984.
388. O'Neill, P. G., Rokey, R., Greenberg, S., and Pacifico, A., Resolution of ventricular tachycardia and endocardial tuberculoma following antituberculosis therapy, *Chest*, 100, 1467, 1991.
389. Abaskaron, M., Multiple pseudoaneurysms in a tuberculous patient, *South. Med. J.*, 79, 182, 1986.
390. Sandron, D., Patra, P., Lelann, P., Bouillard, S., and Pioche, D., Tuberculous pseudo-aneurysm of the descending thoracic aorta, *Eur. Respir. J.*, 1, 62, 1988.
391. Felson, B., Akers, P. V., Hall, G. S., Schreiber, J. T., Greene, R. E., and Pedrosa, C. S., Mycotic tuberculous aneurysm of the thoracic aorta, *JAMA*, 237, 1104, 1977.
392. Bacourt, F., Goeau-Brissoniere, O., Lacombe, P., et al., Surgical treatment of a tuberculous thoracoabdominal aneurysm*, Ann. Vasc. Surg., 1,* 378, 1986.
393. Catinella, F. P. and Kittle, C. F., Tuberculous oesophagus with aortic aneurysm fistula, *Ann. Thorac. Surg.*, 4, 87, 1988.
394. Long, R., Guzman, R., Greenberg, H., Safneck, J., and Hershfield, E., Tuberculous mycotic aneurysm of the aorta: review of published medical and surgical experience, *Chest,* 115, 522, 1999.
395. Rupa, V. and Bhanu, T. S., Laryngeal tuberculosis in the eighties — an Indian experience, *J. Laryngol. Otol.*, 103, 864, 1989.
396. Brodovsky, D. M., Laryngeal tuberculosis in an age of chemotherapy, *Can. J. Otol.*, 4, 168, 1977.
397. el-Hakim, I. E. and Langdon, J. D., Unusual presentation of tuberculosis of the head and neck region, *Int. J. Oral Maxillofac. Surg.*, 18, 194, 1989.
398. Sehgal, V. N. and Wagh, S. A., Cutaneous tuberculosis, *Int. J. Dermatol.*, 29, 237, 1990.
399. Beyt, B. E., Jr., Ortbals, D. W., and Santa Cruz, D. J., Cutaneous mycobacteriosis: analysis of 34 cases, *Medicine*, 60, 9, 1981.
400. Beyt, B. E., Cutaneous tuberculosis, in Schlossberg, D., Ed., *Tuberculosis*, Springer Verlag, New York, 1993, 225.
401. Minkowitz, S., Brandt, L. J., Rapp, Y., and Radlauer, C. B., "Prosector's wart" (cutaneous tuberculosis) in a medical student, *Am. J. Clin. Pathol.*, 1, 260, 1969.
402. Michelson, H. E., Scrofuloderma gummosa (tuberculosis colliguativa), *Arch. Dermatol.*, 10, 6, 1924.
403. Forstrom, L., Carcinomatous changes in lupus vulgaris, *Ann. Clin. Res.*, 1, 213, 1969.
404. Rietbrok, R. C., Dahlmans, R. P. M., Smedts, F., Frantzen, P. J., Koopman, R. J. J., and van der Meer, J. W. M., Tuberculosis cutis miliaris disseminata as a manifestation of miliary tuberculosis; literature review and report of a case of recurrent skin lesions, *Rev. Inf. Dis.*, 13, 265, 1991.
405. Rohatgi, P. K., Palazollo, J. V., and Saini, N., Acute miliary tuberculosis of the skin in acquired immunodeficiency syndrome, *J. Am. Acad. Dermatol.*, 26, 36, 1992.
406. Sharma, P. K., Babel, A. L., and Yadav, S. S., Tuberculosis of breast (study of 7 cases), *J. Postgrad. Med.*, 37, 24, 1990.
407. Hutton, M. D., Nosocomial transmission of tuberculosis associated with a draining abscess, *J. Inf. Dis.*, 12, 83, 1990.
408. Zalla, M. J., Su, W. P. D., and Fransway, A. F., Dermatologic manifestations of human immunodeficiency virus infection, *Mayo Clin. Proc.*, 67, 1096, 1992.
409. Frampton, M. W., An outbreak of tuberculosis among hospital personnel caring for a patient with a skin ulcer, *Ann. Int. Med.*, 117, 312, 1992.

410. Degitz, K., Detection of mycobacterial DNA in the skin, *Arch. Dermatol.,* 132, 71, 1996.

411. Sarma, G. R., Immanuel, C., Ramachandran, G., Krishnamurthy, P. V., Kumaraswani, V., and Prabhakar, R., Adrenocortical function in patients with pulmonary tuberculosis, *Tubercle*, 71, 277, 1990.

412. Barnes, D. J., Naraqui, S., Temu, P., and Turtle, J. R., Adrenal function in patients with active tuberculosis, *Thorax*, 44, 422, 1989.

413. Arnstein, A. R., Endocrine and metabolic aspects of tuberculosis, in Schlossberg, D., Ed., *Tuberculosis*, Springer Verlag, New York, 1993, 247.

414. Vita, J. A., Silverberg, S. J., Goland, R. S., Austin, J. H. M., and Knowlton, A. I., Clinical clues to the cause of Addison's Disease, *Am. J. Med.*, 78, 461, 1985.

415. Des Prez, R. M., Mycobacterial infections, in Rogers, D. E., Des Prez, R. M., Cline, M. J., Braunwald, E., Greenberger, N. J., Wilson, J. D., Epstein, F. H., and Malawista, S. E., *The Yearbook of Medicine*, Yearbook Medical Publishers, Inc., Chicago, 1986, 201.

416. Wilkins, E. G. L., Hnizdo, E., and Cope, E., Addisonian crisis induced by treatment with rifampicin, *Tubercle*, 70, 69, 1989.

417. Orth, D. N., Kovacs, W. J., and DeBold, C. R., The adrenal cortex, in Wilson, J. D. and Foster, D. W., Eds., *Williams Textbook of Endocrinology*, W.B. Saunders, Philadelphia, 1992, 2.

418. Barnes, P. and Weatherstone, R., Tuberculosis of the thyroid: two case reports, *Br. J. Dis. Chest*, 73, 187, 1979.

419. Berger, S. A., Edberg, S. C., and David, G., Infectious disease in the sella turcica, *Rev. Inf. Dis.*, 8, 747, 1986.

420. Shenoi, A., Deshpande, S. A., and Marwaha, R. K., Diabetes insipidus and growth hormone deficiency following tubercular meningitis, *Ind. Ped.*, 27, 624, 1990.

421. Lam, K. S. L., Sham, M. M. K., Tam, S. C. F., Ng, M. M. T., and Ma, H. G. T., Hypopituitarism after tuberculous meningitis in childhood, *Ann. Int. Med.*, 118, 701, 1993.

8 Tuberculosis in Childhood and Pregnancy

Jeffrey R. Starke, M.D.

CONTENTS

0-8493-1565-4/97/$0.00+$.50
© 2000 by CRC Press LLC

I. TUBERCULOSIS IN CHILDREN

A. INTRODUCTION

Tuberculosis remains a significant cause of morbidity and mortality for children throughout the world. In many developing countries, tuberculosis infection and disease have remained commonplace among children. The incidence appears to be increasing in many countries also experiencing the epidemic of infection due to the human immunodeficiency virus (HIV).[1] In most industrialized countries, the incidence of childhood tuberculosis declined substantially between the 1920s and the 1980s, due in part to improved social conditions, the widespread use of antituberculosis drugs, and, perhaps, to the use of certain bacille Calmette-Guérin (BCG) vaccines. Unfortunately, several industrialized countries experienced a resurgence in pediatric tuberculosis infection and disease in the late 1980s and in the 1990s.[2,3]

Beyond the profound health consequences for the affected child due to tuberculosis, the occurrence of tuberculosis in children represents a sentinel health marker for ongoing transmission of tuberculosis in a community. Infected children also are a large portion of the pool from which future tuberculosis cases will arise. However, childhood tuberculosis has a limited influence on the immediate epidemiology of the disease because children rarely are a source of infection to others. Programs that target children for treatment of tuberculosis will have few short-term effects on disease rates but will have a profound impact on the long-term control of the disease.[4]

B. EPIDEMIOLOGY

1. Worldwide Tuberculosis Disease

The worldwide scope of tuberculosis in children is difficult to assess because data are scarce and poorly organized. Reports of disease rates usually grossly underestimate the true incidence. The prevalence of tuberculosis infection without disease in children is completely unknown in most areas of the world due to the lack of surveillance testing. In many areas of Africa and Asia, the annual new tuberculosis infection rate for all ages is approximately 2%, which would yield an estimated 220 cases of tuberculosis per 100,000 population per year.[5] Approximately 15 to 20% of these cases occur in children younger than 15 years of age. In addition, between 10 to 20% of deaths caused by tuberculosis in the developing world occur among children. The World Health Organization (WHO) has estimated that the developing world has 1.3 million cases of tuberculosis and 400,000 tuberculosis-related deaths annually among children younger than 15 years of age.[6] There is no indication that tuberculosis rates among children in developing nations are declining; in several surveys it is clear that infection and disease rates are increasing, especially in areas where HIV infection is prevalent.[7]

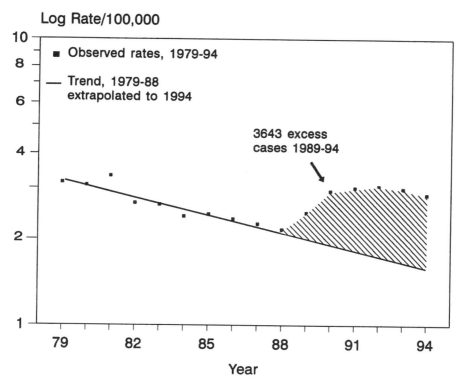

FIGURE 8.1 Observed and expected tuberculosis cases in children younger than 15 years of age in the U.S., 1979–1994.

2. Tuberculosis Disease in the U.S.

Between 1953 and 1980 the number of cases of childhood tuberculosis in the U.S. declined by approximately 6% per year.[8] Case rates declined in a similar fashion, from 10 per 100,000 children less than 15 years of age in 1962 to 2.4 per 100,000 children in 1985. Between 1980 and 1987 the case rates remained relatively flat, but they began to steadily increase in 1988. In 1992, 1800 cases of tuberculosis were reported in children less than 15 years of age, a 39% increase over 1987 cases (Figure 8.1). Factors that contributed to the resurgence of pediatric tuberculosis were (1) the increased occurrence of pulmonary tuberculosis among HIV-infected adults who transmit *M. tuberculosis* to children in their environment;[9] (2) increasing rates of tuberculosis infection and disease in foreign-born individuals;[10] and (3) a decline in the tuberculosis public health infrastructure in many regions and cities, which disproportionately affects the prevention of tuberculosis in children.[11,12] From 1993 to the present, with improved tuberculosis control in the U.S., childhood tuberculosis cases declined to approximately 1100 in 1998.

The source of tuberculosis infection for children usually is an adult in the environment who has infectious pulmonary tuberculosis. Therefore, the risk of a child developing tuberculosis infection or disease depends upon the likelihood that he or she will come in contact with an adult at high-risk for tuberculosis (Table 8.1). Determining the risk level for tuberculosis in a child can be difficult since it is dependent upon determining the risk level of all the adults with whom a child has significant contact. Children with tuberculosis rarely, if ever, infect other children or adults.[13] In tuberculous children, tubercle bacilli are sparse in endobronchial secretions, and cough often is absent. When young children do cough they rarely produce sputum and they lack the tussive force of adults. When transmission of *M. tuberculosis* has been documented in childrens' hospitals, it usually has come from an adult with undiagnosed pulmonary tuberculosis.[14] The Centers for Disease Control and Prevention (CDC) recommend that young children with suspected pulmonary

TABLE 8.1
Adults at Highest Risk for Tuberculosis in the U.S.

Persons with HIV coinfection
Foreign-born persons from high-prevalence countries
Current or former residents of correctional institutions
Homeless persons
Substance abusers
Socioeconomically disadvantaged persons, especially within cities
Healthcare workers in high-risk settings
Persons with immunosuppressive conditions or medications

Source: Friedman, L. N., Ed., *Tuberculosis: Current Concepts and Treatment,* 1st ed., CRC Press LLC, Boca Raton, FL, 1994. With permission.

tuberculosis do not need to be isolated in the hospital unless they have characteristics of adult-type disease (sputum production, cavity on chest radiograph).[15] Adolescents with reactivation forms of pulmonary tuberculosis may be infectious to others. Occasionally, transmission of *M. tuberculosis* from a child may occur by direct contact with infected fluids and discharges such as urine or purulent sinus tract drainage. Fomites such as syringes, gastric lavage tubes, or bronchoscopes are rare sources of infection.[16]

Age and gender are important variables for tuberculosis among children. While there is no evidence that the likelihood of infection with *M. tuberculosis* is influenced by age or gender, both probably influence the risk of developing disease in an infected child. Approximately 60% of the pediatric tuberculosis cases in the U.S. occur in children younger than 5 years of age, the group traditionally at highest risk for disease. The interval between ages 5 and 14 years often has been referred to as the "favored age" since these children have the lowest rates of tuberculosis disease in any population. Age also affects the anatomic site of involvement of tuberculosis.[17,18] Younger children are more likely to develop meningeal, disseminated, or lymphatic tuberculosis, whereas adolescents more frequently present with pleural, genitourinary, or peritoneal disease (Table 8.2).

TABLE 8.2
Major Sites of Extrapulmonary Tuberculosis Among Children in the U.S.

Sites	Percentage (%)	Average Age (Years)
Lymphatic	67	5
Meningeal	13	3
Pleural	6	16
Miliary	5	1
Skeletal	4	5
Other	5	—
	100	

Source: Adapted from Smith, M. H. D., *Clin. Chest Med.,* 10, 381, 1989, and Reider, H. L., Snider, D. E., Jr., and Cauthen, G. M., *Am. Rev. Respir. Dis.,* 141, 347, 1990.

Among younger children, the gender ratio for tuberculosis disease usually is approximately 1:1, but girls have a slightly higher incidence of tuberculosis than boys during adolescence.

Historically, pediatric tuberculosis case rates in the U.S. have been highest between January and June, possibly due to more extensive indoor contact with infectious adults during the colder months. The disease also is geographically focal, with seven states — California, Florida, Georgia, Illinois, New York, New Jersey, and Texas — accounting for 70% of reported cases among children less than 5 years of age. As expected, disease rates among children are highest in cities with more than 250,000 residents.

Childhood tuberculosis case rates in the U.S. are strikingly higher among ethnic and racial minority groups and the foreign-born than among whites. Approximately 85% of cases occur among African-American, Hispanic, Asian, and Native American children, which probably reflects the increased risk of transmission within the living conditions of these children.[2] Although most of these children were born in the U.S., from 1986 to 1994 the proportion of foreign-born children with tuberculosis rose from 13 to 16% among children less than 5 years of age and from 40 to 49% among adolescents aged 15 to 19 years.[2] Foreign-born adoptees are at particularly high risk for tuberculosis infection and disease.[19]

Most children with tuberculosis become infected with *M. tuberculosis* in their home, but outbreaks of childhood tuberculosis centered in elementary and high schools, nursery schools, family daycare homes, churches, school buses, and stores still occur.[20-22] In most cases, a high-risk adult working in the area has been the source of the outbreak. In certain environments, these outbreaks can be quite widespread; during an outbreak in a St. Louis, MO elementary school, almost 50% of the students in the school developed tuberculosis infection and 11% had radiographic evidence of tuberculosis disease after a teacher was found to have extensive pulmonary tuberculosis.

3. Human Immunodeficiency Virus-Related Tuberculosis

The recent epidemic of HIV infection has had a profound effect on the epidemiology of tuberculosis among children in the U.S., by two major mechanisms:[1,23] (1) most important, HIV-infected adults with tuberculosis may transmit *M. tuberculosis* to children, a portion of whom will develop tuberculosis disease; and (2) children with HIV infection may be at increased risk of progressing from tuberculosis infection to disease.[24,25]

The infectiousness of HIV-infected adults with pulmonary tuberculosis depends mostly on the proportion who have acid-fast sputum smear-positive disease. Pulmonary involvement is common among HIV-infected adults with tuberculosis especially when the tuberculosis precedes other opportunistic infections.[26] Although many HIV-infected adults with pulmonary tuberculosis have a positive sputum smear, some studies have shown that they were slightly less likely to have a positive sputum smear than non-HIV-infected adults with pulmonary tuberculosis.[27] However, studies from Africa and New York City have suggested that HIV-seronegative and HIV-infected patients with smear-positive pulmonary tuberculosis infect similar proportions of their contacts with *M. tuberculosis*.[1] One retrospective study in Florida showed that an observed increase in pediatric tuberculosis cases was linked to an increase in pulmonary tuberculosis cases among HIV-infected adults in the same population.[9] Across the U.S., the largest increases in pediatric tuberculosis cases over the last decade have occurred in cities with high rates of HIV infection among the adult population. It appears as though the increased case load of infectious adult tuberculosis associated with the HIV is at least partly responsible for rising tuberculosis case rates among children.

Information about the risk of tuberculosis disease in HIV-infected children has become plentiful in the last 10 years.[28-36] Population-based studies performed in Cote d'Ivoire, Zambia, Brazil, Haiti, and South Africa have demonstrated that HIV-infected pediatric cohorts have a higher risk of developing tuberculosis than non-HIV-infected children living in the same areas. The difficulty encountered in many of the reports is that the diagnosis of tuberculosis is usually established on clinical criteria without microbiologic confirmation, especially in the youngest children in whom the highest rates of HIV infection are found. While overdiagnosis of tuberculosis in HIV-infected children may occur, underdiagnosis also is common because of the similarity of its clinical presentation to other opportunistic infections, and the difficulty in confirming the diagnosis with an acid-fast stain of sputum or gastric washings in young children. When HIV-infected children develop tuberculosis disease, the clinical features are similar to those in immunocompetent children, but with greater severity, more rapid progression, and a higher mortality rate.[25,34,35] There may be an increased tendency for extrapulmonary or disseminated disease. Unusual presentations, such as chronic fever and lobar infiltrates, may be found in HIV-infected children. In the U.S., all children with suspected tuberculosis disease should have HIV serological testing, because the two infections are linked epidemiologically and recommended treatment for tuberculosis may be prolonged for HIV-infected patients.

4. Tuberculosis Infection

While data on tuberculosis disease among children are available, data on tuberculosis infection without disease are lacking. Although there are estimates that approximately 30% of the world's population is infected with *M. tuberculosis*, it is impossible to determine how many children actually have asymptomatic tuberculosis infection.[6] All countries but two (U.S. and The Netherlands) have used BCG vaccine extensively, and population surveys for tuberculosis infection using the tuberculin skin test rarely are performed and may be difficult to interpret. In the U.S., tuberculosis infection without disease is a reportable condition in only three states — Kentucky, Indiana, and Missouri — and national surveys of tuberculosis infection rates in children were discontinued in 1971.

The most efficient method of finding children infected with *M. tuberculosis* is through contact investigation of adults with infectious pulmonary tuberculosis. On average, 30 to 50% of household contacts of an index case will have a reactive skin test, indicating infection with *M. tuberculosis*.[37] Even among children who have received a BCG vaccine, a positive tuberculin skin test in a child who has had close contact with an adult with suspected tuberculosis probably represents infection with *M. tuberculosis*, and therapy to halt progression of infection to disease should be given.

In the U.S., most children have a risk of less than 1% of acquiring asymptomatic tuberculosis infection. However, in some urban populations the risk appears to be much greater. In a 1990 study of Boston public schools, 5.1% of 7th graders and 8.9% of 10th graders were tuberculin skin test positive; approximately 85% of the infections occurred among foreign-born children.[38] Similar studies in Los Angeles[39] and Houston[40] revealed tuberculosis infection rates between 2 and 10% for elementary and high school children. However, surveys in some other large cities have revealed infection rates in public schools of less than 1%.

The performance of optimal contact investigations should have a large impact on the incidence of tuberculosis disease among children since these investigations identify recently infected children who are most likely to develop disease within a short time period. In general, community programs of tuberculin testing for school aged children are unlikely to have a significant impact on the incidence of childhood tuberculosis since most childhood cases occur in children less than 5 years of age and many of the "positive" tuberculin skin test reactions found among low-risk children in large screening programs actually represent false-positive cross reactions.[41,42] For high-incidence populations, especially foreign-born children who have immigrated from high tuberculosis prevalence countries, targeted testing and chemotherapy programs will be necessary to diminish the pool of infected children and prevent future adolescent and adult cases of tuberculosis disease.

C. CLINICAL MANIFESTATIONS

1. Asymptomatic Infections

The vast majority of children with tuberculosis infection develop no signs or symptoms, nor radiographic abnormalities at any time. Occasionally, the initiation of the infection is marked by several days of low-grade fever and mild cough. The child rarely experiences clinically significant disease with high fever, cough, malaise, and flu-like symptoms which resolve within 1 to 2 weeks. Other children, at the onset of tissue hypersensitivity, experience a fever and mild systemic symptoms that resolve over 1 to 3 weeks. The asymptomatic presentation of tuberculosis infection is more common among school-aged children than among younger infants. Approximately 80 to 90% of infected older children have completely asymptomatic infection, whereas only 50 to 60% of infected infants less than 1 year of age remain free of symptoms or radiographic abnormalities with tuberculosis infection.[43]

2. Intrathoracic Disease

a. Pulmonary

The primary pulmonary complex includes the lung parenchymal focus and regional lymphadenopathy. Approximately 70% of primary foci are subpleural, and localized pleurisy is a common part of the primary complex. During the initial infection, all lobar segments are at equal risk of being involved, and 25% of cases have multiple primary lung foci.[44] The initial parenchymal inflammation usually is not visible on chest radiograph but a localized, nonspecific infiltrate may be seen. Within days, the infection spreads to regional lymph nodes. As tuberculin hypersensitivity develops, within 3 to 10 weeks after infection, the inflammatory reaction in the lung tissue and lymph nodes often intensifies. The hallmark of primary tuberculosis is the relatively large size and importance of the hilar, mediastinal, or subcarinal adenitis compared with the relatively small size of the initial lung focus.

In most children, the parenchymal infiltrate and adenitis resolve early, often by the time the chest radiograph is obtained. In some children, particularly infants, the lymph nodes continue to enlarge (Figure 8.2). Bronchial obstruction caused by external compression may begin as the nodes impinge on the neighboring regional bronchus, compressing it and causing diffuse inflammation of its outer wall.[45] If the inflammation intensifies, the lymph nodes may erode through the bronchial wall leading to perforation and formation of thick caseous material within the lumen. This process may result in partial or complete obstruction of the bronchus.[46,47] The common radiographic sequence is adenopathy followed by localized hyperinflation and, eventually, atelectasis.[48] These radiographic shadows have been called "collapse-consolidation" or "segmental" lesions (Figure 8.3). The radiographic picture is similar to that caused by aspiration of a foreign body but usually

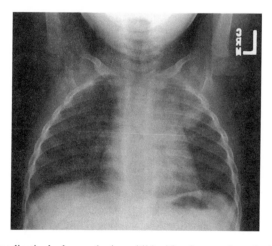

FIGURE 8.2 Hilar and mediastinal adenopathy in a child with primary tuberculosis. (From Friedman, L. N., Ed., *Tuberculosis: Current Concepts and Treatment,* 1st ed., CRC Press LLC, Boca Raton, FL, 1994. With permission.)

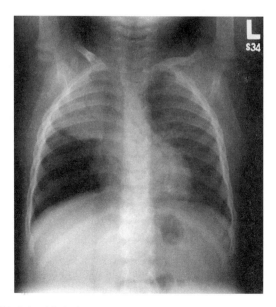

FIGURE 8.3   A child with right-sided adenopathy and a collapse-consolidation lesion of the right upper lobe due to tuberculosis. (From Friedman, L. N., Ed., *Tuberculosis: Current Concepts and Treatment,* 1st ed., CRC Press LLC, Boca Raton, FL, 1994. With permission.)

is quite different from a bacterial or viral pneumonia. In pulmonary tuberculosis, the lymph nodes act as the foreign body.

Obstructive emphysema of a lobar segment may accompany bronchial obstruction.[49] This rare complication occurs most often in children younger than 2 years of age. The obstruction usually resolves spontaneously but this may take several months. Rarely is surgical removal of the lymph nodes necessary to hasten the clinical improvement. The most common complication of bronchial obstruction is the fan-shaped segmental lesion which results from a combination of the primary pulmonary focus, the caseous material from an eroded bronchus, the host inflammatory response, and the subsequent atelectasis. Up to 45% of children younger than 1 year of age, who are infected with *M. tuberculosis,* develop a segmental lesion compared with 25% of children aged 1 to 10 years and 16% of children aged 11 to 15 years.[43] Usually a single segmental lesion is present but lesions may occur simultaneously in several different pulmonary lobes.

The symptoms and physical signs of pulmonary tuberculosis in children usually are surprisingly meager considering the degree of radiographic changes often seen. The physical manifestations of disease tend to differ by the age of onset. Young infants and adolescents are more likely to have significant signs and/or symptoms while school-aged children usually have clinically silent disease. More than 50% of infants and children with radiographically moderate to severe pulmonary tuberculosis have no symptoms or physical findings, and they are discovered only via contact tracing of an adult with pulmonary tuberculosis.[44,50] Infants are more likely to experience signs and symptoms probably because of their smaller airway diameters relative to the parenchymal and lymph node changes in pulmonary tuberculosis.[51,52] Nonproductive cough and mild dyspnea are the most common symptoms in infants. Systemic complaints such as fever, night sweats, anorexia, and decreased activity are less common. Some infants present with difficulty gaining weight or failure to thrive and these signs may not improve significantly until several months into therapy. Pulmonary signs are even less common. Some infants and young children with bronchial obstruction show signs of air trapping such as localized wheezing or decreased breath sounds that may be accompanied by tachypnea or, rarely, respiratory distress. A double-headed stethoscope may reveal delayed exhalation of air on the affected side. Occasionally these nonspecific symptoms and signs are alleviated by antibiotics, suggesting that bacterial superinfection distal to the focus of tuberculous bronchial obstruction contributes to the clinical presentation of disease.

Enlargement of other groups of intrathoracic lymph nodes can cause additional clinical manifestations. Enlarged subcarinal nodes, which cause splaying of the large bronchi, may impinge on the esophagus causing difficulty swallowing or leading to the development of a bronchoesophageal fistula. Enlarged nodes may compress the subclavian vein producing edema of the hand or arm. Occasionally, nodes rupture into the mediastinum causing left or right sided supraclavicular adenitis.

The majority of cases of pulmonary tuberculosis in children resolve radiographically with or without antituberculosis chemotherapy. In the pretreatment era, up to 60% of children had residual anatomic sequelae not apparent on radiographs. With delayed or no treatment, calcification of the caseous lesions is common but usually takes at least 6 months to occur. Healing of the pulmonary segment can be complicated by scarring or contraction associated with cylindrical bronchiectasis or bronchostenosis. When these complications occur in the upper lobes, they often are clinically silent. They appear to be rare in children who have successfully completed current regimens of chemotherapy.

A rare but serious complication of primary pulmonary tuberculosis occurs when the parenchymal focus enlarges and develops a large caseous center. The radiographic and clinical picture of progressive primary tuberculosis is closest to that of bronchial pneumonia, the child having high fever, moderate to severe cough, night sweats, dullness to percussion, rales, and decreased breath sounds. Liquefaction in the center of the lesion may result in formation of a thin-walled cavity, which may become a tension cavity as a result of a valve-like mechanism allowing air to enter but not escape (Figure 8.4). The enlarging focus may slough debris into adjacent bronchi leading to intrapulmonary dissemination of infection. Rupture of this cavity into the pleural space causes a bronchopleural fistula or pyopneumothorax. Rupture into the pericardium can cause acute pericarditis with constriction. Prior to the advent of antituberculosis chemotherapy, the mortality of progressive primary pulmonary tuberculosis in children was 30 to 50%; with current treatment the prognosis is excellent for full recovery.

Older children and adolescents may develop chronic reactivation pulmonary tuberculosis that resembles disease in adults. Even before the discovery of antituberculosis drugs, chronic

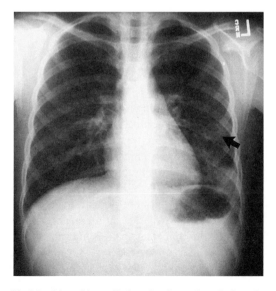

FIGURE 8.4 A 12-year-old girl with a thin-walled cavity (arrow) and pleural reaction due to tuberculosis. (From Friedman, L. N., Ed., *Tuberculosis: Current Concepts and Treatment,* 1st ed., CRC Press LLC, Boca Raton, FL, 1994. With permission.)

pulmonary tuberculosis complicated infection in only 6 to 7% of pediatric patients.[53] Children with a healed primary tuberculosis infection acquired before 2 years of age rarely develop chronic pulmonary disease. Chronic pulmonary tuberculosis is more common among children who acquire the initial infection after 7 years of age, particularly if they become infected close to the onset of puberty. The most common sites of chronic pulmonary tuberculosis are the original parenchymal focus, the regional lymph nodes, or the apical seedings (Simon foci). Typical symptoms are fever, anorexia, malaise, weight loss, night sweats, productive cough, chest pain, and hemoptysis. However, the findings on physical examination usually are minor or absent even when cavities or large infiltrates are present. Most signs and symptoms improve within several weeks of starting effective treatment, although a cough may last for several months. This form of tuberculosis disease usually remains localized to the lungs because the presensitization of tissue to tuberculin evokes an immune response that prevents further lymphohematogenous spread. Older children and adolescents with this form of tuberculosis may be sources of transmission of *M. tuberculosis* to other children.[54]

b. Pleural

Tuberculous pleural effusions are caused by the hypersensitivity response to the discharge of bacilli into the pleural space from a subpleural pulmonary focus or from subpleural caseous lymph nodes.[55] The discharge usually is small and the subsequent pleuritis is localized and asymptomatic. Occasionally, a larger discharge causes a generalized pleural effusion, usually within 6 months after initial infection. The effusion usually is unilateral in children.[56] A clinically significant pleural effusion occurs in 10 to 30% of tuberculosis cases in young adults but is infrequent in children younger than 6 years of age and extremely rare in children below 2 years of age.[18] It is most common among adolescents. It virtually is never associated with a segmental pulmonary lesion and occurs only rarely with miliary tuberculosis.

The onset of symptoms and signs usually is abrupt with fever, chest pain, shortness of breath, dullness to percussion, and diminished breath sounds on the affected side. Fever can be high and may last for several weeks even after antituberculosis chemotherapy has been started. The diagnosis may be difficult to make as the acid-fast stain of the pleural fluid virtually is always negative and the culture is positive in only 30 to 50% of cases. The best material for diagnosis is a biopsy of the pleura which will reveal caseating granulomas in up to 90% of cases and a positive culture in up to 70% of cases.[57]

c. Cardiac

Involvement of the myocardium may occur during miliary tuberculosis. Direct extension of tuberculosis into the myocardium from adjacent lymph nodes or lung parenchyma is rare. Tuberculous endocarditis has been described in several children.

The most common form of cardiac tuberculosis is pericarditis, which occurs in 0.4 to 4% of tuberculosis cases in children.[58,59] Pericarditis usually arises by direct invasion or lymphatic drainage from subcarinal lymph nodes. Early in the course, the pericardial fluid is serofibrinous or, occasionally, hemorrhagic. Echocardiography often reveals thin strands of fibrinous material in the pericardial space. In approximately 10 to 20% of cases, fibrosis leads to obliteration of the pericardial sac with development of constrictive pericarditis over a period of months to years. The presenting symptoms of serofibrinous pericarditis are nonspecific and include low-grade fever, malaise, and weight loss; in children, chest pain is unusual. A pericardial friction rub with distant heart sounds and with pulsus paradoxicus may be present, especially if constrictive changes have occurred. The acid-fast smear of the pericardial fluid rarely reveals the organism, but cultures of the fluid are positive in 30 to 70% of cases. Pericardial biopsy may be necessary to confirm the diagnosis; typical findings of caseating granulomas are present in 50 to 75% of cases. Partial or complete pericardiectomy may be required where constrictive pericarditis is present.

3. Lymphohematogenous

Tubercle bacilli are disseminated to distant anatomic sites virtually in all cases of asymptomatic tuberculosis infection. Autopsy cultures from people who died of other causes within days to weeks after initial infection with *M. tuberculosis* have demonstrated the organisms in many tissues, most commonly liver, spleen, skin, and lung apices. The clinical picture produced by lymphohematogenous dissemination depends upon the quantity of organisms released from the primary focus and the host immune response. Individuals who have a diminished immune response, such as infants and those with HIV infection, are more likely to develop severe forms of disseminated disease.[60]

The occult dissemination of tubercle bacilli during the initial infection usually produces no symptoms, but it is the event that results in extrapulmonary foci that can become the site of disease months to years after the initial infection. Rare patients experience protracted hematogenous tuberculosis caused by the intermittent release of tubercle bacilli as a caseous focus erodes through the wall of a blood vessel in the lung. The clinical picture may be acute but often is indolent and prolonged, with spiking fevers accompanying the release of organisms into the blood stream. Multiple organ involvement is common, often leading to hepatomegaly, splenomegaly, lymphadenitis in superficial or deep nodes, or papulonecrotic tuberculids appearing in crops on the skin. Bones and joints or the kidneys may become involved. Meningitis occurs only late in the course and often was the cause of death in the prechemotherapy era. Pulmonary involvement is surprisingly mild early in the course, but diffuse lung involvement usually becomes apparent if treatment is not given early. Culture confirmation of this complication can be difficult; bone marrow or liver biopsy with appropriate stains and cultures may be necessary and should be performed if the diagnosis is considered and other tests are unrevealing. The tuberculin skin test usually is reactive.

The most common clinically significant form of disseminated tuberculosis is miliary disease, which occurs when massive numbers of tubercle bacilli are released into the bloodstream causing disease in two or more organs. Miliary tuberculosis usually is an early complication of the primary infection occurring within 3 to 6 months of the primary inoculation.[61] While this form of disease is most common among infants and young children, it also is common in older adults as a result of the breakdown of a previously healed or calcified primary pulmonary lesion that formed years earlier.

The clinical manifestations of miliary tuberculosis are protean and depend upon the load and the final location of disseminated organisms.[60,61] Tissues have varying susceptibility to infection. Lesions usually are larger and more numerous in the lungs, spleen, liver, and bone marrow than other organs. The distribution may be caused both by blood supply and by the numbers of reticuloendothelial cells and tissue phagocytes.

The onset of clinical disease may be explosive with the patient becoming gravely ill over several days. More often, the onset is insidious and the patient may not be able to accurately pinpoint the time of initial symptoms. Early systemic signs include malaise, anorexia, weight loss, and low grade fever. At this time abnormal physical signs usually are absent. Within several weeks, hepatosplenomegaly and generalized lymphadenopathy develop in approximately 50% of patients. The fever may become higher and more sustained although the chest radiograph usually is normal and respiratory symptoms are few. Within several weeks the lungs often become filled with tubercles, accompanied by the onset of dyspnea, cough, rales, or wheezing.[60,61] As the pulmonary disease progresses, an alveolar air block syndrome may result in frank respiratory distress, hypoxia, and pneumothorax or pneumomediastinum. Signs or symptoms of meningitis or peritonitis are found in only 20 to 40% of patients with advanced disease. Chronic or recurrent headache in a child with miliary tuberculosis usually indicates the presence of meningitis, while the onset of abdominal pain or tenderness often heralds tuberculous peritonitis. Cutaneous lesions such as papulonecrotic tuberculids or nodules often occur in crops. Choroid tubercles occur in 13 to 87% of patients and are highly specific for miliary tuberculosis.

The early diagnosis of miliary tuberculosis can be difficult, requiring a high index of suspicion by the clinician. Up to 30% of children have a negative tuberculin skin test.[60,61] A biopsy of liver or bone marrow may facilitate a rapid diagnosis. In one recent review, the diagnosis could be confirmed by culture in only 33% of cases in children.[60] With proper treatment, the prognosis of miliary tuberculosis in children is excellent. However, resolution of signs and symptoms may be slow with fever declining in 2 to 3 weeks and chest radiograph abnormalities persisting for several months.

4. Lymphatic

Tuberculosis of the superficial lymph nodes — historically referred to as scrofula — is the most common form of extrapulmonary tuberculosis among children, accounting for approximately 67% of cases.[18,62] Historically, scrofula was often caused by drinking unpasteurized cow's milk laden with *Mycobacterium bovis*. However, through effective veterinary control, *M. bovis* has been nearly eliminated from North America.

Most current cases of tuberculous lymphadenitis occur within 6 to 9 months of the initial tuberculosis infection, although some cases arise years later. The tonsillar, anterior cervical and submandibular nodes become involved secondary to extension of a primary lesion of the upper lung fields or abdomen. Infected lymph nodes in the inguinal, epitrochlear, or axillary regions are rare in children and result from regional adenitis associated with tuberculosis of the skin or skeletal system.[63]

In the early stages of infection, the lymph nodes usually enlarge gradually. The nodes are firm but not hard and they are discrete and nontender. The nodes usually feel fixed to underlying or overlying tissues. The disease most often is unilateral but bilateral involvement may occur because of crossover drainage patterns of lymphatic vessels in the chest and lower neck. As infection progresses, multiple nodes usually become involved, often resulting in a mass of matted nodes. Other than low grade fever, systemic signs and symptoms usually are absent. The tuberculin skin test usually is reactive. Although a primary pulmonary focus virtually always is present, it is visible radiographically in only 30 to 70% of cases. Pulmonary signs and symptoms usually are lacking. Occasionally the illness is more acute with rapid enlargement of lymph nodes associated with high fever, tenderness, and fluctuance. Rarely, the initial presentation will be a fluctuant mass with overlying cellulitis and skin discoloration.

If left untreated, the lymph node infection may resolve, but more often progresses to caseation and necrosis of the node.[64] The capsule of the node breaks down leading to spread of infection to adjacent nodes. The skin overlying the mass of nodes becomes thin, shiny, and erythematous. Rupture through the skin results in a draining sinus tract that may require surgical removal.

The most difficult issue in the differential diagnosis of tuberculous adenitis is distinguishing this condition from adenitis due to nontuberculous mycobacteria, which are especially prevalent in the southern U.S.[62,65] Both conditions tend to cause chronic, nontender adenopathy with overlying skin changes and the eventual creation of tissue breakdown and sinus tracts. The chest radiograph often is negative in both conditions and skin test reactions may be positive in either condition. The most important diagnostic clue for tuberculous lymphadenitis is the identification of an adult source case in the child's environment. Often, excisional biopsy and culture of the lymph nodes is required to definitively establish the etiology; however, the cultures are negative in approximately 50% of reported cases of both tuberculous and nontuberculous mycobacterial lymphadenitis.

5. Central Nervous System

a. Meningitis

Central nervous system tuberculosis is the most serious complication in children and is uniformly fatal without effective treatment. It usually arises from the formation of a metastatic caseous lesion in the cerebral cortex or meninges that is established during the occult lymphohematogenous dissemination of the primary infection.[66] This lesion, often called a Rich focus, increases in size and discharges small numbers of tubercle bacilli into the subarachnoid space. The resulting gelatinous exudate may infiltrate the cortical or meningeal blood vessels producing inflammation, obstruction, and subsequent infarction of the cerebral cortex. The brain stem is the area most commonly affected, accounting for the frequent involvement of cranial nerves III, VI, and VII. This exudate interferes with the normal flow of cerebrospinal fluid (CSF) in and out of the ventricular system at the level of the basilar cisterns, leading to a communicating hydrocephalus. This combination of vasculitis, infarction, cerebral edema, and hydrocephalus results in the severe damage that can occur gradually or rapidly with this disease. Profound abnormalities in electrolyte metabolism, especially hyponatremia secondary to the inappropriate secretion of antidiuretic hormone, are common and may contribute to the pathophysiology.[67] Salt wasting may make correction of the electrolyte disturbances difficult.

Tuberculous meningitis complicates approximately 0.5% of untreated primary infections.[68] It is extremely rare in infants less than 4 months of age because it usually takes that long for the pathologic events to take place. It is most common among children between 6 months and 4 years of age. Since it is an early manifestation of the primary infection, the adult source case usually can be identified fairly quickly.

The clinical progression of tuberculous meningitis may be rapid or gradual.[69-72] Rapid progression tends to occur more often among infants and young children who may experience symptoms for only days before the onset of acute hydrocephalus, seizures, or cerebral edema. More often, the signs and symptoms progress slowly over several weeks and can be divided into three stages.[73] The first stage typically lasts 1 to 2 weeks and is characterized by nonspecific symptoms such as fever, headache, irritability, drowsiness, and malaise. Focal neurologic signs are absent but infants may experience a stagnation or loss of developmental milestones. The second stage usually begins more abruptly with lethargy, nuchal rigidity, Kernig or Brudzinsky signs, seizures, hypertonia, vomiting, cranial nerve palsies, and other focal neurologic signs. The clinical picture usually correlates with the early development of hydrocephalus with subsequent increased intracranial pressure and vasculitis. Some children do not have signs of meningeal irritation but have signs of encephalitis such as disorientation, abnormal movements, and speech impairment.[74] The third stage is marked by coma, hemiplegia or paraplegia, hypertension, decerebrate posturing, deterioration in vital signs, and, eventually, death. The prognosis of tuberculous meningitis correlates most closely with the clinical stage of illness at the time antituberculosis chemotherapy is started;[73,75] the vast majority of patients in the first stage have an excellent outcome, while most patients in the third stage who survive have permanent disabilities which include blindness, deafness, paraplegia, diabetes insipidus, and mental retardation. It is imperative that antituberculosis treatment be considered strongly for any child who develops basilar meningitis or meningitis in association with hydrocephalus, cranial nerve palsies or ischemic infarct with no other apparent etiology. Early use of surgical shunting of ventricular CSF improves the outcome when hydrocephalus and increased intracranial pressure are present.[76] The key to the diagnosis in children often is identifying the adult source case.

The initial diagnosis of tuberculous meningitis may be extremely difficult. The tuberculin skin test is negative in up to 40% of cases and the chest radiograph is normal in up to 50% of cases.[77] The CSF leukocyte cell count ranges from 10 cells/mm^3 to 500 cells/mm^3. Polymorphonuclear cells may be the major cell type early, but a lymphocyte preponderance is more typical. The CSF glucose level usually is between 20 and 40 mg/dl, whereas the CSF protein concentration is elevated and occasionally markedly high (>400 mg/dl). The success of microscopic examination of stained CSF and mycobacterial cultures is directly related to the size of the CSF sample. When 10 ml of CSF are available, the acid-fast stain is positive in up to 30% of cases and the culture is positive in up to 70% of cases. Computed tomography or magnetic resonance scans may help establish the diagnosis of tuberculous meningitis and can aid in evaluating the success of therapy.[78-80] Both aid in the recognition of hydrocephalus, an infarct or vasculitis, or a tuberculoma, which may suggest the correct diagnosis.

b. Tuberculoma

Another manifestation of central nervous system tuberculosis is the tuberculoma, which usually presents clinically as a brain tumor. They occur most often in children less than 10 years of age and are usually singular. While the lesions in adults are most often supratentorial, in children they are often infratentorial, located at the base of the brain near the cerebellum. Tuberculomas account for up to 40% of brain "tumors" in some areas of the world, but they are rare in North America. The most common symptoms are headache, fever, and convulsions. The tuberculin skin test usually is reactive but the chest radiograph often is unremarkable. Surgical excision may be necessary to distinguish tuberculoma from other causes of brain tumors.

A phenomenon which has been recognized since the advent of computerized tomography is the paradoxical development of tuberculomas in patients with tuberculous meningitis while on ultimately effective chemotherapy.[81-83] The cause and nature of these tuberculomas are poorly understood, but are thought to be related to the immune response to infection. Their development is not thought to be a failure of drug treatment and does not necessitate a change in the therapeutic regimen. This phenomenon should be considered whenever a child with tuberculous meningitis deteriorates or develops focal neurologic findings while on treatment.[71] Corticosteroids may help alleviate the occasionally severe clinical signs and symptoms these lesions cause. They may be very slow to resolve, persisting for months or even years. It is unclear how long antituberculosis treatment or corticosteroids should be given when these lesions appear.

6. Skeletal

Skeletal tuberculosis usually results from lymphohematogenous seeding of tubercle bacilli during the primary infection. Bone infection also may originate from direct extension of a caseous regional lymph node or by extension from a neighboring infected bone. The time interval between infection and disease can be as short as 1 month in cases of tuberculous dactylitis or 30 months or longer for tuberculosis of the hip. The infection usually begins in the metaphysis (Figure 8.5). Granulation tissue and caseation develop which destroy bone both by direct infection and pressure necrosis. Soft tissue abscess and extension of the infection through the epiphysis into the nearby joint often complicate the bone lesion. Frequently, the infection becomes clinically apparent when the joint involvement progresses. Weight bearing bones and joints are affected most commonly.[84] Most cases of bone tuberculosis occur in the vertebrae causing tuberculosis of the spine, known as Pott's disease.[85] Although any vertebral body can be involved, there is a predilection for the lower thoracic and upper lumbar vertebrae. Involvement of two or more vertebrae is common; they are usually contiguous but there may be skip areas between lesions.[86] The infection is in the body of the vertebra leading to bony destruction and collapse. The usual progression of tuberculous spondylitis is from initial narrowing of one or several disc spaces to collapse and wedging of the vertebral body with subsequent angulation of the spine (gibbus) or kyphosis. The infection may extend out from the bone causing a paraspinal (Pott's), psoas, or retropharyngeal abscess.

The most frequent clinical signs and symptoms of tuberculous spondylitis in children are low-grade fever, irritability and restlessness (especially at night), back pain usually without significant tenderness, and abnormal positioning and gait or refusal to walk. Rigidity of the spine may be caused by profound muscle spasm resulting from the patient's involuntary effort to immobilize the spine.

Other sites of skeletal tuberculosis, in approximate order of frequency, are the knee, hip, elbow, and ankle.[87] The degree of involvement ranges from joint effusion without bone destruction to frank destruction of bone and restriction of the joint caused by chronic fibrosis of the synovial membrane. The process usually evolves over months to years, most commonly causing mild pain, stiffness, limping, and restricted movement. The tuberculin skin test is reactive in 80 to 90% of cases. Culture of joint fluid or bone biopsy usually yields the organism. Tuberculosis should be considered in any child with a persistent bone or joint lesion.

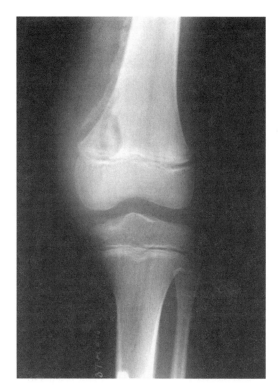

FIGURE 8.5   Tuberculosis in a long bone of a child. (From Friedman, L. N., Ed., *Tuberculosis: Current Concepts and Treatment,* 1st ed., CRC Press LLC, Boca Raton, FL, 1994. With permission.)

One form of bony tuberculosis peculiar to infants is tuberculous dactylitis.[88] Affected children develop distal endarteritis followed by painless swelling and cystic bone lesions. Abscesses are rare but the tuberculin skin test usually is reactive.

D. Diagnostic Tests

1. General Approach

Many children with tuberculosis are discovered via contact investigations of adults with infectious pulmonary tuberculosis. Many of these children have asymptomatic disease that would have progressed or escaped detection if the contact tracing had not occurred. Some children are discovered after a symptomatic illness begins. A strong index of suspicion for tuberculosis is required to correctly identify the cause of illness in children since the signs and symptoms of most forms of tuberculosis are similar to those of many other infections and conditions. The importance of the epidemiologic setting of the child in establishing the diagnosis of tuberculosis cannot be overemphasized.

Routine laboratory tests such as a complete blood count and cell differential, erythrocyte sedimentation rate, urinalysis, and blood chemistries are usually normal in children with tuberculosis disease. Abnormalities in liver enzymes or function tests may indicate hepatic involvement in miliary tuberculosis.

2. Tuberculin Skin Test

The principles for tuberculin skin testing for children are the same as those for adults.[89] A positive tuberculin skin test is the hallmark of the primary infection with *M. tuberculosis*. In children, the tuberculin reaction persists for many years, even after successful completion of chemotherapy.[90]

However, young infants generally produce less induration and response to tuberculin than do older children and adults. A variety of factors common in children such as malnutrition, viral infections (especially varicella, influenza, and measles) and, perhaps, administration of live virus vaccines, can lower tuberculin reactivity. Approximately 10% of immunocompetent children with culture documented tuberculosis initially do not react to tuberculin although most become reactive after several months of therapy.[40,91] Parents should not be allowed to interpret their children's skin test results because of unreliable interpretation and reporting.

Two techniques are used for tuberculin skin testing in children — multiple puncture tests and the Mantoux test. The multiple puncture tests utilize either purified protein derivative (PPD) or Old Tuberculin as the antigen which is delivered intradermally via metal or plastic prongs. Unfortunately, several technical and practice-related problems severely limit their usefulness. First, the exact dose of tuberculin introduced into the skin cannot be precisely controlled so interpretation of the reaction size is difficult to standardize. As a result, a reactive test cannot be considered diagnostic of infection unless a vesicular reaction occurs. The need to verify a positive multiple puncture test with a Mantoux test leads to the second problem, called boosting.[92] Boosting is an increase in the reaction size to a skin test in a person already sensitized to mycobacterial antigens caused by repetitive tests. This phenomenon is caused in older adults by stimulation of a waned immunologic response to *M. tuberculosis* and in children and young adults by cross-reactions due to nontuberculous mycobacteria or prior vaccination with BCG.[93] The booster reaction may occur for tuberculin tests performed several days to 12 or more months apart, resulting in a subsequent positive Mantoux skin test that may not represent infection with *M. tuberculosis*.

The third problem with multiple puncture skin tests is that the sensitivity and specificity compared with the Mantoux test is quite variable and in some studies quite low. False-positive rates may be as high as 30% or greater and false-negative results may be greater than 10%.[94] The final problem is that many clinicians allow parents and families to interpret their own tuberculin skin tests, a practice that should be condemned.[95]

In general, multiple puncture skin tests should not be used in children. They are absolutely contraindicated for children who have had BCG vaccine, known contacts of persons with infectious tuberculosis, ill children, or testing of children in high-risk groups for tuberculosis.

The effect of BCG vaccination on the subsequent Mantoux skin test in children is highly variable, and is partly dependent on the strain of BCG used.[96] Several studies have shown that at least 50% of infants who received BCG vaccine do not convert their tuberculin skin test to reactive, and 80 to 90% of those who react initially become tuberculin skin test negative within 2 to 3 years after BCG vaccination.[97,98] Prior BCG vaccination in a child is never a contraindication to subsequent tuberculin skin testing and, in general, the results of the skin test should be interpreted as if the child had never received BCG vaccination.

In general, the interpretation of the Mantoux tuberculin skin test should be the same for children as it is for adults.[92] One recent study implied that pediatricians tend to underread or underreport the amount of induration present in reaction to a tuberculin test.[99]

3. Acid-Fast Stain and Culture

Generally, the most important laboratory tests for the diagnosis and management of tuberculosis are the acid-fast stain and mycobacterial culture. The best culture specimen for children with suspected pulmonary tuberculosis is the early morning gastric aspirate obtained before the child has arisen and peristalsis has emptied the stomach of the pooled, swallowed overnight respiratory secretions. Unfortunately, even under optimal conditions three consecutive morning gastric aspirates yield the organism in less than 50% of cases; negative cultures never exclude the diagnosis of tuberculosis in a child. The yield from culture obtained via flexible bronchoscopy is significantly less than that from properly obtained gastric aspirates.[100]

Fortunately, there may not be a need for culture confirmation for many children with suspected pulmonary tuberculosis. If the child has a positive tuberculin skin test, clinical and/or radiographic findings suggestive of tuberculosis, and previous contact with an adult source case with infectious tuberculosis, the child should be treated for tuberculosis disease. The drug susceptibility test results from the source case isolate can be used to determine the best therapeutic regimen for the child. However, cultures should be obtained and susceptibility tests performed on specimens from the child with suspected tuberculosis under four conditions:

1. The source case is unknown.
2. The source case has a drug-resistant organism.
3. The child has extrapulmonary tuberculosis (since the differential diagnosis for the condition is somewhat broader than it usually is for pulmonary tuberculosis).
4. The diagnosis is in doubt, especially in a child with HIV infection or another cause of immune suppression.

The yield from gastric aspirate acid-fast stains is much lower than for culture, but a markedly positive result from gastric fluid usually is indicative of pulmonary tuberculosis. Unfortunately, while acid-fast stains of gastric contents may have a specificity for tuberculosis greater than 90%, the sensitivity usually is below 25%.[101] Acid-fast stain and mycobacterial culture of urine may be helpful for children with suspected miliary tuberculosis or in some cases of primary pulmonary tuberculosis.

4. New Techniques

The serodiagnosis of tuberculosis has been envisioned since 1898, when the first agglutination test was developed. In the past 15 years, there have been numerous studies using both whole-cell and specific antigens in various antibody detection systems. For adults, most serologic tests have a sensitivity and specificity approaching those of a sputum acid-fast smear. Several studies have used samples from children. One study of a small number of children with pulmonary tuberculosis in Argentina, which used a specific mycobacterial antigen in an enzyme-linked immunosorbent assay (ELISA) system, found a sensitivity of 86% and specificity of 100%.[102] Another study of children with tuberculosis, using whole-cell *M. tuberculosis* as the antigen in an ELISA test, found a sensitivity of 62% and specificity of 98%.[103] However, a different study that used various whole mycobacterial sonicates had a sensitivity of only 26% and specificity of 40%.[104] Recent studies have examined the use of ELISA tests for detecting antibodies against antigen A60, but the results in children were variable and the sensitivity and specificity were too low for routine use.[105,106] It is unlikely that serodiagnosis will make a substantial contribution to the diagnosis of tuberculosis in children in the near future.

The predominant method of nucleic acid amplification used to detect the presence of mycobacterial DNA in studies of children with tuberculosis is the polymerase chain reaction (PCR). Compared with a clinical diagnosis of pulmonary tuberculosis in children, the sensitivity of PCR using the insertion element IS6110 has varied from 25 to 83%, and the specificity has varied from 80 to 100%.[107-109] However, PCR of gastric aspirates may be positive in recently infected children with no clinical or radiographic signs of disease, demonstrating the occasional arbitrary nature of the distinction between tuberculosis infection and disease. PCR may have a useful but limited role in evaluating children. A negative PCR never eliminates tuberculosis as a diagnostic possibility, and a positive result does not confirm it. PCR may be useful in evaluating immunocompromised children with pulmonary disease, although published reports of its performance in such children are lacking. PCR also may aid in confirming the diagnosis of extrapulmonary tuberculosis in children, although only a few case reports have been published.[110,111]

E. Treatment

1. Principles

The general principles that have determined the development of antituberculosis chemotherapy regimens in adults generally apply to infants and children. However, there are several special considerations for children with tuberculosis based on microbiology, natural history of the disease, and product availability. First, children usually develop tuberculosis disease as an immediate complication of the primary infection. They typically have closed caseous lesions with relatively few mycobacteria. The large bacterial populations found within cavities or infiltrates that are characteristic of adult reactivation pulmonary tuberculosis usually are absent in children. Since the likelihood of developing resistance to any antimycobacterial drug is proportional to the size of the bacillary population, children generally are less likely than adults to develop secondary drug resistance while receiving therapy, even if adherence is poor.[112]

A related problem concerns the natural history of primary tuberculosis in children. All children with tuberculosis infection have involvement of the hilar or mediastinal lymph nodes; however, the involvement is visible radiographically in less than 20% of children. While asymptomatic infection and pulmonary disease usually are easily distinguishable events in adults, the range of microbiologic and host response events lays more on a continuum in children. Pediatric radiographs can be difficult to interpret and there are no standards for what constitutes significant intrathoracic adenopathy in a child. In general, the clinician considers the child to have tuberculosis disease if adenopathy is readily visible on the chest radiograph, even if the child has no signs or symptoms of tuberculosis. When determining the best treatment regimen for a child, it usually is safer to overestimate rather than underestimate the extent of disease, particularly in a child known to be at high risk for recent acquisition of tuberculosis infection.

Third, children have a higher propensity than adults to develop extrapulmonary forms of tuberculosis, especially disseminated disease and meningitis. It is important that antituberculosis drugs for children penetrate into a variety of tissues and fluids, especially across the meninges. Isoniazid, rifampin, pyrazinamide, and ethionamide cross both inflamed and uninflamed meninges adequately to kill virtually all strains of drug-susceptible *M. tuberculosis*.

Fourth, the pharmacokinetics of antituberculosis drugs differ between children and adults.[113] In general, children tolerate larger doses per kg of body weight and have fewer adverse reactions than adults.[114,115] It is unclear whether the higher serum concentration of drugs achieved in children have any therapeutic advantage.[116] The lower rates of toxicity in children usually mean that fewer interruptions in treatment will occur. In general, children with more severe forms of tuberculosis, especially disseminated disease and meningitis, experience more significant hepatotoxic effects than less severely ill children treated with the same doses per kg of isoniazid and rifampin, especially if the isoniazid dose exceeds 10 mg/kg per day.[117] However, many hepatotoxic "reactions" in children taking antituberculosis medications really are caused by intercurrent infections with hepatitis A and B viruses or other viruses.[118]

Finally, an important difference between children and adults concerns the administration of medications. Most available dosage forms were designed for use in adults. Giving these preparations to children may involve crushing pills or making suspensions that are neither standardized nor well studied. Some dosage forms may lead to inadequate absorption of oral medications.[119] Many children experience difficulty taking the several antituberculosis medications required at the beginning of therapy. If these problems are not anticipated and addressed, they may cause significant delays and interruptions of treatment. Currently, fixed dose combination preparations are not readily usable in children. Technical problems may be difficult to solve; one recent study demonstrated a marked decline in rifampin concentration over time in suspensions also containing isoniazid or pyrazinamide.[120]

2. Antituberculosis Drugs for Children (Table 8.3)

Isoniazid is familiar to pediatricians as it is effective and well tolerated by children. Although it is metabolized by acetylation in the liver, there is no correlation in children between acetylation rate and either efficacy or adverse reactions.[121] The major toxic effects of isoniazid in adults are very rare in children. Pyridoxine levels are decreased in children taking isoniazid, but peripheral neuritis is exceedingly rare.[122] However, certain children — especially teenagers with inadequate diets, children from ethnic groups with low meat and milk intake, and breast feeding babies — should receive pyridoxine supplementation. Hepatotoxicity among children taking isoniazid also is rare with only 3 to 10% experiencing transiently elevated serum liver enzyme levels; clinically significant hepatitis occurs in far less than 1% of children.[115] Adolescents are more likely than younger children to experience hepatotoxicity.[123] For most children and adolescents, toxicity can be monitored using only clinical signs and symptoms; routine biochemical monitoring is not necessary.

Rifampin is well tolerated by children. Hepatotoxicity is infrequent and other adverse reactions that occur in adults, such as leukopenia, thrombocytopenia, and the immunologically mediated

TABLE 8.3
Antituberculosis Drugs in Children

Drugs	Dosage Forms	Daily Dose (mg/kg)	Twice-Weekly Dose (mg/kg/dose)	Maximum Dose
Isoniazid[a]	Scored tablets: 100 mg 300 mg Syrup: 10mg/ml[b]	10–15	20–40	Daily: 300 mg; twice-weekly: 900 mg
Rifampin[a]	Capsules: 150 mg 300 mg Syrup: formulated in syrup from capsules[c]	10–20	10–20	600 mg
Pyrazinamide	Scored tablets: 500 mg	20–40	50–70	2 g
Streptomycin	Vials: 1 g, 4 g	20–40 (IM)	20–40 (IM)	1 g
Ethambutol	Scored tablets: 100 mg 400 mg	15–25	50	2.5 g
Ethionamide	Tablets: 250 mg	10–20		1 g
Kanamycin	Vials: 1 g	15 (IM)	15–25 (IM)	1 g
Cycloserine	Capsules: 250 mg	10–20		1 g

[a] Rifamate is a capsule containing 150 mg of isoniazid and 300 mg of rifampin. Two capsules provide the usual adult (more than 50 kg) daily dose of each drug.

[b] Many experts recommend not using isoniazid syrup, as it is unstable and is associated with frequent gastrointestinal complaints, especially diarrhea.

[c] Merrill Dow issues directions for preparation of this "extemporaneous" syrup.

Source: Friedman, L. N., Ed., *Tuberculosis: Current Concepts and Treatment,* 1st ed., CRC Press LLC, Boca Raton, FL, 1994. With permission.

flu-like syndrome, are rare. Pyrazinamide has been used extensively in children over the past decade. Formal pharmacokinetic studies in children have not been reported but a daily dose of 30 mg/kg results in adequate CSF levels, is well tolerated, produces little toxicity, and appears to be effective.[124] Hepatitis and complications of hyperuricemia are exceedingly rare among children. Streptomycin is used less frequently than in the past but is well tolerated by children. Although safe in infants, it cannot be given to pregnant women because it causes damage to the eighth cranial nerve of the fetus.

Ethambutol has not been used widely among children because of its potential toxicity to the eye and the relative difficulty monitoring ophthalmological signs and symptoms in young children. However, there is no published evidence of optic toxicity in children and there is no damage to the fetus when the pregnant woman takes ethambutol.[125,126] Ethambutol is not recommended for general use in children, but should be considered strongly for children with suspected drug-resistant tuberculosis. Ethionamide is well tolerated by children and is probably underutilized in this population. Children experience much less gastrointestinal distress than adults. Ethionamide can be used as a fourth antituberculosis medication for initial treatment in children with possible or suspected resistance to either isoniazid or rifampin, or for children with tuberculous meningitis.[127]

3. Specific Treatment

a. Thoracic Disease

During the past decade, several treatment trials for tuberculosis for children have been reported. One study from Arkansas reported successful treatment of 50 children with tuberculosis using isoniazid and rifampin daily for 1 month, then twice weekly for 8 months, a total treatment duration of 9 months.[128] Some patients with only hilar adenopathy were successfully treated with a 6-month regimen of isoniazid and rifampin.[129] One study from Brazil reported successful treatment of 117 children with pulmonary tuberculosis using isoniazid and rifampin daily for 6 months.[130] Although these results are impressive, this 6-month regimen in children has not been adopted widely because of limited data and the growing problem of isoniazid and rifampin resistance in many areas of the world. The Brazilian study also demonstrated the difficult problem of nonadherence among children since, even with this fairly simple regimen, 17% of the patients did not complete treatment.

There have been several studies of 6-month duration of antituberculosis therapy in children using at least three drugs initially for drug-susceptible tuberculosis.[131-135] Although the exact regimens used in these trials differed slightly, the most common was a 6-month regimen of isoniazid and rifampin supplemented during the first 2 months with pyrazinamide. The success of these regimens was the same whether or not streptomycin also was given. Most trials used daily therapy for the first 1 to 2 months followed by daily or twice weekly, directly observed therapy for the last 4 months. Regimens using twice weekly therapy under the direct observation of a healthcare worker were as safe and effective as those using daily self-administered therapy. In all trials, the overall success rate was greater than 95% for complete clinical and radiographic cure and 99% for significant radiographic improvement during a 2-year period of follow-up. The incidence of clinically significant adverse reactions, most commonly gastrointestinal upset or mild skin rash, was less than 2%.

The current recommendations of the American Academy of Pediatrics,[136] Centers for Disease Control and Prevention, and the International Union Against Tuberculosis and Lung Disease,[4] suggest that standard therapy for drug-susceptible thoracic tuberculosis in children should be 6 months of isoniazid and rifampin supplemented during the first 2 months with pyrazinamide. Although daily administration of medications during the first 2 months is preferable, two studies have shown that 6 months of twice or thrice weekly medications yielded results equivalent to regimens that used an initial phase of daily self-administered treatment.[132,134] If the risk of initial isoniazid or rifampin resistant tuberculosis is significant for a child, a fourth drug, usually ethambutol, streptomycin, or ethionamide, should be given initially until drug susceptibility patterns can be established.

b. Extrathoracic Disease

Controlled trials comparing treatment regimens for various forms of extrapulmonary tuberculosis in children are virtually nonexistent. Several of the 6-month, three-drug regimen trials in children included cases of lymph node and disseminated tuberculosis, both of which responded favorably to these regimens.[133,134] Most data come from series of extrathoracic tuberculosis in adults. In general, the 6-month regimen using isoniazid, rifampin, and pyrazinamide initially is recommended for most forms of extrathoracic tuberculosis. One exception may be bone and joint tuberculosis which may require a treatment duration of 9 to 12 months, especially if surgical intervention has not been undertaken.[137]

Tuberculous lymphadenitis responds well to antituberculosis chemotherapy although involved nodes may remain enlarged for months to years.[138] Surgical removal alone is not adequate treatment since the lymph node disease is only part of a systemic infection. However, surgical biopsy and culture may be necessary to distinguish tuberculous adenitis from other entities, especially cat-scratch disease or infection due to nontuberculous mycobacteria. Excisional biopsy is preferred over incisional biopsy because of an increased risk of subsequent sinus tract formation or severe scarring with the latter procedure.

Tuberculous meningitis has not been included in trials of extrapulmonary tuberculosis because of its serious nature and low incidence. As with other forms of extrapulmonary tuberculosis, the number of mycobacteria causing disease usually is small. Treatment with isoniazid and rifampin daily for 12 months generally is effective for drug-susceptible disease.[139] Several recent reports have suggested that 6 to 9 months of therapy is effective if isoniazid, rifampin, and pyrazinamide are administered during the initial phase of treatment.[140] At present, there probably are not sufficient data to recommend the 6-month treatment duration for most children with tuberculous meningitis. The recommendation of the American Academy of Pediatrics for tuberculous meningitis is 12 months of treatment that includes at least isoniazid and rifampin and usually one or two other drugs during the initial phase of treatment.[136] However, some experts believe that a treatment duration of 6 to 9 months is adequate if pyrazinamide is included in the initial treatment. Many experts add a fourth drug during initial treatment — usually streptomycin or another aminoglycocide, ethambutol or ethionamide — to protect against unsuspected initial drug resistance.

c. Human Immunodeficiency Virus-Related

The optimal treatment of tuberculosis in HIV-infected children has not been established. Adults with tuberculosis who are HIV-infected usually can be treated successfully with standard regimens that include isoniazid, rifampin, and pyrazinamide, if the total duration of therapy is extended to 9 months, or to 6 months after cultures of sputum become sterile, whichever is longer.[141] It may be difficult to determine whether a pulmonary infiltrate is due to *M. tuberculosis* in an HIV-infected child who has a positive tuberculin reaction or history of exposure to an adult with infectious tuberculosis. It is likely, as in immunocompetent children, that gastric aspirate or bronchoscopy cultures may be sterile even when tuberculosis disease is present. The radiographic appearance of other pulmonary complications of HIV infection in children, such as lymphoid interstitial pneumonitis, may be similar to that of tuberculosis. Treatment usually is empiric, based upon epidemiologic and radiographic information, and it should be considered when tuberculosis cannot be excluded.

Most experts believe that HIV-infected children with drug-susceptible tuberculosis disease should receive isoniazid, rifampin, and pyrazinamide for 2 months followed by isoniazid and rifampin to complete a total treatment duration of 9 to 12 months. All children with tuberculosis disease should be evaluated for HIV infection since its presence may necessitate a longer duration of treatment.

d. Drug-Resistant Tuberculosis

The incidence of drug-resistant tuberculosis appears to be increasing in North America, particularly in large cities such as New York and Miami, and along the Mexican border.[142] For the entire U.S., approximately 10% of isolates of *M. tuberculosis* are resistant to at least one drug, while many countries in Latin America and Asia routinely report drug resistance rates of 20 to 30%. Patterns of drug resistance among children tend to mirror those found among adults in the same population.[143,144] Certain epidemiologic factors such as being an Asian or Latin American immigrant, being homeless, or having a history of prior antituberculosis treatment, correlate with drug resistance in adults and their childhood contacts.

Treatment for drug-resistant tuberculosis is successful only when at least two bactericidal drugs to which the infecting strain of *M. tuberculosis* is susceptible are given. When a child has possible drug-resistant tuberculosis at least three and usually four or five drugs should be given initially until the exact susceptibility pattern is determined and a more specific regimen can be designed. The specific regimen must be individualized for each patient according to the results of susceptibility testing on the isolates from the child or the adult source case.[145,146] Although primary resistance to pyrazinamide is rare, pyrazinamide may not be effective in preventing the emergence of rifampin resistance during treatment when isoniazid resistance initially is present. Therefore, the combination of isoniazid, rifampin, and pyrazinamide may not be adequate for children if initial isoniazid or rifampin resistance is present. A fourth drug — usually streptomycin, ethambutol, or ethionamide — also should be given initially. When isoniazid or rifampin resistance is present, the total duration of therapy usually is extended to 9 to 12 months. Optimal treatment regimens for these children with multidrug-resistant tuberculosis disease can be determined only after complete drug susceptibility information from their, or the adult source case, isolate is available.

e. Corticosteroids

Corticosteroids are useful in the treatment of some children with tuberculosis but only when used with effective antituberculosis drugs. They are beneficial for tuberculosis in children when the host inflammatory reaction is contributing significantly to tissue damage or impairment of organ function (Table 8.4). There is convincing evidence that corticosteroids decrease mortality rates and long-term neurologic sequelae in children with tuberculous meningitis by reducing vasculitis, inflammation, and, ultimately, intracranial pressure.[147] Lowering the intracranial pressure not only limits tissue damage but also favors the circulation of antituberculosis drugs through the brain and meninges. Short courses of corticosteroids may be effective for children with enlarged hilar lymph nodes that compress the tracheobronchial tree causing respiratory distress, localized emphysema, or segmental pulmonary lesions.[148,149] There also is evidence that corticosteroids can help ameliorate the chronic sequelae associated with acute tuberculous pericardial effusion.[150] In patients with tuberculous

---

TABLE 8.4
Manifestations of Tuberculosis Which
May Benefit from Corticosteroid Therapy

Tuberculous meningitis
Tuberculoma with edema
Endobronchial disease
Miliary disease with alveolar-capillary block
Constrictive pericarditis
Massive pleural effusion
Pott's disease with nerve compression

Source: Friedman, L. N., Ed., *Tuberculosis: Current Concepts and Treatment*, 1st ed., CRC Press LLC, Boca Raton, FL, 1994. With permission.

pleural effusion in whom there is shift of the mediastinum and acute respiratory compromise, corticosteroids may cause dramatic improvement in symptoms; although, the long-term course probably is unaffected.[55] Some children with severe miliary tuberculosis have dramatic improvement with corticosteroids if the inflammatory reaction is so severe that alveolocapillary block is present. There is no convincing evidence that one corticosteroid is better than another. The most commonly prescribed regimen is prednisone at 1 to 2 mg/kg/d for 4 to 6 weeks, with gradual tapering.

f. Asymptomatic Tuberculosis Infection

The treatment of children with asymptomatic tuberculosis infection to prevent the development of tuberculosis disease is an established practice. The effectiveness of isoniazid-preventive therapy in children has approached 100% and the effect has lasted for at least 30 years.[151] Tuberculin-positive children with contact to an infectious adult are at the highest risk of developing disease and always should be given therapy. Almost all tuberculin-positive children without known contact also should receive therapy, especially adolescents and children younger than 6 years of age.

Children who are tuberculin negative, including newborn infants, who have had contact with an infectious adult should receive isoniazid therapy until 10 to 12 weeks after contact has been broken by either physical separation from the source case or chemotherapy. If the repeat tuberculin skin test is negative, isoniazid can be discontinued; if the test is positive, a full course of isoniazid therapy should be given. The American Academy of Pediatrics recommends treatment with isoniazid for 9 months[136] (see also Chapter 13). Rifampin is recommended for therapy in children with asymptomatic infection due to an isoniazid-resistant strain of *M. tuberculosis*. Although controlled trials are lacking, either isoniazid or rifampin probably will be effective if given twice weekly under direct supervision when adherence with daily therapy cannot be assured. There are no available data concerning the effectiveness of any therapy regimen in children infected with isoniazid and rifampin resistant strains of *M. tuberculosis*.

g. Supportive and Follow-Up Care

In the prechemotherapy era, supportive care was all the clinician was able to offer children with tuberculosis. With proper chemotherapy, supportive care plays a small role in the management of the child with tuberculosis. Activity need not be restricted unless the child develops respiratory embarrassment or immobilization is necessary for treatment, as in some cases of vertebral tuberculosis. Adequate nutrition is important although many small children with tuberculosis who present with failure to thrive will not begin to gain weight until several months after effective chemotherapy has been started.

Nonadherence with treatment is a major problem in tuberculosis control due to the long-term nature of treatment and sometimes difficult social circumstances of the patients.[152] Several factors may influence adherence among children with tuberculosis. Many children with significant disease have relatively few symptoms and, therefore, do not receive the feedback of improvement in symptoms as treatment progresses. Since the initial diagnosis often cannot be confirmed by a positive culture, there is no opportunity to inform the patient and family that the cultures have gone from positive to negative during treatment. Many children in socially disrupted families have multiple caregivers and assurance of administration of medications is lacking. Finally, the lack of dosage preparations suitable for use in children makes the administration of several medications difficult, especially for small infants and toddlers.

An assessment of potential nonadherence should be made at the initiation of therapy. During treatment, if the physician suspects any chance of nonadherence with daily self-administered medications, directly observed therapy should be instituted with the help of the local health department. Responsible adults in the child's environment such as teachers, school nurses, or church workers often can be used to help ensure that medication is given properly. Twice weekly directly observed therapy is extremely effective in children and most experts would consider it part of standard antituberculosis treatment.

It is important that the physician and other healthcare workers take an active role in the care of children with tuberculosis. Children should be followed carefully to ensure adherence with treatment, to monitor for toxic reactions to medications, and to ensure that the tuberculosis is coming under adequate control. It is extremely important for the family that a single healthcare provider be identified as the person primarily responsible for care. Nonadherence rates are significantly higher in clinical situations where several physicians care for the child on a rotating basis, as frequently occurs in teaching hospitals with housestaff clinics. In general, children on treatment should be seen at monthly intervals and should be given enough medication at each visit to last until the next scheduled visit.

Anticipatory guidance in taking the several antituberculosis medications is crucial when treating children. Children may receive little medication in the first several days due to vomiting and difficult administration until the family develops a dosing scheme that works for them. Commercially available preparations of antituberculosis medications may be difficult to administer to small children. A liquid suspension of isoniazid is available but its stability is variable and many children have diarrhea and gastrointestinal upset while taking this preparation. Rifampin can be made into a stable suspension by a pharmacist, which is helpful for treating small children who cannot swallow capsules. Isoniazid, pyrazinamide, and other pills can be crushed and given with small amounts of food, but rifampin should be taken on an empty stomach, if possible.

The rates of adverse reactions to antituberculosis medications are low enough in children that routine biochemical monitoring is not necessary. If there is any history of previous hepatitis or other chronic illness, it is advisable to obtain a baseline set of serum liver enzyme and uric acid levels. If the patient or family reports any symptoms that could be toxic reactions to antituberculosis medications, the child should have a complete physical examination and a set of serum hepatic enzymes and bilirubin determinations. Serum liver enzyme elevations of two to three times normal are fairly common and do not necessitate discontinuation of medications if all other findings are normal. Mild arthralgias or arthritis could be due to pyrazinamide but usually are transient even when pyrazinamide is continued. All children taking ethambutol should have regular monitoring of visual acuity and color discrimination.

Radiographic changes with intrathoracic tuberculosis in children occur very slowly and frequent chest radiography is not necessary. A common practice is to obtain a chest radiograph at diagnosis and 1 to 2 months after the beginning of treatment to be sure that no unusual changes in radiographic appearance have occurred. If these radiographs are satisfactory, it is not necessary to repeat a chest radiograph until the completion of 6 months of treatment. A normal chest radiograph at this time is not necessary to discontinue treatment. The majority of children with significant intrathoracic adenopathy have abnormal radiographic findings for 1 to 3 years, long after effective antituberculosis treatment has been stopped. If improvement has occurred after 6 months of treatment, medications can be discontinued and the child can be followed at intervals of 3 to 6 months with appropriate chest radiographs to determine continued improvement in radiographic appearance.

II. TUBERCULOSIS IN PREGNANT WOMEN AND THE NEWBORN

A. INTRODUCTION

Before 1985, tuberculosis in the pregnant woman and her newborn infant had become an infrequent event in the U.S. Although specific statistics concerning tuberculosis in pregnancy are not reported, the recent increase in total cases and the shift to young adults and children imply that tuberculosis in pregnancy may become an increasing problem. This problem should disproportionately affect minority urban populations because this group has very high tuberculosis rates, a greater relative shift in cases to childbearing-aged adults, and, in general, poor access to prenatal care and testing for tuberculosis disease and infection.

The influence of pregnancy on the incidence and prognosis of tuberculosis has been debated since antiquity.[153] At various times, pregnancy has been thought to improve, worsen, or have no effect on the prognosis of tuberculosis. This controversy has lost some of its importance since the advent of effective antituberculosis chemotherapy. Although it is generally accepted that with adequate treatment a pregnant woman with tuberculosis has a prognosis equivalent to that of a comparable nonpregnant woman, debate remains about the use of preventive therapy for tuberculosis infection during pregnancy and the postpartum period.

B. Pathogenesis

The pathogenesis of pulmonary tuberculosis during pregnancy is similar to that for nonpregnant individuals. Shortly after the initiation of infection, some organisms enter the lymphatic and blood vessels and disseminate throughout the body. During this phase of infection, the genitalia, endometrium, or placenta may become involved. Tuberculous endometritis and salpingeal tuberculosis have become rare in the U.S. Genital tuberculosis is most likely to start around the time of menarche and can have a very long and relatively asymptomatic course. The fallopian tubes most often are involved (90 to 100%), followed by the uterus (50 to 60%), ovaries (20 to 30%), and cervix (5 to 15%).[154] Sterility is often the presenting complaint of tuberculous endometritis which diminishes the likelihood of congenital tuberculosis occurring.[155] When infection of the placenta occurs, it results more frequently from disseminated tuberculosis in the mother than from a local endometritis. However, tuberculous endometritis can lead to congenital infection in the newborn.[156-158]

The potential modes of inoculation of the newborn infant with tuberculosis from the mother are shown in Table 8.5. Infection of the neonate through the umbilical cord has been rare with fewer than 300 cases reported in the English language literature.[159] These infants' mothers frequently suffer from tuberculous pleural effusion, meningitis, or disseminated disease during pregnancy or soon after.[160-163] However, in some series of congenital tuberculosis, fewer than 50% of the mothers were known to be suffering from tuberculosis at the time of delivery.[162,163] In most of these cases, diagnosis of the child led to the discovery of the mother's tuberculosis. The intensity of lymphohematogenous spread during pregnancy is one of the factors that determines if congenital tuberculosis will occur. Hematogenous dissemination in the mother leads to infection of the placenta with subsequent transmission to the fetus. Tubercle bacilli have been demonstrated in the decidua, amnion, and chorionic villi of the placenta.[155] However, even massive involvement of the placenta with tuberculosis does not always give rise to congenital infection. It is not clear whether the fetus can be directly infected from the mother's bloodstream without a caseous lesion forming first in the placenta, although this phenomenon has been reported in experimental animal models.[164]

TABLE 8.5
Potential Modes of Inoculation of the
Newborn with *Mycobacterium tuberculosis*

Maternal Focus	Mode of Spread
Pneumonitis	Airborne
Placentitis	Hematogenous (umbilical vessel)
Amniotic	Aspiration of infected fluid
Cervicitis	Direct contact, aspiration

Source: Friedman, L. N., Ed., *Tuberculosis: Current Concepts and Treatment,* 1st ed., CRC Press LLC, Boca Raton, FL, 1994. With permission.

In hematogenous congenital tuberculosis, *M. tuberculosis* reaches the fetus via the umbilical vein. If some bacilli infect the liver, a primary focus develops with involvement of the periportal lymph nodes. However, the bacilli can pass through the liver into the main circulation leading to a primary focus in the fetus' lung. The tubercle bacilli in the lung often remain dormant until after birth when oxygenation and circulation increase significantly, leading to pulmonary tuberculosis in the young infant.

Congenital infection of the infant also might occur via aspiration or ingestion of amniotic fluid.[165] If the caseous lesion in the placenta ruptures directly into the amniotic cavity, the fetus can inhale or ingest the tubercle bacilli. Inhalation or ingestion of infected amniotic fluid is the most likely cause of tuberculosis if the infant has multiple primary foci in the lung, gut, or middle ear.[166]

The pathology of tuberculosis in the fetus and newborn usually demonstrates the predisposition to dissemination and fatal disease.[167] The liver and lungs are the primary involved organs with bone marrow, bone, the gastrointestinal tract, adrenal glands, spleen, kidney, abdominal lymph nodes, and skin also involved frequently.[168] The histologic patterns of involvement are similar to those in adults; tubercles and granulomas are common. Central nervous system involvement occurs in fewer than 50% of cases. In most recent series, the mortality of congenital tuberculosis has been close to 50% due primarily to the failure to suspect the correct diagnosis. Most fatal cases are diagnosed at autopsy.[159,162,163]

Postnatal acquisition of tuberculosis via airborne inoculation is the most common route of infection for the neonate. It may be impossible to differentiate postnatal infection from prenatal acquisition on clinical grounds alone. It is important to remember that any adult in the neonate's environment can be a source of airborne tuberculosis. Since newborns infected with tuberculosis are at extremely high risk of developing severe forms of disease, investigation of an adult with tuberculosis whose household contains a pregnant woman or newborn infant should be considered a public health emergency. In addition, all adults in contact with an infant suspected of having tuberculosis infection or disease should undergo a thorough investigation for tuberculosis.

C. Epidemiology: Interaction of Tuberculosis and Pregnancy

The current epidemiology of tuberculosis in pregnant women and the newborn largely is unknown. From 1966 to 1972, the incidence of tuberculosis during pregnancy at New York Lying-In Hospital ranged from 0.6% to 1%.[154] During this time, 2.3% of the patients with culture-proven pulmonary tuberculosis were diagnosed first during pregnancy, a rate equal to that of nonpregnant women of comparable age. There have been only two reported series of pregnant women with tuberculosis in the last two decades.[169,170]

From ancient times, medical opinions regarding the interaction of pregnancy and tuberculosis have varied considerably. Hippocrates believed that pregnancy had a beneficial effect on tuberculosis, a view that persisted virtually unchallenged into the 19th century, when an opposite view emerged. In 1850, Grisolle reported 24 cases of tuberculosis that developed during pregnancy.[171] In all patients the progression of tuberculosis during pregnancy was more severe than usually seen in nonpregnant individuals of the same age. Shortly thereafter, several papers were published that implied that pregnancy had a deleterious effect on tuberculosis. This view gained so much support that by the early 20th century, the concept of induced abortion to deal with the consequences of tuberculosis during pregnancy became widely accepted.

The opinion that pregnancy had a deleterious effect on tuberculosis predominated until the late 1940s. In 1943, Cohen detected no increased rate of progression of tuberculosis among 100 pregnant women with abnormal chest radiographs.[172] In 1953, Hedvall presented a comprehensive review of published studies concerning tuberculosis in pregnancy in the prechemotherapy era.[173] He cited studies totaling over 1000 cases that reported negative effects of pregnancy on tuberculosis. However, he discovered a nearly equal number of reported cases in which a neutral or favorable relationship between pregnancy and tuberculosis was observed. In his own study of 250 pregnant women with abnormal chest radiographs consistent with tuberculosis, he noted that 9% improved, 7% worsened, and 84% remained unchanged during pregnancy. During the first postpartum year, 9% improved, 15% worsened, and 76% were stable. Crombie noted that 31 of 101 pregnant women with quiescent tuberculosis experienced a relapse after delivery; 20 of the 31 relapses occurred in the first postpartum year.[174] Several other investigators observed a higher risk of relapse during the puerperium. However, other studies failed to support an increased risk of progression of tuberculosis in the postpartum period.[175] Cohen's study failed to show a major increase in activity of tuberculosis during pregnancy or any postpartum interval.[172] Other studies had similar results and, although they did not have control populations, it was estimated that the rates of progression would be comparable to nonpregnant age-matched control subjects.[176,177] From these and other studies it became clear that the anatomic extent of disease, the radiographic pattern, and the susceptibility of the individual patient to tuberculosis are more important than pregnancy itself in determining the course and prognosis of the pregnant woman with tuberculosis.

The controversy concerning the effect of pregnancy or the postpartum period on tuberculosis has lost most of its importance since the advent of effective chemotherapy. With adequate treatment, pregnant women with tuberculosis have the same excellent prognosis as nonpregnant women. Several studies could document no adverse affects of pregnancy, birth, the postpartum period, or lactation on the course of tuberculosis in women receiving chemotherapy.[154,178]

Most of the studies cited previously deal with the risk of reactivation of tuberculosis among women with abnormal chest radiographs but no evidence of active tuberculous lesions. It is not as clear if women with asymptomatic tuberculosis infection but no radiographic disease are at increased risk of developing tuberculosis disease during pregnancy or the postpartum period. In 1959, Pridie and Stradling found that the incidence of pulmonary tuberculosis among pregnant women was the same as in the nonpregnant female population of the area.[179] From 1966 to 1972, Schaefer et al. found that the annual pulmonary tuberculosis case rate among pregnant women at New York Lying-In Hospital was 18 to 29 per 100,000 population, comparable to the incidence during the same period in women of child-bearing age in New York City of 19 to 39 per 100,000.[154] Although no definitive study has been reported, it appears unlikely that progression from asymptomatic tuberculosis infection to tuberculosis disease is accelerated during pregnancy or the postpartum period.

In the prechemotherapy era, active tuberculosis at an advanced stage carried a poor prognosis for both mother and child. Schaefer et al. reported that the infant and maternal mortality from untreated tuberculosis was between 30 and 40%.[154] In the chemotherapy era, the outcome of pregnancy rarely is altered by the presence of tuberculosis in the mother, except in the rare cases of congenital tuberculosis. One study from Norway revealed a higher incidence of toxemia, postpartum hemorrhage, and difficult labor in mothers with tuberculosis compared with control subjects.[180] The incidence of miscarriage was almost 10 times higher in tuberculous mothers, but there was no significant difference in the rate of congenital malformations between children born to mothers with and without tuberculosis. One study reported an incidence of prematurity among infants born to untreated mothers in a tuberculosis sanitarium ranging from 23 to 64%, depending upon the severity of tuberculosis in the mother.[181] However, most experts now believe that with adequate treatment of the pregnant tuberculous woman, the prognosis of pregnancy should not be adversely affected by the presence of tuberculosis. Because of the excellent prognosis for both mother and child, the recommendation for therapeutic abortion has been abandoned.

D. CLINICAL MANIFESTATIONS

1. The Pregnant Woman

In general, the clinical manifestations of tuberculosis in the pregnant woman are the same as those in nonpregnant individuals of the same age and with the same disease severity. In one series of 27 pregnant and postpartum women with pulmonary tuberculosis, the most common clinical findings were cough, weight loss, fever, malaise, fatigue, and hemoptysis.[170] Almost 20% of the patients had no significant symptoms; the tuberculin skin test was positive in 26 of 27 patients. Other studies have found less significant symptoms in pregnant women with tuberculosis.[169] Diagnosis was established in all cases by culture of sputum for *M. tuberculosis*. A total of 16 of these patients had drug-resistant tuberculosis and their clinical course was marked by more extensive pulmonary involvement, higher incidence of pulmonary complications, longer sputum conversion times, and a higher incidence of death. In other series, approximately 5 to 10% of pregnant women with tuberculosis have had extrapulmonary disease, a rate comparable to the nonpregnant population. [169,182]

The indications for treatment and the basic principles for management of tuberculosis disease in the pregnant woman are really no different from those in the nonpregnant patient. However, the recommended regimens and drugs used are slightly different, mostly due to possible effects of several drugs on the developing fetus. There is no doubt that untreated tuberculosis disease represents a far greater risk to the pregnant woman and her fetus than does appropriate treatment of the disease.[183] The recommended treatment for drug-susceptible tuberculosis in pregnancy is 9 months of isoniazid and rifampin daily, with ethambutol added to the initial regimen until the drug susceptibility pattern is known. Pyridoxine also should be given because of increased requirements for this vitamin in pregnancy.[184] Extensive experience with isoniazid, rifampin, and ethambutol has shown that they are safe to both the mother and fetus.[185,186] Streptomycin should be avoided during pregnancy, if possible, since almost 20% of infants will have eighth nerve damage if the drug is given to their mothers during pregnancy.[187,188] The safety of pyrazinamide during pregnancy is unknown, although it appears to be used safely by many experts. Nonspecific teratogenic effects attributed to ethionamide have been observed in animal models.[189] Treatment of drug-resistant tuberculosis in pregnancy is difficult because some of the "contraindicated" or unknown safety drugs may be required for adequate treatment; under these conditions, an expert in tuberculosis should be consulted.

3. Newborn

The clinical manifestations of tuberculosis in the fetus or newborn are shown in Table 8.6. Most patients have an abnormal chest radiograph and approximately 50% have a miliary pattern. Some

TABLE 8.6
Most Frequent Signs and Symptoms of Congenital Tuberculosis

Sign or Symptom	Frequency (%)
Respiratory distress	77
Fever	62
Hepatic and/or splenic enlargement	62
Poor feeding	46
Lethargy or irritability	42
Lymphadenopathy	35
Abdominal distention	27
Failure to thrive	19
Ear discharge	15
Skin lesions	12

Source: Adapted from Hageman, J., Shulman, S., Schreiber, M., Luck, S., and Rogeu, R., *Pediatrics*, 66, 980, 1980.

infants with a normal chest radiograph early in the course develop profound radiographic abnor-malities as the disease progresses. The most common findings are adenopathy and parenchymal infiltrates. Occasionally, the pulmonary involvement progresses very rapidly, leading to develop-ment of a thin-walled cavity.

The clinical presentation of tuberculosis in the newborn is similar to that caused by bacterial sepsis and other congenital infections such as syphilis and cytomegalovirus. The diagnosis of congenital tuberculosis should be suspected in any infant with appropriate signs and symptoms who does not respond to vigorous antibiotic therapy and whose evaluation for other congenital infections is unrevealing. Of course, suspicion also should be high if the mother has or has had tuberculosis or if she is in a high-risk group for tuberculosis.

The timely diagnosis of congenital or neonatal tuberculosis often is difficult. The tuberculin skin test reaction usually is negative initially although it may become positive after 1 to 3 months. The diagnosis must be established by finding acid-fast bacilli in body fluids or tissue and by culturing *M. tuberculosis*. A positive acid-fast smear of an early morning gastric aspirate in a newborn should be considered indicative of tuberculosis, although false-positive smears occur. Direct acid-fast smears from middle ear fluid, bone marrow, tracheal aspirate, or biopsy tissue can be useful and should be attempted more frequently. One study found positive cultures for *M. tuberculosis* in 10 of 12 gastric aspirates, 3 of 3 liver biopsies, 3 of 3 lymph nodes biopsies, and 2 of 4 bone marrow aspirations from children with congenital tuberculosis.[162] Open lung biopsy also has been used to establish the diagnosis.[190] The cerebrospinal fluid should be examined and cultured, although the yield for isolating *M. tuberculosis* is low.[162,163]

The most important clue to rapidly establish the diagnosis of congenital or neonatal tuberculosis is the maternal and family history. Suspicion should increase if the mother or other family members suffer from unexplained pneumonia, bronchitis, pleural effusion, meningeal disease, or endometritis during, shortly before, or after pregnancy. Testing of both parents and other family members can yield important clues about the presence of tuberculosis within the family. The importance of this epidemiologic information cannot be overemphasized. The need for thorough investigation of the mother was emphasized by Hageman et al., who found that only 10 of 26 mothers who gave birth to neonates with congenital tuberculosis were diagnosed prior to their infants; the other 16 were discovered as part of the investigation of the infant.[162]

The Beitzke criteria for distinguishing true congenital from postnatally acquired tuberculosis were appropriate in the prechemotherapy era as they required autopsy study of the infant. Cantwell et al., based on a review of congenital tuberculosis cases published after 1980, proposed the criteria that the infant have proven tuberculosis and at least one of the following:

1. Lesions in the first week of life.
2. A primary hepatic complex or caseating hepatic granulomas.
3. Tuberculosis infection of the placenta or mother's genital tract.
4. Exclusion of postnatal transmission by a thorough contact investigation.[159]

The optimal treatment of congenital tuberculosis has not been established since the rarity of the condition precludes formal treatment trials. It would appear that the basic principles for treatment of other children and adults also apply to the treatment of congenital tuberculosis. Although the optimal duration of therapy has not been established, many experts would treat infants with congenital tuberculosis for a total duration of 9 to 12 months due to the decreased immunologic capability of the young infant. Isoniazid given alone is known to be safe in the neonate.[159,162] There are no comparable data for isoniazid given in combination with other drugs or for other drugs alone. Rifampin, pyrazinamide, streptomycin, and kanamycin appear to be safe in neonates. Young infants taking these drugs should have biochemical monitoring of serum liver enzymes and uric acid performed on a regular basis. Although the pharmacokinetics of antituberculosis drugs in the neonate are basically unknown, the doses listed in Table 8.3 appear to be effective and relatively safe.

E. Testing for Tuberculosis During Pregnancy

For all pregnant women, the history obtained in an early visit should include questions about a previously positive tuberculin skin test, previous treatment for tuberculosis, current symptoms compatible with tuberculosis, and known exposure to other adults with the disease. Membership in a high-risk group is a sufficient reason for a tuberculin skin test. For many high-risk women, prenatal or peripartum care represents their only contact with the healthcare system and the opportunity to test them for tuberculosis infection or disease should not be lost. Some experts believe that all pregnant women should receive a tuberculin skin test. However, it must be emphasized that women coinfected with HIV and *M. tuberculosis* may show no reaction to a tuberculin skin test. Pregnant women at high risk for or with known HIV infection should have a thorough investigation for tuberculosis.

The effect of pregnancy on tuberculin hypersensitivity as measured by the tuberculin skin test is controversial.[191] Some studies have shown a decrease in *in vitro* lymphocyte reactivity to PPD during pregnancy.[192] However, *in vivo* studies using patients as their own controls have demonstrated no effect of pregnancy on cutaneous delayed hypersensitivity to tuberculin.[193,194] Most experts believe the tuberculin test by the Mantoux technique is valid throughout pregnancy. There is no evidence that the tuberculin skin test has adverse affects on the pregnant mother or fetus or that skin testing reactivates quiescent foci of tuberculosis infection.

Routine chest radiography is not currently advisable as a screening test for pregnant women because the prevalence of tuberculosis remains fairly low.[195] However, with appropriate shielding, pregnant women with a positive tuberculin skin test result should have a chest radiograph to rule out active tuberculosis. In addition, a thorough review of systems and physical examination should be carried out to exclude extrapulmonary tuberculosis.

The principles of treatment of asymptomatic tuberculosis infection are similar for pregnant women and other adults of comparable age. Although treatment of tuberculosis disease during pregnancy is unquestioned, the treatment of the pregnant woman who has an asymptomatic tuberculosis infection is more controversial. Some clinicians prefer to delay therapy until after delivery because pregnancy does not seem to increase the risk of developing tuberculosis disease. Others believe that because recent infection can be accompanied by hematogenous spread to the placenta, it is preferable to treat without delay or to wait until the second trimester to start chemotherapy.[196] Certainly, the benefits of immediate treatment are greater in high-risk patients such as HIV-positive women or close contacts who are recent skin test convertors.

Recent reports suggest that the risk of isoniazid-associated hepatitis and death is higher in women than men, and that women in the postpartum period are especially vulnerable to isoniazid hepatotoxicity.[197,198] The authors of these studies suggest that it might be prudent to avoid isoniazid during the postpartum period or at least to monitor postpartum women taking isoniazid with frequent examinations and laboratory studies. The possible increased risk of isoniazid hepatotoxicity must be weighed against the risk of developing tuberculosis disease as well as the consequences to both mother and baby should tuberculosis disease develop in the mother.

Because treatment of tuberculosis in pregnant women often continues after delivery, the question arises whether it is safe for the mother to breastfeed her infant. Snider and Powell[199] concluded that a breastfeeding infant would receive no more than 20% of the usual therapeutic dosage of isoniazid for infants and less than 11% for other antituberculosis drugs. Potential toxic effects of drugs delivered via breast milk have not been reported. However, because pyridoxine deficiency in the neonate can cause seizures,[200] and breast milk has relatively low levels of pyridoxine, an infant whose breastfeeding mother is taking isoniazid probably should receive supplemental pyridoxine.

F. Management When the Mother Has a Positive Tuberculin Skin Test

1. Negative Chest Radiograph

If the mother is well, no separation of infant and mother is needed. The child needs no special evaluation or therapy if he remains asymptomatic. Because the mother's skin test result may be a marker that there is infectious tuberculosis within the household, all other household members should receive a Mantoux skin test and further evaluation as indicated. The mother usually is a candidate for therapy for tuberculosis infection.

2. Abnormal Chest Radiograph

In general, the newborn should be separated from the mother until the chest radiograph is taken, hopefully a matter of only hours. If the mother's radiograph is abnormal, separation should be maintained until the mother has been thoroughly evaluated. Examination of the mother's sputum always is necessary even if obtaining a sample requires vigorous measures.

If the mother's chest radiograph is abnormal but the history, physical examination, sputum examination, and evaluation of the radiograph reveal no evidence of tuberculosis disease, it is reasonable to assume that the infant is at low risk. The radiographic abnormality is due to another cause or a quiescent focus of past tuberculosis. However, if the mother remains untreated, she may develop active tuberculosis and expose her infant.[201,202] The untreated mother should receive appropriate treatment, and she and her infant receive careful follow-up care. In addition, all household members should be evaluated for tuberculosis.

If the mother's chest radiograph or acid-fast sputum smear reveal evidence of tuberculosis disease, additional steps will be necessary to protect the infant. Isoniazid therapy for newborn infants has been so efficacious that separation of the mother and infant no longer is considered mandatory.[203,204] Separation should occur only if the mother is ill enough to require hospitalization, she has been or is expected to become nonadherent with her treatment, or she has or is suspected of having a resistant strain of *M. tuberculosis*. Because isoniazid resistance is increasing, it is not always clear that isoniazid therapy for the neonate will be effective. If, due to epidemiologic factors, isoniazid resistance is suspected or the mother's adherence with medication is in question, rigorous separation of the infant from the mother must be considered. The duration of separation will vary but must be at least as long as it takes to render the mother noninfectious. Although modern chemotherapy often eliminates infectivity within several weeks, it takes several more weeks to document sterility of the mother's sputum culture. A conservative suggestion for duration of separation would be 6 to 12 weeks of culture negativity for the mother.[164] In cases where the organism is drug susceptible, isoniazid should be continued in the infant at least until the mother has been shown to be sputum culture negative for 3 months. At that time, a Mantoux tuberculin skin test is placed on the child; if positive, isoniazid is continued for a total duration of 9 to 12 months, but if negative, isoniazid can be discontinued.

If a family member has tuberculosis and cannot be relied upon to receive proper treatment, then BCG vaccination of the infant should be considered.[202,205] Vaccination with BCG appears to decrease the risk of tuberculosis in the infant but the effect is variable. Kendig reported 117 infants born to mothers with active tuberculosis around the time of delivery; none of the 30 BCG vaccinated infants developed tuberculosis, while 38 cases of tuberculosis and 3 deaths occurred among the 75 infants who received neither BCG vaccine nor isoniazid.[202] Similar studies in England and Canada also described the apparent efficacy of BCG given to neonates.[205,206] BCG has some protective effect against the development of tuberculosis in newborns and appears to decrease the incidence of life-threatening forms of disease. Many experts recommend that the child be kept out of the household until the skin test becomes reactive, although there is poor correlation between skin test status and the presence or absence of infection. While routine BCG vaccination of newborns is not appropriate in the U.S., it should be considered for the neonate whose household is chaotic and cannot be made free from tuberculosis, or who is likely to be lost to follow-up. For further information on this matter, please refer to Chapter 15.

REFERENCES

1. Braun, M. M. and Cauthen, G., Relationship of the human immunodeficiency virus epidemic to pediatric tuberculosis and bacille Calmette-Guerin immunization, *Pediatr. Infect. Dis. J.*, 11, 220, 1992.
2. Ussery, X. T., Valway, S. E., McKenna, M., and McCray, E., Epidemology of tuberculosis among children in the United States, *Pediatr. Infect. Dis. J.*, 15, 704, 1966.
3. Starke, J. R., Jacobs, R. F., and Jereb, J., Resurgence of tuberculosis in children, *J. Pediatr.*, 120, 839, 1992.
4. International Union Against Tuberculosis and Lung Disease, Tuberculosis in children: guidelines for diagnosis, prevention and treatment, *Bull. Int. Union Tuberc. Lung Dis.*, 66, 61, 1991.
5. Murray, C. J. L., Styblo, K., and Rouillon, A., Tuberculosis in developing countries: burden, intervention, and cost, *Bull. Int. Union Tuberc. Lung Dis.*, 65, 6, 1990.
6. Kochi, A., The global tuberculosis situation and the new control strategy of the World Health Organization, *Tubercle*, 72, 1, 1991.
7. Klausner, J. D., Ryder, R., Baende, E., et. al., *Mycobacterium tuberculosis* in household contacts of human immunodeficiency virus-type-1-seropositive patients with active pulmonary tuberculosis in Kinshosa, Zaire, *J. Infect. Dis.*, 168, 106, 1993.
8. Snider, D. E., Rieder, H. L., Combs, D., Bloch, A. B., Hayden, C. H., and Smith, M. H. D., Tuberculosis in children, *Pediatr. Infect. Dis. J.*, 7, 271, 1988.
9. Jones, D., Malecki, J., Bigler, W., et al., Pediatric tuberculosis and human immunodeficiency virus infection in Palm Beach County, FL, *Am. J. Dis. Child.*, 146, 1166, 1992.
10. McKenna, M. T., McCray, E., and Onorato, I. M., The epidemiology of tuberculosis among foreign-born persons in the United States, 1986 to 1993, *N. Engl. J. Med.*, 332, 1071, 1995.
11. Mehta, J. B. and Bentley, S., Prevention of tuberculosis in children: missed opportunities, *Am. J. Prev. Med.*, 8, 283, 1992.
12. Nolan, R., Jr., Childhood tuberculosis in North Carolina: a study of the opportunities for intervention in the transmission of tuberculosis in children, *Am. J. Public Health*, 76, 26, 1986.
13. Wallgren, A., On contagiousness of childhood tuberculosis, *Acta Paediatr. Scand.*, 22, 229, 1937.
14. Weinstein, J., Barrett, C., Baltimore, R., et al., Nosocomial transmission of tuberculosis from a hospital visitor on a pediatrics ward, *Pediatr. Infect. Dis. J.*, 14, 232, 1995.
15. Centers for Disease Control and Prevention, Guidelines for preventing the transmission of *Mycobacterium tuberculosis* in healthcare facilities, 1994, *MMWR*, 43 (RR-13), 1, 1994.
16. Smith, M. H. D. and Marquis, J. R., Tuberculosis and other mycobacterial diseases, *Textbook of Pediatric Infectious Diseases*, 2nd ed., Feigin, R. D. and Cherry, J. D., Eds., W.B. Saunders, Philadelphia, 1987.
17. Smith, M. H. D., Tuberculosis in children and adolescents, *Clin. Chest Med.*, 10, 381, 1989.
18. Reider, H. L., Snider, D. E., Jr., and Cauthen, G. M., Extrapulmonary tuberculosis in the United States, *Am. Rev. Respir. Dis.*, 141, 347, 1990.
19. Lange, W. R., Wornock-Eckhart, E., and Bean, M. E., *Mycobacterium tuberculosis* infection in foreign-born adoptees, *Pediatr. Infect. Dis. J.*, 8, 625, 1989.
20. Lincoln, E. M., Epidemics of tuberculosis, *Adv. Tuberc. Res.*, 14, 157, 1965.
21. Nolan, C. M., Barr, H., Elarth, A. M., and Boase, J., Tuberculosis in a daycare home, *Pediatrics*, 79, 630, 1987.
22. Braden, C. R. and an investigative team, Infectiousness of a university student with laryngeal and cavitary tuberculosis, *Clin. Infect. Dis.*, 21, 565, 1995.
23. Gutman, L., Moye, J., Zimmer, G., et al., Tuberculosis in human immunodeficiency virus-exposed or -infected United States children, *Pediatr. Infect. Dis. J.*, 13, 963, 1994.
24. Luo, C., Chinto, C., Bhat, G., et al., Human immunodeficiency virus type-1 infection in Zambian children with tuberculosis, *Tuberc. Lung Dis.*, 75, 110, 1994.

25. Khouri, Y., Mastrucci, M., Hutto, C., et. al., *Mycobacterium tuberculosis* in children with human immunodeficiency virus type 1 infection, *Pediatr. Infect. Dis. J.*, 11, 950, 1992.

26. Chaisson, R. E. and Slutkin, G., Tuberculosis and human immunodeficiency virus infection, *J. Infect. Dis.*, 159, 96, 1989.

27. Klein, N. C., Duncanson, F. P., Lenox, T. H., Pitta, A., Cohen, S. C., and Wormser, G. P., Use of mycobacterial smears in the diagnosis of pulmonary tuberculosis in AIDS/ARC patients, *Chest*, 95, 1190, 1989.

28. Moss, W. J., Dodyo, T., Suarez, M., Nicholas, S. W., and Abrams, E., Tuberculosis in children infected with human immunodeficiency virus: a report of five cases, *Pediatr. Infect. Dis. J.*, 10, 114, 1992.

29. Chintu, C., Bhat, G., Luo, C., Raviglione, M., Diwan, V., Dupont, H. L., and Zumla, A., Seroprevalence of human immunodeficiency virus type 1 infection in Zambian children with tuberculosis, *Pediatr. Infect. Dis. J.*, 12, 499, 1993.

30. Jeena, P. M., Mitha, T., Bamber, S., Wesley, A., Cortsoudis, A., and Coovadia, H. M., Effects of human immunodeficiency virus on tuberculosis in children, *Tuberc. Lung Dis.*, 77, 437, 1996.

31. Sassan-Morokra, M., de Cock, K. M., and Ackah, A., Tuberculosis and HIV infection in children in Agidjan, Cote d'Ivoire, *Trans. R. Soc. Trop. Med. Hyg.*, 88, 178, 1994.

32. Coovadia, H. M., Jeena, P., and Wilkinson, D., Childhood human immunodeficiency virus and tuberculosis co-infections: reconciling conflicting data, *Int. J. Tuberc. Lung Dis.*, 2, 844, 1998.

33. Schaaf, H. S., Geldenduys, A., Gie, R. P., and Cotton, M. F., Culture positive tuberculosis in human immunodeficiency virus type 1 infected children, *Pediatr. Infect. Dis. J.*, 17, 599, 1998.

34. Chan, S. P., Binbaum, J., and Rao, M., Clinical manifestations and outcome of tuberculosis in children with acquired immunodeficiency syndrome, *Pediatr. Infect. Dis. J.*, 15, 443, 1996.

35. Mukadi, Y. D., Wiktor, S. Z., Laulibaly, I. M., et al., Impact of HIV infection on the development, clinical presentation and outcome of tuberculosis among children in Abidjan, Cofe d'Ivoire, *AIDS*, 11, 1151, 1997.

36. Garay, J. E., Clinical presentation of pulmonary tuberculosis in under 10's and differences in AIDS related cases: a cohort study of 115 patients, *Trop. Doctor*, 27, 139, 1997.

37. Hsu, K. H. K., Contact investigation: a practical approach to tuberculosis eradication, *Am. J. Public Health*, 53, 1761, 1963.

38. Barry, M. A., Shirley, L., Grady, M. T., Etkind, S. W., Almeida, C., Bernardo, J., and Lamb, G. A., Tuberculous infection in urban adolescents: results of a school-based testing program, *Am. J. Public Health*, 80, 439, 1990.

39. Davidson, P. T., Ashkar, B., and Salem, N., Tuberculosis testing of children entering school in Los Angeles County, CA, *Am. Rev. Respir. Dis.*, 141 (Suppl.), 336, 1990.

40. Starke, J. R., Taylor, K. T., Martindill, C. A., Pyle, N. D., and Herrin, C. M., Extremely high rates of tuberculin reactivity among young school children in Houston, *Am. Rev. Respir. Dis.*, 137 (Suppl.), 22, 1988.

41. Mohle-Boetani, J. C., Miller, B., Halpan, M., et al., School-based screening for tuberculosis infection: a cost benefit analysis, *JAMA*, 274, 613, 1995.

42. Driver, C. R., Valway, S. E., Cantwell, M. E., et al., Tuberculosis skin test screening of school children in the United States, *Pediatrics*, 98, 97, 1996.

43. Miller, F. J. W., Seale, R. M. E., and Taylor, M. D., *Tuberculosis in Children*, Little Brown and Co., Boston, 1963.

44. Starke, J. R. and Taylor-Watts, K. T., Tuberculosis in the pediatric population of Houston, TX, *Pediatrics*, 84, 28, 1989.

45. Daly, J. F., Brown, D. S., Lincoln, E. M., and Wilkins, V. N., Endobronchial tuberculosis in children, *Dis. Chest*, 22, 380, 1952.

46. Lorriman, G. and Bentley, F. J., The incidence of segmental lesions in primary tuberculosis of childhood, *Am. Rev. Tuberc.*, 79, 756, 1959.

47. Morrison, J. B., Natural history of segmental lesions in primary pulmonary tuberculosis, *Arch. Dis. Child.*, 48, 90, 1973.

48. Stansberry, S. D., Tuberculosis in infants and children, *J. Thorac. Imaging*, 5, 17, 1990.

49. Giammona, S. T., Poole, C. A., Zelowitz, P., and Skrovan, C., Massive lymphadenopathy in primary pulmonary tuberculosis in children, *Am. Rev. Respir. Dis.*, 100, 480, 1969.

50. Lobato, M. N., Cummings, K., Will, D., and Royce, S., Tuberculosis in children and adolescents: California, 1985 to 1995, *Pediatr. Infect. Dis. J.*, 17, 407, 1998.
51. Schaaf, H., Gie, R. P., Beyers, N., et al., Tuberculosis in infants less than three months of age, *Arch. Dis. Child.*, 69, 371, 1993.
52. Vallejo, J., Ong, L., and Starke, J., Clinical features, diagnosis and treatment of tuberculosis in infants, *Pediatrics*, 94, 1, 1994.
53. Lincoln, E. M., Gilbert, L., and Morales, S. M., Chronic pulmonary tuberculosis in individuals with known previous primary tuberculosis, *Dis. Chest*, 38, 473, 1960.
54. Ridzon, R., Kent, J. H., Valway, S., et al., Outbreak of drug resistant tuberculosis with second-generation transmission in a high school in California, *J. Pediatr.*, 131, 863, 1997.
55. Smith, M. H. D. and Matsaniotis, N., Treatment of tuberculous pleural effusions with particular reference to adrenal corticosteroids, *Pediatrics*, 22, 1074, 1958.
56. Lincoln, E. M., Davies, P. A., and Bovornkitti, S., Tuberculous pleurisy with effusion in children. A study of 202 children with particular reference to prognosis, *Am. Rev. Tuberc.*, 77, 271, 1958.
57. Levine, H., Metzger, W., and Lacera, S., Diagnosis of tuberculosis pleurisy by culture of pleural biopsy specimen, *Arch. Intern. Med.*, 126, 269, 1970.
58. Boyd, G. L., Tuberculous pericarditis in children, *Am. J. Dis. Child.*, 86, 293, 1953.
59. Hugo-Hammon, C. T., Scher, H., and DeMoor, M. M. A., Tuberculosis pericarditis in children: a review of 44 cases, *Pediatr. Infect. Dis. J.*, 13, 13, 1994
60. Hussey, G., Chisholm, T., and Kibel, M., Miliary tuberculosis in children: a review of 94 cases, *Pediatr. Infect. Dis. J.*, 10, 832, 1991.
61. Schuitt, K. E., Miliary tuberculosis in children. Clinical and laboratory manifestations in 19 patients, *Am. J. Dis. Child.*, 133, 583, 1979.
62. Margileth, A. M., Chandra, R., and Altman, R. P., Chronic lymphadenopathy due to mycobacterial infection. Clinical features, diagnosis, histopathology and management, *Am. J. Dis. Child.*, 138, 917, 1984.
63. Dandapat, M. C., Mishra, B. M., Dash, S. P., et al., Peripheral lymph node tuberculosis: review of 80 cases, *Br. J. Surg.*, 77, 911, 1990.
64. Appling, D. and Miller, R. H., Mycobacterial cervical lymphadenopathy: 1981 update, *Laryngoscope*, 91, 1259, 1981.
65. Lai, K. K., Stottmeier, K. D., Sherman, I. H., et al., Mycobacterial cervical lymphadenopathy: relation of etiologic agents to age, *JAMA*, 251, 1286, 1984.
66. Rich, A. R. and McCordock, H. A., The pathogenesis of tuberculous meningitis, *Bull. Johns Hopkins Hosp.*, 52, 5, 1933.
67. Cotton, M. F., Donald, P. R., Schoeman, J. F., Aalbers, C., VanZyl, L. E., and Lombard, C., Plasma arginine vasopressin and the syndrome of inappropriate antidiuretic hormone secretion in tuberculous meningitis, *Pediatr. Infect. Dis. J.*, 10, 837, 1991.
68. Jaffe, I. P., Tuberculous meningitis in childhood, *Lancet*, 1, 738, 1982.
69. Waecker, N. J., Jr. and Conners, J. D., Central nervous system tuberculosis in children: a review of 30 cases, *Pediatr. Infect. Dis. J.*, 9, 539, 1990.
70. Idriss, Z. H., Sinno, A., and Kronfol, N. M., Tuberculous meningitis in childhood: 43 cases, *Am. J. Dis. Child.*, 130, 364, 1976.
71. Doerr, C. A., Starke, J. R., and Ong, L. T., Clinical and public health aspects of tuberculosis meningitis, *J. Pediatr.*, 127, 27, 1995.
72. Yaramis, A. Gurkan, F., Eleveli, M., Soker, M., Hospolaf, K., Kirbas, G., and Tas, M. A., Central nervous system tuberculosis in children: a review of 214 cases, *Pediatrics*, 102, 249, 1998.
73. Humphries, M. J., Teoh, R., Lav, J., et al., Factors of prognostic significance in Chinese children with tuberculous meningitis, *Tubercle*, 71, 161, 1990.
74. Udani, P. M., Parekh, U. C., and Dastur, D. K., Neurologic and related syndromes in CNS tuberculosis: clinical features and pathogenesis, *J. Neurol. Sci.*, 14, 341, 1971.
75. Ramachandran, P., Duraipandian, M., Nagarajan, M., Probhakar, R., Ramakrishnan, C. V., and Tripathy, S. P., Three chemotherapy studies of tuberculous meningitis in children, *Tubercle*, 67, 17, 1986.
76. Palur, R., Rajohelchar, U., Chandy, M. J., et al., Shunt surgery for hydrocephalus in tuberculous meningitis: a long-term follow-up study, *J. Neurosurg.*, 74, 64, 1991.
77. Zarabi, M., Sane, S., and Girdany, B. R., Chest roentgenogram in the early diagnosis of tuberculous meningitis in children, *Am. J. Dis. Child.*, 121, 389, 1971.

78. Gupta, R., Gupta, S., Dingh, D., et al., MR imaging and angiography in tuberculous meningitis, *Neuroradiology*, 36, 87, 1994.
79. Jinkins, J. R., Computed tomography of intracranial tuberculosis, *Neuroradiology*, 33, 126, 1991.
80. Curless, R. G. and Mitchell, C. D., Central nervous system tuberculosis in children, *Pediatr. Neurol.*, 7, 270, 1991.
81. Chambers, S. T., Hendrickse, W. A., Record, C., Rudge, P., and Smith, H., Paradoxical expansion of intracranial tuberculomas during chemotherapy, *Lancet*, 2, 181, 1984.
82. Teoh, R., Humphries, M. J., and O'Mahony, S. G., Symptomatic intracranial tuberculoma developing during treatment of tuberculosis: a report of 10 patients and review of the literature, *Quart. J. Med.*, 63, 449, 1987.
83. Afghani, B. and Lieberman, J. M., Paradoxical enlargement or development of intracranial tuberculosis during therapy: case report and review, *Clin. Infect. Dis.*, 19, 1092, 1994.
84. Vallejo, J., Ong, L. T., and Starke, J. R., Tuberculous osteomyelitis of the long bones in children, *Pediatr. Infect. Dis. J.*, 14, 542, 1995.
85. Janssens, J. P. and deHaller, R., Spinal tuberculosis in a developed country, *Clin. Ortho. Rel. Res.*, 257, 67, 1990.
86. Hoffman, E. B., Crosier, J. H., and Cremin, B. J., Imaging in children with spinal tuberculosis. *J. Bone Joint Surg.*, 75 (B), 233, 1993.
87. Bavadekar, A., Osteoarticular tuberculosis in children, *Prog. Pediatr. Surg.*, 15, 131, 1982.
88. Hardy, J. B. and Hartmann, J. R., Tuberculous dactylitis in childhood, *J. Pediatr.*, 30, 146, 1947.
89. Centers for Disease Control and Prevention, Screening for tuberculosis and tuberculosis infection in high-risk populations, *MMWR*, 44 (RR-11), 19, 1995.
90. Hsu, K. H. K., Tuberculin reaction in children treated with isoniazid, *Am. J. Dis. Child.*, 137, 1090, 1983.
91. Steiner, P., Rao, M., Victoria, M. S., Jabbar, H., and Steiner, M., Persistently negative tuberculin reactions: their presence among children culture positive for *Mycobacterium tuberculosis*, *Am. J. Dis. Child.*, 134, 747, 1980.
92. Huebner, R. E., Schein, M. F., and Bass, J. B., The tuberculin skin test, *Clin. Infect. Dis.*, 17, 968, 1993.
93. Sepulveda, R. L., Burr, C., Ferrer, X., and Sorensen, R. U., Booster effect of tuberculin testing in healthy 6-year-old school children vaccinated with bacille Calmette-Guerin at birth in Santiago, Chile, *Pediatr. Infect. Dis. J.*, 7, 578, 1988.
94. Catanzaro, A., Multiple-puncture skin test and Mantoux test in Southeast Asian refugees, *Chest*, 87, 346, 1985.
95. Howard, T. P. and Soloman, D. A., Reading the tuberculin skin test: who, when and how? *Arch. Intern. Med.*, 148, 2457, 1988.
96. Ashley, M. J. and Siebenmann, C. O., Tuberculin skin sensitivity following BCG vaccination with vaccines of high and low viable counts, *Can. Med. Assoc. J.*, 97, 1335, 1967.
97. Lifschitz, M., The value of the tuberculin skin test as a screening test for tuberculosis among BCG-vaccinated children, *Pediatrics*, 36, 264, 1965.
98. Karalliede, S., Katugha, L. P., and Uragoda, C. G., The tuberculin response of Sri Lankan children after BCG vaccination at birth, *Tubercle*, 68, 33, 1987.
99. Kendig, E. L., Kirkpatrick, B. U., Carter, W. H., Hill, F. A., Caldwell, K., and Entwistle, M., Under reading of the tuberculosis skin test reaction, *Chest*, 113, 1175, 1998.
100. Abadco, D. L. and Steiner, P., Gastric lavage is better than bronchoalveolar lavage for isolation of *Mycobacterium tuberculosis* in childhood pulmonary tuberculosis, *Pediatr. Infect. Dis. J.*, 11, 735, 1992.
101. Klotz, S. A. and Penn, R. L., Acid-fast staining of urine and gastric contents is an excellent indicator of mycobacterial disease, *Am. Rev. Respir. Dis.*, 136, 1197, 1987.
102. Alde, S. L. M., Pinasco, H. M., Pelosi, F. R., Budani, H. F., Palma-Beltran, O. H., and Gonzalez-Montaner, L. J., Evaluation of an enzyme-linked immunosorbent assay using an IgG antibody to *Mycobacterium tuberculosis* antigens in the diagnosis of active tuberculosis in children, *Am. Rev. Respir. Dis.*, 139, 748, 1989.
103. Hussey, G., Kibel, M., and Dempster, W., The serodiagnosis of tuberculosis in children: an evaluation of an ELISA test using IgG antibodies to *Mycobacterium tuberculosis*, strain H37RV, *Ann. Tropic. Med.*, 11, 113, 1991.

104. Rosen, E. U., The diagnostic value of an enzyme-linked immune sorbent assay using absorbed mycobacterial sonicates in children, *Tubercle*, 71, 127, 1990.

105. Delacourt, C., Gobin, J., and Gaillard, J. L., Value of ELISA using antigen 60 for the diagnosis of tuberculosis in children, *Chest*, 104, 393, 1993.

106. Turneer, M., Van Nerom, E., Nyabenda, J., et al., Determination of humoral immunoglobulin M and G directed against mycobacterial antigen 60 failed to diagnose primary tuberculosis and mycobacterial adenitis in children, *Am. J. Respir. Crit. Care Med.*, 150, 1508, 1994.

107. Pierre, C., Oliver, C., Lecossier, D., Boussougont, Y., Yeni, P., and Hance, A. J., Diagnosis of primary tuberculosis in children by amplification and detection of mycobacterial DNA, *Am. Rev. Respir. Dis.*, 147, 420, 1993.

108. Delacourt, C., Proveda, J. D., Churean, C., et al., Use of polymerase chain reaction for improved diagnosis of tuberculosis in children, *J. Pediatr.*, 126, 703, 1995.

109. Smith, K. C., Starla, J. R., Eisenach, K., et al., Detection of *Mycobacterium tuberculosis* in chemical specimens from children using a polymerase chain reaction, *Pediatrics*, 97, 155, 1996.

110. Mancao, M. Y., Nolte, F. S., Nahmias, A. S., et al., Use of polymerase chain reaction for diagnosis of tuberculous meningitis, *Pediatr. Infect. Dis. J.*, 13, 154, 1994.

111. Miorner, H., Sjobring, U., Nayak, P., et al., Diagnosis of tuberculous meningitis: a comparative analysis of 3 immuno assays, an immune complex assay and the polymerase chain reaction, *Tubercle Lung Dis.*, 76, 381, 1995.

112. Starke, J. R., Multidrug therapy for tuberculosis in children, *Pediatr. Infect. Dis. J.*, 9, 785, 1990.

113. Reed, M. D. and Blumer, J. L., Clinical pharmacology of antitubercular drugs, *Pediatr. Clin. North Am.*, 30, 177, 1983.

114. Stein, M. T. and Liang, D., Clinical hepatotoxicity of isoniazid in children, *Pediatrics*, 64, 499, 1979.

115. O'Brien, R. J., Long, M. W., Cross, F. S., Lyle, M. A., and Snider, D. E., Jr., Hepatotoxicity from isoniazid and rifampin among children treated for tuberculosis, *Pediatrics*, 72, 491, 1983.

116. Olson, W. A., Pruitt, A. W., and Dayton, P. G., Plasma concentrations of isoniazid in children with tuberculous infections, *Pediatrics*, 67, 876, 1981.

117. Tsagarpoulou-Stinga, H., Mataki-Emmanouilidou, T., Karida-Kavalioti, S., and Manios, S., Hepatotoxic reactions in children with severe tuberculosis treated with isoniazid-rifampin, *Pediatr. Infect. Dis. J.*, 4, 270, 1985.

118. Kumar, A., Misra, P. K., Mehotra, R., Govil, Y. C., and Rana, G. S., Hepatotoxicity of rifampin and isoniazid: is it all drug-induced hepatitis? *Am. Rev. Respir. Dis.*, 143, 1350, 1991.

119. Notterman, D. A., Nardi, M., and Saslow, J. G., Effect of dose formulation on isoniazid adsorption in two young children, *Pediatrics*, 77, 850, 1986.

120. Seifart, H. I., Parkin, D. P., and Donald, P. R., Stability of isoniazid, rifampin and pyrazinamide in suspensions used for the treatment of tuberculosis in children, *Pediatr. Infect. Dis. J.*, 10, 827, 1991.

121. Martinez-Roig, A., Roig, A., Cami, J., Llorens-Terol, J., de la Torre, R., and Perich, F., Acetylation phenotype and hepatotoxicity in the treatment of tuberculosis in children, *Pediatrics*, 77, 912, 1986.

122. Pellock, J. M., Howell, J., Kendig, E. L., Jr., and Baker, H., Pyridoxine deficiency in children treated with isoniazid, *Chest*, 87, 658, 1985.

123. Litt, I. F., Cohen, M. I., and McNamara, H., Isoniazid hepatitis in adolescents, *J. Pediatr.*, 89, 133, 1976.

124. Donald, P. R. and Seifart, H., Cerebrospinal fluid pyrazinamide concentrations in children with tuberculous meningitis, *Pediatr. Infect. Dis. J.*, 7, 469, 1988.

125. Treburg, A., Should ethambutol be recommended for routine treatment of tuberculosis in children? *Int. J. Tuberc. Lung Dis.*, 1, 12, 1997.

126. Snider, D. E., Jr., Layde, P. M., and Johnson, M. W., Treatment of tuberculosis during pregnancy, *Am. Rev. Respir. Dis.*, 122, 65, 1980.

127. Donald, P. R. and Siefart, H. I., Cerebrospinal fluid concentrations of ethionamide in children with tuberculous meningitis, *J. Pediatr.*, 115, 483, 1989.

128. Abernathy, R. S., Dutt, A. K., Stead, W. W., and Doers, D. L., Short-course chemotherapy for tuberculosis in children, *Pediatrics*, 72, 801, 1983.

129. Jacobs, R. F. and Abernathy, R. S., The treatment of tuberculosis in children, *Pediatr. Infect. Dis. J.*, 4, 513, 1985.

130. Reis, F. J. C., Bedran, M. R. M., Moura, J. A. R., Assis, I., and Rodrigues, M. E., Six-month isoniazid-rifampin treatment for pulmonary tuberculosis in children, *Am. Rev. Respir. Dis.*, 142, 996, 1990.

131. Ibanez, S. and Ross, G., Quimioterapia abreviado de 6 meses en tuberculosis pulmonar infantil, *Rev. Chil. Pediatr.*, 51, 249, 1980.

132. Varudkar, B. L., Short-course chemotherapy for tuberculosis in children, *Indian J. Pediatr.*, 52, 593, 1985.

133. Biddulph, J., Short-course chemotherapy for childhood tuberculosis, *Pediatr. Infect. Dis. J.*, 9, 794, 1990.

134. Kumar, L., Dhand, R., Singhi, P. D., Rao, K. L. N., and Katariya, S., A randomized trial of fully intermittent and daily followed by intermittent short-course chemotherapy for childhood tuberculosis, *Pediatr. Infect. Dis. J.*, 9, 802, 1990.

135. Tsakalidis, D., Pratsidou, P., Hitoglou-Makedou, A., Tzouvelekis, G., and Sofroniadis, I., Intensive short course chemotherapy for treatment of Greek children with tuberculosis, *Pediatr. Infect. Dis. J.*, 11, 1036, 1992.

136. American Academy of Pediatrics Committee on Infectious Diseases, Chemotherapy for tuberculosis in infants and children, *Pediatrics*, 89, 161, 1992.

137. Dutt, A. K., Doers, D., and Stead, W. W., Short-course chemotherapy for extrapulmonary tuberculosis, *Ann. Intern. Med.*, 107, 7, 1986.

138. Jawahar, M. S., Sivasubramanian, S., Vijayan, V. K., Ramakrishnan, C. V., Paramasivan, C. N., Selvakumar, V., Paul, S., Tripathy, S. P., and Prabhakar, R., Short-course chemotherapy for tuberculous lymphadenitis in children, *Br. Med. J.*, 301, 359, 1990.

139. Visudhiphan, P. and Chiemchanya, S., Tuberculous meningitis in children: treatment with isoniazid and rifampin for twelve months, *J. Pediatr.*, 114, 875, 1989.

140. Jacobs, R. F., Sunakorn, P., Chotpitayasunonah, T., Pope, S., and Kelleher, K., Intensive short-course chemotherapy for tuberculous meningitis, *Pediatr. Infect. Dis. J.*, 11, 194, 1992.

141. Barnes, P. F., Bloch, A. B., Davidson, P. T., and Snider, D. E., Jr., Tuberculosis in patients with human immunodeficiency virus infection, *N. Engl. J. Med.*, 324, 1644, 1991.

142. Pablos-Mendez, A., Raviglione, M. C., Loszlo, A., et al., Global surveillance for antituberculosis drug resistance, 1994–1997, *N. Engl. J. Med.*, 338, 1641, 1998.

143. Steiner, P., Rao, M., Victoria, M. S., Hunt, J., and Steiner, M., A continuing study of primary drug-resistant tuberculosis among children observed at Kings County Hospital Medical Center between the years 1961-1980, *Am. Rev. Respir. Dis.*, 128, 425, 1983.

144. Steiner, P., Rao, M., Mitchell, M., and Steiner, M., Primary drug-resistant tuberculosis in children. Correlation of drug-susceptibility patterns of matched patient and source case strains of *Mycobacterium tuberculosis*, *Am. J. Dis. Child.*, 139, 780, 1985.

145. Swanson, D. S. and Starla, J. R., Drug resistant tuberculosis in pediatrics, *Pediatr. Clin. North Am.*, 42, 553, 1995.

146. Steiner, P. and Rao, M., Drug resistant tuberculosis in children, *Semin. Pediatr. Infect. Dis.*, 4, 275, 1993.

147. Girgis, N. I., Farid, Z., Kilpatrick, M. E., Sultan, Y., and Mikhail, I. A., Dexamethasone adjunctive treatment for tuberculous meningitis, *Pediatr. Infect. Dis. J.*, 10, 179, 1991.

148. Nemir, R. L., Cordova, J., Vaziri, F., and Toledo, F., Prednisone as an adjunct in the chemotherapy of lymph node-bronchial tuberculosis in childhood: a double-blinded study. II. Further term observation, *Am. Rev. Respir. Dis.*, 95, 402, 1967.

149. Toppet, M., Malfroot, A., Derde, M. P., Toppet, V., Spehl, M., and Dab, I., Corticosteroids in primary tuberculosis with bronchial obstruction, *Arch. Dis. Child.*, 65, 1222, 1990.

150. Strang, J. I. G., Kakaza, H. H. S., Gibson, D. G., Allen, B. W., Mitchison, D. A., Evans, D. J., Girling, D. J., Nunn, A. J., and Fox, W., Controlled clinical trial of complete open surgical drainage and prednisolone in treatment of tuberculous pericardial effusion in Transkei, *Lancet*, 2, 759, 1988.

151. Hsu, K. H. K., Thirty years after isoniazid. Its impact on tuberculosis in children and adolescents, *JAMA*, 251, 1283, 1984.

152. Sbarbaro, J. A., Compliance: inducements and enforcements, *Chest*, 76 (Suppl.), 750, 1979.

153. Snider, D. E., Jr., Pregnancy and tuberculosis, *Chest*, 86, 11, 1984.

154. Schaefer, G., Zervoudakis, I. A., and Fuchs, F. F., Pregnancy and pulmonary tuberculosis, *Obstet. Gynecol.*, 46, 706, 1975.

155. Bazaz-Malik, G., Maheshwari, B., and Lal, N., Tuberculous endometritis: a clinicopathologic study of 1000 cases, *Br. J. Obstet. Gynaecol.*, 90, 84, 1983.

156. Hallum, J. L. and Thomas, H. E., Full term pregnancy after proved endometrial tuberculosis, *J. Obstet. Gyneaecol. Br. Emp.*, 62, 548, 1955.

157. Kaplan, C., Benirschke, K., and Tarzy, B., Placental tuberculosis in early and late pregnancy, *Am. J. Obstet. Gynecol.*, 137, 858, 1980.

158. Cooper, A. R., Heneghan, W., and Mathew, J. D., Tuberculosis in a mother and her infant, *Pediatr. Infect. Dis. J.,* 4, 181, 1985.

159. Cantwell, M.F., Shehab, Z.M., Costello, A.M., et al., Brief report: congenital tuberculosis, *N. Engl. J. Med.,* 330, 1051, 1994.

160. Centeno, R. S., Winter, J., and Bentson, J. R., Central nervous system tuberculosis related to pregnancy, *J. Comput. Tomogr.*, 6, 141, 1982.

161. Grenville-Mathers, R., Harris, W. C., and Trenchard, H. J., Tuberculous primary infection in pregnancy and its relation to congenital tuberculosis, *Tubercle*, 41, 181, 1960.

162. Hageman, J., Shulman, S., and Schreiber, M., Congenital tuberculosis: critical reappraisal of clinical findings and diagnostic procedures, *Pediatrics*, 66, 980, 1980.

163. Nemir, R. L. and O'Hare, D., Congenital tuberculosis, *Am. J. Dis. Child.*, 139, 284, 1985.

164. Smith, M. H. D. and Teele, D. W., *Tuberculosis, Infectious Diseases of the Fetus and Newborn*, 3rd ed., Remington, J. S. and Klein, J. O., Eds., W.B. Saunders, Philadelphia, 1990.

165. Hertzog, A. J., Chapman, S., and Herring, J., Congenital pulmonary aspiration-tuberculosis, *Am. J. Clin. Pathol.*, 19, 1139, 1940.

166. Hughesdon, M. R., Congenital tuberculosis, *Arch. Dis. Child.*, 21, 131, 1946.

167. Jacobs, R. F. and Abernathy, R. S., Management of tuberculosis in pregnancy and the newborn, *Clin. Perinatol.*, 15, 305, 1988.

168. Siegel, M., Pathologic findings and pathogenesis of congenital tuberculosis, *Am. Rev. Tuberc.*, 29, 297, 1934.

169. Carter, F. J. and Mates, S., Tuberculosis during pregnancy: the Rhode Island experience, 1987 to 1991, *Chest,* 106, 1466, 1994.

170. Good, J. T., Jr., Iseman, M. D., and Davidson, P. T., Tuberculosis in association with pregnancy, *Am. J. Obstet. Gynecol.*, 140, 492, 1981.

171. Grisolle, A., De l'influence que la grossesse et la phthisie pulmonaire excercent reciproquement l'une sur l'autre, *Arch. Gener. de Med.*, 22, 41, 1850.

172. Cohen, R. C., Effect of pregnancy and parturition on pulmonary tuberculosis, *Br. Med. J.*, 2, 775, 1943.

173. Hedvall, E., Pregnancy and tuberculosis, *Acta Med. Scand.*, 147 (Suppl 286), 1, 1953.

174. Crombie, J. B., Pregnancy and pulmonary tuberculosis, *Br. J. Tuberc.*, 48, 97, 1954.

175. Rosenbach, L. M. and Gangemi, C. R., Tuberculosis and pregnancy, *JAMA*, 161, 1035, 1956.

176. Cohen, J. D., Patton, E. A., and Badger, T. L., The tuberculous mother, *Am. Rev. Respir. Dis.*, 65, 1, 1952.

177. Edge, J. R., Pulmonary tuberculosis and pregnancy, *Br. Med. J.*, 2, 845, 1952.

178. De March, P., Tuberculosis and pregnancy, *Chest*, 68, 800, 1975.

179. Pridie, R. B. and Stradling, P., Management of pulmonary tuberculosis during pregnancy, *Br. Med. J.*, 3, 78, 1961.

180. Bjerkedal, T., Bahna, S. L., and Lehmann, E. H., Course and outcome of pregnancy in women with pulmonary tuberculosis, *Scand. J. Respir. Dis.*, 56, 245, 1975.

181. Ratner, B., Rostler, A. E., and Salgado, P. S., Care, feeding and fate of premature and full term infants born of tuberculous mothers, *Am. J. Dis. Child.*, 81, 471, 1951.

182. Wilson, E. A., Thelin, T. J., and Dilts, P. V., Tuberculosis complicated by pregnancy, *Am. J. Obstet. Gynecol.*, 115, 526, 1972.

183. Lowe, C. R., Congenital defects among children born to women under supervision or treatment for pulmonary tuberculosis, *Br. J. Prev. Soc. Med.*, 18, 14, 1964.

184. Atkins, J. N., Maternal plasma concentration of pyridoxal phosphate during pregnancy: adequacy of vitamin B_6 supplementation during isoniazid therapy, *Am. Rev. Respir. Dis.*, 126, 714, 1982.

185. Lewit, T., Nebel, L., and Terracina, S., Ethambutol in pregnancy: observations on embryogenesis, *Chest*, 68, 25, 1974.

186. Snider, D. E., Pregnancy and tuberculosis, *Chest,* 86 (Suppl.), 105, 1984.

187. Robinson, G. C. and Cambon, K. G., Hearing loss in infants of tuberculous mothers treated with streptomycin during pregnancy, *N. Engl. J. Med.*, 271, 949, 1964.

188. Donald, P. R. and Sellars, S. L., Streptomycin ototoxicity in the unborn child, *S. Afr. Med. J.,* 60, 316, 1981.

189. Potworowska, M., Sianozecka, E., and Szufladowicz, R., Ethionamide treatment and pregnancy, *Polish Med. J.,* 5, 1152, 1966.

190. Stallworth, J. R., Brasfield, D. M., and Tiller, R. E., Congenital miliary tuberculosis proven by open lung biopsy specimen and successfully treated, *Am. J. Dis. Child.,* 134, 320, 1980.

191. Gillum, M. D. and Maki, D. G., Brief report: tuberculin testing, BCG in pregnancy, *Infect. Control Hosp. Epidemiol.,* 9, 119, 1988.

192. Smith, J. K., Caspary, E. A., and Field, E. J., Lymphocyte reactivity to antigen in pregnancy, *Am. J. Obstet. Gynecol.,* 113, 602, 1972.

193. Montgomery, W. P., Young, R. C., Jr., and Allen, M. P., The tuberculin test in pregnancy, *Am. J. Obstet. Gynecol.,* 100, 829, 1968.

194. Present, P. A. and Comstock, G. W., Tuberculin sensitivity in pregnancy, *Am. Rev. Respir. Dis.,* 112, 413, 1975.

195. Bonebrake, C. R., Noller, K. L., and Loehnen, P. C., Routine chest radiography in pregnancy, *JAMA,* 240, 2747, 1978.

196. Vallejo, J. G. and Starke, J. R., Tuberculosis and pregnancy, *Clin. Chest Med.,* 13, 693, 1992.

197. Franks, A. L., Binkin, N. J., and Snider, D. E., Jr., Isoniazid hepatitis among pregnant and postpartum hispanic patients, *Public Health Rep.,* 104, 151, 1989.

198. Snider, D. E., Jr. and Caras, G. J., Isoniazid-associated hepatitis deaths: a review of available information, *Am. Rev. Respir. Dis.,* 145, 494, 1992.

199. Snider, D. E., Jr. and Powell, K. E., Should mothers taking antituberculosis drugs breast-feed?, *Arch. Intern. Med.,* 144, 589, 1984.

200. McKenzie, S. A., Macnab, A. J., and Katz, G., Neonatal pyridoxine responsive convulsions due to isoniazid therapy, *Arch. Dis. Child.,* 51, 567, 1976.

201. Kendig, E. L. and Rogers, W. L., Tuberculosis in the neonatal period, *Am. Rev. Tuberc.,* 77, 418, 1958.

202. Kendig, E. L., The place of BCG vaccine in the management of infants born to tuberculous mothers, *N. Engl. J. Med.,* 281, 520, 1969.

203. Dormer, B. A., Swarit, J. A., and Harrison, I., Prophylactic isoniazid protection of infants in a tuberculosis hospital, *Lancet,* 2, 902, 1959.

204. Light, I. J., Saidleman, M., and Sutherland, J. M., Management of newborns after nursery exposure to tuberculosis, *Am. Rev. Respir. Dis.,* 109, 415, 1974.

205. Young, T. K. and Hershfield, E. S., A case-control study to evaluate the effectiveness of mass neonatal BCG vaccination among Canadian Indians, *Am. J. Public Health,* 76, 783, 1986.

206. Curtis, H. M., Bamford, F. N., and Leck, I., Incidence of childhood tuberculosis after neonatal BCG vaccination, *Lancet,* 1, 145, 1984.

9 Nontuberculous Mycobacteria

David L. Lakey M.D., Paul W. Wright M.D., and Richard J. Wallace, Jr., M.D.

CONTENTS

0-8493-1565-4/97/$0.00+$.50
© 2000 by CRC Press LLC

I. INTRODUCTION

The family of bacteria called Mycobacteriaceae, of the order Actinomycetales, contains the single genus, *Mycobacterium*. This group of aerobic, nonmotile, nonspore-forming rods are resistant to decolorization by acid-alcohol decolorizing agents (acid-fast), are slow growers (generation time of 2 to over 20 h compared to 20 min for *Escherichia coli*), and have high lipid concentrations in their cell walls.

The first description of the mycobacteria occurred in 1873 when the Norwegian physician, G. H. Armauer Hansen, described rod-shaped bodies (*Mycobacterium leprae)* in skin preparations of leprosy patients. In 1882, the German physician, Robert Koch, isolated the tubercle bacillus, *Mycobacterium tuberculosis*. Three years later Alvarez and Tavel described the smegma bacillus.[1] Following these discoveries, many other mycobacteria were discovered, most of which were not pathogenic in animal models, e.g., the guinea pig. Only *M. tuberculosis, M. bovis,* and *M. leprae* were consistently considered pathogenic to humans until the 1940s and 1950s. Currently, more than 80 species of mycobacteria have been described.[2] Approximately half of these species are associated with human disease. The remainder are saprophytic or are associated with animal disease only. Some of these mycobacteria, such as *M. genavense* and *M. haemophilum,* are relatively new and their pathogenicities are yet to be well defined. Rapid advancements in the taxonomic separation of mycobacterial species have occurred with the development of nucleic acid probes, rapid DNA sequencing including 16S ribosomal DNA, high performance liquid chromatography (HPLC) of mycolic acid esters, and other laboratory techniques that facilitate more rapid and accurate identification.

In 1954, Timpe and Runyon[3] classified the nontuberculous mycobacteria into four groups according to their colony growth rate, morphology, and pigmentation. The first three groups contain slowly growing organisms whose colonies show yellow pigmentation when grown in light (Group I, photochromogens), yellow to orange pigmentation when grown in darkness (Group II, scotochromogens), and little or no pigmentation when grown in light or dark (Group III, nonphotochromogens). Group IV, the rapid growers, are similar to the nonphotochromogens except that individual colonies grow in less than 5 to 7 days instead of 10 to 21 days. Runyon's classification was quite helpful in developing a global understanding of the mycobacteria by relating the morphologic qualities of the mycobacteria to their clinical presentation. However, with increased understanding of the complex taxonomy and pathogenicity of the mycobacteria, it is evident that a number of mycobacteria species do not fit well into the Runyon classification. Consequently, it has been replaced and the mycobacteria are now classified according to their species designation and grouped by the clinical disease syndromes they produce, i.e., pulmonary, cutaneous, disseminated disease, or lymphadenitis (Table 9.1). This newer organ-system grouping provides a more clinical and pathologic basis for understanding the etiology, diagnosis, clinical course, and management of mycobacterial disease.

II. NONTUBERCULOUS MYCOBACTERIA: NON-HIV

A. EPIDEMIOLOGY

1. Microbiology of Human Disease

In the early 1980s, nontuberculous mycobacteria (NTM) accounted for approximately one third of all mycobacteria isolated by state laboratories, with *M. avium* complex (MAC) comprising 61% of

TABLE 9.1
Clinical Sites of Infection with the Nontuberculous Mycobacteria

	Common Organism	Less Common Organism
Lung	*M. avium* complex	*M. gordonae*
	M. kanasasii	*M. simiae*
	M. abscessus	*M. szulgai*
	M. malmoense[a]	*M. smegmatis*
	M. xenopi[a]	*M. fortuitum*
Skin/soft tissue	*M. marinum*	*M. avium* complex
	M. fortuitum	*M. kansasii*
	M. abscessus	*M. smegmatis*
	M. chelonae	*M. nonchromogenicum*
	M. ulcerans[a]	(*M. terrae* complex)
	M. haemophilum[a]	
Lymph node disease	*M. avium* complex	*M. kansasii*
	M. scrofulaceum	*M. fortuitum*
		M. abscessus
		M. chelonae
		M. marinum
Postoperative catheter-related	*M. fortuitum*	*M. chelonae*
	M. abscessus	*M. mucogenicum*
Disseminated	*M. avium* complex	*M. xenopi*
	M. kansasii	*M. genavense*
	M. chelonae	
	M. abscessus	
	M. haemophilum	
Bone/joint	*M. avium* complex	*M. kansasii*
	M. marinum	
	M. abscessus	
	M. fortuitum	

[a] These organisms are common only in certain geographic regions, as described in the text.

Source: Adapted from Friedman, L. N., Ed., *Tuberculosis: Current Concepts and Treatment,* 1st ed., CRC Press LLC, Boca Raton, FL, 1994. With permission.

the NTM isolates.[4-6] Other commonly isolated species of NTM include *M. fortuitum* complex (19%), *M. kansasii* (10%), and *M. scrofulaceum, M. marinum,* and *M. xenopi.* Unpublished data currently (i.e., 1990s) suggest that NTM isolates (primarily MAC) now are more common than *M. tuberculosis* isolates in most large private and state laboratories, especially in areas of high endemicity for MAC. The majority of these isolates are respiratory and are considered to be non-HIV-related based on the usual patient populations evaluated by nonhospital laboratories. In laboratories that see HIV-related opportunistic infections, MAC also is the most common mycobacterial isolate.

MAC includes several phenotypically similar species: *M. avium, M. intracellulare, M. paratuberculosis,* and *M. lepraemurium.* These organisms are serologically different, but have been considered collectively as one entity because of the difficulty in separating them in the laboratory.[7] Separate commercial DNA probes now are available for *M. avium* and *M. intracellulare* which allow for rapid and accurate separation of these two species. *M. avium* strains appear to be more virulent than *M. intracellulare,*[8] but both organisms can cause significant human illness. *M. lepraemurium* is associated with animal illness only. Some include *M. scrofulaceum* in this group, calling the group "MAIS,"[9] but we will consider *M. scrofulaceum* separately. MAC contains at least 28 separate serovars which can be differentiated by seroagglutination testing.[10] Such serotyping is not readily available and has no utility in the evaluation of individual patients.

Clinical disease due to rapidly growing mycobacteria (RGM) is almost always due to a member of *M. fortuitum* complex or the *M. smegmatis* complex. The clinically important members of the *M. fortuitum* complex are *M. fortuitum, M. fortuitum* third biovariant complex, *M. chelonae* (formerly *M. chelonae* subspecies *chelonae*), and *M. abscessus* (formerly *M. chelonae* subspecies *abscessus*). *M. fortuitum* complex is responsible for the majority of mycobacterial skin and soft tissue infections as well as an increasing number of pulmonary infections. The *M. smegmatis* complex consists of *M. smegmatis, M. goodii*, and *M. wolinskyi*. There are 23 other RGM species including pigmented species such as *M. gadium, M. thermoresistible, M. vaccae, M. flavescens*, and *M. neoaurum*; and nonpigmented species such as *M. peregrinum* and *M. mucogenicum* (formerly *M. chelonae*-like organisms or MCLO), which rarely are associated with human disease.[11]

2. Prevalence and Incidence

The prevalence and incidence of the NTM are difficult to define because infections due to the NTM rarely cause death in non-AIDS patients and are not routinely reported to public health departments. Although state laboratories provide data concerning the isolation of the NTM, many private laboratories isolate these organisms without referring the specimens to the state laboratories for further identification. This results in the lack of documentation of these infections. Furthermore, it is often difficult from single cultures to determine whether the isolation of NTM indicates a state of disease, infection without apparent disease (i.e., colonization), or environmental contamination. Nevertheless, much work is being accomplished on our understanding of the epidemiology of NTM infections, not only with studies of the organism as it exists in the environment (primarily for *M. avium* complex), but also in our ability to separate different strains of the same species. These techniques primarily utilize DNA fingerprinting methods such as large restriction fragment (LRF) pattern analysis using pulse field gel electrophoresis.[12] Studies using this identification system have shown that isolates of a specific NTM such as *M. fortuitum, M. abscessus*, or *M. avium* complex, recovered from a single individual, maintain the same LRF pattern, even from different body fluids cultured several years apart.[13]

Skin tests with complex mixtures of mycobacterial soluble antigens demonstrate that the prevalence of infection due to NTM is very high.[14] Unfortunately, these skin test antigens do not offer a reliable picture of the rate of infection for any given species because of cross reactivity to various specific antigens.[15] One interesting aspect of the skin-test reactivity to MAC, as measured by PPD-B (intradermal skin test for MAC), is that it tends to be lower in older age groups for reasons that are unclear. This contrasts to reactivity to PPD-S (standard tuberculin skin test) which tends be higher in older age groups.[16]

Despite these limitations, surveillance studies from the Centers for Disease Control and Prevention (CDC) have indicated that the prevalence of NTM disease might be increasing. State laboratory reports from 1979 to 1980 demonstrated that NTM comprised approximately one third of the 32,000 mycobacterial isolates. The most recent CDC survey showed that from 1991 to 1992, more than two thirds of mycobacterial isolates were NTM (unpublished data). The average yearly incidence of NTM disease in past studies has varied from 0.7 per 100,000 in South Carolina[17] to an estimated annual incidence of 2 per 100,000 per year in Australia.[18] MAC was the most commonly isolated NTM species in studies from South Carolina (86%),[17] the U.S. (60%),[4,5] and British Columbia (73%).[19]

Infection due to *M. kansasii* occurs most commonly in the central and southern U.S.; the more common states include Texas, Louisiana, Illinois, and Florida. Infection from this organism has been reported in England and Wales.[20] Its incidence in Japan has increased to 0.34 per 100,000 per year.[21]

M. xenopi was the most commonly isolated NTM causing mycobacterial disease in southeast England from 1977 to 1984.[22] In a 1992 study from Brooklyn, *M. xenopi* was the second (MAC was first) most common pathogenic NTM isolated from 86 hospitalized patients of whom only 41% were seropositive for HIV.[23] Simor et al.[24] have noted that most isolates of this organism are from the respiratory tract. In his study, only 9 of 28 isolates of *M. xenopi* recovered were considered to be causing disease.

M. malmoense, a slow-growing pathogen first isolated in 1977, has been infrequently reported in North America.[25] The incidence in Europe, however, seems to be increasing.[26] Although similar to MAC, *M. malmoense* seems to be more sensitive to the decontamination process for samples and grows more slowly, which may explain the difficulty in isolating this organism.

M. ulcerans skin and soft tissue infections have not been reported in the U.S. They are, however, endemic and relatively common in parts of Asia, Africa, Mexico, and Australia.

The incidence of pulmonary NTM cases secondary to RGM, especially *M. abscessus*, is also thought to be increasing. From 1981 to 1983, the CDC identified 441 pulmonary cases secondary to RGM. The majority of these isolates were *M. abscessus*, which also has caused several recent nosocomial outbreaks linked to contaminated water.

Other NTM species, including *M. scofulaceum, M. gordonae, M. haemophilium, M. genavense, M. celatum, M. conspicuum, M. simiae,* and *M. szulgai,* also have been known to cause pulmonary and/or disseminated disease, but the majority of these cases have been in immunocompromised/AIDS patients.

3. Patient Characteristics

a. Pulmonary Disease

The classic non-HIV-infected patient with MAC pulmonary disease is an older (late 50s to 60s) white male living in a rural area of the southeastern U.S. with a long history of cigarette abuse and resultant pulmonary disease. Alcohol abuse in this group also is common.[27] This cavitary form of pulmonary MAC disease was recently shown to have a female-to-male ratio of 2:7.[28a] In this study the mean age of the patients was 51.9 years, 78% abused alcohol, 89% smoked (mean, 56 pack/year history), and none had other pathogens recovered from their sputum. All patients had cavitary disease in at least one upper lobe.

The second phenotype consists of patients who are typically female, white, nonsmokers, average age over 60 years, living in a rural area, and with associated bronchiectasis involving primarily the right middle lobe and lingula. Some patients have thoracic skeletal abnormalities, including scoliosis and pectus excavatum. Iseman has hypothesized that these thoracic abnormalities, through unknown mechanisms, make an individual more susceptible to environmental pathogens.[28b] Reich and Johnson[29] described six elderly female patients with MAC pulmonary infection involving the middle lobe or lingula portions of the lung. They suggested that these females became ill due to their reluctance to cough, and thus developed nonspecific inflammation in areas of the lung with poor drainage. They labeled this the "Lady Windermere's syndrome." This form of pulmonary MAC disease is currently referred to as nodular bronchiectesis. Nodular bronchiectesis was recently shown to have a 13:4 female-to-male ratio, and occurs at a mean age of 66 years.[28] None of the 17 patients in this study had a history of alcohol abuse, and only 5 smoked cigarettes (mean, 5.1 pack/year). Almost half (8 of 17) of these patients had other possible pathogens recovered from their sputum. The chest radiographic pattern was interstitial and nodular, predominantly either in the right middle lobe or in the lingula. Chest CT scan demonstrated multifocal bronchiectasis in 12 of 12 patients.

The third group to develop NTM pulmonary disease is cystic fibrosis (CF) patients.[30] The emergence of NTMs in the CF population recently was reviewed by Olivier and coworkers.[31] Prior to 1990, NTM infection in CF patients was rare, with only 16 reported cases. Recently, however, NTM disease has been increasingly recognized in this patient population for reasons that are unknown. A recent review demonstrated that 84 (13%) of 644 patients with CF who were screened for NTMs had positive cultures.[31] Possible explanations include increased physician concern and, thus, increased screening; increased survival and, thus, an increased average age of CF patients; improved culture techniques that prevent overgrowth by pseudomonas; increased transmission in

CF centers; and overall emergence of NTMs as pathogens. In a recent study by Kilby et al.,[32] the only distinguishing feature that predicted positive NTM cultures in CF patients was older age.

Occupation does not seem to be a risk factor for MAC infection, although its rural association puts farmers and ranchers at higher risk. As noted above, smoking is a risk factor for cavitary MAC disease.[28] Other potential pulmonary risk factors are previously treated mycobacterial disease, including tuberculosis, cystic fibrosis, and some forms of pneumoconiosis. In Wales, for example, MAC disease occurs more often in coal miners[33] and, along with tuberculosis, is found more often in patients with silicosis ("sand-blaster's" disease). However, at the time of diagnosis, as many as one third of patients with MAC disease (especially women) have no definable predisposing condition.[34]

Similar to patients with nodular bronchiectasis and MAC, typical patients with RGM pulmonary disease are female nonsmokers without underlying lung disease. In a 1993 study of 154 patients with RGM pulmonary disease, most patients were white (83%), female (65%), and nonsmokers (66%), with a mean age of 54 years.[35] As many as 15% of these patients are coinfected with MAC, and radiographic features are similar to patients with MAC and nodular bronchiectasis.

The average age of patients with *M. kansasii* is 50 years for males and 42 years for females.[36] The male-to-female ratio is 3:1[36] to 2:1.[6] In the U.S., the ethnic distribution of this disease corresponds to that of the population being studied, with more disease usually found in white rather than in African Americans or Hispanic populations. The typical patient is a 50-year-old white male living in an urban area of one of the states mentioned above.[6] Underlying lung disease, 95% of which is chronic obstructive pulmonary disease, is present in 62% of patients with *M. kansasii*.[37] Patients who develop *M. kansasii* disease seem to have less underlying disease than those infected with MAC. Occupation has not been established as a risk factor, but some studies suggest that *M. kansasii* disease occurs more commonly in the setting of both nonindustrial and industrial dust exposure,[21,33,38,39] including patients with clinical silicosis. In a bacteriological survey of gold miners, NTM were recovered from 8 to 12% of collected sputums, with *M. kansasii* the commonest NTM isolated (67 to 79%).[38] NTM were isolated from 16.9% of sputums from gold miners with silicosis, but only 5.7% of those without silicosis.[38]

Pulmonary disease due to *M. xenopi* has been reported predominantly in England and Canada.[22,24,40,41] It typically occurs in the elderly male patient who has a history of chronic obstructive pulmonary disease (COPD), past tuberculosis, or a similar underlying condition.

b. Cutaneous Disease

Patients infected with *M. marinum* often are young (mean age, approximately 36 years) men (male-to-female ratio of 1.5:1) who present with a history of skin trauma prior to exposure and infection.[42] They typically present with an indolent papule, nodule, or ulcerated skin lesion on an extremity with no systemic symptoms. Ascending nodules (lymphocutaneous syndrome), as with sporotrichosis and nocardia, occasionally is seen. Most patients are in excellent health before acquiring this infection, only a few with a history of immunosuppression from HIV infection or renal transplantation therapy.

M. haemophilum infection of the skin and subcutaneous tissues recently has been recognized, almost exclusively in immunocompromised patients such as organ transplant patients or patients with AIDS.[43] The incidence of infection, the natural habitat, and route of infection are unknown. The organism has been isolated in patients from widely diverse geographic areas, (e.g., Australia, Israel, and the U.S.), but has yet to be isolated from the environment. *M. haemophilum* requires growth media enriched with iron (ferric) salts (hence, its name), a feature which may explain its previous lack of growth and attention.

4. Sources of Infection and Transmission

Although the method of initial infection with NTM is poorly understood, these opportunistic pathogens probably enter the human host from environmental sources. There is little evidence to support human-to-human transmission. Support for environmental sources of infection derives from serotype matching of MAC soil isolates with isolates from patients living in areas where the soil was sampled.[44,45] Support for animal-to-human infection comes from West Germany,[44] but similar studies from South Africa failed to support the concept of this mode of transmission.[46]

MAC commonly is found in water sources, demonstrated by Wolinsky and Rynearson[47] who isolated at least one species of NTM from 86% of soil samples collected from the eastern U.S. MAC has been recovered from soil,[47] fresh and brackish water,[48] house dust,[49] chickens,[50] birds,[51] food,[52] and animals.[53] MAC tends to grow better in warmer water with low salinity, low pH, and low dissolved oxygen.[54] Water, including tap water, is considered to be a major reservoir for these organisms. Both MAC and *M. scrofulaceum*, have been recovered from one third of sampled aquatic environments in the southeastern U.S.[55] Waters, aerosols, and soils associated with the acidic swamp waters of the southeastern U.S. are optimal sources for MAC recovery.[54] Correspondingly, the greatest number of human isolates of MAC and the highest prevalence of skin-test reactivity to a MAC-purified protein derivative come from this same geographic area.[55]

M. fortuitum complex species are commonly recovered from water and soil samples.[6] They also have been isolated from such nosocomial sources as procedural instruments,[56,57] tap water, surgical marking solutions, ice, distilled water, and surgical cleansing solutions,[58] with water the almost universal common denominator. In a series of 125 cases of RGM infection reported in 1983, 74 cases (59%) were cutaneous infections and over half of these followed surgical procedures.[59] The mode of transmission of *M. fortuitum* complex lung disease is unclear but probably parallels that of MAC, both commonly recovered from the environment. Direct inoculation is the usual mode of transmission for localized cutaneous, and/or bone disease, while nosocomial infections usually relate to contamination from colonized distilled water or tap water.

M. kansasii is only rarely recovered from the natural environment (no isolations from soil and only one from fresh water).[60] It has been isolated from samples of municipal water supplies,[48] biofilm from water treatment plants, domestic water supply systems, aquaria,[61] and tap waters sources.[60,62] (These sites of isolation fit well with the general urban character of clinical disease.) Rarely, *M. kansasii* has been recovered from dust[63] and animals (cattle and swine).[64] The mode of transmission of *M. kansasii* is unclear, but infection probably originates from inhaled environmental sources. In spite of the limited recovery of this organism in the environment, and the major concentration of disease within the urban setting, there has been little evidence for human-to-human transmission of this organism.

M. xenopi has been recovered from hot water systems almost exclusively, most often in hospitals where the species has been associated with nosocomial outbreaks. It has not been isolated from intake water pipes, but only from hot water pipe systems. It grows optimally in temperatures of 43 to 45°C and is one of the most heat stable of the mycobacterial species.[58]

M. marinum skin infections have been reported from the U.S.,[65] Europe,[66] Japan,[67] Israel,[42] Hong Kong,[68] New Zealand,[69] Australia,[70] and Canada.[71] This infection occurs typically in patients exposed to water, particularly saltwater activities and the cleaning of freshwater fish tanks.[66] It also has been associated with saltwater and freshwater fish[48], soil,[48] natural bathing pools, dolphins, shrimp, snails, water fleas, and rarely fresh water sources such as tributaries, lakes, and wells.[42] *M. marinum* exhibits powerful fucosidase activity[48] which may enable it to derive its carbon requirement from aquatic algae containing fucose. This may explain its recovery in certain types of waters such as aquaria, swimming pools, and biofilms.[48]

M. malmoense has been isolated from soil in Zaire and natural water in Finland. *M. ulcerans'* natural reservoir and mode of transmission are unknown. Likewise the sources of infection for other NTM, including *M. haemophilium*, *M. szugai*, *M. celatum*, *M. genavense*, and *M. conspicuum* are unknown, although they are all thought to be acquired from the environment.

5. Pathogenesis

The pathogenesis of NTM infection is unclear but may be similar to tuberculosis. Pulmonary patients are thought to inhale the aerosolized organisms from infected soil, dust, and natural water supplies such as estuaries. The source may be nosocomial, as MAC of the serotype causing human disease has been found in the hot water systems of hospitals.[72] Mycobacterial organisms in desiccated water droplets (so called droplet nuclei) are thought to localize in the heavily ventilated portions of the lung, namely the middle or lower lung zones or the anterior segments of the upper lobes.[73] Following this primary infection, there is lymphohematogenous dissemination of NTM to the lungs and (perhaps) to the rest of the body, causing a mild self-limited disease in most nonimmunocompromised patients.[74] It is not known whether NTM disease occurs soon after infection or develops after a period of latency.

Ingestion of NTM provides a second possible mode for disease entry, especially in patients with extrapulmonary infection. The sources may be water or foodstuffs contaminated with NTM. Direct entry across protective skin barriers is a third method of infection seen in penetrating skin and soft tissue injuries, as well as postoperative wounds.

Very little is known about the pathogenesis of *M. kansasii*. Some evidence suggests that the organism is inhaled by the susceptible human host with potable (tap) water as a likely source.

Although most pathogenic bacteria produce toxins that are important in their pathogenesis, none have been isolated from *M. tuberculosis* or *M. leprae*. Recently, however, a toxin was isolated from *M. ulcerans*, the causative agent of the Buruli ulcer.[75] A polyketide derived macrolide, named mycolactone, produces reversible cytopathic effects on L929 cells at concentrations as low as 25 pg/ml. Guinea pigs injected with mycolactone develop an ulcerative lesion consistent with a Buruli ulcer. Furthermore, avirulent strains of *M. ulcerans* seem to have lost their ability to produce this compound. The implications of mycolactone as a virulence determinant may extend to other mycobacteria besides *M. ulcerans,* since other mycobacteria have similar polyketide genes.

Transmission of *M. marinum* occurs when susceptible hosts are exposed to penetrating skin trauma in an aquatic environment containing the organism, or place their hands in such water before a cutaneous injury heals (e.g., cleaning a household fish tank). Eighty-five percent of *M. marinum* patients in an outbreak at Glenwood Springs, CO had reactive skin tests to PPD-S, with 91% of these patients having negative PPD skin tests within 2 years prior to their illness.[76] In a study of 12 patients with culture proven *M. marinum* infection of deep tissues, 11 had antigen-specific T-cell anergy to *M. marinum* with normal responses to other antigens.[77] This study suggests that patients may have had a narrow immune defect causing susceptibility to *M. marinum* infection.

B. CLINICAL MANIFESTATIONS AND DIAGNOSTIC CRITERIA

In the HIV-negative populations, pulmonary disease accounts for almost 90% of disease due to NTM (Figure 9.1), followed by lymph node, skin, bone and joint, and disseminated illness.[6] MAC and *M. kansasii* are the most frequently isolated species in patients with NTM pulmonary disease in the U.S.[5,6]

1. Pulmonary

The presentation of pulmonary MAC disease is partially dependent on the phenotype of the disease, as described above in the epidemiology section. Ahn and colleagues reported that 76.5% of 226 patients with MAC pulmonary disease had cavitary disease.[78] Cavitary MAC disease typically presents with nonspecific signs and symptoms that may include productive cough, weakness, dyspnea, and hemoptysis. Patients usually present with less fever and weight loss than patients with pulmonary tuberculosis.

Patients with nodular bronchiectasis are most likely to present with a chronic cough associated with severe fatigue. Less common symptoms include hemoptysis, low grade fever, dyspnea, and weight loss.

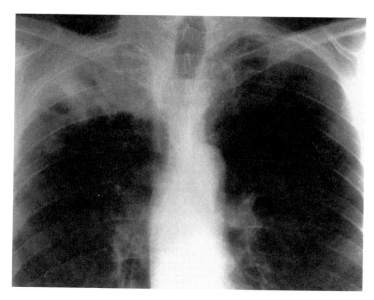

FIGURE 9.1   Chest x-ray of patient with MAC disease, right upper lobe fibronodular infiltrate. (From Friedman, L. N., Ed., *Tuberculosis: Current Concepts and Treatment,* CRC Press LLC, Boca Raton, FL, 1994. With permission.)

The presentation of pulmonary NTM disease in CF is very similar to the presentation of CF lung disease.[31] Patients frequently present with increased cough and sputum, dyspnea, weight loss, anorexia, night sweats, and fever. This is similar to bacterial exacerbations in CF patients, thus making diagnosis difficult.[79] Nodular shadows, thin-walled cavities, and hilar retraction have been described on radiographic evaluation. These findings were seen in patients with advanced NTM disease and, therefore, the presentation of less severe disease is less well described.

Pulmonary disease is the most common presentation of *M. kansasii* infection, followed by disseminated disease, lymph node disease, bone and joint disease, and skin and soft tissue disease. Patients with pulmonary infection with *M. kansasii* typically present with a clinical picture indistinguishable from pulmonary tuberculosis. Cavitary disease is found in 85[37] to 95%[78] of patients with *M. kansasii*, and 20% have bilateral cavitary disease.[37] Clinical symptoms are similar to that of pulmonary tuberculosis, except that they are generally less intense. Pulmonary disease due to *M. kansasii* or other NTM is rarely seen in children.[80]

Pulmonary disease due to RGM is not uncommon and involves primarily *M. abscessus* (approximately 80% of cases).[35,59] In a 1993 study of 154 patients with RGM pulmonary disease, cough was the most common presenting symptom and constitutional symptoms appeared only after disease progression. Other symptoms included recurrent episodes of acute bronchitis, fatigue, mild fever, weight loss, and occasional hemoptysis. The radiographic appearance differed from tuberculosis or pulmonary disease due to MAC or *M. kansasii* in that cavitary disease was rare (16% of cases).[35] The commonly seen interstitial (37%), reticulonodular (36%), or interstitial/alveolar (40%) infiltrates typically involved three or four lobes (>50%) and was bilateral in 77% of cases.[35] Upper lobe disease was seen more frequently in the right upper lobe (77%) than the left upper lobe (61%).[35] The disease may be easily confused clinically and/or radiographically with fibrotic lung disease or bronchiectasis. The diagnosis is confirmed in patients who have compatible radiographic abnormalities and multiple sputum cultures that are positive for the same organism.

In a study of 19 patients with *M. xenopi* pulmonary illness, 12 presented with mild symptoms of cough, fever, and increased sputum production.[41] Three patients had hemoptysis and seven were asymptomatic, having only a change on chest film. Roentgenographic features included, either singly or in combination, a nodular or mass shadow (14/19), single or multiple cavities (9/19), and a tuberculosis-type presentation with multifocal, nodular densities.

Diagnostic criteria for pulmonary disease due to MAC and other NTM have been somewhat controversial. Recent American Thoracic Society criteria[58] suggest that anyone with two of more positive respiratory cultures containing moderate numbers of organisms determined by positive AFB smears and/or culture and an abnormal chest x-ray not explained by other diseases should be considered to have NTM lung disease. Tsukamura suggests that patients with a new pulmonary cavitary with two or more (and perhaps only one) sputum culture positive for MAC should be considered to have MAC pulmonary disease.[81] This latter criteria is more specific, but excludes the more than one third of current patients with noncavitary disease (especially nodular bronchiectasis).

2. Extrapulmonary

a. Lymph Node

Lymph node disease due to NTM infection in the non-HIV-infected patient is typically seen in young children, from 1 to 10 years of age. The unilateral rapidly enlarging (often painless) lymph node or group of nodes usually are the only presenting complaint, with occasional low-grade fever and malaise. The lymph nodes most frequently encountered are the submandibular, submaxillary, cervical, and preauricular nodes. The majority of infections are currently due to MAC (80%) and *M. scrofulaceum; M. kansasii, M. fortuitum,* and *M. abscessus* are only occasionally cultured from infected lymph nodes. Only 10% of mycobacterial lymphadenitis in children is due to *M. tuberculosis,* whereas it is responsible for 90% of adult mycobacterial lymphadenitis.[82]

The differential diagnosis includes cat-scratch disease, tuberculosis, drug reactions, malignancies, nocardiosis, brucellosis, mononucleosis, sarcoidosis, toxoplasmosis, and others. Distinguishing between tuberculosis and NTM lymphadenitis is very important, as tuberculosis requires drug therapy and public health measures, while NTM does not. The presumptive diagnosis of NTM can be made from the patient's history, a negative tuberculin skin test, and the histopathologic appearance of a lymph node demonstrating caseating granulomata with or without acid-fast bacilli (AFB). A definitive diagnosis of mycobacterial lymphadenitis is made by culturing the organism from the lymph node, a procedure which yields a positive culture in cervical lymph nodes in only 50 to 85% of cases.[83] The reason for the high false-negative rate is unknown, but could reflect the presence of more fastidious mycobacterial species such as *M. haemophilum* or *M. genavense.* Some culture-negative samples have been shown to be positive for *M. avium* by PCR.

The majority of children with NTM lymphadenitis react to *M. avium* skin test antigens, such as PPD-B. Some children, however, will have a blistering reaction to PPD-B. A less potent, protein weight standardized *M. avium* skin test material called "sensitin" and a dual skin-test technique to determine *M. avium*–dominant vs. PPD-dominant reactions seems to have increased the specificity. However, no commercial NTM skin product is currently available for clinical use in the U.S., and this procedure is not recommended for diagnosis of NTM. Therefore, all children should be tested with the standard PPD. Most of these children will have a weak reaction (5 to 9 mm) to the intermediate strength PPD due to cross reactivity with NTM. Some children, however, with NTM lymphadenitis may be negative, while one third of the patients will have induration of 10 mm or more.

Fine-needle aspiration has been utilized to obtain diagnostic material from lymph nodes, but its role is controversial. Incomplete or incisional biopsies of lymphadenitis due to mycobacteria should be avoided to prevent problems with fistulae and chronic drainage. Lymph nodes infected with NTM should be excised to facilitate both diagnosis and therapy. Without treatment, spontaneous drainage usually occurs, but spontaneous resolution may be more common than reported, especially in children.

b. Cutaneous Disease

Cutaneous disease due to NTM is caused most commonly by *M. fortuitum, M. abscessus, M. chelonae, M. marinum, M. haemophilum,* and *M. ulcerans.* Patients with cutaneous manifestations of NTM infection usually present with local symptoms; systemic symptoms and disease are uncommon. In the immunocompetent patient, these skin lesions usually are the site of primary disease (as opposed to disseminated disease) and typically occur after trauma to the skin.

M. marinum skin disease commonly presents as a nodular or ulcerative sporotrichosis-like lesion on the elbows, fingers, hands, or knees. Systemic disease, lymphadenitis, and disseminated disease are uncommon in the immunocompetent host. The time interval between exposure and the appearance of lesions varied from 10 days to 2 years with an average of 3 to 8 weeks.[76] Without treatment the lesions usually persist for 14 or 15 months. Most lesions (80%) resolve spontaneously by 36 months.[84]

RGM infections present most commonly in the skin or soft tissue. Although sporadic disease is more common than clustered outbreaks, 80% of these infections occur in the southern coastal states.[85] Most community-acquired infections produce lesions of the lower extremity in healthy hosts, usually following trauma such as nail or other puncture wounds. In community-acquired skin infections due to RGM, one third involve *M. chelonae* and *M. abscessus*, with the remainder due to *M. fortuitum*.[85] Typically there is a long incubation period averaging 1 month and extending up to 6 months. Symptoms include pain, local swelling, and serous-bloody drainage. Disseminated skin disease, usually due to *M. chelonae* in the setting of low dose corticosteroid therapy, may occur but is uncommon. Nosocomial infections due to RGM can occur in association with the use of indwelling catheters, especially long-term intravenous catheters, and certain surgical procedures such as augmentation mammaplasty and cardiac bypass surgery. *M. fortuitum* has been associated with 80% of breast and sternum wound infections due to RGM. Diagnosis is made by culturing the organism from the wound, which usually can be accomplished without a tissue biopsy by the use of a vigorously applied swab.

M. haemophilum skin infection is a newly described cause of rash, papules, nodules, and draining sinuses in immunocompromised patients. Most infections have occurred in patients who are post renal transplantation or who are infected with HIV. One case presented as a chronic erythematous papular eruption, mimicking tinea corporis, in a patient who underwent coronary artery bypass surgery who was otherwise healthy.[86]

The typical *M. ulcerans* patient is a child, 5 to 8 years old, who develops a painless nodule on his leg without other signs or symptoms. This nodule will develop into a shallow ulcer with a necrotic base. Spontaneous resolution may occur in 6 to 9 months, but others will persist, spread, and eventually cause serious deformity. Other satellite nodules may develop, but lymphadenitis is absent.[87]

c. Osteomyelitis and Septic Arthritis

Posttraumatic, localized bone and joint infections due to mycobacteria are occasionally due to the *M. fortuitum* complex, MAC, and *M. kansasii*. In a review of 25 non-HIV-infected patients with granulomatous synovitis and bursitis, mycobacteria were identified in 20 patients. The isolates were *M. tuberculosis* (four cases), *M. kansasii* (six cases), MAC (two cases), and one case each of *M. marinum, M. chelonae,* and *M. gordonae*.[88] MAC infection also has been reported in patients with reactive arthritis,[89] and acute mastoiditis.[90] Synovitis of the hands, fingers, and wrists due to infection with *M. marinum* are common.[91] Sternal wound and osteomyelitis following cardiac surgery occurs in both sporadic and outbreak forms due to *M. fortuitum* and *M. abscessus*.

d. Ocular Disease

Corneal infections due to NTM were first described by Turner and Stinson in 1965.[92] The majority of these infections are caused by *M. abscessus* and *M. chelonae*, although keratitis caused by *M. flavescens*, MAC, *M. gordonae*, and *M. marinum* have been reported. In a review of 22 cases of culture positive NTM keratitis, 19 were caused by *M. chelonae*, and 3 were caused by *M. fortuitum*.[93] In 20 of these 22 patients, antecedent trauma (18) or surgery (2) occurred. Trauma frequently involved superficial corneal foreign body injuries, the majority with metallic agents. Infection also has been associated with anterior segment surgery, corneal suture abscesses, and contact lenses.

The time interval between injury and infection ranges from 3 days to 3 weeks. Symptoms included ocular pain, photophobia, and visual blurring. On exam these patients have corneal epithelial defects and underlying inflammatory stromal infiltrates. Only approximately 50% of culture positive cases have positive Ziehl-Neelson AFB stains.

e. Disseminated Disease

Disseminated disease due to NTM was rare before 1970. Today most cases occur in AIDS patients, less frequently in other immunosuppressed patients, and rarely in normal children or adults. Organisms causing disseminated disease include MAC, *M. kansasii, M. chelonae,*[94] *M. scrofulaceum, M. abscessus,*[59] *M. haemophilum,*[95] and most recently, *M. genavense.* In 1984, Horsburgh et al. described 37 non-AIDS patients with disseminated MAC infection and found 20 to have immunosuppression, mostly from corticosteroid therapy.[96] The clinical presentation of these patients included fever, bone pain, weight loss, lymphadenopathy, hepatosplenomegaly, and cutaneous lesions. Disseminated disease due to *M. kansasii, M. chelonae,* and *M. haemophilum* generally presents with cutaneous disease such as nodules or abscesses rather than the systemic disease presentation of MAC.

Disseminated disease due to RGM usually involves immunosuppressed patients with chronic renal failure, renal transplantation, those treated with low-dose corticosteroids, but not from HIV infection.[85] Ninety percent of disseminated cutaneous RGM infection is due to *M. chelonae* or *M. abscessus.* Initial reports that included approximately 10 patients suggested that most infections were due to *M. abscessus.*[59] However, recently, 52 cases of cutaneous disease due to disseminated *M. chelonae* have been reported,[97] suggesting that this species is responsible for most of the current cases. The majority of these patients have disseminated cutaneous disease only, with little or no systemic symptoms. The remainder, especially those with dialysis-dependent renal failure, have systemic disease, positive blood cultures, and are seriously ill.

Diagnosis of disseminated disease is made when the organism is isolated from closed sterile sites such as blood, bone marrow, liver, or from multiple skin sites. Mortality due to disseminated NTM disease depends upon the organism and the status of the underlying disease. In 1972, Lincoln and Gilbert reported 12 fatal cases of disseminated NTM (most were MAC) disease in children.[98] They also describe nine cases of meningitis due to NTM with at least four fatalities.

C. Diagnosis

The cornerstone of diagnosis of NTM disease is isolation of the organism from sputum, tissue, or body fluid in patients presenting with histories, physical examinations, and radiographic findings suggestive of NTM disease.[58] A single positive sputum culture, usually with a low number of organisms, may occur as a consequence of transient contamination or colonization of the respiratory tract, or even from specimen contamination. Therefore, the diagnosis of lung disease caused by MAC or other NTM (with the possible exception of *M. kansasii*) requires more than one positive acid-fast sputum smear and/or culture positivity (moderate or heavy growth) for acid-fast bacteria. However, recovery of *M. kansasii* from sputum and other human tissue and fluids usually indicates infection because this organism is rarely a contaminant.[47] Nonetheless, a minimum of two positive cultures is preferred.[58] Other causes of lung disease such as tuberculosis, fungal disease, and malignancy should be excluded. Bronchial washings seem to have greater sensitivity and less specificity in diagnosing NTM lung disease than routinely expectorated sputums.[58] Suggested criteria for the diagnosis for NTM disease are shown in Table 9.2.

D. Laboratory Evaluation of Mycobacterial Specimens

NTM are differentiated from *M. tuberculosis* by colony morphology and pigment, nucleic acid composition, growth rate, biochemical behavior, and pathogenicity. They are readily stained with

TABLE 9.2

Diagnostic Criteria for Skin and Lung Nontuberculous Mycobacterial Disease

	Usual History	Minimum Number of Cultures	Chest X-Ray
Non-HIV Related			
Cutaneous			
M. marinum	Water/fish tank exposure, typical skin lesions	1	NA
M. fortuitum	Penetrating/open trauma or prior surgery	1	NA
M. abscessus	Same as *M. fortuitum*	1	NA
M. chelonae	On low dose steroids	1	NA
Pulmonary			
MAC	Rural male smoker, female over age 50 with chronic cough	2	2/3 cavitary; abnormal, not explained by other diseases (bronchiectasis not an acceptable explanation)
M. abscessus	Adult, no prior lung disease; prior granulomatous lung disease; or cystic fibrosis	2	Same as above except 10–20% cavitary
M. kanasasii	Urban male smoker over age 50	2	Same as above
Lymph node disease			
MAC	Child, age 1–10 years, cervical node	0–1 Compatible histopathology, negative culture for *M. tuberculosis*	Should be negative
M. scrofulaceum	Cervical node	Same as above	Same as above
M. fortuitum	Regional drainage from trauma/surgical site	Same as above	Same as above
M. chelonae	Regional drainage from trauma/surgical site	Same as above	Same as above
HIV Related			
Pulmonary			
M. kansasii	Not helpful	(?) 2	Cavitary upper lobe disease, miliary disease, some nonspecific
MAC	Not helpful	(?) 2	Cavitary upper lobe disease, miliary disease, some nonspecific
Disseminated			
MAC	Blood, bone marrow, liver; sputum and stool are not diagnostic	1	NA

Source: Friedman, L. N., Ed., *Tuberculosis: Current Concepts and Treatment,* 1st ed., CRC Press LLC, Boca Raton, FL, 1994. With permission.

acid-fast dye techniques (Kinyoun or Ziehl-Neelsen) and also the fluorochrome procedure. However, only *M. kansasii* and *M. marinum* can be occasionally distinguished from other mycobacteria on stain identification alone by their larger and more beaded appearance.

1. Processing and Culturing Specimens

Clinical sputum samples for NTM are digested and decontaminated using a technique similar to that used for *M. tuberculosis*. Although specific recommendations for mycobacterial laboratory methods are explained in detail in Chapter 4, several specific points concerning NTM cultures need to be reemphasized. First, NTM are more susceptible than *M. tuberculosis* to killing by NaOH during the decontamination and digestion of clinical samples.[58] Therefore, extra care must be taken not to exceed the recommended concentration and time guidelines. Second, since many patients with NTM lung disease have associated bronchiectesis (especially those with nodular bronchiectasis and cystic fibrosis), their sputum cultures also may contain other species such as *Pseudomonas aeruginosa*, aspergillus, yeast, and other gram-negative rods that can overgrow the sample. This overgrowth can be minimized by processing the samples with the conventional N-acetyl-L-cysteine-sodium hydroxide (NALC-NaOH) solution followed by a second processing with 5% oxalic acid. This should be considered when one or more specimens are contaminated in a patient suspected of having NTM lung disease. At least three sputum cultures should be sent for the initial evaluation of NTM pulmonary disease. These cultures should be inoculated onto both solid and liquid media, because liquid media has a greater recovery rate for all mycobacteria. Furthermore, quantification of growth on solid media is important to help determine the clinical significance of an isolate and the response to therapy. Mycobacterial blood cultures may be either inoculated into BACTEC (Becton-Dickinson) 13A broth or plated onto 7H10 or 7H11 agar after lysis centrifugation. Most slow-growing NTM are detectable in 2 to 4 weeks on the solid media and within 1 to 2 weeks by the BACTEC or similar broth culture systems. Cultures usually are grown at 35 to 37°C for 6 weeks.

All the currently recognized NTM pathogens will grow under the above conditions except *M. haemophilum*, *M. genavense*, and *M. conspicuum*. If *M. haemophilum* is suspected, a commercial paper disk containing hemin (factor X) should be added to the surface of the 7H10 or 7H11 plate, or hemin or ferric ammonium citrate should be added to the media.[58] *M. genavense* requires a minimum of 8 weeks to grow, and often only grows from the blood in BACTEC 13A media. Acidic (pH 6) radiometric Middlebrook broth media (pyrazinamide test media) may enhance its growth. *M. conspicuum* will grow in BACTEC media at 35 to 37°C, but will not grow on solid media unless the temperature is 22 to 31°C. Thus, if solid media cultures are negative from patients with AFB smear-positive sputum, these three NTM must be considered.

All skin and soft tissue NTM cultures need to be incubated at both 35° and 28 to 32°C, because many of the common NTM that cause these infections may only grow at the lower temperature on primary isolation. These NTM include *M. haemophilum*, *M. ulcerans*, *M. marinum*, and *M. chelonae*. *M. marinum* forms a yellow colony when exposed to light and grows more rapidly (within 5 days) than other slow growers at lower temperature.

2. Identification of NTMs

Biochemical tests, growth rates, and colony morphologies traditionally were used to identify NTMs, e.g., the niacin test distinguishes *M. tuberculosis* from NTMs. *M. tuberculosis* is niacin positive, while most NTMs are negative. Growth rates and colony morphology can then be used to further characterize the NTM. These traditional tests, however, are slow and most larger laboratories are using more rapid technologies to identify mycobacteria.

Currently three rapid methods are in use. These methods include high performance liquid chromatography (HPLC), commercial DNA probes, and PCR-based technologies. Since the type and amount of mycolic acids of the NTMs vary according to species, the HPLC mycolic acid fingerprints of mycobacterial isolates can be used for identification and applied to the specimen or to a positive culture. Recent improvements in HPLC technology now allow the identification of mycobacteria directly from sputum samples in 50% of AFB smear-positive samples. HPLC generally is not helpful with AFB smear-negative samples, and cannot distinguish between many of the pathogenic rapid growing mycobacteria.

Mycobacterial species-specific DNA probes are commercially available to identify *M. tuberculosis, M. gordonae, M. kansasii, M. avium,* and *M. intracellulare.* These DNA probes specifically bind to the mycobacterial ribosomal RNA. These probes are highly specific and sensitive.[99] Using these probes, mycobacteria growing in a BACTEC broth can be identified in less than 4 h.

Several laboratories also have developed PCR-based procedures to identify *M. tuberculosis* and MAC. These procedures are based on either the 16s rRNA hypervariable sequence[100] or on the 65 hsp restriction analysis.[101]

Finally, the BACTEC TB 460 system utilizes a selective growth inhibitor called NAP (*p*-nitro-α-acetylamino-β-hydroxypropiophenone) at a concentration of 5 µg/ml to inhibit *M. tuberculosis* complex growth. The NAP test takes 5 days to complete, and does not further identify the NTMs. *M. genavense,* unlike other NTM, is inhibited by NAP. *M. genavense* can be presumptively identified based on its morphology on AFB smear (small coccobacillary forms), failure to grow on subculture in solid media, a negative nucleic acid test for *M. avium* complex, and a positive NAP test.[58]

3. Antimicrobial Susceptibility Testing

The role of antimicrobial susceptibility testing for slow growing NTMs is controversial.[58] Routine testing of all NTMs is discouraged, but testing is appropriate for certain circumstances. The methodology of susceptibility testing is not yet standardized and will not be discussed in this chapter.

Susceptibility testing for *M. avium* to the primary antituberculous drugs (isoniazid, rifampin, and pyrazinamide) has not been shown to be beneficial, and is not recommended by the American Thoracic Society[58] (similar recommendations are under discussion by the National Committee for Clinical Laboratory Standards). Alterations in rifabutin minimal inhibitory concentrations (MICs) following treatment or prophylaxis has been difficult to demonstrate and, therefore, rifabutin susceptibility testing is not recommended. The relevance of testing sensitivities to amikacin, ciprofloxacin, ethambutol, ethionamide, rifampin, and streptomycin is uncertain at this time; hence, testing with these agents also is not recommended. Newer macrolides such as clarithromycin and azithromycin have been shown to undergo changes in MICs associated with clinical and microbiologic relapse. These strains have a point mutation at adenine 2058 or 2059 in the 23S ribosomal DNA not evident in macrolide susceptible strains.[102] Therefore, although pretreatment clarithromycin susceptibility testing is not recommended, it should be performed for all isolates from patients on prior or concurrent macrolide therapy.

Treatment of rifampin-susceptable *M. kansasii* is empiric and not influenced by the susceptibility to drugs other than rifampin. Therefore, all initial isolates (and isolates following relapse) of *M. kansasii* should have susceptibility testing to rifampin.[58] If the isolate is susceptible to 1 µg/ml of rifampin, no further testing is recommended. If the isolate is rifampin resistant, susceptibility testing to ciprofloxacin, ofloxacin, clarithromycin, ethambutol, streptomycin, and a sulfonamide may be helpful (these are the current recommendations of the American Thoracic Society[58]).

The role of susceptibility testing for slowly growing mycobacteria other than MAC or *M. kansasii* is uncertain due to limited knowledge of their susceptibility patterns.[58] These include such species as *M. xenopi, M. simiae, M. gordonae,* and *M. terrae* complex. Susceptibility testing to ethambutol, isoniazid, rifampin, clarithromycin, and ciprofloxacin may be beneficial. Routine susceptibility testing of *M. marinum* appears unnecessary since its drug susceptibility pattern is predictable and includes susceptibility to rifampin, ethambutol, doxycycline or tetracycline, clarithromycin, and sulfonamides.

The role of susceptibility testing for the rapidly growing mycobacteria is better defined.[58] Antimicrobial susceptibilities vary between, and within, species of the rapid-growing mycobacteria. Therefore, susceptibility testing should be performed on all initial clinically significant rapid-growing mycobacterial isolates, and on isolates following relapse or treatment failure. Initial testing should include amikacin, cefoxitin, ciprofloxacin, clarithromycin, doxycycline, imipenem, a sulfonamide, and (for *M. chelonae* only) tobramycin. As with the slowly growing species, methods for such testing have yet to be standardized by the National Committee for Clinical Laboratory Standards.

E. Treatment

Therapy for NTM disease is both difficult and controversial, and there are few prospective clinical trials of antibiotic therapy. A summary of the authors' recommended therapy for NTM disease is shown in Table 9.3.

1. *Mycobacterium avium* Complex Pulmonary Disease

Therapy for MAC infection is challenging because of the increasing number of patients who require therapy and the resistance of MAC to first-line antituberculous agents. Antituberculous drugs such as cycloserine and ethionamide have excellent *in vitro* activity against MAC but are seldom used because of their toxicity. Prior to the release of the newer macrolides, relapses after medical therapy were so common that surgical resection was frequently required for optimal outcome.[103] Recent advances, however, may now allow effective treatment with medicine alone. Recent studies have demonstrated excellent *in vivo* clinical activity of the newer macrolides: azithromycin and clarithromycin.[104] This activity is likely secondary to the high levels these antibiotics achieve in tissues and phagocytes. Short-term initial treatment studies using these agents as monotherapy have demonstrated effective significant sterilization activity.[105,106] Although monotherapy is not appropriate for patients with MAC disease, these studies are the first to demonstrate *in vivo* activity for any agent against MAC pulmonary disease. These newer macrolides now are the cornerstone of effective therapy for MAC pulmonary disease.[58]

Rifabutin is more active than rifampin *in vitro* against MAC.[107] Although peak rifabutin serum concentrations are much lower than rifampin, rifabutin achieves higher levels in tissues than in serum.[108] Clinically, rifabutin provides effective prophylaxis against MAC disease in AIDS patients,[109] and may improve the clinical response in MAC pulmonary disease in HIV-negative patients.

In non-AIDS patients with MAC pulmonary disease, the American Thoracic Society[58] currently recommends triple drug therapy with clarithromycin (500 mg twice a day) or azithromycin (250 mg/day), rifabutin (300 mg/day) or rifampin (600 mg/day), and ethambutol (25 mg/kg per day for 2 months, followed by 15 mg/kg per day). For patients over 70 years old or in patients of small body mass, the macrolides may not be well tolerated. In these patients, clarithromycin may be decreased to 250 mg twice a day. Recent studies suggest that intermittent therapy may work as well as daily therapy.[58] Drug doses are clarithromycin (500 mg twice daily); ethambutol (25 mg/kg); and rifampin 600 or rifabutin (150 to 300 mg, given on Monday, Wednesday, and Friday). Rifabutin is the preferred rifamycin due to the increased *in vivo* activity noted above,[107] but it may cause more adverse effects (fever, chills, uveitis, leukopenia).[108] The risk of adverse events is relatively high for patients on the above triple regimen. Sputum conversion rates for patients who tolerate the above medical regimens are approximately 90%.[105,106]

Patients with extensive disease (primarily upper lobe fibrocavitary disease) should receive intermittent streptomycin therapy for at least the first 2 months of therapy in addition to the above

TABLE 9.3
Therapy[a]

Organism	First Line (Oral, Except Where Specified)	Injectable or Alternative Drugs (Oral Except Where Specified)	Surgery Potentially Beneficial
Therapy for Non-HIV-Related Disease			
Cutaneous			
M. marinum	Doxycycline (100 mg bid); or minocycline (100 mg bid); or TMP (160 mg)/SMX (800 mg bid); or rifampin (600 mg qd) + ethambutol (15 mg/kg qd)	Clarithromycin (500 mg bid)	+
M. fortuitum	Doxycycline (100 mg bid) or minocycline (100 mg bid): 50% susceptible; or sulfamethoxazole (1.0 g bid); or ciprofloxacin (750 mg bid); or ofloxacin (400 mg bid); or clarithromycin (500 mg bid): 80% susceptible	Amikacin (7.5–10 mg/kg qd) IM/IV, imipenem-cilastin (0.5 g qid) IV, cefoxitin (3.0 g q 6 h) IV	+
M. chelonae	Clarithromycin (500 mg bid); or doxycycline (100 mg bid): 25% susceptible	Tobramycin (3.0–5.0 mg/kg qd) IM/IV, imipenem-cilastin (0.5 g qid) IV	++
M. abscessus	Clarithromycin (500 mg bid)	Amikacin (7.5–10 mg/kg qd) IM/IV, imipenem-cilastin (0.5 g qid) IV, cefoxitin (3.0 g q 6 h) IV	++
Pulmonary Disease			
MAC	Clarithromycin (500 mg bid) + ethambutol (15 mg/kg qd) + rifampin (600 mg qd); or [clarithromycin (500 mg bid) + ethambutol (25 mg/kg) + rifampin (600 mg)] Mon-Wed-Fri	Azithromycin (250 mg qd), rifabutin (150–300 mg qd), ciprofloxacin (750 mg bid), streptomycin (0.5–1.0 g TIW) IM, amikacin (7.5–10 mg/kg TIW) IM/IV	++
M. abscessus	Clarithromycin (500 mg bid)	Amikacin (7.5–10 mg/kg qd for 2–4 weeks) IM/IV, imipenem-cilastin (0.5 g qid) IV, cefoxitin (3.0 g q 6 h) IV	++
M. kansasii	INH (300 mg qd) + rifampin (600 mg qd) + ethambutol (15 mg/kg qd)	Clarithromycin (500 mg bid), sulfamethoxazole (1.0 g bid), TMP (160 mg)/SMP (800 mg) bid, streptomycin (0.5–1.0 g qd) IM	–
M. xenopi	INH (300 mg qd) + rifampin (600 mg qd) + ethambutol (15 mg/kg qd) + clarithromycin (500 mg bid),	Streptomycin (0.5–1.0 g TIW) IM	++
M. fortuitum	Same as cutaneous, except a combination of drugs should be used	Same as cutaneous	++
M. simiae	Clarithromycin (500 mg bid)	Unknown	Unknown

TABLE 9.3 *(continued)*
Therapy[a]

Organism	First Line (Oral, Except Where Specified)	Injectable or Alternative Drugs (Oral Except Where Specified)	Surgery Potentially Beneficial
Lymph Node			
M. scrofulaceum	Surgery	Clarithromycin (500 mg bid)	+++
MAC	Surgery	Clarithromycin (500 mg bid) + rifampin, rifabutin, or ethambutol	+++
M. fortuitum	Same as cutaneous	Same as cutaneous	+
M. chelonae	Same as cutaneous	Same as cutaneous	++
M. abscessus	Same as cutaneous	Same as cutaneous	++
Disseminated			
M. chelonae	Same as cutaneous, except drug combinations should be considered for first 4–8 weeks	Same as cutaneous	
M. abscessus	Same as cutaneous, except drug combinations should be considered for first 4–8 weeks	Same as cutaneous	
M. haemophilum	Clarithromycin (500 mg bid) + rifampin (600 mg qd)	Sulfamethoxazole (1.0 g bid), TMP (160 mg)/SMP (800 mg bid), Ciprofloxacin (750 mg bid), Ofloxacin (400 mg bid), Rifabutin (150–300 mg qd)	
M. kansasii	Same as pulmonary	Same as pulmonary	
Therapy for HIV-Related Disease[b]			
MAC (prophylaxis)	Azithromycin (1200 mg qw)	Clarithromycin (500 mg bid), rifabutin (150–300 mg qd), azithromycin (1200 mg qw) + rifabutin (150–300 mg qd)	
MAC (disease)	Clarithromycin (500 mg bid) + ethambutol (15 mg/kg qd) ± rifabutin (300 mg qd)	Azithromycin (500 mg qd), streptomycin (0.5–1.0 g qd) IM, amikacin (7.5 mg/kg qd) IM or IV	
M. chelonae	Same as non-HIV	Same as non-HIV	
M. kansasii	INH (300 mg qd) + rifabutin (150 mg qd) + ethambutol (15 mg/kg qd)	Same as non-HIV	
M. haemophilum	Clarithromycin (500 mg bid) + rifabutin (150–300 mg qd)	Same as non-HIV	
M. abscessus	Same as non-HIV	Same as non-HIV	

a See text for clarification of dosing schedules.
b If protease inhibitors or nonnucleoside reverse transcriptase inhibitors are used, an expert should be consulted for rifabutin dosage adjustments.

Source: Adapted from Friedman, L. N., Ed., *Tuberculosis: Current Concepts and Treatment*, 1st ed., CRC Press LLC, Boca Raton, FL, 1994.

oral regimen.[58] The exact dose of streptomycin is dependent on the patient's age, weight, and renal function. Ototoxicity due to streptomycin often is not reversible and, therefore, patients must be instructed on the signs and symptoms of this toxicity at the beginning of therapy and at each visit.

The optimal duration of therapy for MAC lung disease has not been established. Prior to the macrolide era, the recommended duration was 18 to 24 months. [107] With macrolide therapy, shorter courses seem appropriate. Two recent studies indicate that treating 10 to 12 months after culture negativity is adequate for patients on a clarithromycin-containing regimen.[110,111] Patients treated for MAC pulmonary disease should have sputum sent for AFB smear and culture monthly during therapy, and periodically after the completion of therapy. Positive cultures containing low numbers of MAC after sputum conversion that are the same as the infecting strain will necessitate restarting the time clock.[58] All patients should clinically and/or microbiologically improve within 3 to 6 months and should clear their sputum within 12 months on a macrolide-containing regimen.

Failure to respond to a macrolide-containing regimen may be secondary to *in vitro* resistance, nonadherence, or drug intolerance. Patients that fail to respond, have progressive disease, and are found to have macrolide-resistant isolates should be placed on an alternative regimen, such as the combination of rifabutin (300 to 600 mg daily), ethambutol, and streptomycin.[58] Other possible components include cycloserine, ethionamide, clofazimine, the newer fluoroquinolones, amikacin, and capreomycin. Patients intolerant of one macrolide should be tried on the other. Little clinical efficacy data are available for many of these alternative medications in MAC pulmonary disease. Regimens containing only two of the above medications are not likely to be effective and are strongly discouraged, especially in patients with extensive disease. The risk of drug toxicity is substantial for patients on these regimens and, therefore, patients may be best served by physicians experienced in the treatment of MAC pulmonary disease. The role of immunotherapy in the treatment of patients with MAC pulmonary disease following drug failure is unknown at this time.

The use of surgery in conjunction with chemotherapy has been highly effective in some patients with MAC lung disease but the timing is not well defined. Surgery should be considered in patients with localized disease (such as a unilateral cavity) and adequate cardiopulmonary reserve. In one recent series (1998), the major indications for surgery in the macrolide era were drug failure without macrolide resistance (60%), macrolide resistance (25%), symptomatic bronchiectasis, and massive hemoptysis.[112] Resectional surgery for MAC pulmonary disease can be associated with significant morbidity. In one report from a thoracic surgeon experienced in mycobacterial surgery, postoperative bronchopleural fistulas occurred in 8 of 17 (47%) of patients who underwent pneumonectomy, although none occurred in those who underwent lobectomy.[113] Bronchopleural fistulas are more common following right pneumonectomy. Their incidence (on both sides) has been reduced since these initial reports because of the routine use of muscle flaps to wrap the bronchial stump. Whenever possible, this surgery should be performed by surgeons with substantial experience in this type of surgery. Ideally, patients should be culture negative for several months prior to resection. With expanded future knowledge of rifabutin and clarithromycin, surgery to prevent disease relapse/recurrence may be indicated less often or may no longer be necessary.

Due to the number of medications needed to treat MAC pulmonary disease and the advanced age of most patients with this disease, side effects occur frequently during therapy. Monitoring patients for such adverse events, therefore, is essential. Monitoring should include visual acuity (ethambutol and rifabutin); red-green discrimination (ethambutol); liver enzymes (macrolides, rifabutin, rifampin, isoniazid, ethionamide); ototoxicity (streptomycin, amikacin, macrolides); renal function (streptomycin, amikacin); leukocyte and platelet counts (rifabutin); gastrointestinal (all drugs except aminoglycosides); and central nervous system (cycloserine).[58] Combining clarithromycin with rifabutin increases the incidence of uveitis, while rifamycins lower clarithromycin serum levels.

2. Extrapulmonary *Mycobacterium avium*

The current treatment of choice for cervical lymphadenitis due to MAC in HIV-negative hosts is excisional surgery without chemotherapy. This has been the standard of care for more than 30 years, and usually establishes the diagnosis as well as yielding a 95% cure rate.[114] Incisional biopsy or chemotherapy alone (with antituberculous drugs) frequently results in the formation of sinus tract formation with chronic drainage or persistent clinical disease. Curettage has been suggested by some investigators because it requires only a small incision, but excision of all necrotic tissue may be difficult and require more than one surgery. In children with recurrent disease following excisional surgery, a second surgery usually is performed. Although clinically unproven, a course of clarithromycin with rifampin, rifabutin, or ethambutol also may be considered in children with limited disease, with recurrent lymph node disease after surgical resection, or in those in whom the surgical risk is high.

Adults with extrapulmonary localized MAC disease involving skin, soft tissue, tendons, joints, or bones are usually treated with a combination of surgical debridement and chemotherapy. Chemotherapy should include at least three drugs. The duration of therapy usually is 6 to 12 months, but the optimal duration has not been determined.[58]

3. *Mycobacterium kansasii*

Untreated wild strains of *M. kansasii* are susceptible to the antituberculous drug concentrations used to test rifampin (1 µg/ml) and ethambutol (5 µg/ml), are moderately susceptible to isoniazid (MICs 1 to 5 µg/ml) and are resistant to pyrazinamide. Currently, rifampin is the cornerstone of multiple drug therapy. Prior to rifampin therapy, the 6-month sputum conversion rates for pulmonary patients infected with *M. kansasii* were only 52 to 81% with a 10% relapse rate.[115,116] With multidrug therapy using rifampin, 100% of sputums converted within 4 months of therapy with only a 1.1% relapse rate.[116] The current recommendation of the American Thoracic Society for pulmonary infection caused by *M. kansasii* is the regimen of isoniazid (300 mg), rifampin (600 mg), and ethambutol (25 mg/kg for the first 2 months, then 15 mg/kg) given daily for 18 months with at least 12 months of negative sputum cultures.[58] Susceptibilities of untreated strains of *M. kansasii* are highly predictable and routine susceptibility testing (except for rifampin) is not needed.

In patients unable to tolerate one of the above medications, clarithromycin is an alternative, but its effectiveness has not been established by clinical trial. Addition of streptomycin at a dose of 1 g twice weekly for 3 months to the above regimen resulted in cure in 39 of 40 patients, and its addition may be of benefit in patients intolerant to the above regimen.[58]

In patients who develop rifampin-resistant *M. kansasii*, a daily regimen, lasting 18 to 24 months, of isoniazid (900 mg plus pyridoxine), ethambutol (25 mg/kg for the duration), trimethoprim-sulfamethoxazole (160/800 mg three times/day), and streptomycin (3 to 6 months only) has been used with excellent success.[117] The follow-up report from this study indicates that long-term sputum conversion can be accomplished in 90% of patients (mean onset of negative cultures, 11 weeks) using the above therapy.[118] Caution should be exercised, and symptoms and liver function tests should be monitored very closely when using these high doses of isoniazid; higher doses of pyridoxine should be used liberally. Recent data indicates that clarithromycin is highly active against both rifampin-susceptible and rifampin-resistant strains of *M. kansasii* with mean MICs of ≤ 0.25 µg/ml. Given its success with other mycobacterial diseases, clarithromycin would seem to be a reasonable agent to include in future retreatment regimens, perhaps in place of the more toxic streptomycin.

4. Rapidly Growing Mycobacteria

More than 90% of clinical disease caused by the RGM is caused by *M. fortuitum, M. abscessus,* and *M. chelonae*.[58] These three mycobacteria are resistant to most antituberculous agents, but are variably susceptible (*M. fortuitum* is more susceptible than *M. abscessus* which is more susceptible than *M. chelonae*) to a number of traditional antibiotics including amikacin, fluorinated quinolones, sulfonamides, cefoxitin, imipenem, and doxycycline. Isolates of *M. fortuitum* are susceptible or intermediate to clarithromycin (80%),[119] ciprofloxacin, ofloxacin (100%), amikacin (100%), sulfonamides (90%), imipenem (100%), cefoxitin (95%), and doxycycline (50%). Isolates of *M.*

abscessus are less susceptible than *M. fortuitum,* and 20% or fewer of *M. chelonae* isolates were susceptible to doxycycline, ciprofloxacin, ofloxacin, and sulfamethoxazole. However, 100% of both *M. chelonae* and *M. abscessus* are susceptible *in vitro* to low concentrations of clarithromycin,[119] and this agent has been proven highly successful in the treatment of localized and disseminated skin and soft tissue disease. Resistance to clarithromycin due to a point mutation at adenine 2058 or 2059 in the 23S ribosomal DNA occurs in approximately 10% of cases on monotherapy in disseminated disease caused by these two species,[102] but has not been seen with therapy of localized wound infections. The new drug, linezolid, offers some promise for treatment of *M. fortuitum* and *M. chelonae* (unpublished data). Due to the variability in drug susceptibility between and within species of the RGM, drug susceptibility testing should be performed on all initial isolates. As noted, mutational resistance during therapy can occur with clarithromycin, the newer quinolones, and the aminoglycosides with *M. abscessus,* so repeat testing of treatment failures also is indicated.[58]

5. *Mycobacterium marinum*

M. marinum disease has been treated using several different approaches:

1. Simple observation for minor cutaneous infection.
2. Surgical excision.
3. Single and multiple drug therapy.

Isolates of *M. marinum* are susceptible to antituberculous concentrations of rifampin and ethambutol. They have intermediate susceptibility to sulfonamides (including trimethoprim-sulfamethoxazole), doxycycline, amikacin, kanamycin, and streptomycin, and are resistant to isoniazid.[120-122] Recent studies have shown 100% of isolates to be susceptible to 4 µg/ml or less of clarithromycin.[104] Acceptable single-drug regimens include minocycline or doxycycline at 100 mg twice a day, trimethoprim-sulfamethoxazole at 160/800 mg two to three times a day, and perhaps clarithromycin. Acceptable dual-drug therapy is rifampin (600 mg) and ethambutol (15 mg/kg) daily. The optimal duration of therapy is unknown, but a minimum of 3 months, or 4 weeks after clearing of symptoms, seems acceptable.[58] Surgical debridement sometimes is indicated and most prescribe antibiotics during the perioperative period. Since the clinical response rate varies, additional therapeutic options should not be started any earlier than 3 weeks following initiation of therapy. As many as 80% of skin lesions may spontaneously resolve without therapy within 36 months.[123]

6. Other Mycobacteria

Most *M. xenopi* isolates show varying resistance to first-line antituberculous agents, but are susceptible to streptomycin, kanamycin, ethionamide, cycloserine,[124] the macrolides,[125] and the fluorinated quinolones (ciprofloxacin and ofloxacin).[126] Because drug susceptibilities are predictable, routine susceptibility testing with this species is not recommended.[58] Results from drug therapy in the premacrolide era were unpredictable, sometimes poor, and not related to the results of *in vitro* drug susceptibility tests.[127] A recent study which included a clarithromycin containing regimen demonstrated an excellent sputum conversion rate compared to previous studies, although the duration of therapy and relapse rates are not known.[128] Therefore, most patients with *M. xenopi* infection should be started on a macrolide, rifampin or rifabutin, ethambutol, and possibly streptomycin. Patients that fail therapy might be considered for surgery. Parrot and Grosset[127] studied the outcome of surgery in 57 patients with *M. xenopi* disease who failed to respond adequately to chemotherapy (the premacrolide era). Only 21 of these patients were cured of their *M. xenopi* infection without experiencing significant complications.

Skin infections due to *M. haemophilum* are typically the result of disseminated disease often involving the extremities. Isolates of *M. haemophilum* have shown *in vitro* resistance to most drugs tested with the exception of rifampin and rifabutin, the newer quinolones, and clarithromycin. A current treatment regimen includes one of each of these three drug groups.[58] Drugs tested include rifampin, isoniazid, streptomycin, ethambutol, *p*-aminosalicylic acid, capreomycin, kanamycin, gentamicin, amikacin, cefoxitin, sulfamethoxazole, ciprofloxacin, and clofazimine.[129]

M. malmoense isolates usually are susceptible to ethambutol and many are susceptible to streptomycin and rifampin. Treatment with the four-drug regimen of isoniazid, rifampin, ethambutol, and streptomycin has resulted in clinical responses in most cases. The role of the newer macrolides and rifabutin in treating *M. malmoense* infections has not been determined.[58]

M. simiae isolates are resistant to all first-line antituberculosis medications. Patients with progressive pulmonary disease should have their isolate sent for antimicrobial susceptibility testing to guide therapy. Initial therapy could include clarithromycin, ethambutol, and streptomycin despite *in vitro* results. They are one of the few slow growing NTM with high level resistance (>32 µg/ml) to both rifampin and rifabutin. Many isolates are treatable with clarithromycin, but the MICs often range from 8 to 32 µg/ml.[58]

Susceptibilities to *M. szulgai* are similar to the closely related *M. kansasii. M. szulgai* is usually susceptible to rifampin and higher concentrations of isoniazid, ethambutol, and streptomycin. Although infection is very rare, isolation of *M. szulgai* indicates true infection.[58]

III. NONTUBERCULOUS MYCOBACTERIA: HIV

A. EPIDEMIOLOGY

Since the advent and recognition of the AIDS epidemic in the early 1980s, the prevalence of mycobacterial disease has risen concurrently with the proliferation of patients infected with HIV. In 1985, the incidence of disease due to *M. tuberculosis* in the U.S. increased for the first time in more than 2 decades.[130] Infection due to MAC likewise has risen in a spectacular fashion. Before the AIDS epidemic, MAC disease was essentially limited to lymph node disease in children and chronic pulmonary disease in elderly patients with underlying lung disease. Extrapulmonary MAC disease and, in particular, disseminated MAC disease, was rare. Before 1980, only 24 cases of disseminated MAC disease had been reported in the medical literature.[131] By the end of 1990, 7.6% (12,202 of 161,073) of all AIDS patients reported to the CDC had disseminated nontuberculous mycobacterial infection.[131]

During the mid 1990s, however, two significant medical advances helped control the emerging epidemic. First, effective antiretroviral therapy (specifically, the use of protease inhibitors) dramatically improved the care of HIV-infected individuals. Although the number of HIV-infected individuals continued to rise, the number of patients with AIDS stabilized or decreased. Thus, fewer patients were at risk for developing disseminated MAC. The second advance was the advent of effective prophylaxis for MAC.[109,132] Studies published in 1996 demonstrated that clarithromycin prophylaxis decreased the incidence of disseminated *M. avium* from 16 to 6% in patients with CD4 cell counts below 100, and significantly decreased overall mortality.[132] However, with an increasing incidence of retroviral-resistant HIV and macrolide-resistant MAC, the future of this benefit is uncertain.

Disseminated MAC disease (D-MAC) in AIDS patients accounts for over 96% of NTM disseminated illness, followed by *M. kansasii* (2.9%), *M. gordonae, M. fortuitum, M. chelonae,*[133] *M. xenopi, M. haemophilum,*[133] and newer mycobacteria such as *M. genavense.*

Case-surveillance information may markedly underestimate the true prevalence of D-MAC infection in AIDS patients because reporting often occurs only at the time of diagnosis. Premortem diagnosis rates for this illness vary from 18 to 28% and postmortem prevalences range above 50%, especially during the early years of the AIDS epidemic when the significance of the organism was not appreciated.[134-136] Figure 9.2 shows by month the percentage of patients developing MAC bacteremia after the diagnosis of AIDS has been made.[137] In the U.S. and other developed countries, MAC is the most commonly isolated mycobacteria in patients infected with HIV.[134] The incidence

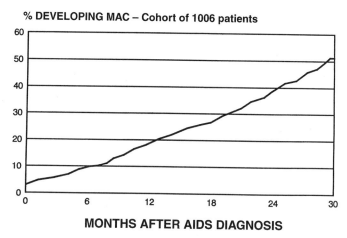

FIGURE 9.2   The percentage of patients developing MAC bacteremia by month after the diagnosis of AIDS. (From Nightingale, S. D., et al., *J. Infect. Dis.*, 165, 1082, 1992. With permission.)

of D-MAC has fallen dramatically over the past several years with the use of highly active antiretroviral therapy.

The distribution of D-MAC among AIDS patients in the U.S. appears to be fairly uniform in that it relates to the distribution of AIDS cases and not the geographic location of the cases. This is in striking contrast to the localized geographic distribution seen in non-AIDS patients with lung disease. The latter parallels the environmental recovery of the organism (e.g., commonly recovered in the southeastern coastal states). In Europe and Australia a similar pattern of distribution is seen in the AIDS patient populations. Only in Africa has there been a dearth of reported AIDS cases with disseminated MAC. In a 1990 report from Uganda, all of 50 severely ill AIDS patients were blood culture negative for MAC.[138]

A CD4 cell count of less than 60 cells per cubic millimeter is the major risk factor for this illness (Figure 9.3).[131,135,137] The majority of patients have CD4 counts less than 20 at the time of D-MAC diagnosis. This corresponds to the late development of MAC infection in patients with AIDS and to a shortened survival time (median, 7.5 months) compared with other AIDS patients (median, 13.3 months).[133] Disseminated NTM disease has been seen less in AIDS cases with

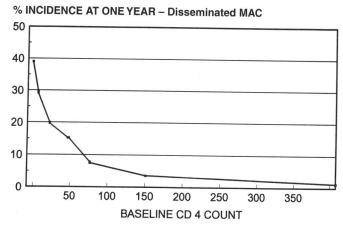

FIGURE 9.3   The incidence of MAC bacteremia at 1 year in relationship to the baseline CD4 cell count. (From Nightingale, S. D., et al., *J. Infect. Dis.*, 165, 1082, 1992. With permission.)

Kaposi's sarcoma than in other AIDS cases.[133] The frequency of D-MAC infection is similar for both sexes and for persons with various HIV risk factors. Overall, Hispanics have less infection than non-Hispanic whites and Blacks. This infection is more common in younger age groups and the frequency of infection decreases with age.[131]

Based on the use of the species-specific DNA probe, more than 90% of AIDS patients in the U.S. with D-MAC are infected with strains of *M. avium;* these isolates most commonly are serotypes 4 and 8.[131,139] This is in contrast to pulmonary disease, where *M. intracellulare* is the current predominant species and includes numerous different serotypes. The *M. avium* strains recovered from AIDS patients tend to be more virulent than other MAC isolates in animal models.[140]

The second most common NTM in AIDS patients is *M. kansasii*. Two retrospective studies[141,142] describe a total of 28 AIDS patients infected with *M. kansasii*, 22 with pulmonary disease, 4 with pulmonary and extrapulmonary disease, 5 with extrapulmonary disease only, and 10 with positive blood cultures or disseminated disease. The extrapulmonary disease involved one case of osteo-myelitis and two cases of gastrointestinal involvement. Only three patients had normal chest x-rays. Thin-walled cavitary lesions were present in 9 of 19 patients in one study and in none of 9 patients in the other study. Other chest film patterns were heterogeneous with focal upper lobe infiltrates or diffuse interstitial infiltrates being somewhat common. The infection occurred late in the AIDS illness with a median CD4 lymphocyte count of 49 in the larger study.[142]

A more recent study from Louisiana of 49 HIV-infected patients with *M. kansasii* demonstrated that the average patient had a CD4 count of 62/mm^3, and a mean interval of 17 months from the diagnosis of AIDS. Of these 49 patients, 17 had disseminated disease, 29 had AFB-positive sputum smears, 35 were cigarette smokers, and only 1 was thought to have *M. kansasii* colonization without disease. At the time of initial diagnosis, 13 had concurrent pulmonary infiltrates and 15 had another NTM isolated from the sputum. Antimycobacterial therapy decreased mortality in these patients.[143] It is unknown if the number of drugs or duration of therapy for *M. kansasii* should differ in AIDS patients vs. non-AIDS patients. Rifampin is replaced with rifabutin (150 mg daily) or clarithromycin (500 mg BID) in patients on protease inhibitors.[58]

In a study from Brooklyn, NY, 23 patients with AIDS and pulmonary *M. xenopi* infection were described briefly.[23] Only one of these patients had bacteremia due to *M. xenopi*. Six of these patients had clearing of pulmonary symptoms without therapy; none were treated for their pulmonary infections due to *M. xenopi*. In this same study, only 5 (15%) of 34 patients with disease due to *M. fortuitum* or *M. chelonae* had concomitant HIV infection.[143] Another study from Buffalo, NY evaluated 35 HIV-positive patients with pulmonary disease due to NTMs other than MAC and *M. kansasii*. Of these 35 patients, 66% were infected with *M. xenopi*.[144] These patients were more likely than the HIV-negative patients to present with fever. Adenopathy was not a feature and was thought suggestive of an alternative diagnosis. Chest radiographs showed a tendency toward inter-stitial infiltrates. No specific radiographic pattern was diagnostic for any particular NTM. In two patients, pulmonary disease preceded disseminated disease.

Infection due to *M. haemophilum* occurs primarily in immunocompromised hosts, but initially only a few cases (less than 20) were reported in patients infected with HIV. In 1992 a larger number of patients were recognized in New York City. In the reported cases, the median age at diagnosis was 34 years old.[145] The organisms were isolated in this group of patients from multiple sites and blood, suggesting disseminated disease. CD4 cell counts were markedly depressed with *M. hae-mophilum* infection being the AIDS-defining illness in only one case. Therapy using a variety of antimycobacterial agents showed a favorable response to therapy with decreased symptoms, but all relapsed shortly after discontinuation of antibiotic therapy.

M. genavense is a recently described mycobacterium which has been isolated from the blood, bone marrow, liver, spleen, lymph nodes, and intestinal cultures in 2,[146] 7,[147] and 18[148] patients with AIDS in Australia, Seattle, and Europe, respectively. The first patients were from Geneva, Swit-zerland; hence, the organism's name. These patients had advanced AIDS with low CD4 counts and typically presented with fever, weight loss, and diarrhea, indistinguishable from the presentation of D-MAC.

B. Pathogenesis

While the pathogenesis of D-MAC infection in AIDS patients is not fully understood, it appears that this infection results from primary infection rather than reactivation. The portal of entry for MAC infection in the AIDS patients appears to be the gastrointestinal tract rather than the respiratory tract. Common gastrointestinal symptoms in AIDS patients such as nausea, diarrhea, abdominal pain, and biliary tract obstruction lend support to this notion. Further support comes from studies in which MAC is recovered more frequently from lymphoid tissue in the gastrointestinal tract than from respiratory tissues.[149,150] The reservoir for MAC is presumed to be the usual soil and natural water supplies implicated in MAC lung disease, although as many as 10% of isolates in some series match hospital water supply isolates and may well be nosocomial.

Since AIDS patients are uniquely and highly vulnerable to MAC infection, cell-mediated immunity is considered to be the main defense against infection with this organism. Phagocytosis seems to be intact while macrophage-mediated killing seems to be defective. This may be related to the role of lymphokines such as interleukin-2, tumor necrosis factor, and granulocyte-macrophage colony-stimulating factor.[131]

Autopsies of cases with advanced disease show that the infected organ is enlarged, and it is yellow because of pigmentation from great quantities of the organisms (nearly 10^{10} colony-forming units per gram).[131] Microscopic exam reveals many organisms, reduced inflammatory reaction, and few and poorly formed granulomas.

C. Clinical Manifestations

Early in the AIDS epidemic the clinical presentation of D-MAC was variable and often mimicked other signs and symptoms associated with AIDS. Persistent fever, weight loss, night sweats, abdominal pain, and diarrhea were the most common and significant presenting symptoms. Today, however, clinicians are better at recognizing MAC disease in AIDS patients, and most patients with MAC are diagnosed after presenting with fever. Although localized disease is uncommon in AIDS patients, pulmonary nodules, pulmonary infiltrates, soft tissue abscesses, osteomyelitis, lymphad-enitis, and skin infections are well described. Gastrointestinal manifestations include diarrhea, abdominal pain, malabsorption, and obstructive jaundice. Severe anemia, often requiring transfusions, and neutropenia also may be present in advanced disease.[150] A few patients with positive blood cultures for MAC may (at least initially) be asymptomatic.

D. Diagnosis

Diagnosis of MAC or other NTM disease in the AIDS patient typically is made when the organism is cultured from normally sterile body fluid or tissue. Blood is now the most common site of positive cultures. Less common sites include bone marrow, liver, lymph nodes, spleen, eyes, brain, meninges, cerebrospinal fluid, tongue, skin, heart, stomach, lungs, thyroid, breasts, parathyroids, adrenals, kidneys, pancreas, prostate, testes, and urine.[149,150] Because of the ease of acquisition and almost uniform positivity in D-MAC, blood cultures for MAC are the usual method for making or excluding the diagnosis. When the organism is cultured from nonsterile sites such as feces or sputum, colonization or localized disease must be differentiated from D-MAC disease. Direct examination of blood films can provide rapid diagnosis of mycobacteremia in some AIDS patients with high-grade bacteremia. Eng and colleagues[151] found 13 of 15 patients who were culture positive for mycobacteria (14 with MAC, 1 with *M. tuberculosis)* and had identifiable organisms on Kinyoun- or auramine-stained buffy coat blood smears.

A retrospective analysis of abdominal computed tomography (CT) scans in 24 patients with MAC-positive blood cultures demonstrated that 42% had enlarged intraabdominal mesenteric and/or retroperitoneal lymph nodes.[152] Hepatomegaly, splenomegaly, and small bowel thickening were found in 50%, 46%, and 14% of patients respectively. Normal abdominal CT scans were seen in 25% of patients, thus demonstrating that a normal CT scan does not exclude the diagnosis of D-MAC. This study was performed prior to our current understanding of MAC disease in AIDS patients and, therefore, likely represents patients with high-grade bacteremia and long-standing disease. Thus, the high incidence of lymphadenopathy, hepatomegaly, and splenomegaly seen in this study may overestimate the current incidence.

E. TREATMENT

Therapy for D-MAC has been difficult because the organism is resistant to standard antimycobacterial agents, and controlled studies have been difficult to perform. This is especially true when antiretroviral agents or drugs for other opportunistic infections are used concurrently. Early trials of therapy for D-MAC were discouraging, in part because the organism burden was very high and the expected response times were probably unrealistic.

A dramatic improvement in early clinical and microbiologic responses was seen in trials containing the newer macrolides, azithromycin[153] and clarithromycin.[154] In a randomized, double-blind, placebo-controlled trial, Dautzenberg et al. showed that clarithromycin alone was more effective against D-MAC than placebo plus four other drugs (Figure 9.4).[154] A dose response study comparing daily doses of 1, 2, and 4 g of clarithromycin showed that patients cleared their mycobacteremia more rapidly at higher doses, but limiting side effects (gastrointestinal and hepatic) were greater.[155] Furthermore, unexplained early mortality was observed in patients receiving higher doses of clarithromycin, a trend that was repeated in several subsequent studies (see paragraph below on clarithromycin dosing). The development of MAC resistance to clarithromycin with clinical and microbiologic relapse occurs in most patients who receive macrolide monotherapy. This contrasts with approximately 20% of isolates from patients who receive clarithromycin as part of a multidrug regimen.[156]

Several different multidrug regimens have been used for therapy. Initially, regimens included ciprofloxacin (750 mg twice daily), ethambutol (1000 mg or 15 mg/kg daily), and rifampin (600 mg daily) with either amikacin (7.5 mg/kg daily),[157] or clofazimine (100 mg once daily),[158] or all five drugs.[159]

The effectiveness of macrolide-based antimycobacterial therapy in AIDS patients was recently confirmed by a randomized prospective clinical trial. A study published by Shafran et al. in 1996 demonstrated the effectiveness of macrolide-based therapy over quinolone-based therapy.[160] In this study, 229 patients were randomly assigned to receive either rifampin, ethambutol, and clarithromycin, or rifampin, ethambutol, clofazimine, and ciprofloxacin. Patients on the three-drug, macrolide-based, regimen were more likely to clear their bacteremia (69 vs. 29%), and had an increased median survival (8.6 vs. 5.2 months). Late treatment failure was associated with the emergence of clarithromycin resistance in the initial MAC strain.

The optimal dose for clarithromycin in combination chemotherapy was recently evaluated. In a prospective randomized trial by Cohn et al., AIDS patients with culture confirmed disseminated MAC were placed on either 500 mg or 1000 mg of clarithromycin twice a day plus rifabutin (300 mg daily) and ethambutol (800 mg or 1200 mg per day depending on the patients size).[161] In another arm of the study, clofazamine (100 mg per day) was substituted for rifabutin. This study was discontinued by the Data and Safety Monitoring Board because of increased mortality (10 vs. 43%) in patients receiving the higher clarithromycin dose. No difference was demonstrated between rifabutin and clofazamine. This confirmed the findings of the earlier monotherapy trial of Chaison et al.[155] Thus, in treating MAC disease in AIDS patients, the maximum dose of clarithromycin should be 500 mg twice a day.

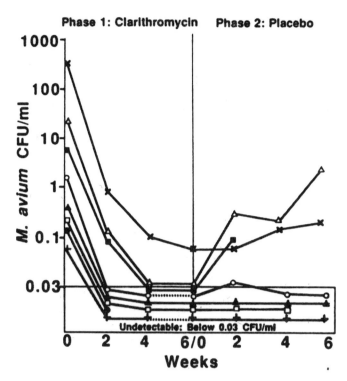

FIGURE 9.4 Changes in levels of *M. avium* bacteremia (colony-forming units, CFU) in eight patients initially receiving clarithromycin alone for 6 weeks (phase 1) and then receiving placebo plus a four-drug regimen (rifampin, isoniazid, ethambutol, and clofazimine) for 6 more weeks (phase 2). (From Dautzenberg, B., et al., *Am. Rev. Resp. Dis.,* 144, 564, 1991. With permission.)

Macrolide resistance appears to occur more readily to clarithromycin than azithromycin in both prophylaxis and treatment of D-MAC,[162] despite the fact that the same two mutations in the 23S ribosomal DNA (adenine 2058 and 2059) produce resistance to both drugs.[102] Mice infected with MAC were recently shown to be more likely to develop macrolide-resistant MAC when treated with clarithromycin than when treated with azithromycin. Although both medications demonstrated the ability to initially reduce the MAC burden in mice, macrolide resistance emerged in all of the clarithromycin-treated mice and none of the azithromycin-treated mice. The relevance of this study on human populations has not been determined at this time. The development of macrolide resistance was lower for azithromycin than clarithromycin in noncomparative prophylaxis trials as well.[163]

Ethambutol has been shown to decrease the development of MAC resistance to clarithromycin in AIDS patients. In patients treated with clarithromycin and clofazimine, the addition of ethambutol decreased the relapses at 36 weeks from 68 to 12%. All relapses were secondary to macrolide-resistant MAC.[156]

Clofazimine is now thought to have no value in the treatment of D-MAC. In fact, clofazimine has been shown by Chaisson et al. to increase the mortality of AIDS patients treated with clarithromycin and ethambutol.[163] In that study, 106 AIDS patients with D-MAC were randomized to receive clarithromycin, 500 mg twice daily, and ethambutol, 800 to 1000 mg daily, with or without clofazimine, 100 mg daily. During the study, 61% of the patients that received the three-drug regimen and 38% of the patients that received the two-drug regimen died.

Rifabutin has been shown to be efficacious against D-MAC. Sullam et al. compared rifabutin, 600 mg per day, to a placebo, each combined with clofazimine and ethambutol in a prospective D-MAC treatment trial.[164] At the end of 4 weeks of therapy, 7 of 11 patients receiving rifabutin and 0 of 13 patients receiving the placebo responded to therapy. Furthermore, *in vitro* data demonstrated a synergistic effect between rifabutin and clarithromycin against clinical MAC isolates. Ribabutin also has been shown to be effective in MAC prophylaxis,[109] and in a treatment trial when combined with clarithromycin and ethambutol.[160] However, a recent trial failed to demonstrate a beneficial effect of rifabutin over clofazimine when combined with clarithromycin and ethambutol.[156]

The potential role of highly active antiretroviral therapy in the treatment HIV-positive patients infected with D-MAC was demonstrated recently.[165] Four AIDS patients with D-MAC were treated with at least 12 months of macrolide-based antimycobacterial therapy in addition to effective protease inhibitor-based antiretroviral therapy. After completion of the antimycobacterial therapy, the patients remained asymptomatic and blood culture negative for mycobacteria. Thus, in patients with sustained CD4 lymphocyte increases following highly active antiretroviral therapy, D-MAC can be cured by a prolonged antimycobacterial regimen.

The interactions between antiretroviral medications and the standard tuberculosis medications are well outlined in Chapters 6, 11, and 13. The medications used to treat D-MAC, likewise, can interact with antiretroviral therapy. Ritonavir significantly inhibits the formation of 14-(R)-hydrox-yclarithromycin from clarithromycin, and increases the half life from 5 to 14 h.[166] The effect of clarithromycin on ritonivir levels is minimal, increasing the half life from 3.5 to 3.9 h. In patients with normal renal function, no adjustment in the doses of either medication is recommended. Clarithromycin increases rifabutin levels by almost 100% in AIDS patients, which may explain the increased frequency of uveitis observed with the concomitant use of these drugs.[167] Uveitis also has been demonstrated to correlate with patient size, with 14% of patients on clarithromycin, ethambutol, and rifabutin weighing over 65 kg developing uveitis, compared to 64% of patients weighing less than 55 kg.[168]

Despite combination antimycobacterial therapy, approximately one third of patients will remain bacteremic and some patients will relapse with macrolide-resistant organisms. Patients with AIDS and D-MAC can have progressive disease. Recently, the utility of adjunctive corticos-teroids for patients with refractory symptoms despite combination antimycobacterial therapy was examined.[169] This retrospective review examined 12 consecutive patients who failed MAC che-motherapy and who subsequently received low-dose oral corticosteroids in addition to continued combination antimycobacterial therapy. Eleven of 12 patients experienced a rapid improvement in symptoms, with diminished or resolved fevers and night sweats, and an increased sense of well-being and energy. Ten of 12 patients gained weight, and the weights achieved were similar to baseline weights prior to the development of MAC infection. However, new opportunistic pro-cesses developed in seven patients during corticosteroid therapy, which may or may not be related to the corticosteroid therapy.

Little information is currently available on the discontinuation of chronic maintenance therapy for patients who have been treated for D-MAC disease. Current recommendations are that these patients should continue on full therapeutic doses of antimycobacterial agents for life.

In summary, the cornerstone of current therapy for D-MAC in AIDS patients is macrolide therapy, usually consisting of clarithromycin dosed at 500 mg twice a day. Azithromycin (500 mg daily) also is effective. Ethambutol, dosed at 15 mg/kg (800 to 1000 mg) daily, is essential to prevent the development of macrolide resistance. Rifabutin (300 mg daily) is currently recom-mended in combination with the macrolide and ethambutol. Finally, initial data indicates that the addition of highly active antiretroviral therapy to D-MAC therapy may allow for cures of D-MAC.

F. PREVENTIVE THERAPY

Given the problems with therapy, the ideal or preferred approach to D-MAC would be disease prevention. Prophylactic chemotherapy currently is recommended for all HIV-infected adults and adolescents with CD4+ counts less than 50 cells/μl.[170] Three medications — rifabutin, clarithro-mycin, and azithromycin — have been shown to prevent D-MAC disease.

A randomized, double-blind, placebo-controlled trial of rifabutin (300 mg/day) in patients with CD4 counts of less than 200 showed that this drug was highly effective both in delaying and preventing D-MAC.[171] None of the breakthrough bacteremic isolates were resistant to rifabutin.

In 1996, the utility of macrolide-based chemoprophylaxis was demonstrated in a randomized, double-blinded, placebo-controlled trial.[132] Only 19 (6%) of 333 of AIDS patients with CD4+ counts less than 100 cells per μl, who were given clarithromycin prophylaxis, developed MAC infection, while 53 (16%) of 334 patients receiving a placebo developed MAC. Furthermore, mortality at 10 months decreased from 41 to 32% with prophylaxis. However, 11 of the 19 patients in the clarithromycin treatment arm who developed MAC had isolates resistant to clarithromycin.

Weekly azithromycin therapy (1200 mg once weekly) also was demonstrated recently to prevent D-MAC in AIDS patients with CD4 counts less than 100/mm^3.[172] A double-blind, placebo-controlled trial showed that 10.6% of patients on weekly azithromycin, and 24.7% of patients on placebo, developed D-MAC. No difference, however, was demonstrated in the total number of deaths, or the total time to death. Gastrointestinal side effects were common, occurring in 78.9% of the azithromycin group and 27.5% of the placebo group.

Recently, a double-blinded, randomized trial compared primary prophylaxis with azithromycin (1200 mg weekly), rifabutin (300 mg daily), or both drugs in 693 HIV-infected patients with CD4+ counts less than 100 cells per μl.[109] The incidence of D-MAC at 1 year was 7.6% in the azithromycin-treated patients, 15.3% in the rifabutin-treated patients, and 2.8% in patients receiving both medications. The combination therapy, however, was less well tolerated than monotherapy with azithromycin.

The currently preferred prophylatic regimen for D-MAC is macrolide therapy. Azithromycin is preferred over clarithromycin due to the absence of significant drug interactions, once-a-week dosing, and a lower incidence of resistance among breakthrough isolates. The addition of rifabutin to clarithromycin does not increase the effectiveness, is associated with a higher incidence of side effects, and should not be used routinely.[168] Rifabutin plus azithromycin, however, may be more effective than azithromycin alone.[109] This combination is not currently recommended because of the additional cost, increased number of side effects, and absence of survival benefit. It should be considered in patients with very low CD4 counts (<10) because the incidence of macrolide resistance with breakthrough bacteremia is high with macrolide monotherapy. If patients do not tolerate macrolide therapy, rifabutin may be used as an alternative. Before prophylaxis is started, disseminated MAC should be ruled out by clinical assessment and, possibly, a mycobacterial blood culture.

Currently there are no firm recommendations concerning discontinuing MAC prophylaxis for patients who respond well to antiretroviral therapy. Patients who achieve a sustained increase in their CD4+ cells to over 100 cell per μl seem to have a low rate of developing D-MAC. Some authorities suggest that, although optimal criteria have not yet been developed (1999), it is reasonable to consider discontinuing prophylaxis in these patients if they also have sustained suppression of their HIV plasma RNA.

IV. DISEASE DUE TO *MYCOBACTERIUM BOVIS* AND *M. BOVIS* BACILLUS CALMETTE-GUÉRIN (BCG)

Technically, *M. bovis* BCG and *M. bovis* are not NTMs, but are part of the tuberculosis spectrum of diseases.

A. *MYCOBACTERIUM BOVIS*

Although common 100 years ago, disease with *Mycobacterium bovis* is rare today, due to the pasteurization of milk, the slaughter of infected cattle, and the absence (especially in the U.S.) of common wild animal hosts. In the recent past, reports from various hospitals have shown only a handful of cases.[173-178] However, England and Wales have had a slightly higher percentage of cases, and from January 1986 to October 1991, 117 isolates, or 1.2% of the total number of mycobacterial isolates were identified as *M. bovis*.[178] Furthermore, in San Diego, Dankner et al. reported 73 cases (48 adults, 25 children) of *M. bovis* during the 12-year period from 1980 to 1991, accounting for almost 3% of all mycobacterial cases in San Diego during that time period.[179] Hispanics comprised the majority of cases, and Mexican cattle were thought to be a likely source. AIDS was present in 25% of adults and 4% of children with *M. bovis* disease. Pulmonary disease was present in 25 (52%) of adults and 3 (12%) of children.

Humans can become infected by drinking contaminated milk or by sharing a closed air space with a group of cows with pulmonary disease.[179] In cattle, the respiratory route is thought to be the primary route of infection.[180]

Extrapulmonary tuberculosis is present in a higher percentage of persons diseased with *M. bovis* than in those diseased with *M. tuberculosis*. The disease is not difficult to cure, but the treatment regimen cannot utilize pyrazinamide because the organism is resistant to this drug. There has been some confusion on this issue because of the similarity between *M. bovis* and *M. africanum*, and there has been discussion about whether *M. africanum* actually is a subvariant of *M. bovis*. Collins et al., in a series of 137 cases from southeast England, divided *M. bovis* into "classical" strains (n = 63), resistant to pyrazinamide, and "Afro-Asian" strains (n = 74), sensitive to pyrazinamide, and stated that the organisms in the "Afro-Asian" group that were also nitrate positive might be considered *M. africanum*.[181]

In general, treatment of this disease should be based on a nonpyrazinamide-containing regimen. It would be wise to use 9-month therapy starting with initial isoniazid, rifampin, and ethambutol followed by isoniazid and rifampin. Finally, recently, a strain of multidrug-resistant *M. bovis* was identified.[182] Thus, antibiotic susceptibility testing should be considered on clinical *M. bovis* isolates.

B. *M. bovis* Bacillus Calmette-Guérin

Immunization and cancer therapy with bacillus Calmette-Guérin (BCG) has produced localized lymphadenitis with and without abscess formation, pulmonary infection, osteomyelitis, cutaneous nodules, and other disseminated disease sometimes referred to as "BCGosis" or "BCGitis." BCG vaccine, a live attenuated vaccine derived from *M. bovis* is used worldwide (except in the U.S.) to prevent tuberculosis.

Intravesical instillation of BCG for bladder cancer therapy can produce localized cystitis, as well as disseminated disease involving the lungs and liver and, less frequently, the bone marrow, brain, kidney, prostate, and spleen.[183] There are 45,000 new cases of bladder cancer each year in the U.S.[183] From retrospective studies, it is estimated that as much as 1% of these cases treated with BCG therapy may experience BCGosis.[183] Only a small number of treated cases have been reported, but some have responded well to standard two-drug antituberculous therapy (isoniazid 300 mg/day and rifampin 600 mg/day). BCG, like wild strains of *M. bovis*, is resistant to pyrazinamide.

When BCG is administered to young infants, 0.5 to 5.0% will experience a localized injection abscess or regional (axillary) lymphadenitis.[184] This complication usually is benign, but often persists for 6 to 12 months. Therapy may, in some cases, shorten the duration of disease. Therapeutic options for infants include erythromycin (50 mg/kg/day in four divided doses) for 1 month, INH 5 to 10 mg/kg/day for 1 to 3 months, surgical removal, or local INH instillation (50 mg) into the abscess.[185] Disseminated disease occurs rarely (3.4 per 1 million) in newborns immunized with BCG, but when it does occur, it often is resistant to therapy and often is fatal.[186] Apparently, infants born to women infected with HIV are not at appreciably higher risk of adverse effects to BCG vaccine.[187] However, infants with other immunodeficiency syndromes probably are at severe risk of BCGosis and death from BCG vaccination.[186] Further information may be found in Chapter 15.

REFERENCES

1. Alvarex, E. and Tavel, E., Recherches sur le bacille de Lustgarten, *Arch. Physiol. Norm. Pathol.*, 3, 303, 1885.

2. Metchock, B. G., Nolte, F. S., and Wallace, R. J., Jr., 1999, Mycobacteria, in *Manual of Clinical Microbiology,* Murray, P. R., Baron, E. J., Pfaller, M. A., Tenover, F. C., and Yolken, R. H., Eds., Manual of Clinical Microbiology, ASM Press, Washington, D.C.

3. Timpe, A. and Runyon, E. H., The relationship of "atypical acid-fast" bacteria to human disease: a preliminary report, *J. Lab. Clin. Med.,* 44, 202, 1954.

4. Good, R. C., Isolation of nontuberculous mycobacteria in the United States, 1979, *J. Infect. Dis.*, 142, 779, 1980.

5. Good, R. C. and Snider, D. E. Jr., Isolation of nontuberculous mycobacteria from the United States, 1980, *J. Infect. Dis.,* 146, 829, 1982.

6. O'Brien, R. J., Geiter, L. J., and Snider, D. E., Jr., The epidemiology of nontuberculous mycobacterial diseases in the United States, *Am. Rev. Respir. Dis.*, 135, 1007, 1987.

7. Wayne, L. G. and Sramek, H. A., Agents of newly recognized or infrequently encountered mycobacterial diseases, *Clin. Microbiol. Rev.,* 5, 1, 1992.

8. Yamori, S. and Tsukamura, M., Comparison of prognosis of pulmonary diseases caused by *Mycobacterium avium* and by *Mycobacterium intracellulare*, *Chest,* 102, 89, 1992.

9. Tsang, A. Y., Drupa, I., Goldberg, M., McClatchy, J. K., and Brennan, P. J., Use of serology and thin-layer chromatography for the assembly of an authenticated collection of serovars within the *Mycobacterium-avium-Mycobacterium intracellulare-Mycobacterium scrofulaceum* complex, *Int. J. Syst. Bacteriol.,* 33, 285, 1983.

10. Shaefer, W. B., Serologic identification and classification of the atypical mycobacteria by their agglutination, *Am. Rev. Tuberc.,* 96, 115, 1967.

11. Wayne, L. G. and Sramek, H. A., Agents of newly recognized or infrequently encountered mycobacterial disease, *Clin. Microbiol. Rev.,* 5, 1, 1992.

12. Hector, J. S. R., Pang, Y., Mazurek, G. H., Zhang, Y., Brown, B., and Wallace, R. J., Jr., Large restriction fragment patterns of genomic *Mycobacterium fortuitum* DNA strain-specific markers and their use in epidemiologic investigation of four nosocomial outbreaks, *J. Clin. Microbiol.,* 30, 1250, 1992.

13. Mazurek, G. H., Hartman, S. L., Zhang, Y., Brown, B. A., Hector, J. S. R., Murphy, D., and Wallace, R. J., Jr., Large DNA restriction fragment polymorphism in the *Mycobacterium avium-M. intracellulare* complex: a potential epidemiologic tool, *J. Clin. Microbiol.,* 31, 390, 1993.

14. Edwards, L. B., Acquaviva, F. A., Livesay, V. T., and Palmer, C. E., An atlas of sensitivity to tuberculin, PPD, and histoplasmin in the United States, *Am. Rev. Respir. Dis.,* 99, 1, 1969.

15. Huebner, R. E., Schein, M. F., Cauthen, G. M., Geiter, L. J., Selin, M. J., Good, R. C., and O'Brien, R. J., Evaluation of the clinical usefulness of mycobacterial skin test antigens in adults with pulmonary mycobacterioses, *Am. Rev. Respir. Dis.,* 145, 1160, 1992.

16. Wijsmuller, G. and Erickson, P., The reaction to PPD-Battey: a new look, *Am. Rev. Respir. Dis.,* 29, 109, 1974.

17. Krajnack, M. A. and Dowda, H., Nontuberculous mycobacteria in South Carolina, 1971–1980, *J. S.C. Med. Assoc.,* 77, 551, 1981.

18. Edwards, F. G. B., Disease caused by "atypical" (opportunistist) mycobacteria: a whole population review, *Tubercle,* 51, 285, 1970.

19. Issac-Renton, J. L., Allen, E. A., Chao, C. W., Grzybowski, E., and Black, W. A., Isolation and geographic distribution of *Mycobacterium* other than *M. tuberculosis* in British Columbia, 1972–1981, *Can. Med. Assoc. J.,* 133, 573, 1985.

20. Banks, J., Hunter, A. M., Campbell, I. A., Jenkins, P. A., and Smith, A. P., Pulmonary infection with *Mycobacterium kansasii* in Wales, 1970–9: review of treatment and response, *Thorax,* 38, 271, 1983.

21. Tsukamura, M., Kita, N., Shimoide, H., Arakawa, H., and Kuze, A., Studies on the epidemiology of nontuberculous mycobacteriosis in Japan, *Am. Rev. Respir. Dis.,* 137, 1280, 1988.

22. Yates, M. D., Grange, J. M., and Collins, C. H., The nature of mycobacterial disease in southeast England, 1977–84, *J. Epidemiol. Comm. Health*, 40, 295, 1986.

23. Shafer, R. W. and Sierra, M. F., *Mycobacterium xenopi, Mycobacterium fortuitum, Mycobacterium kansasii,* and other nontuberculous mycobacteria in an area of endemicity for AIDS, *Clin. Infect. Dis.,* 15, 161, 1992.

24. Simor, A. E., Salit, I. E., and Vellend, H., The role of *Mycobacterium xenopi* in human disease, *Am. Rev. Respir. Dis.,* 129, 435, 1984.

25. Buchholz, U. T., McNeil, M. M., Keyes, L. E., and Good, R. C., *Mycobacterium malmoense* infections in the United States, January 1993 through June 1995, *Clin. Infect. Dis.,* 27, 551, 1998.

26. Henriques, B., Hoffner, S. E., Petrini, B., Juhlin, I., Wahlen, P., and Kallenius, G., Infection with *Mycobacterium malmoense* in Sweden: report of 221 cases, *Clin. Infect. Dis.,* 18, 596, 1994.

27. Yeager, H. and Raleigh, J. W., Pulmonary disease due to *Mycobacterium intracellulare, Am. Rev. Respir. Dis.,* 108, 547, 1979.

28a. Wright, P. W., Wallace, R. J., Jr., Wright, N. W., Brown, B., and Griffith, D. E., Sensitivity of fluorochrome microscopy for detection of *Mycobacterium tuberculosis* versus nontuberculous mycobacterium, *J. Clin. Microbiol.,* 36, 1046, 1998.

28b. Iseman, M. D., Buschman, D. L., and Ackerson, L. M., Pectus excavation and scoliosis: thoracic anomalies associated with pulmonary disease caused by *Mycobacterium avium* complex, *Am. Rev. Respir. Dis.,* 144, 914, 1991.

29. Reich, J. M. and Johnson, R. E., *Mycobacterium avium* complex pulmonary disease presenting as an isolated lingular or middle lobe pattern, *Chest,* 101, 1605, 1992.

30. Torrens, J. K., Dawkins, P., Conway, S. P., and Moya, E., Non-tuberculous mycobacteria in cystic fibrosis, *Thorax,* 53, 182, 1998.

31. Olivier, K. N., Yankaskas, J. R., and Knowles, M. R., Nontuberculous mycobacterial pulmonary disease in cystic fibrosis, *Sem. Respir. Infect.,* 11, 272, 1996.

32. Kilby, J. M., Gilligan, P. H., Yankaskas, J. R., Highsmith, W. E., Jr., Edwards, L. J., and Knowles, M. R., Nontuberculous mycobacteria in adult patients with cystic fibrosis, *Chest,* 102, 70, 1992.

33. Kamat, S. R., Rossiter, C. E., and Gilson, J. C., A retrospective clinical study of pulmonary disease due to "anonymous mycobacteria in Wales," *Thorax,* 16, 297, 1961.

34. Rosenzweig, D. Y., Pulmonary mycobacterial infections due to *Mycobacterium intracellulare-avium* complex: clinical features and course in 100 consecutive cases, *Chest,* 75, 115, 1979.

35. Griffith, D. E., Girard, W. M., and Wallace, R. J., Jr., Clinical features of pulmonary disease caused by rapidly growing mycobacteria: an analysis of 154 patients, *Am. Rev. Respir. Dis.,* 147, 1271, 1993.

36. Mammo, A., Epidemiologic trends of lung disease due to *Mycobacterium kansasii* and *Mycobacterium avium-intracellulare* in Texas, 1977–1983, Doctoral thesis, University of Texas Health Science Center at Houston, 1, 1983.

37. Johanson, W., Jr. and Nicholson, D., Pulmonary disease due to *Mycobacterium kansasii, Am. Rev. Respir. Dis.,* 99, 73, 1969.

38. Cowie, R. L., The mycobacteriology of pulmonary tuberculosis in South African gold miners, *Tubercle,* 71, 39, 1990.

39. Chapman, J. S., *The Atypical Mycobacteria and Human Mycobacteriosis,* Plenum Medical Book Co., New York, 1977, Chap. 5.

40. Thomas, P., Liu, F., and Weiser, W., Characteristics of *Mycobacterium xenopi* disease, *Bull. Int. Union Tuberc. Lung Dis.,* 6, 12, 1988.

41. Costrini, A. M., Mahler, D. A., Gross, W. M., Hawkins, J. E., Yesner, R., and D'Esposo, E., Clinical and roentgenographic features of nosocomial pulmonary disease due to *Mycobacterium xenopi, Am. Rev. Respir. Dis.,* 123, 104, 1981.

42. Huminer, D., Pitlik, S. D., Block, C., Kaufman, L., Amit, S., and Rosenfeld, J. B., Aquarium-borne *Mycobacterium marinum* skin infection, *Arch. Dermatol.,* 122, 698, 1986.

43. Dever, L. L., Martin, J. W., Seaworth, B., and Jorgensen, J. H., Varied presentations and responses to treatment of infections caused by *Mycobacterium haemophilum* in patients with AIDS, *Clin. Infect. Dis.,* 14, 1195, 1992.

44. Meissner, G. and Anz, W., Sources of *Mycobacterium avium* complex infection resulting in human diseases, *Am. Rev. Respir. Dis.,* 116, 1057, 1977.

45. Reznikov, M. and Dawson, D. J., Mycobacteria of the *intracellulare-scrofulaceum* group in soils from the Adelaide area, *Pathology,* 12, 525, 1980.

46. Nel, E. E., *Mycobacterium avium-intracellulare* complex serovars isolated in South Africa from humans, swine, and the environment, *Rev. Infect. Dis.*, 3, 1013, 1981.

47. Wolinsky, E. and Rynearson, T. K., Mycobacteria in soil and their relation to disease-associated strains, *Am. Rev. Respir. Dis.*, 97, 1032, 1968.

48. Collins, C. H., Grange, J. M., and Yates, M. D., Mycobacteria in water, *J. Appl. Bacteriol.*, 57, 193, 1984.

49. Reznikov, M., Leggo, J. H., and Dawson, D. J., Investigation by seroagglutination of strains of the *Mycobacterium intracellulare-M. scrofulaceum* group from house dusts and sputum in southeastern Queensland, *Am. Rev. Respir. Dis.*, 104, 951, 1974.

50. Thoen, C. O. and Karson, A. G., Tuberculosis, in Hoffstead, M. S., Calnek, B. W., and Helmboldt, C. F., Eds., *Disease of Poultry*, 7th ed, Iowa State University Press, Ames, 209, 1978.

51. Montali, R. J., Bush, M., Thoen, C. O., and Smith, E., Tuberculosis in captive exotic birds, *J. Am. Vet. Med. Assoc.*, 169, 920, 1976.

52. Chapman, J. S., Isolation of atypical mycobacteria from pasteurized milk, *Am. Rev. Respir. Dis.*, 98, 1052, 1968.

53. Engbaek, H. C., Vergmann, B., Baiss, I., and Bentzon, M. W., *Mycobacterium avium:* a bacteriological and epidemiological study of *M. avium* isolated from animals and man in Denmark. II. Strains isolated from man, *Acta Pathol. Microbiol. Scand.*, 72, 295, 1968.

54. Kirschner, R. A., Parker, B. C., and Falkinham, J. O., III., Epidemiology of infection by nontuberculous mycobacteria, *Am. Rev. Respir. Dis.*, 145, 271, 1992.

55. Falkinham, J. O., III., Parker, B. C., and Gruft, H., Epidemiology of infection by nontuberculous mycobacteria. I. Geographic distribution in the eastern United States, *Am. Rev. Respir. Dis.*, 121, 931, 1980.

56. Fraser, V. J., Jones, M., Murray, P. R., Medoff, G., Zhang, Y., and Wallace, R. J., Jr., Contamination of flexible fiberoptic bronchoscopes with *Mycobacterium chelonae* linked to an automated broncho-scope disinfection machine, *Am. Rev. Respir. Dis.*, 145, 853, 1992.

57. Raad, I. I., Vartivarian, S., Khan, A., and Bodey, G. P., Catheter-related infections caused by the *Mycobacterium fortuitum* complex: 15 cases and review, *Rev. Infect. Dis.*, 13, 1120, 1991.

58. Wallace, R. J., Jr., Glassroth, J., Griffith, D. E., Olivier, K. N., Cook, J. L., and Gordin, F., Diagnosis and treatment of disease caused by nontuberculous mycobacteria (an official statement of the ATS), *Am. J. Respir. Crit. Care Med.*, 156, S1, 1997.

59. Wallace, R. J., Jr., Swenson, J. M. , Silcox, V. A., Good, R. C., Tschen, J. A., and Stone, M. S., Spectrum of disease due to rapidly growing mycobacteria, *Rev. Infect. Dis.*, 5, 657, 1983.

60. Engel, H. W. B., Berwald, L. G., and Havelaar, A. H., The occurrence of *Mycobacterium kansasii* in tap water, *Tubercle,* 61, 21, 1980.

61. Janning, R. S. B. and Fischeder, J. R., Occurrence of mycobacteria in biofilm samples, *Tubercle Lung Dis.*, 73, 141, 1992.

62. Bailey, R. K., Wyles, S., Dingley, M., Hesse, F., and Kent, G. W., The isolation of high catalase *Mycobacterium kansasii* from tap water, *Am. Rev. Respir. Dis.*, 101, 430, 1970.

63. Reznikow, M., Leggo, J. H., and Dawson, D. J., Investigation by Sero-agglutination of strains of *Mycobacterium intracellulare-Mycobacterium scrofulaceum* group house dusts and sputum in south-eastern Queensland, *Am. Rev. Respir. Dis.*, 104, 951, 1971.

64. Wolinsky, E., State of the art — nontuberculous mycobacteria and associated diseases, *Am. Rev. Respir. Dis.*, 199, 107, 1979.

65. Philpott, J. A., Woodburne, A. R., Philpott, O. S., Schaefer, O. S., and Mollohan, C. S., Swimming pool granuloma: a study of 290 cases, *Arch. Dermatol.*, 88, 94, 1963.

66. Keczkes, K., Tropical fish tank granuloma, *Br. J. Dermatol.*, 91, 709, 1974.

67. Arai, H., Nakajima, H., and Nagai, R., *Mycobacterium marinum* infections of the skin in Japan, *J. Dermatol.*, 11, 37, 1984.

68. Chow, S. P., Stroebel, A. B., Lau, J. K., and Collins, R. J., *Mycobacterium marinum* infection of the hand involving deep structures, *J. Hand. Surg.*, 8, 568, 1983.

69. Faoagali, J. L., Muir, A. D., Sears, P. J., and Paltridge, G. P., Tropical fish tank granuloma, *N. Z. Med. J.*, 85, 332, 1977.

70. MacLellan, D. G. and Moon, M., Fish tank granuloma: a diagnostic dilemma, *Aust. N. Z. J. Surg.*, 8, 568, 1982.

71. Brown, J., Kelm, M., and Bryan, L. E., Infection of the skin by *Mycobacterium marinum*: report of five cases, *Can. Med. Assoc. J.*, 117, 912, 1989.

72. Du Moulin, G. C., Stottmeier, K. D., Pelletier, P. A., Tsang, A. Y., and Hedley-Whyte, J., Concentration of *Mycobacterium avium* by hospital hot water system, *JAMA*, 260, 1599, 1988.

73. Geppert, E. F. and Feff, A., The pathogenesis of pulmonary and miliary tuberculosis, *Arch. Intern. Med.*, 139, 1381, 1979.

74. Woodring, J. H. and MacVandiviere, H., Pulmonary disease caused by nontuberculous mycobacteria, *J. Thorac. Imag.*, 5, 64, 1990.

75. George, K. M., Chatterjee, D., Gunawardana, G., Welty, D., Hayman, J., Lee, R., and Small, P. L. C., Mycolactone: a polyketide toxin from *Mycobacterium ulcerans* required for virulence, *Science*, 283, 854, 1999.

76. Johnston, J. M. and Izumi, A. K., Cutaneous *Mycobacterium marinum* infection ("swimming pool granuloma"), *Clin. Dermatol.*, 5, 68, 1987.

77. Dattwyler, R. J., Thomas, J., and Hurst, L. C., Antigen-specific T-cell anergy in progressive *Mycobacterium marinum* infections in humans, *Ann. Intern. Med.*, 107, 675, 1987.

78. Ahn, C. H., McLarty, J. W., Ahn, S. S., Ahn, S. I., and Hurst, G. A., Diagnostic criteria for pulmonary disease caused by *Mycobacterium kansasii* and *Mycobacterium intracellulare*, *Am. Rev. Respir. Dis.*, 125, 388, 1982.

79. Konstan, M. W. and Berger, M., Infection and inflamation of the lung in cystic fibrosis, in Davis, P. B., Ed., *Cystic Fibrosis*, Marcel Dekker, New York, 219, 1993.

80. Herrod, H. G., Rourk, M. H., Jr., and Spock, A., Pulmonary disease in children caused by nontuberculous mycobacteria, *J. Pediatr.*, 94, 915, 1979.

81. Tsukamura, M., Diagnosis of disease caused by *Mycobacterium avium* complex, *Chest*, 99, 667, 1991.

82. Lai, K. K., Stottmeir, K. D., Sherman, I. H., and McCabe, W. R., Mycobacterial cervical lymphadenopathy: relation of etiologic agents to age, *JAMA*, 251, 1286, 1984.

83. Schaad, H. B., Votteler, P., McCracken, G. H., Jr., and Nelson, J. D., Management of atypical mycobacterial lymphadenitis in childhood: a review based on 380 cases, *J. Pediatr.*, 95, 356, 1979.

84. Feingold, D., *Mycobacterium marinum* granuloma, *Arch. Dermatol.*, 114, 1564, 1978.

85. Wallace, R. J., Jr., The clinical presentation, diagnosis, and therapy of cutaneous and pulmonary infections due to the rapidly growing mycobacteria, *M. fortuitum* and *M. chelonae*, *Clin. Chest Med.*, 10, 419, 1989.

86. McBride, M. E., Rudolph, A. H., Tschen, J. A., Cernoch, P., Davis, J., Brown, B. A., and Wallace, R. J., Jr., Diagnostic and therapeutic considerations for cutaneous *Mycobacterium haemophilum* infections, *Arch. Dermatol.*, 127, 276, 1991.

87. Radford, A. J., *Mycobacterium ulcerans* in Australia, *Aust. N. Z. J. Med.*, 5, 162, 1975.

88. Sutker, W. L., Lankford, L. L., and Tompsett, R., Granulomatous synovitis: the role of atypical mycobacteria, *Rev. Infect. Dis.*, 1, 729, 1979.

89. Maricic, M. J. and Alepa, E. P., Reactive arthritis after *Mycobacterium avium-intracellulare* infection: Poncet's disease revisited, *Am. J. Med.*, 88, 549, 1990.

90. Wardrop, P. A. and Pillsbury, H. C., III, *Mycobacterium avium* acute mastoiditis, *Arch. Otolaryngol.*, 110, 686, 1984.

91. Beckman, E. N., Pankey, G. A., and McFarland, G. B., The histopathology of *Mycobacterium marinum* synovitis, *J. Clin. Pathol.*, 83, 457, 1985.

92. Turner, L. and Stinson, I., Mycobacterium fortuitum as a cause of corneal ulcer, *Am. J. Ophthalmol.*, 60, 329, 1965.

93. Huang, S. C. M., Soong, H. K., Chang, J. S., and Liang Y. S., Nontuberculous mycobacterial keratitis: a study of 22 cases, *Br. J. Ophthalmol.*, 80, 962, 1996.

94. Bennett, C., Vardiman, J., and Golomb, H., Disseminated atypical mycobacterial infection in patients with hairy cell leukemia, *Am. J. Med.*, 80, 891, 1986.

95. Lichtenstein, I. H. and MacGregor, R. R., Mycobacterial infections in renal transplant recipients: report of five cases and review of the literature, *Rev. Infect. Dis.*, 5, 216, 1983.

96. Horsburgh, C. R., Jr., Mason, U. G., III, Farhi, D. C., and Iseman, M. D., Disseminated infection with *Mycobacterium avium-intracellulare*: a report of 13 cases and a review of the literature, *Medicine*, 64, 36, 1985.

97. Wallace, R. J., Jr., Brown, B. A., and Onyi, G. O., Skin, soft tissue, and bone infections due to *Mycobacterium chelonae*: importance of prior corticosteroid therapy, frequency of disseminated infections, and resistance to oral antimicrobials other than clarithromycin, *J. Infect. Dis.*, 166, 405, 1992.

98. Lincoln, E. M. and Gilbert, L. A., Disease in children due to Mycobacteria other than *Mycobacterium tuberculosis, Am. Rev. Respir. Dis.*, 105, 683, 1972.

99. Ichiyama, S., Ito, Y., Sugiura, F., Iinuma, Y., Yamori, S., Shimojima, M., Hasegawa, Y., Shimokata, K., and Nakashima, N., Diagnostic value of the strand displacement amplification method compared to those of Roche Amplicor PCR and culture for detecting mycobacteria in sputum samples, *J. Clin. Microbiol.*, 35, 3082, 1997.

100. Sansila, A., Hongmanee, P., Chuchottaworn, C., Reinthong, S., Reinthong, D., and Palittapongarnpim, P., Differentiation between *Mycobacterium tuberculosis* and *Mycobacterium avium* by amplification of the 16 S-23S ribosomal DNA spacer, *J. Clin. Microbiol.*, 36, 2399, 1998.

101. Eriks, I. S., Munck, K. T., Besser, T. E., Cantor, G. H., and Kapur, V., Rapid differentiation of *Mycobacterium avium* and *M. paratuberculosis* by PCR and restriction enzyme analysis, *J. Clin. Microbiol.*, 34, 734, 1996.

102. Sander, P., Prammananan, T., Meier, A., Frischkorn, K., and Bottger, E. C., The role of ribosomal RNAs in macrolide resistance, *Mol. Microbiol.*, 26,469, 1997.

103. Corpe, R. F., Surgical management of pulmonary disease due to *Mycobacterium-avium-intracellulare, Rev. Infect. Dis.*, 35, 597, 1981.

104. Brown, B. A., Wallace, R. J., Jr., and Onyi, G. O., Activities of clarithromycin against eight slowly growing species of nontuberculous mycobacteria, determined by using a broth microdilution MIC system, *Antimicrob. Agents Chemother.*, 36, 1987, 1992.

105. Wallace, R. J., Brown, B. A., Griffith, D. E., Girard, W. M., Murphy, D. T., Onyi, G. O., Steingrube, V. A., and Mazurek, G. H., Initial clarithromycin monotherapy for *Mycobacterium avium-intracellulare* complex lung disease, *Am. J. Respir. Crit. Care Med.*, 149, 1335, 1994.

106. Griffith, D. E., Brown, B. A., Girard, W. M., Murphy, D. T., and Wallace, R. J., Jr., Azithromycin activity against *Mycobacterium avium* complex lung disease in patients who were not infected with human immunodeficiency virus, *Clin. Infect. Dis.*, 23, 983, 1996.

107. Woodley, C. L. and Kilburn, J. O., *In vitro* susceptibility of *Mycobacterium avium* complex and *Mycobacterium tuberculosis* strains to spiro-piperidyl rifamycin, *Am. Rev. Resp. Dis.*, 126, 586, 1982.

108. Heifets, L. B., Iseman, M. D., Linhold-Levy, P. F., and Kanes, W., Determination of ansamycin MICs for *Mycobacterium avium* complex in liquid medium by radiometric and conventional methods, *Antimicrob. Agents Chemother.*, 28, 570, 1985.

109. Havlir, D. V., Dube, M. P., Sattler, F. R., Forthal, D. N., Kemper, C. A., Dunne, M. W., Parenti, D. M., Lavelle, J. P., White, A. C., Jr., Witt, M. D., Bozzette, S. A., and McCutchan, J. A., Prophylaxis against disseminiated *Mycobacterium avium* complex with weekly azithromycin, daily rifabutin, or both, *N. Engl. J. Med.*, 335, 292, 1996.

110. Wallace, R. J., Jr., Brown, B. A., Griffith, D. E., Girad, W. M., and Murphy, D. T., Clarithromycin regimens for pulmonary *Mycobacterium avium* complex: the first 50 patients, *Am. J. Crit. Care Med.*, 153, 1766, 1996.

111. Dautzenberg, B., Piperno, D., Diot, P., Truffot-Pernot, C., Chauvin, J.-P., and the Clarithromycin study group of France, Clarithromycin in the treatment of *Mycobacterium avium* lung infections in patients without AIDS, *Chest*, 107, 1035, 1995.

112. Nelson, K. G., Griffith, D. E., Brown, B., and Wallace, R. J., Jr., Results of operation in *Mycobacterium avium-intracellulare* lung disease, *Ann. Thorac. Surg.*, 66, 325, 1998.

113. Pomerantz, M., Madsen, L., Goble, M., and Iseman, M., Surgical management of resistant *Mycobacterium tuberculosis* and other mycobacterial pulmonary infections, *Ann. Thorac. Surg.*, 52, 1108, 1991.

114. Taha, A. M., Davidson, P. T., and Bailey, W. C., Surgical treatment of atypical mycobacterial lymphadenitis in children, *Pediatr. Infect. Dis.*, 111, 816, 1985.

115. Pezzia, W., Raleigh, J. W., Bailey, M. C., Toth, E. A., and Sliverblatt, J., Treatment of pulmonary disease due to *Mycobacterium kansasii*: recent experience with rifampin, *Rev. Infect. Dis.*, 3, 1035, 1981.

116. Jenkins, D. E., Bahar, D., and Chofuas, I., Pulmonary disease due to atypical mycobacteria: current concepts, *Trans. 19th Conf. Chemotherapy of Tuberculosis*, 224, 1960.

117. Ahn, C. H., Wallace, R. J., Jr., Steele, L. C., and Murphy, D. T., Sulfonamide-containing regimens for disease caused by rifampin-resistant *Mycobacterium kansasii, Am. Rev. Respir. Dis.*, 135, 10, 1987.

118. Wallace, R. J., Jr., Dunbar, D., Brown, B. A., Onyi, G., Dunlap, R., Ahn, C. H., and Murphy, D. T., Rifampin-resistant *Mycobacterium kansasii, Clin. Infect. Dis.*, 18, 736, 1994.

119. Brown, B. A., Wallace, R. J., Jr., Onyi, G. O., de Rosas, V., and Wallace, R. J., III, Activities of four macrolides, including clarithromycin, against *Mycobacterium fortuitum, Mycobacterium chelonae,* and *M. chelonae*-like organisms, *Antimicrob. Agents Chemother.*, 36, 180, 1992.

120. Donta, S. T., Smith, P. W., Levitz, R. E., and Quinitiliani, R., Therapy of *Mycobacterium marinum* infections use of tetracyclines vs. rifampin, *Arch. Intern. Med.*, 146, 902, 1986.

121. Sanders, W. J. and Wolinsky, E., *In vitro* susceptibility of *Mycobacterium marinum* to eight antimicrobial agents, *Antimicrob. Agents Chemother.*, 18, 529, 1980.

122. Stone, M. S., Wallace, R. J., Jr., Swenson, J. M., Thornsberry, C., and Christensen, L. A., Agar disk elution method for susceptibility testing of *Mycobacterium marinum* and *Mycobacterium fortuitum* complex to sulfonamides and antibiotics, *Antimicrob. Agents Chemother.*, 4, 486, 1983.

123. Santa Cruz, D. J. and Strayer, D. S., The histologic spectrum of the cutaneous mycobacterioses, *Hum. Pathol.*, 13, 485, 1982.

124. Thomas, P., Liu, F., and Weiser, W., Characteristics of *Mycobacterium xenopi* disease, *Bull. Int. Union Tuberc. Lung Dis.*, 6, 12, 1988.

125. Maugein, J., Fourche, J., Mormede, M., and Pellegrin, J. L., Sensibliite *in vitro* de *Mycobacterium avium* et *Mycobacterium xenopi* a l'erythromycine, roxithromycine et doxycycline, *Pathol. Biol.*, 37, 565, 1989.

126. Leysen, D. C., Haemers, A., and Pattyn, S. R., Mycobacteria and the new quinolones, *Antimicrob. Agents Chemother.*, 33, 1, 1989.

127. Parrot, R. G. and Grosset, J. H., Post-surgical outcome of 57 patients with *Mycobacterium xenopi* pulmonary infection, *Tubercle*, 69, 47, 1988.

128. Dautzenberg, B., Papillon, F., Lepitre, M., Truffot-Pernod, C., and Chauvin, J. P., *Mycobacterium xenopi* infections treated with clarithromycin-containing regimens, Annual Meeting, 33rd Interscience Conference on Antimicrobial Agents and Chemotherapy, New Orleans, LA, Abstract 1125, 1993.

129. Kristjanson, M., Bieluch, V. M., and Byeff, P. D., *Mycobacterium haemophilum* infection in immunocompromised patients: case report and review of the literature, *Rev. Infect. Dis.*, 13, 906, 1991.

130. Centers for Disease Control, Tuberculosis — United States, 1985 — and the possible impact of human T-lymphotropic virus type III/lymphadenopathy-associated virus infection, *MMWR*, 35, 74, 1986.

131. Horsburgh, C. R., Jr., Current concepts: *Mycobacterium avium* complex infection in the acquired immunodeficiency syndrome, *N. Engl. J. Med.*, 324, 1332, 1991.

132. Pierce, M., Crampton, S., Henry, D., Heifets, L., LaMarca, A., Montecalvo, M., Wormser, G. P., Jablonowski, H., Jemsek, J., Cynamon, M., Yangco, B. G., Notaria, G., and Craft, J. C., A randomized trial of clarithromycin as prophylaxis against disseminated *Mycobacterium avium* complex infection in patients with advanced acquired immunodeficiency syndrome, *N. Engl. J. Med.*, 335, 384, 1996.

133. Horsburgh, C. R. and Selik, R. M., The epidemiology of disseminated nontuberculous mycobacterial infection in the acquired immunodeficiency syndrome (AIDS), *Am. Rev. Respir. Dis.*, 139, 4, 1989.

134. Pitchenik, A. E. and Fertel, D., Medical management of AIDS patients: tuberculosis and nontuberculous mycobacterial disease, *Med. Clin. N. Am.*, 76, 121, 1992.

135. Hoy, J., Mijch, A., Sandland, M., Grayson, L., Lucas, R., and Dwyer, B., Quadruple-drug therapy for *Mycobacterium avium-intracellulare* bacteremia in AIDS patients, *J. Infect. Dis.*, 161, 801, 1990.

136. Meduri, G. U. and Stein, D. S., Pulmonary manifestations of acquired immunodeficiency syndrome, *Clin. Infect. Dis.*, 14, 98, 1992.

137. Nightingale, S. D., Byrd, L. T., Southern, P. M., Jockusch, J. D., Cal, S. X., and Wynne, B. A., Incidence of *Mycobacterium avium-intracellulare* complex bacteremia in human immunodeficiency virus-positive patients, *J. Infect. Dis.*, 165, 1082, 1992.

138. Okello, D. O., Sewankambo, N., Goodgame, R., Aisu, T. O., Kwezi, M., Morrissey, A., and Ellner, J. J., Absence of bacteremia with *Mycobacterium avium-intracellulare* in Ugandan patients with AIDS, *J. Infect. Dis.*, 162, 208, 1990.

139. Yakrus, M. A., Reeves, M. W., and Hunter, S. B., Characterization of isolates of *Mycobacterium avium* serotypes 4 and 8 from patients with AIDS by multilocus enzyme electrophoresis, *J. Clin. Micro.*, 30, 1474, 1992.

140. Gangadharam, P. R. J., Perumal, V. K., Crawford, J. T., and Bates, J. H., Association of plasmids and virulence of *Mycobacterium avium* complex, *Am. Rev. Respir. Dis.*, 137, 212, 1988.

141. Carpenter, J. L. and Parks, J. M., *Mycobacterium kansasii* infections in patients positive for human immunodeficiency virus, *Rev. Infect. Dis.*, 13, 789, 1990.

142. Levine, B. and Chaisson, R. E., *Mycobacterium kansasii:* a cause of treatable pulmonary disease associated with advanced human immunodeficiency virus (HIV) infection, *Ann. Intern. Med.*, 114, 861, 1991.

143. Witzig, R. S., Fazal, B. A., Mera, R. M., Mushatt, D. M., Dejace, P. M. J. T., Greer, D. L., and Hyslop, N. E., Jr, Clinical manifestations of coinfection with *Mycobacterium kansasii* and human immunodeficiency virus type 1, *Clin. Infect. Dis.*, 21, 77, 1995.

144. El-Solh, A. A., Nopper, J., Abdul-Khoudoud, M. R., Sherif, S. M., Aquilina, A. T., and Grant, B. J., Clinical and radiographic manifestations of uncommon pulmonary nontuberculous mycobacterial disease in AIDS patients, *Chest*, 114, 138, 1998.

145. Armstrong, D., Kiehn, T., Boone, N., White, M., Pursell, K., Lewin, S., Sordillo, E. M., Schneider, N., Grieco, M. H., et al., *Mycobacterium haemophilum* infections — New York City metropolitan area, 1990–1991, *MMWR*, 40, 636, 1991.

146. Jackson, K., Sievers, A., Ross, B. C., and Dwyer, B., Isolation of a fastidious *Mycobacterium* species from two AIDS patients, *J. Clin. Microbiol.*, 30, 11, 1992.

147. Wald, A., Coyle, M. B., Carlson, L. C., Thompson, R. L., and Hooten, T. M., Infection with a fastidious mycobacterium resembling *Mycobacterium simiae* in seven patients with AIDS, *Ann. Intern. Med.*, 7, 586, 1992.

148. Bottger, E. C., Teske, A., Kirschner, P., Bost, S., Chang, H. R., Beer, V., and Hirshcel, B., Disseminated "*Mycobacterium genavense*" infection in patients with AIDS, *Lancet*, 340, 76, 1992.

149. Klatt, E. C., Jensen, D. F., and Meyer, P. R., Pathology of *Mycobacterium avium-intracellulare* infection in acquired immune deficiency syndrome (AIDS), *Hum. Pathol.*, 18, 709, 1987.

150. Wallace, J. M. and Hannah, J. B., *Mycobacterium avium* complex infection in patients with the acquired immunodeficiency syndrome, *Chest*, 93, 926, 1988.

151. Eng, R. H. K., Bishburg, E., Smith, S. M., and Mangia, A., Diagnosis of *Mycobacterium* bacteremia in patients with acquired immunodeficiency syndrome by direct examination of blood films, *J. Clin. Microbiol.*, 27, 768, 1989.

152. Pantongrag-Brown, L., Krebs, T. L., Daly, B. D., Wong-You-Cheong, J. J., Beiser, C., Ktause, B., and Brown, A. E., Frequency of abdominal CT findings in AIDS patients with *M. avium* complex bacteraemia, *Clin. Radiol.*, 53, 816,1998.

153. Young, L. S., Wiviott, L., Wu, M., Kolonoski, P., Bolan, R., and Inderlied, B. B., Azithromycin for treatment of *Mycobacterium avium-intracellulare* complex infection in patients with AIDS, *Lancet*, 338, 1107, 1991.

154. Dautzenberg, B., Truffot, C., Legris, S., Meyohas, M., Berlie, H. C., Mercat, A., Chevret, S., and Grosset, J., Activity of clarithromycin against *Mycobacterium avium* infection in patients with the acquired immune deficiency syndrome, *Am. Rev. Respir. Dis.*, 144, 564, 1991.

155. Chaisson, R. E., Benson, C. A., Dube, M. P., Korvick, J. S., Elkin, S., Smith, T., Craft, J. C., and Sattler, F. R., and the AIDS Clinical Trial Group Protocol 157 Study Team, Clarithromycin therapy for bacteremic *Mycobacterium avium* complex disease: a randomized, double-blind, dose-ranging study in patients with AIDS, *Ann. Intern. Med.*, 121, 905, 1994.

156. Dube, M. P., Sattler, F. R., Torriani, F. J., See, D., Havlir, D. V., Kemper, C. A., Dezfuli, M. G., Bozzette, S. A., Bartok, A. E., Leedom, J. M., Tilles, T. G., and McCutchan, J. A., A randomized evaluation of ethambutol for prevention of relapse and drug resistance during treatment of *Mycobacterium avium* complex bacteremia with clarithromycin-based combination therapy, California Collaborative Treatment Group, *J. Infect. Dis.*, 176, 1225, 1997.

157. Chiu, J., Nussbaum, J., Bozzette, S., Tilles, J. G., Young, L. S., Leedom, J., Heseltine, N. R., McCutchan, J. A., and the California Collaborative Treatment Group, Treatment of disseminated *Mycobacterium avium* complex infection in AIDS with amikacin, ethambutol, rifampin, and ciprofloxacin, *Ann. Intern. Med.*, 113, 358, 1990.

158. Kemper, C. A., Meng, T., Nussbaum, J., Chiu, J., Feigal, D. F., Bartok, A. E., Leedom, J. M., Tilles, J. G., Deresinski, S. C., McCutchan, J. A., and the California Collaborative Treatment Group, Treatment of *Mycobacterium avium* complex bacteremia in AIDS with a four-drug oral regimen, *Ann. Intern. Med.,* 116, 466, 1992.

159. Benson, C. A., Kessler, H. A., Pottage, J. C., and Trenholme, G. M., Successful treatment of acquired immunodeficiency syndrome-related *Mycobacterium avium* complex disease with a multiple drug regimen including amikacin, *Arch. Intern. Med.*, 151, 582, 1991.

160. Shafran, S. D., Singer, J., Zarowny, D. P., Phillips, P., Salit, I., Walmsley, S. L., Fong, I. W., Gill, M. J., Rachlis, A. R., Lalonde, R. G., Fanning, M. M., and Tsoukas, C. M., A comparison of two regimens for the treatment of *Mycobacterium avium* complex bacteremia in AIDS: rifabutin, ethambutol, and clarithromycin versus rifampin, ethambutol, clofazimine, and ciprofloxacin, Canadian HIV Trials Network Protocol 010 Study Group, *N. Engl. J. Med.*, 335, 377, 1996.

161. Cohn, D. L., Fisher, E. J., Peng, G. T., Hodges, J. S., Chesnut, J., Child, C. C., Franchino, B., Giobert, C. L., El-Sadr, W., Hafner, R., Korvick, J., Ropka, M., Heifets, R., Clotfelter, J., Munroe, D., and Horsburgh, C. R., A prospective randomized trail of four three-drug regimens in the treatment of disseminated *Mycobacterium avium* complex disease in AIDS patients: excess mortality associated with high-dose clarithromycin, *Clin. Infect. Dis.*, 29, 125, 1999.

162. Bermudez, L. E., Petrofsky, M., Kolonski, P., and Young, L. S., Emergence of *Mycobacterium avium* populations resistant to macrolides during experimental chemotherapy, *Antimicrob. Agents Chemother.*, 42, 180, 1998.

163. Chaisson, R. E., Keiser, P., Pierce, M., Fessel, W. J., Ruskin, J., Lahart, C., Benson, C. A., Meek, K., Siepman, N., and Craft, J. C., Clarithromycin and ethambutol with or without clofazimine for the treatment of bacteremic *Mycobacterium avium* complex disease in patients with HIV infection, *AIDS,* 11, 311, 1997.

164. Sullam, P. M., Gordin, F. M., and Wynne, B. A., Efficacy of rifabutin in the treatment of disseminated infection due to *Mycobacterium avium* complex, the Rifabutin Treatment Group, *Clin. Infect. Dis.,* 19, 84, 1994.

165. Aberg, J. A., Yajko, D. M., and Jacobson, M. A., Eradication of AIDS-related disseminated *Mycobacterium avium* complex infection after 12 months of antimycobacterial therapy combined with highly active antiretroviral therapy, *J. Infect. Dis.,* 178,1446, 1998.

166. Oullet, D., Hsu, A., Granneman, G. R., Carlson, G., Cavenaugh, J., Guenther, H., and Leonard, J. M., Pharmacokinetic interaction between ritonavir and clarithromycin*, Clin. Pharmacol. Ther.*, 64, 355, 1998.

167. Hafner, R., Bethel, J., Power, M., Landrey, B., Banach, M., Mole, L., Standiford, H. C., Follansbee, S., Kumar, P., Raasch R., Cohn, D., Mushatt, D., and Drusano, G., Tolerance and pharmacokinetic interactions of rifabutin and clarithromycin in human immunodeficiency virus-infected volunteers, *Antimicrob. Agents Chemother.*, 42, 631, 1998.

168. Shafran, S. D., Singer, J., Zarowny, D. P., Deschenes, J., Phillips, P., Turgeon, F., Aoki, F. Y., Toma, E., Miller, M., Duperval, R., Lemieux, C., and Schlech, W. F., III, Determinants of rifabutin-associated uveitis in patients treated with rifabutin, clarithromycin, and ethambutol for *Mycobacterium avium* complex bacteremia: a multivariate analysis, Canadian HIV Trials Network Protocol 010 Study Group, *J. Infect. Dis.*, 177, 252, 1998.

169. Dorman, S. E., Heller, H. M., Basgoz, N. O., and Sax, P. E., Adjunctive corticosteroid therapy for patients whose treatment for disseminated *Mycobacterium avium* complex infection has failed, *Clin. Infect. Dis.*, 26, 611, 1998.

170. Masur, H. and the members of the USPHS/IDSA prevention of oppotunistic infections working group, 1999 USPHS/IDSA guidelines for the prevention of opportunistic infections in persons infected with human immunodeficiency virus, *MMWR*, 48 (RR-10), 1, 1999.

171. Nightingale, S. D., Cameron, D. W., Gordin, F. M., Sullam, P. M., Cohn, D. L., Chaisson, R. E., Eron, L. J., Sparti, P. D., Bihari, B., Kaufman, D. L., et al., Two controlled trials of rifabutin prophylaxis against *Mycobacterium avium* complex infection in AIDS, *N. Engl. J. Med.,* 329, 828, 1993.

172. Oldfield, E. C., III, Fessel, W. J., Dunne, M. W., et al., Once weekly azithromycin therapy for prevention of *Mycobacteriam avium* complex infection in patients with AIDS: a randomized, double-blind, placebo-controlled multicenter trial, *Clin. Infect. Dis.,* 26, 611, 1998.

173. Karlson, A. G. and Carr, D. T., Tuberculosis caused by *Mycobacterium bovis:* report of six cases: 1954–1968, *Ann. Intern. Med.,* 73, 979, 1970.

174. Wilkins, E. G. L., Griffiths, R. J., and Roberts, C., Pulmonary tuberculosis due to *Mycobacterium bovis, Thorax*, 41, 685, 1986.

175. Damsker, B., Bottone, E. J., and Schneierson, S. S., Human infections with *Mycobacterium bovis, Am. Rev. Respir. Dis.*, 110, 446, 1974.

176. Wigle, W. D., Ashley, M. J., Killough, E. M., and Cosens, M., Bovine tuberculosis in humans in Ontario: the epidemiologic features of 31 active cases occurring between 1964 and 1970, *Am. Rev. Respir. Dis.*, 106, 528, 1972.

177. Sauret, J., Jolis, R., Ausina, V., Castro, E., and Cornudella, R., Human tuberculosis due to *Mycobacterium bovis:* report of 10 cases, *Tubercle*, 73, 388, 1992.

178. Hardie, R. M. and Watson, J. M., *Mycobacterium bovis* in England and Wales: past, present and future, *Epidemiol. Infect.*, 109, 23, 1992.

179. Dankner, W. M., Waecker, J. J., Essey, M. A., Moser, K., Thompson, M., and Davis, C. E., *Mycobacterium bovis* infections in San Diego: a clinicoepidemiologic study of 73 patients and a historical review of a forgotten pathogen, *Medicine*, 72, 11, 1993.

180. Collins, C. H. and Grange, J. M., A review: the bovine tubercle bacillus, *J. Appl. Bacteriol.*, 55, 13, 1983.

181. Collins, C. H., Yates, M. D., and Grange, J. M., A study of bovine strains of *Mycobacterium tuberculosis* isolated from humans in southeast England, 1977–1979, *Tubercle*, 62, 113, 1981.

182. Long, R., Nobert, E., Chomye, S., van Embden, J., McNamee, C., Duran, R.R., Talbot, J., and Fanning, A., Transcontinental spread of multidrug resistant *Mycobacterium bovis, Am. J. Respir. Crit. Care Med.*, 159, 2014, 1999.

183. McParland, C., Cotton, D. J., Gowda, K. S., Hoeppner, V. H., Martin, W. T., and Weckworth, P. F., Miliary *Mycobacterium bovis* introduced by intravesical Bacillus Calmette-Guérin immunotherapy, *Am. Rev. Respir. Dis.*, 146, 1330, 1992.

184. Lotte, A., Wasz-Hockert, P., Poisson, N., Dumitresau, N., Venon, M., and Couvet, E., BCG complications, *Adv. Tuberc. Res.*, 21, 107, 1984.

185. Noah, P. K., Pande, D., Johnson, B., and Ashley, D., Evaluation of oral erythromycin and local isoniazid instillation therapy in infants with Bacillus Calmette-Guérin lymphadenitis and abscesses, *Pediatr. Infect. Dis. J.*, 12, 136, 1993.

186. Gonzalez, B., Moreno, S., Burdach, R., Valenzuela, M. T., Henriquez, A., Ramos, M. I., and Sorenson, R. U., Clinical presentation of Bacillus Calmette-Guérin infections in patients with immunodeficiency syndromes, *Pediatr. Infect. Dis. J.*, 8, 201, 1989.

187. Braun, M. M. and Cauthen, G., Relationship of the human immunodeficiency virus epidemic to pediatric tuberculosis and Bacillus Calmette-Guérin immunization, *Pediatr. Infect. Dis. J.*, 11, 220, 1992.

10 Radiology of Mycobacterial Disease

Anne McB. Curtis, M.D.

CONTENTS

I. PRIMARY TUBERCULOSIS

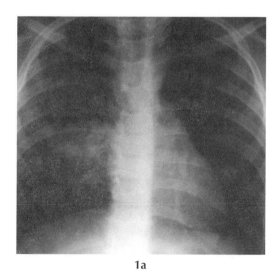
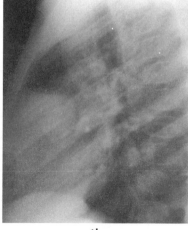

1a   1b

FIGURE 10.1a,b A 12-year-old female who presented with a fever and cough. Her grandmother had active tuberculosis. The location of the infiltrate and the adenopathy are typical for primary infection.

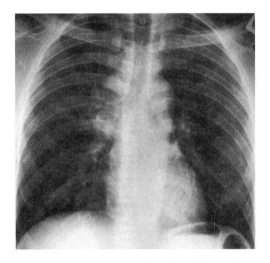

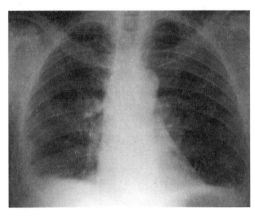

FIGURE 10.2 A 43-year-old male with carpal tunnel syndrome and right paratracheal and hilar adenopathy. The carpal tunnel syndrome was the result of caseating granulomas found at surgery. In the non-HIV-positive population, adenopathy is more common in children and noncaucasian adults, particularly in African-Americans and persons from India. Although asymmetric adenopathy is uncommon in sarcoidosis, the patterns of tuberculous adenopathy may mimic exactly those of sarcoid and lymphoma.

FIGURE 10.3 A 25-year-old male with fever and weight loss. The pleural effusion and adenopathy (arrows) are characteristic of primary infection.

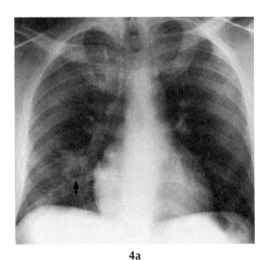

4a

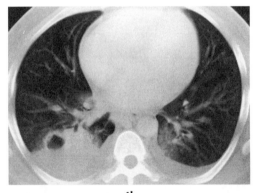

4b

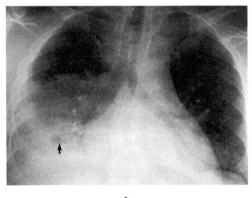

FIGURE 10.4a–c A 40-year-old male diabetic with fever, chills, and cough of 3 weeks duration. An ill-defined infiltrate with a cavity is present on the admission film (a) and is seen easily on computed tomography (b). A tuberculous pleural effusion developed as well (c). The patient was anergic at admission and the diagnosis was made initially by a positive smear at bronchoscopy. He then remembered that a friend had been sick with tuberculosis several months earlier (Figure 10.11).

4c

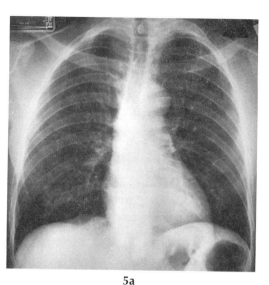

5a

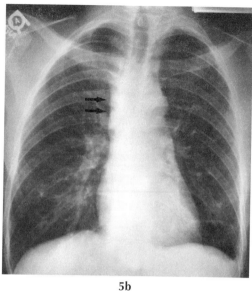

5b

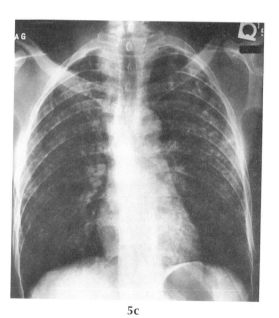

5c

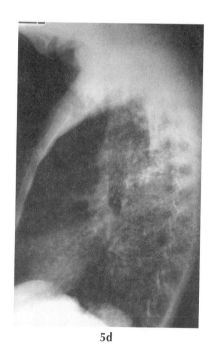

5d

FIGURE 10.5a–d A 25-year-old male presenting with cough and fever in February 1977 (b). In comparison with an earlier film in November 1976 (a), there now is right paratracheal, right hilar, and aortopulmonary adenopathy as well as a left pleural effusion (b). All of these findings favor primary infection. The patient was lost to follow-up until he returned in April 1977 with continued fevers and a 30 lb weight loss. The adenopathy and pleural effusion resolved, but nodules disseminated throughout both lungs (c, d); the sputum was positive for AFB. No apparent cavitary focus is present and nodules, now larger than 3 mm, are too big to be considered miliary. Presumably, this represents progression of the hematogenously disseminated primary disease.

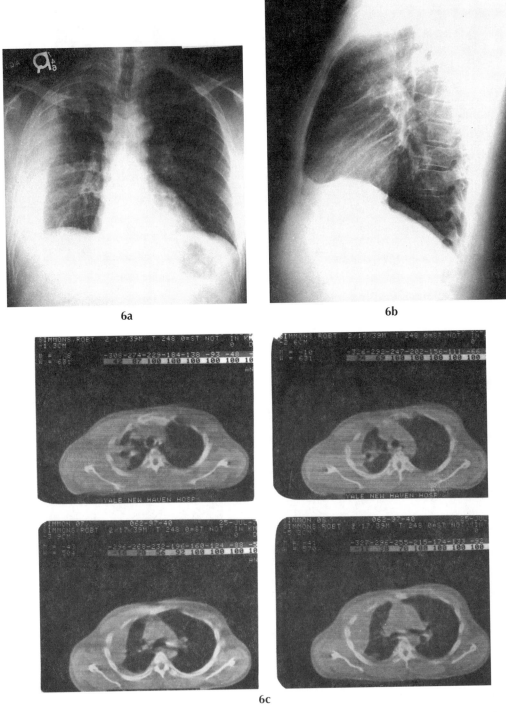

6a

6b

6c

FIGURE 10.6a–c A 32-year-old male with an asymptomatic routine chest radiograph. No parenchymal focus is evident on posteroanterior and lateral chest radiographs in the presence of a large effusion (a, b). Computed tomography of the chest shows an apical focus of parenchymal disease (c). *Mycobacterium tuberculosis* was found on pleural biopsy and culture. In cases of pleural effusion, a parenchymal lesion that ruptures into the pleural space to produce the effusion usually may be found on computed tomography. Effusions are more frequent with primary infection.

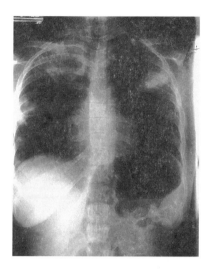

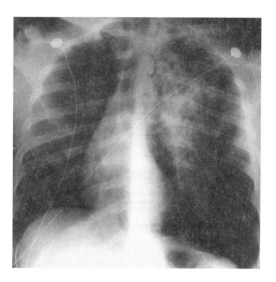

FIGURE 10.7 A 23-year-old female, 7 weeks postpartum presented with fever. The tuberculin skin test was negative and septic emboli were suspected. Angiography was negative and the diagnosis of tuberculosis was made at open lung biopsy. The skin test converted 6 weeks after admission.

FIGURE 10.8 A 32-year-old male presented with chest pain, fever, and a 20 lb weight loss the day his sister was discharged from the hospital for treatment of active pulmonary tuberculosis. Multiple areas of cavitation are noted in the left lung, which is partially collapsed in the presence of a pneumothorax. The pneumothorax probably resulted from rupture of a necrotic focus into the pleural space. Smear and culture were positive for *M. tuberculosis*.

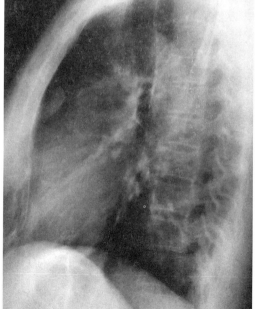

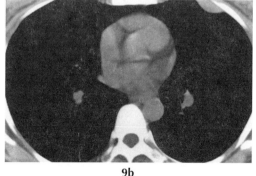

9a

9b

FIGURE 10.9a,b Residual pleural focus. A 45-year-old female with a history of fever and pleurisy 7 years earlier treated in China for 3 months with streptomycin, isoniazid, and penicillin. A lateral chest film and computed tomography show a pleural-based soft tissue mass without evidence of bony destruction. No parenchymal lesions or adenopathy were evident. A needle biopsy was negative; caseating granulomas were found at surgery, and *M. tuberculosis* was cultured. The differential diagnosis includes pleural tumors, both benign and malignant.

II. REACTIVATION TUBERCULOSIS

A. PULMONARY

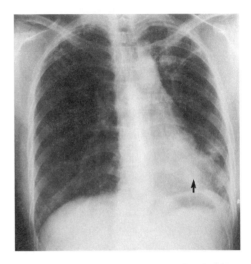

FIGURE 10.10 A 28-year-old laboratory worker with chronic cough. Bilateral upper lobe volume loss with nodular opacities of varying sizes are seen. Poorly marginated larger opacities are noted in the left lower lobe with a central lucency (arrow) representing cavitary disease. This lesion probably is of bronchogenic origin with proliferation of inflammatory foci.

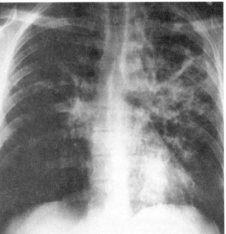

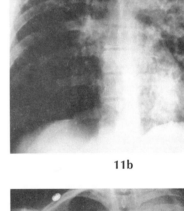

11b

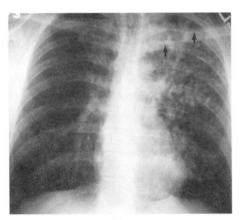

11a

FIGURE 10.11a–c Bronchogenic spread. A 31-year-old male with fever and cough. Cavities at the left apex (arrow) were not observed initially and the patient was treated for a presumed community acquired infection (a). Progressive cavitation developed with bronchogenic spread to both lungs (b, c). The sputum smear was markedly positive for *M. tuberculosis*. This patient is the contact for Figure 10.4.

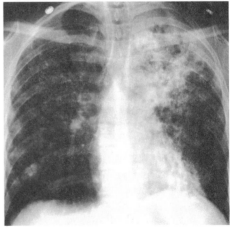

11c

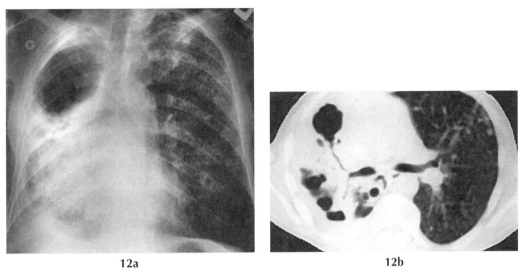

12a 12b

FIGURE 10.12a,b Multiple cavities with bronchogenic spread. A 52-year-old alcoholic male with cough and weight loss. The sputum smear was markedly positive for *M. tuberculosis*. There is extensive destruction of the right upper lobe with consolidation of the rest of the right lung and bronchogenic spread to the left lung (a). Computed tomography demonstrates much more destruction with multiple irregular cavities in the right lung, as well as bronchogenic spread to the left lung (b). If untreated, destruction of the lung can be complete, with gangrene resulting.

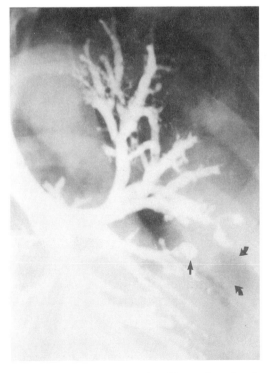

FIGURE 10.13 Bronchogram. Extensive bronchiectasis with small cavity formation (arrows). Note the lucency peripherally which represents a cavity that did not fill (curved arrows). The smear was markedly positive for *M. tuberculosis*.

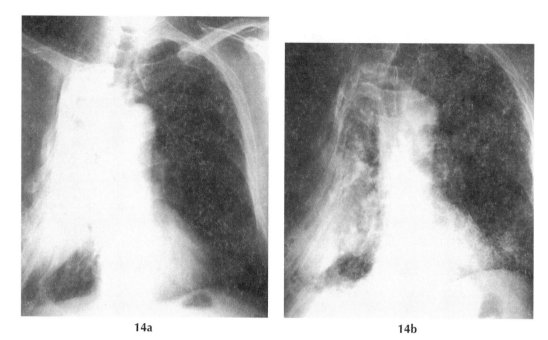

14a   14b

FIGURE 10.14a,b   A 60-year-old male who had had a thoracoplasty for tuberculosis 30 years earlier (a). He presented with a fever in January 1978. Miliary dissemination had occurred (b).

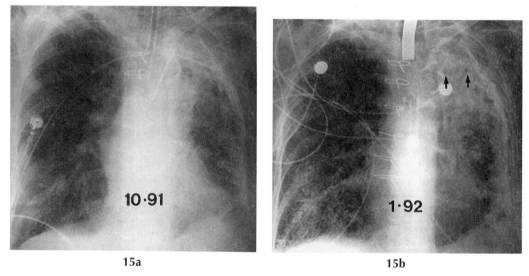

15a   15b

FIGURE 10.15a,b   A 55-year-old female with diabetes who underwent a therapeutic pneumothorax for tuberculosis in 1944. Multiple complications followed a coronary artery bypass graft in October 1991 (a). In January 1992, the patient developed a relentless fever and the sputum was positive for *M. tuberculosis*. On the film of January 1992 (b), lucencies in the left upper lobe represent necrotic foci from which bronchogenic spread occurred (arrow).

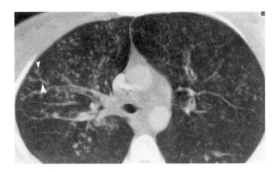

FIGURE 10.16   Tree-in-bud pattern. A 31-year-old Asian female presented with cough, fever, and a positive smear for *M. tuberculosis*. The buds, or tufts (small arrowhead), represent impacted material in the lobular bronchioles and alveolar ducts, while the stem represents impaction in the last order bronchus of the secondary pulmonary lobule (large arrowhead).

B. EXTRAPULMONARY

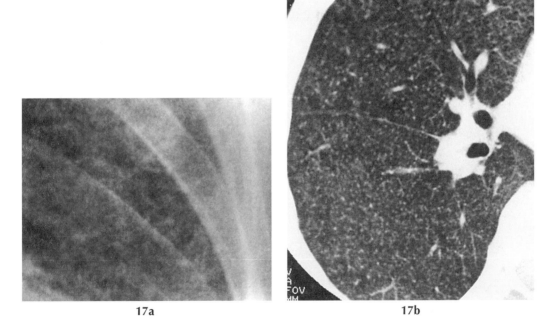

17a   17b

FIGURE 10.17a,b   A 43-year-old male with multiple abdominal fistulae and abscesses as a result of a gunshot wound. One year following the initial injury, he developed miliary lesions in the lung. Bronchoscopy demonstrated caseating granulomas, *M. tuberculosis* was grown from the lungs, and multiple abscesses were visualized in the abdomen. Miliary lesions are seen on a chest radiograph (a) and to better advantage on computed tomography (b).

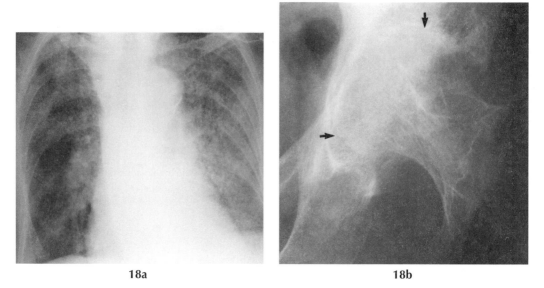

18a   18b

FIGURE 10.18a,b   A 50-year-old female with a history of congestive heart failure and hip pain who was treated with steroids. The chest radiograph initially was thought to suggest congestive heart failure (a). However, typical miliary lesions are noted throughout both lungs. Such miliary spread may occur either in primary or reactivation tuberculosis. The left hip film demonstrates narrowing and destruction of the joint space (arrows) (b). Lack of marginal erosions of the joint are unusual. Aspiration of the hip demonstrated *M. tuberculosis*. Presumably, the steroids led to the breakdown of preexisting tuberculous foci.

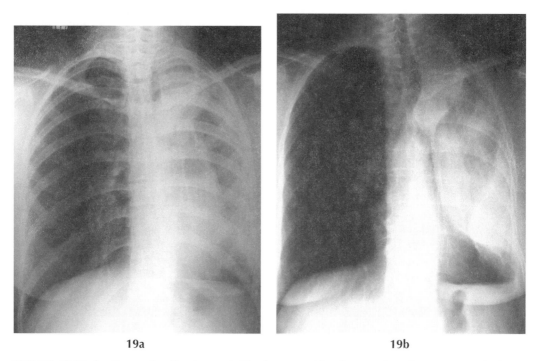

19a   19b

FIGURE 10.19a,b   Progressive fibrothorax. A fibrothorax resulting from a tuberculous empyema is shown with progressive contraction and calcification over 26 years. Computed tomography occasionally may demonstrate fluid within areas of the "fibrothorax." Viable organisms may be present as well, predisposing to reactivation.

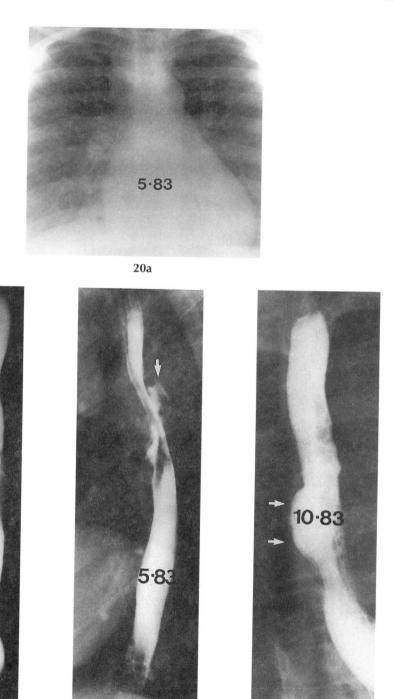

20a

20b

20c

20d

FIGURE 10.20a–d A 35-year-old female with cough. A chest radiograph in May 1983 demonstrates paratracheal adenopathy on the right (a). A barium swallow shows ulceration of the esophagus with extravasation of contrast at the level of the subcarinal lymph nodes (arrows) (b, c). Follow-up in October demonstrates healing with a residual esophageal diverticulum (arrows) (d). Fistulization occurred from erosion of tuberculous lymph nodes into the esophagus.

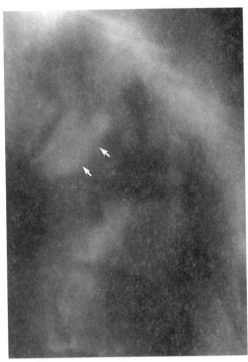

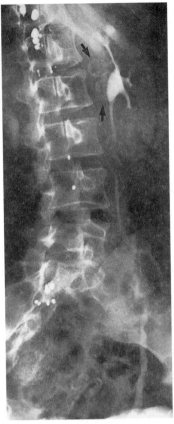

21a   21b

FIGURE 10.21a,b   Tuberculosis of the spine and cavitary tuberculosis of kidney. Destruction of the inferior portion of an upper thoracic vertebral body and complete destruction of the vertebral body below resulted in a gibbus deformity (a). The initial infection usually results from hematogenous spread. Spread from one vertebral body to the next may occur across the disc space or beneath the anterior and posterior longitudinal ligaments. The cavitary lesions in the kidney (arrows) are filled with debris (b). Stricture formation may occur with healing, and careful follow-up with intravenous pyelography is warranted to avoid obstruction. (Photo courtesy of Arthur Rosenfield, M.D.)

III. HEALING

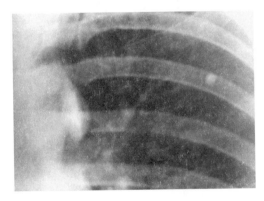

FIGURE 10.22   Formation of Rhanke complex. Calcified nodule associated with a calcified mediastinal lymph node.

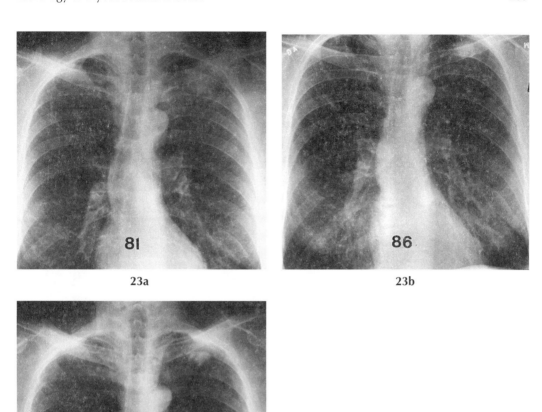

23a

23b

23c

FIGURE 10.23a–c Tuberculoma formation in a 40-year-old male. A 1981 radiograph shows a poorly marginated opacity in the left upper lobe and some scarring (stable over several years) in the right upper lobe (a). *M. tuberculosis* was grown on culture. Films in 1986 (b) and 1989 (c) demonstrate contraction of the left upper lobe infiltrate with increasing density to form a smooth lobulated mass, typical of a tuberculoma. At autopsy, tuberculomas may contain viable organisms.

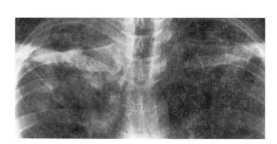

FIGURE 10.24 Biapical cavities as well as nodules in a 39-year-old alcoholic male. Complete resolution occurred after 1 year of therapy.

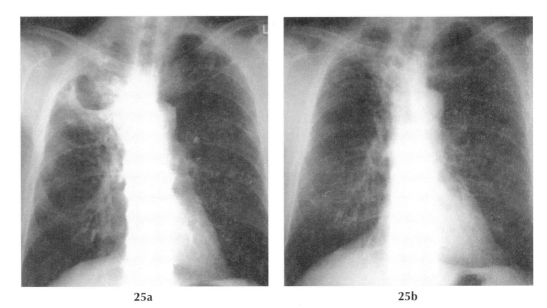

25a   25b

FIGURE 10.25a,b Healing with cavity closure. A large cavity in the right upper lobe in October has an air fluid level (a). Note the calcified nodule in the left perihilar region. Twelve months following treatment the cavity has closed with right upper lobe volume loss and residual apical nodular opacities (b). In cavitary tuberculosis, air fluid levels are slightly unusual, but do occur. Cavities may or may not close completely. Radiographic stability for 6 months must be documented to describe "inactive" tuberculosis.

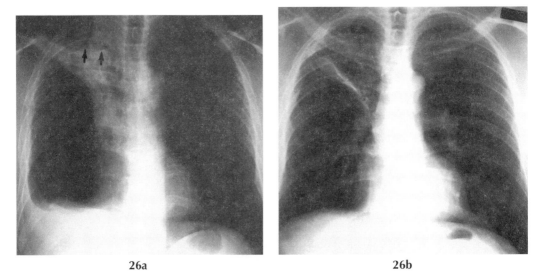

26a   26b

FIGURE 10.26a,b Healing of cavitary disease. The right upper lobe infiltrate with multiple lucencies representing cavities is seen in association with a pleural effusion (a). Considerable resolution was demonstrated 6 months later with clearing of the pleural effusion and volume loss of the right upper lobe (b).

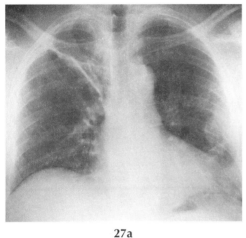

27a

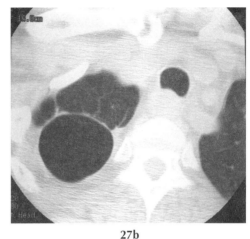

27b

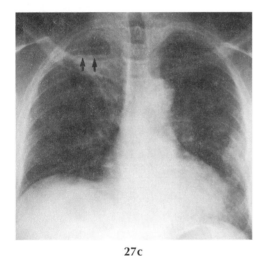

27c

FIGURE 10.27a–c   A 55-year-old male alcoholic with cavitary tuberculosis diagnosed in October 1982 (a) that healed with contraction and residual cystic spaces by April 1983 (b). He presented in December 1992 with weakness, seizures, and vomiting. A posteroanterior chest radiograph demonstrates an air fluid level in the right upper lobe (c). Although tuberculosis was suspected, it was not found at bronchoscopy and the infiltrate healed with antibiotic therapy. This demonstrates that air fluid levels may occur in preexisting spaces and do not necessarily reflect necrosis with cavitation, as would be seen in active tuberculosis.

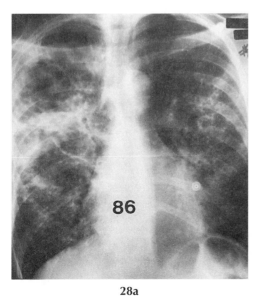

28a

FIGURE 10.28a–c   A 32-year-old male with active tuberculosis and a positive sputum smear. Over a 2-year period, healing occurs with progressive destruction of the parenchyma and extensive bullous formation in the right lung. Minimal nodular changes are seen on the left. (See following page for 28b and c.)

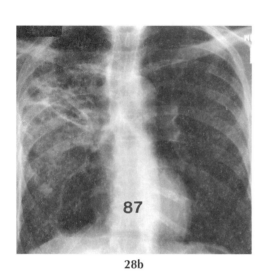

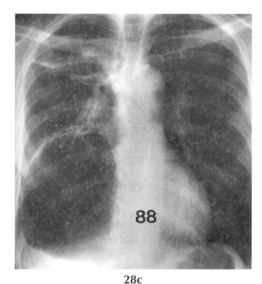

28b   28c

IV. TUBERCULOSIS OR CANCER?

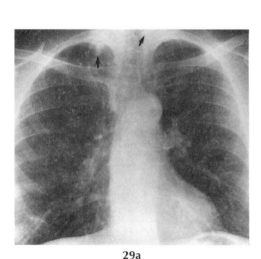

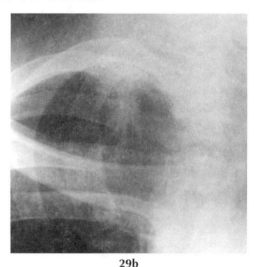

29a   29b

FIGURE 10.29a,b A 60-year-old male with a 50 pack/year smoking history and an apical density at the right apex. The skin test was negative and old films were not available. The irregular margins of this lesion are highly suspicious for a neoplasm, but at resection the lesion proved to be tuberculous.

FIGURE 10.30 A 54-year-old male nonsmoker who had computed tomography of the lung performed to evaluate the pulmonary hilum. The hilum is shown to be normal, but nodular opacities are noted peripherally at both bases. These are too small to evaluate for density using the computed tomography phantom technique because they are less than 4 mm in size. At surgery, multiple subpleural nodules were found that were nonnecrotic granulomas. A lymph node resected at the same time was culture positive for *M. tuberculosis*.

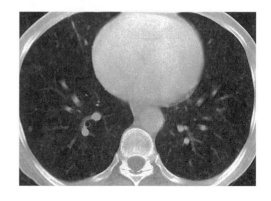

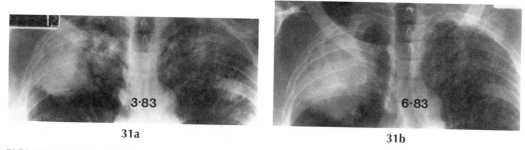

31a   31b

FIGURE 10.31a,b A 50-year-old male with cough and weight loss. His sputum was positive on culture for *M. tuberculosis*. A large mass in the right upper lobe was found to be an adenocarcinoma on needle biopsy (a). A film in June demonstrates some resolution of the tuberculous foci, but progression of the neoplasm (b). Presumably, these are concurrent problems rather than a scar carcinoma in association with long-standing tuberculosis.

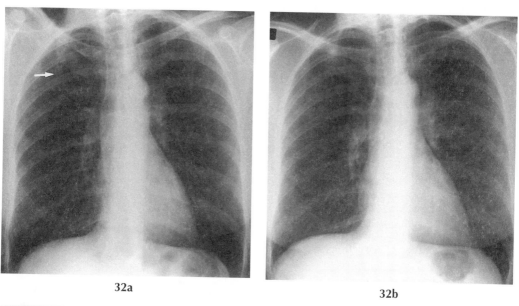

32a   32b

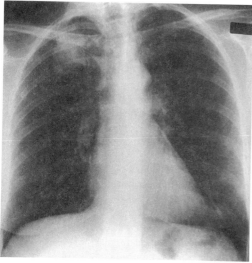

32c

FIGURE 10.32a–c A 44-year-old white female with a history of incomplete treatment for tuberculosis. The patient was followed for several years, and a growing mass was resected and proved to be an adenocarcinoma. Multiple granulomas were noted in the specimen as well. The patient had a 40 pack/year smoking history, but stopped 6 years before entry into the clinic. Adenocarcinoma is the most frequently associated "scar" carcinoma, but other cell types have been reported as well. It is important when evaluating serial films to compare films widely separated in time (e.g., 2 years) if they are available. Subtle progressive changes over repeated short intervals (e.g., 3 to 6 months) may be overlooked, as happened to this patient over a 6-year period.

V. TUBERCULOSIS AND NON-HIV-RELATED IMMUNOSUPPRESSION

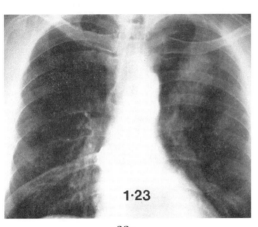

1·23

33a

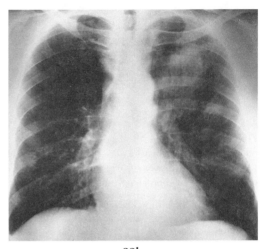

33b

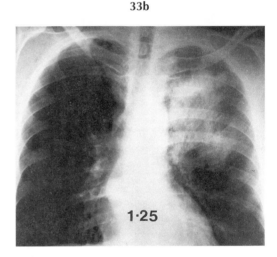

1·25

FIGURE 10.33a–c A 67-year-old male with fever and chronic myelogenous leukemia. Over 3 days, aggressive opacification of the left upper lobe was noted. Sputum smear and culture were positive for *M. tuberculosis*. Rapid progression may be related to immunosuppression.

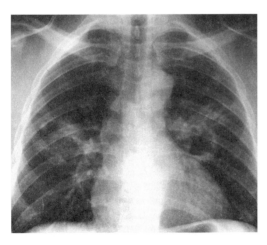

FIGURE 10.34 A 50-year-old male with Wegener's granulomatosis who was completing 1 year of treatment with full doses of cyclophosphamide. He presented with a fever and nasal stuffiness. Recurrence of Wegener's granulomatosis has not been reported once complete remission has occurred in a patient who continues on full doses of chemotherapy. In this case, there was no evidence of relapse, and another cause of cavitary disease was sought. Although tuberculosis is very unusual in patients with Wegener's granulomatosis, the bronchoscopy was positive for *M. tuberculosis*.

VI. HIV-RELATED TUBERCULOSIS

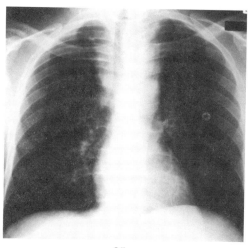

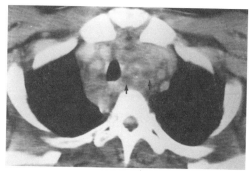

35a
35b

FIGURE 10.35a,b   An HIV-positive intravenous drug abuser with a 3-month history of fever and a mass in the neck. Mediastinal widening extending into the neck with deviation of the trachea to the right is seen on a chest radiograph (a). Computed tomography demonstrates multiple enlarged lymph nodes with low density centers (arrows) (b). *M. tuberculosis* was obtained at mediastinoscopy. Thoracic adenopathy is not a feature of AIDS-related complex, and an infectious or neoplastic cause should be sought to explain the adenopathy.

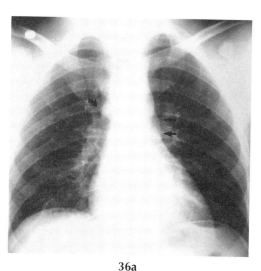

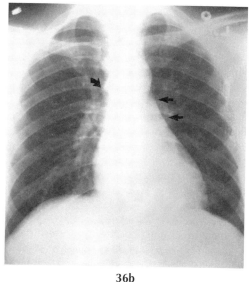

36a
36b

FIGURE 10.36a–c   A 27-year-old HIV-negative intravenous drug abuser, on peritoneal dialysis for 1 year, who presented with fevers. A chest radiograph from September 23, 1986 shows free intraperitoneal air, as well as azygos (curved arrow) and aortopulmonary adenopathy (arrow) (a). Empiric therapy for tuberculosis ensued for 6 weeks but was discontinued when cultures were negative. The chest radiograph from October 25, 1986 demonstrates regression of the aortopulmonary and azygos adenopathy (arrows) (b). A routine chest radiograph from May 11, 1987 demonstrates a mediastinal mass, and the patient was noted to be HIV positive at the same time (c). Thoracotomy demonstrated *M. tuberculosis* of the mediastinal nodes. Adenopathy is far more common in patients with tuberculosis who are HIV positive than those who are HIV negative. Careful comparison with a baseline radiograph is mandatory, as the adenopathy may be subtle. Tuberculosis may be the first manifestation of AIDS. (Photo courtesy of Ernest Moritz, M.D.) (See following page for 36c.)

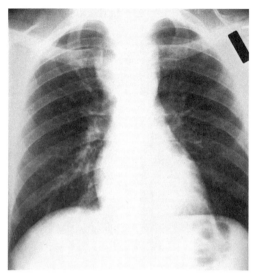

36c

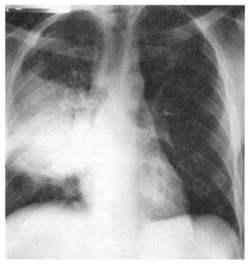

37a

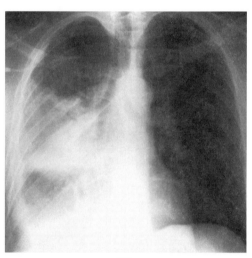

37b

FIGURE 10.37a–c A 37-year-old HIV-positive male intravenous drug abuser with fever and cough. Six months before admission, he had been diagnosed with tuberculosis, but he discontinued therapy after 4 months. There is consolidation of the right upper lobe with bulging of the fissure, as well as paratracheal adenopathy (a). A pleural effusion developed in 5 days (b). Computed tomography demonstrates dense consolidation with a bulging fissure, a pleural effusion, and spread to the right lower lobe (c). The sputum was positive for *M. tuberculosis*. Tuberculosis can be very aggressive in immunocompromised patients, particularly those with low CD4 counts. The infiltrate with a bulging fissure is more typical of staphylococcal and Gram-negative organisms.

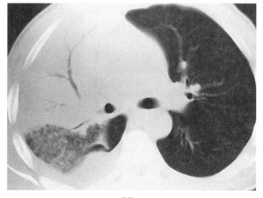

37c

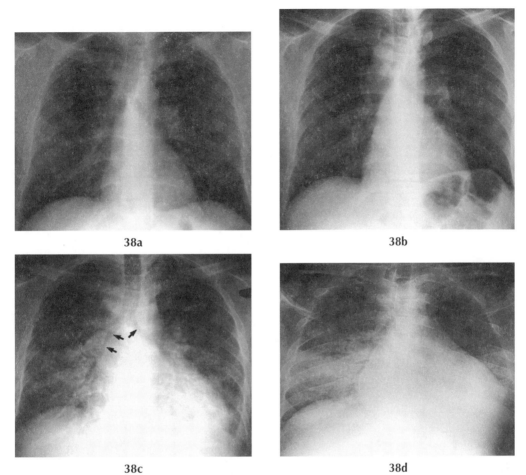

38a

38b

38c

38d

FIGURE 10.38a–d   A 29-year-old intravenous drug abuser with AIDS and a CD4 count of 53 presented with fever and cough. A film of March 29 (a) demonstrates some hilar adenopathy that has progressed to include paratracheal adenopathy by May 3 (b). The film of May 17 demonstrates an impressive increase in the mediastinal and hilar adenopathy with narrowing of the bronchus intermedius as well as the left main stem bronchus (arrows) (c). Diffuse parenchymal infiltrates developed rapidly as well (d). After 12 days, the admission sputum culture was positive for *M. tuberculosis.* The sputum became positive on smear when the parenchymal infiltrates appeared. Rapid clearing resulted after 2 ¹/₂ weeks of therapy, and the patient never required intubation. This is an example of extremely rapid progression of both lymphadenopathy and parenchymal infiltration in an immunocompromised patient. This patient typifies what once was called "galloping consumption."

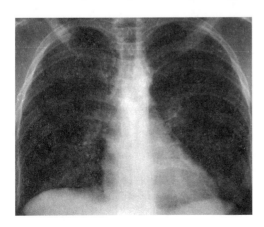

FIGURE 10.39a–c   A 28-year-old HIV-positive female, presenting with cough, fever, abdominal pain, and back pain. Blood cultures were positive for *M. tuberculosis*, and miliary dissemination occurred, followed by ARDS, shown here with three consecutive daily chest radiographs (a–c). Bronchoscopy following intubation demonstrated AFB on smear. Although unusual, tuberculosis is a well-known cause of ARDS. (See following page for 39b and c.)

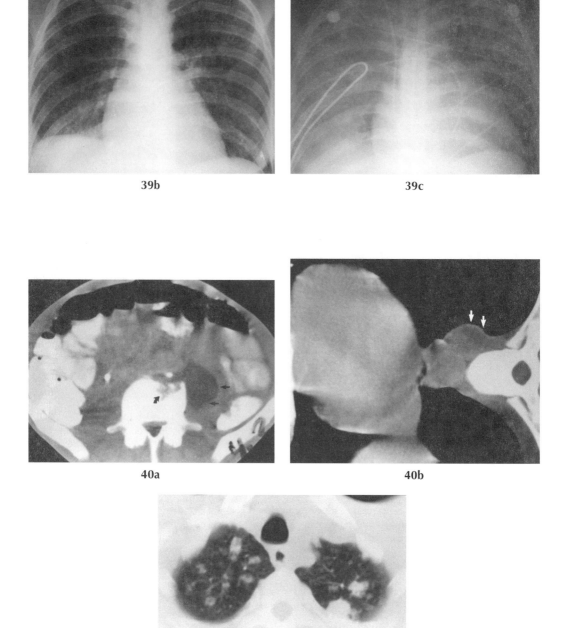

39b   39c

40a   40b

40c

FIGURE 10.40a–c A 32-year-old HIV-positive male with a history of intravenous drug abuse presented with abdominal pain and was found to have a perforated duodenal ulcer. Computed tomography demonstrates destruction of a vertebral body (curved arrow), with a paraspinal fluid collection (arrow) (a). Similar fluid collections were noted elsewhere in the abdomen. Drainage of the paraspinal collection demonstrated *M. tuberculosis*. Mediastinal computed tomography shows a paravertebral mass extending superiorly from the abdomen, representing a tuberculous abscess (arrow) (b). Chest computed tomography shows parenchymal involvement as well (c).

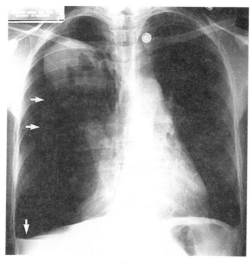

41a

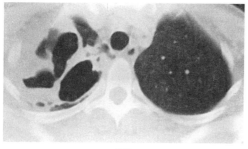

41b

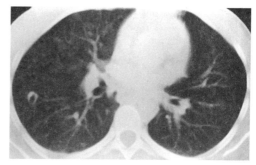

41c

FIGURE 10.41a–c A 27-year-old HIV-positive female intravenous drug abuser presented with a 1-month history of cough and fever followed by the sudden onset of right sided chest pain. A hydropneumothorax is demonstrated (arrows) (a). A sharply marginated mass with multiple air fluid levels is seen in the right upper lobe (a). Extensive cavitation ensued (b), and multiple smaller cavitary lesions were noted on computed tomography (c). Resection of the abscess showed *Pneumocystis carinii* on silver stain, and cultures grew *M. tuberculosis*, *M. avium* complex (MAC), *Klebsiella*, and *Enterobacter*. A portion of a resected rib showed necrotizing granulomas in the marrow. This patient responded well to therapy, but died 3 months later with a severe electrolyte disturbance. The chest radiograph during that admission showed no infiltrates.

VII. ATYPICAL MYCOBACTERIOSIS: HIV- AND NON-HIV-RELATED

A. HIV-RELATED

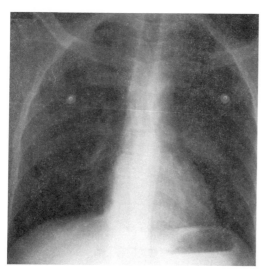

42a

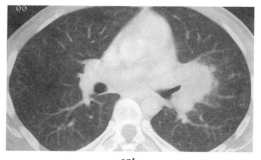

42b

FIGURE 10.42a–d A 36-year-old HIV-positive male with left hilar adenopathy seen on chest radiography (a) and computed tomography (b), followed by lingular consolidation (c, d). At bronchoscopy, an endobronchial mass was found which occluded the lingular bronchus. This was AFB positive on smear and MAC was cultured. (See following page for 42c and d.).

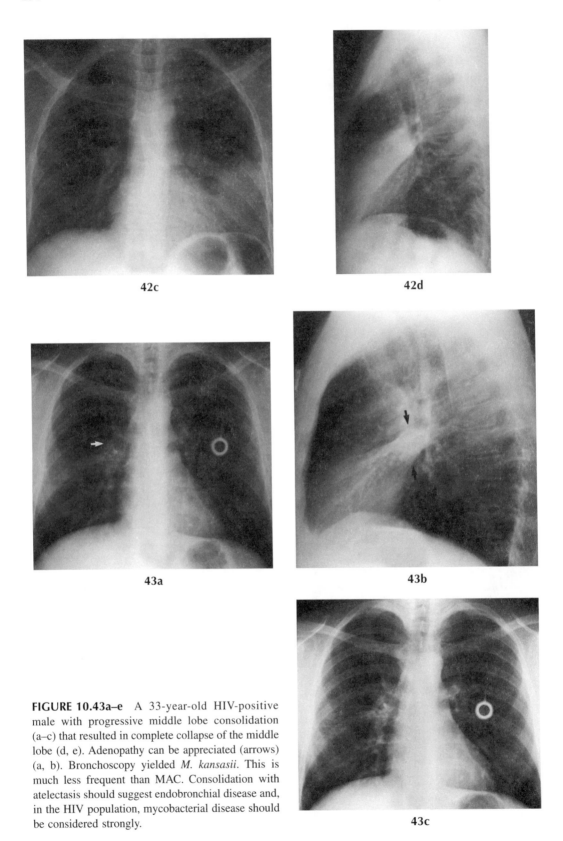

42c

42d

43a

43b

FIGURE 10.43a–e A 33-year-old HIV-positive male with progressive middle lobe consolidation (a–c) that resulted in complete collapse of the middle lobe (d, e). Adenopathy can be appreciated (arrows) (a, b). Bronchoscopy yielded *M. kansasii*. This is much less frequent than MAC. Consolidation with atelectasis should suggest endobronchial disease and, in the HIV population, mycobacterial disease should be considered strongly.

43c

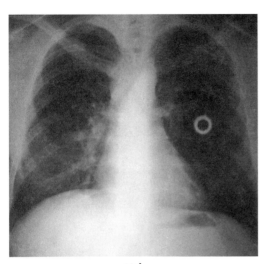

43d

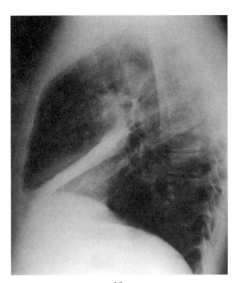

43e

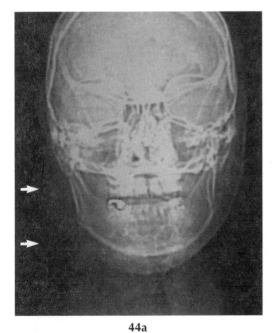

44a

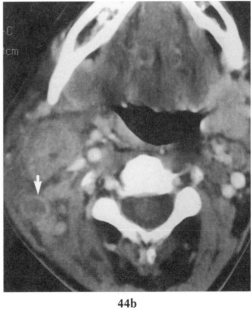

44b

FIGURE 10.44a,b A 37-year-old male with AIDS and a CD4 count of 16 who presented with fever and neck swelling. A digitized radiograph shows massive swelling in the right neck (a) and computed tomography shows large nodes with low-density central areas typical of tuberculous lymphadenitis (arrow) (b). Culture of the biopsied node was positive for MAC.

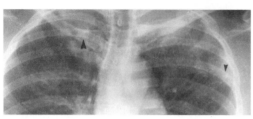 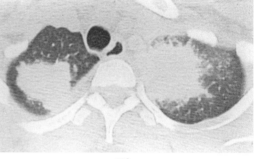

| 45a | 45b |

FIGURE 10.45a,b   HIV with reconstituted immunity. A 35-year-old African-American woman diagnosed 2 months previously with AIDS. After 6 weeks of antiviral treatment, she developed a cough and hemoptysis. The CD4 count had risen from 34 to 490, and the PPD had become positive as had the chest radiograph. The open lung biopsy demonstrated MAC. The chest radiograph (a) shows multiple pleural-based poorly margin-ated apical opacities bilaterally (large arrow) as well as a cavitating parenchymal nodule (small arrow). Computed tomography of the chest shows the poorly marginated pleural-based parenchymal masses (b). Subsequent computed tomography of the abdomen showed necrotic lymph nodes compatible with MAC.

B. Non-HIV-Related

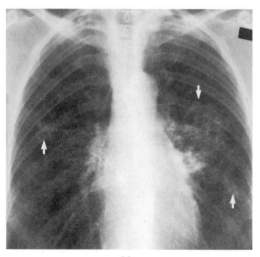 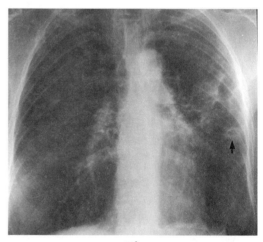

| 46a | 46b |

FIGURE 10.46a–c   A 71-year-old female with a history of whooping cough as a child followed by multiple episodes of pneumonia. Bronchiectasis was diagnosed on bronchography in 1977 and, when required, inter-mittent antibiotics were administered for infection. MAC was seen in increasing concentration in the sputum with the onset of hemoptysis in 1986. A chest radiograph shows cavitary lesions of various sizes in the right and left lungs (a). Over 2 years, the largest cavity on the left has contracted and a new cavity is noted below this (arrow) (b). After 4 years of chemotherapy, the sputum finally became negative and the chest radiograph stabilized (c). Bronchiectasis may be a predisposing factor for infections with atypical mycobacteria.

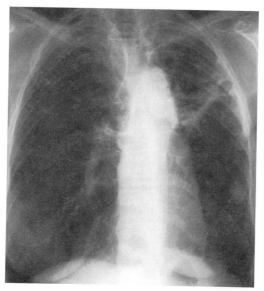

46c

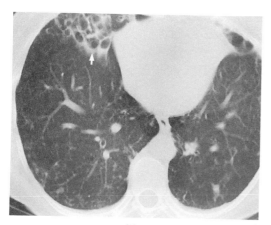

47a

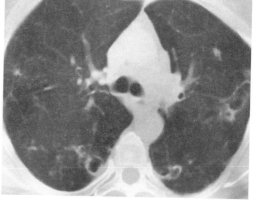

47b

FIGURE 10.47a,b A 54-year-old female with a history of recurrent pneumonias following an episode of whooping cough as a child. She presented with mild hemoptysis and a positive PPD. In 1992 her sputum was positive for acid-fast bacilli which initially were identified by probe as *M. tuberculosis*, then biochemically as *M. xenopi*, and finally as a relatively new mycobacterium, *M. celatum* (for more information on this species, please refer to Chapter 9). Computed tomography demonstrates an area of cystic bronchiectasis in the right middle lobe (arrow) (a). Elsewhere are cavities of varying sizes, some irregularly shaped (b). Smaller cavitary lesions were present on a computed tomographic examination 7 years previously.

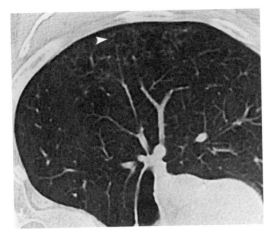

FIGURE 10.48   Tree-in-bud pattern. A 57-year-old woman with a history of several episodes of hemoptysis, diagnosed with MAC. Peripheral branching and nodular opacities (arrow) represent the tree-in-bud pattern. The tree-in-bud pattern can be seen with a wide variety of pulmonary infections as well as cystic fibrosis, allergic bronchopulmonary aspergillosis, asthma, obliterative bronchiolitis, and panbronchiolitis.

VIII. LOOK ALIKES

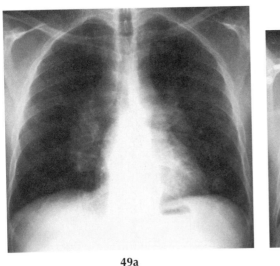

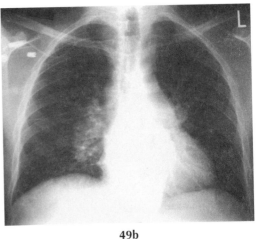

49a   49b

FIGURE 10.49a,b   A 48-year-old HIV-positive male with a history of intravenous drug abuse who presented with a septic groin. A chest radiograph demonstrates extensive bilateral hilar and paratracheal adenopathy (a). A chest radiograph performed 2 years earlier demonstrates that the adenopathy is stable (b). Stable adenopathy is not a feature of tuberculous adenopathy or of HIV disease. A transbronchial biopsy showed noncaseating granulomas compatible with sarcoidosis.

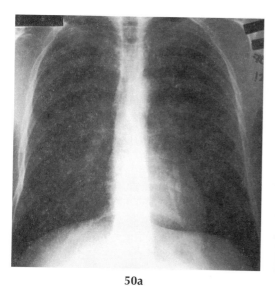

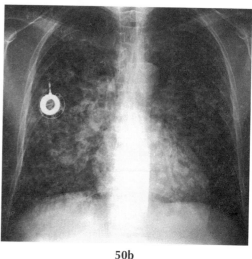

50a

50b

FIGURE 10.50a,b A 24-year-old HIV-positive Puerto Rican male presented with fevers. A chest radiograph from October 1987 demonstrates typical miliary lesions that are the result of histoplasmosis and not tuberculosis (a). Histoplasmosis is endemic in Puerto Rico and this radiograph is thought to represent endogenous reinfection. The patient responded transiently to antifungal therapy but eventually relapsed (b).

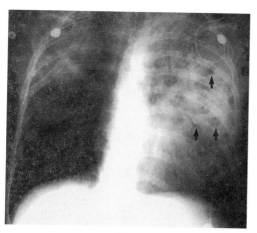

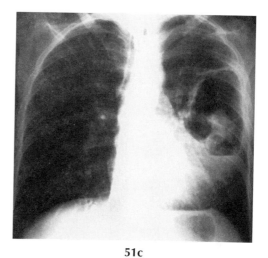

51a

51c

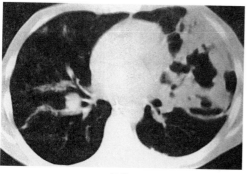

51b

FIGURE 10.51a–c A 53-year-old HIV-positive male presented with fever. Bilateral consolidation is noted, but there also are areas of lucency (arrows) within the consolidated left lung, suggesting cavitation and necrosis (a). Computed tomography shows extensive cavitation with sloughing of lung on the left (b). A chest radiograph from July 8 demonstrates a large cavity with a central mass (c). This gradually resolved and represents pulmonary gangrene. In this instance, *S. pneumoniae* was obtained. Gangrene most frequently results from *Klebsiella*, and less commonly from *S. pneumoniae* infection. Occasionally, tuberculosis will produce a similar appearance.

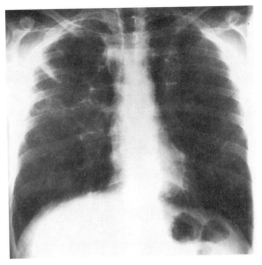

FIGURE 10.52 Multiple thin-walled cystic spaces that are the residua of a previous *Pneumocystis carinii* infection. These may rupture to produce pneumothoraces. The thin walls are fairly smooth and should not be confused with the cavities of mycobacterial disease.

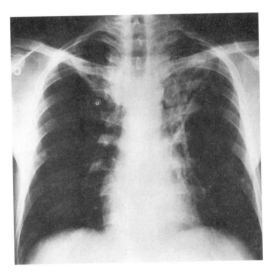

FIGURE 10.53 Atypical distribution of *P. carinii* pneumonia occurs in patients who are on inhaled pentamidine. This appearance may mimic tuberculosis due to its upper lobe distribution, but the history of prophylactic pentamidine should raise the possibility that this is *P. carinii* pneumonia.

ACKNOWLEDGMENTS

Thanks to Michael Brown for photography and to Louise Leader for preparation of the manuscript.

11 Chemotherapeutic Agents for Mycobacterial Infections

Michael H. Cynamon

CONTENTS

I. INTRODUCTION

Chemotherapy for mycobacterial disease began in the late 1940s with the introduction of streptomycin (SM). Rifampin (RIF), the most recent major new therapeutic innovation, was developed in the late 1960s. During the past quarter century there has been little progress in the identification and development of new antituberculosis drugs. Development of new and better agents has been a low priority in developed countries. In addition, the realities of the marketplace have not provided incentives to the pharmaceutical industry to pursue research in this area. In spite of the regrettable lack of research support in the area of mycobacterial disease in general, and of tuberculosis in particular, dramatic improvements in the chemotherapy of tuberculosis have taken place.

Early in the chemotherapy era it became apparent that emergence of resistance during monotherapy could be circumvented with combination therapy. Isoniazid (INH), streptomycin (SM), and para-aminosalicylic acid (PAS) in combination were used in 18- to 24-month regimens. Ethambutol (EMB) subsequently replaced PAS, and RIF replaced SM. Supervised intermittent therapy and short-course therapy were found to be effective strategies in large clinical trials supported by the British Medical Research Council. INH combined with RIF for 9 months or INH, RIF, and pyrazinamide (PZA) for 2 months followed by INH and RIF for 4 months were established as effective short-course regimens. Shorter course regimens will likely require new agents rather than newer combinations.

There has been less study of regimens for the treatment of multidrug-resistant tuberculosis (MDRTB), particularly when resistance to INH, RIF, EMB, and SM is coexistent. Resistance to the so-called primary agents is emerging slowly throughout the world.[1] This was not felt to be a problem in the U.S. until outbreaks of MDRTB in HIV-infected patients occurred in several urban areas in this country.[1-3] These events refocused attention on tuberculosis as a contemporary public health problem here and abroad. There is presently an appreciation of the potential problems of MDRTB associated with a perception that new agents are required to combat the emergence of drug resistance. If we are not to repeat the mistakes of the past, continued emphasis on intermittent supervised or directly observed short-course therapy will be necessary.

Development of new agents for the treatment of slow-growing mycobacteria is difficult because of the long treatment regimens, the use of multidrug therapy, and the need to evaluate relapse rates following the completion of therapy. In addition, there are uncertainties related to the preclinical evaluation of candidate agents. It is unclear whether *in vitro* susceptibility testing coupled with knowledge of pharmacokinetic parameters can predict how an agent will perform in the murine tuberculosis model or in human disease. The murine tuberculosis model may not accurately forecast efficacy in human disease. Additional study of both *in vitro* susceptibility testing and the murine tuberculosis model is needed to validate their ability to predict efficacy in human disease. This is particularly true with regard to organisms judged to be "resistant" to various agents *in vitro*.[4]

II. ISONIAZID, PYRAZINAMIDE, AND ETHIONAMIDE

A. Isoniazid

Chorine reported that nicotinamide had antituberculous activity in a murine model of tuberculosis.[5] Subsequent examination of nicotinamide analogs yielded INH,[6] PZA,[7,8] and ethionamide.

TABLE 11.1
Antituberculosis Agents

Agent	Mechanism of Action	Mechanism(s) of Resistance
Isoniazid	Blocks mycolic acid synthesis by inhibiting InhA (enoyl-ACP reductase) and/or KasA (β-ketoacyl-ACP synthase)	Mutations in KatG (catalase-peroxidase) blocks synthesis of active intermediate of INH Mutations in InhA Mutations in KasA
Ethionamide	Inhibits mycolic acid synthesis	Mutations in InhA and perhaps in enzyme that generates active intermediate of ethionamide
Pyrazinamide	Unknown	Decreased conversion of PZA to pyrazinoic acid by mutations in pyrazinamidase gene (PncA)
Rifampin	Inhibits DNA-dependent RNA-polymerase; suppresses initiation of chain formation	Mutation in rpoβ prevents binding of rifamycin
Ethambutol	Inhibits arabinogalactan and lipoarabinomannan synthesis	Overexpression or mutation of embAB (arabinosyl transferase) facilitates arabinan synthesis
Aminoglycoside	Inhibits protein synthesis by binding to the 30S ribosomal subunit	Reduced affinity for drug by ribosome results from mutations in rpsL (ribosomal protein S12) and rrs (16S rRNA) Possibly reduced transport into cell
Quinolone	Inhibits DNA gyrase subunit A	Mutations in gyrA prevent interactions with fluoroquinolones

Source: Adapted from Friedman, L. N., Ed., *Tuberculosis: Current Concepts and Treatment,* 1st ed., CRC Press LLC, Boca Raton, FL, 1994.

INH continues to be one of the two most important antituberculosis agents. In a recently completed survey, the prevalence of primary resistance to INH ranged from 0 to 17% and the prevalence of acquired resistance to INH varied between 4 and 54%.[9] Victor et al. reported that approximately 50% of the INH-resistant South African isolates that they studied had MICs for INH between 0.2 μg/ml and 5 μg/ml.[10]

The mechanisms of action of this agent has been more clearly defined in the past few years (Table 11.1). INH is thought to inhibit mycolic acid synthesis.[11-14] Other mechanisms of action have been proposed for INH, including action as an antimetabolite for NAD[15] or pyridoxal phosphate.[16] The mechanism of action of INH is complex. INH is a prodrug that is activated by a catalase-peroxidase enzyme (KatG).[17] The activated drug subsequently interacts with one or more targets: Inh A (an NADH-dependent enoyl [acyl carrier protein] reductase)[18] and/or Kas A (a β-ketoacyl [acyl carrier protein] synthase).[19]

Mutations in KatG account for the majority of the INH-resistant clinical isolates.[20] The bulk of the other INH-resistant clinical isolates have mutations in Inh A, Kas A, and Ahp C (alkyl hydroperoxide reductase).[19] Heym et al. found that Ahp C, in contrast to catalase-peroxidase, does not appear to act as a virulence factor in murine infections or to play a direct role in INH resistance.[21]

INH is thought to be bacteriocidal against actively growing tubercle bacilli. This agent is active against *M. tuberculosis* complex. It has variable *in vitro* activity against nontuberculous mycobacteria, perhaps being most reliably active against *M. kansasii*. It is not active *in vitro* against *M. avium* complex or clinically important rapid growers.

1. Absorption, Distribution, and Elimination

INH is well absorbed following oral dosing achieving serum concentrations between 3 and 5 μg/ml (Table 11.2) at 1 to 2 h after a 300 mg dose.[22] Serum concentrations in rapid acetylators are 20 to

TABLE 11.2
Antimicrobial Agents Used to Treat Tuberculosis in Adults[a]

Agent	Daily Dose	Peak Serum Level (m g/ml)	Dose that Corresponds to Peak Serum Level	Maximum Daily Dose	MIC Range in m g/ml (Reference)
Isoniazid	5 mg/kg	3–5	300 mg	300 mg	0.025–0.05 (152)
Ethionamide	0.5–1 g	20	1 g	1 g	2.5–10 (153)
Pyrazinamide	15–30 mg/kg	30–40	1.5 g	2 g	6.25–50 (154)
Rifampin	10 mg/kg	4–32	600 mg	600 mg	0.1–0.5 (155)
Rifabutin	5–10 mg/kg	0.49	300 mg	600 mg	0.04–0.08 (156)
Rifapentine	600 mg twice/week	15	600 mg	600 mg	≤0.125 (153)
Ethambutol	15–25 mg/kg	2–5	25 mg/kg	2.5 g	0.5–2 (157)
Streptomycin	15 mg/kg	25–50	1 g	1 g	0.25–2 (158)
Kanamycin	15 mg/kg	22	7.5 mg/kg	1 g	1.5–3 (159)
Amikacin	15 mg/kg	33	7.5 mg/kg	1 g	0.5–1 (159)
		55	15 mg/kg		
Capreomycin	15 mg/kg	20–47	1 g	1 g	1.25–2.5 (159)
Cycloserine	0.5–1 g	10	250 mg	1 g	6.25–25 (160)
Ciprofloxacin	1–1.5 g	3.4–5.4	1 g	1.5 g	0.12–2 (101)
Ofloxacin	400–800 mg	2.9–5.6	400 mg	800 mg	0.12–2 (101)
PAS	150 mg/kg	9–35	4 g	12 g	1–10 (153)
Levofloxacin	500–1000 mg	5.7	500 mg	1000 mg	0.12–2 (153)

[a] Data abstracted from References 107, 150, 151, as well as from References cited above and in the text.

Source: Revised from Friedman, L. N., Ed., *Tuberculosis: Current Concepts and Treatment,* 1st ed., CRC Press LLC, Boca Raton, FL, 1994.

50% of those in slow acetylators. INH is distributed into all body tissues and fluids including cerebrospinal fluid (CSF). It is minimally bound to plasma proteins, crosses the placenta readily, and achieves levels in milk comparable to those in maternal serum.

INH is metabolized in the liver to acetyl-isoniazid, which is subsequently transformed to the mono- and diacetylhydrazine, isonicotinic acid, and isonicotinyl glycine.[22] Approximately 75 to 95% of the INH is excreted in the urine over 24 h as INH and its metabolites (predominately acetyl-isoniazid and isonicotinic acid).[22] INH can be administered safely at its usual dose to individuals with a serum creatinine less than 12 mg/dl.[23] It also may be administered intramuscularly or intravenously.

2. Adverse Effects

Excretion of pyridoxine is enhanced by isoniazid, resulting in decreased serum pyridoxine levels. Pyridoxine deficiency can manifest itself as peripheral neuropathy which is usually preceded by paresthesias of the hands and feet. This effect occurs in approximately 20% of patients, particularly in those who are malnourished, are alcoholics, or have diabetes mellitus. Although as little as 6 mg/day of pyridoxine is effective in preventing peripheral neuropathy, 25 or 50 mg/day often is given concurrently with INH. Other manifestations of nervous system toxicity that occur rarely are convulsions, optic neuritis, toxic encephalopathy, muscle twitching, ataxia, tinnitus, dizziness, euphoria, memory impairment, and toxic psychosis.

Hepatic dysfunction, manifested by modest increases (less than threefold) in serum AST (SGOT) and ALT (SGPT) occurs in approximately 20% of patients on INH during the initial 4 to 8 weeks of therapy. Patients should be carefully monitored monthly for symptoms of hepatitis (anorexia, malaise, fatigue, nausea, and jaundice). The incidence of INH-associated hepatitis is age-related. It is rare in patients less than 20 years old; occurs in 0.3% of those 20 to 34 years old, increases to 1.2% for patients 35 to 49 years old, and occurs in 2.3% of those individuals older than 50 years of age.[24] Continuation of INH after the appearance of symptoms of hepatic dysfunction increases the severity of hepatic injury and has led to death from fulminant hepatitis in some individuals.[25,26] The mechanism of INH-associated hepatitis has not been clarified.[27] INH should not be given to patients with acute liver disease or with a history of previous INH-associated hepatitis.

INH has been associated with dryness of the mouth, epigastric distress, tinnitus, urinary retention, and methemoglobinemia. Although uncommon, INH also has been associated with a "lupus-like" syndrome consisting of fever, rash, and arthralgias. INH can be used safely to treat clinical tuberculosis during pregnancy. Preventive therapy can usually be initiated during the postpartum period.

Overdose of INH (usually greater than 1.5 g) may lead to coma, severe intractable seizures, metabolic acidosis, and hyperglycemia. The seizures are thought to result from decreased γ-amino butyric acid concentrations due to inhibition of central nervous system (CNS) pyridoxal-5-phosphate activity by INH. Seizures do not respond well to diazepam or phenobarbital; however, pyridoxine hydrochloride intravenously (comparable to dose of INH ingested) has been effective in treating INH-induced seizures.

3. Drug Interactions

INH therapy has been associated with increased serum levels of carbamazepine and symptoms of carbamazepine toxicity (ataxia, headache, vomiting, blurred vision, drowsiness, and confusion). The interaction is thought to result from INH-induced inhibition of the hepatic metabolism of carbamazepine. If INH and carbamazepine are used concurrently, serum concentrations of the anticonvulsant should be monitored. INH inhibits hepatic metabolism of phenytoin resulting in toxicity in some patients. Patients receiving both INH and phenytoin should be observed for development of phenytoin toxicity. Usually, the dose of phenytoin is reduced when it is administered concomitantly with INH.

B. PYRAZINAMIDE

PZA has a narrow spectrum of activity. It is active against *M. tuberculosis* but is not active against *M. bovis* (a closely related member of *M. tuberculosis* complex) or nontuberculous mycobacteria. The mechanism of action of PZA is not known. PZA is converted to pyrazinoic acid by nicotinamidase intracellularly.[28] Some PZA-resistant isolates of *M. tuberculosis* and isolates of *M. bovis* have markedly reduced levels of nicotinamidase activity. Recently, mutations in Pnc A, a gene which encodes pyrazinamidase/nicotinamidase, have been found to correlate with resistance to PZA by *M. tuberculosis*.[29,30] Mutations in this gene account for the majority of PZA resistance.[30] It is likely that PZA is a prodrug of pyrazinoic acid since pyrazinoate esters have been shown to circumvent PZA resistance *in vitro*.[31] PZA is thought to be bacteriostatic. It is unclear whether it inhibits primarily intracellular or extracellular organisms.[32] This agent's clinical importance has been recognized increasingly since its use facilitated 6-month chemotherapy regimens.[33]

1. Absorption, Distribution, and Elimination

PZA is well absorbed within 1 to 2 h after oral administration achieving serum levels between 30 and 40 µg/ml following a 1.5 g dose.[34] It is distributed into body tissues and fluids including the CSF. PZA is approximately 50% bound to plasma proteins. Serum pyrazinoic acid levels peak several hours later than PZA and exceed that of the parent drug. PZA is hydrolyzed primarily in the liver to pyrazinoic acid followed by hydroxylation to 5-hydroxy pyrazinoic acid.[35] A small fraction of PZA is excreted in the urine; however, approximately one third of the dose is excreted as pyrazinoic acid.[34] Pyrazinamide should be used cautiously in patients with renal insufficiency and should be avoided in the presence of severe hepatic dysfunction.

2. Adverse Effects

Transient elevation of serum transaminases, jaundice, hepatitis, fever, anorexia, malaise, or hepatic tenderness are the most common adverse effects of PZA. Liver toxicity is thought to be dose-related and was reported to occur in approximately 15% of patients receiving 3 g/day with jaundice occurring in 3%.[36] The incidence of drug-induced hepatotoxicity in patients receiving 25 to 35 mg/kg of PZA is less than 5%.

Pyrazinoic acid competes with uric acid for renal tubular excretion frequently leading to hyperuricemia and occasionally episodes of acute gout. Rash, arthralgias, vomiting, dysuria, and photosensitivity have rarely been associated with PZA therapy. This agent should be used cautiously in patients with diabetes mellitus because management of diabetes may become difficult. The safety of pyrazinamide during pregnancy has not been established.

3. Drug Interactions

No data are available on drug interactions with PZA.

C. ETHIONAMIDE

Thioisonicotinamide was synthesized in 1952. It was found to be active against *M. tuberculosis in vitro* and in a murine model of tuberculosis; however, it was not effective in human tuberculosis.[37] Ethionamide (ETA), the α-ethyl derivative of thioisonicotinamide, was subsequently synthesized and found to have improved activity.[38] The mechanism of action of ETA is thought to be inhibition of mycolic acid synthesis.[39,40] Cross resistance between ethionamide and INH has been found with some mutations in Inh A.[18] It is likely that other genes are involved for selective resistance to ethionamide.

1. Absorption, Distribution, and Elimination

Peak serum levels of ETA after a 250 mg oral dose is approximately 1.8 μg/ml.[41] The serum $t_{1/2}$ is between 2 and 3 h.[41] This agent is thought to be widely distributed achieving levels comparable to that of serum in various body fluids. The predominant metabolite of ETA is a sulfoxide; a methyl derivative also is found to a lesser extent.[41] The sulfoxide transformation appears to occur in the liver. A small percentage (less than 1%) of ETA is excreted unchanged in the urine.

2. Adverse Effects

The most frequent side effects of ETA are anorexia, nausea, vomiting, diarrhea, and gastrointestinal discomfort.[42] These effects may be managed by changing the time of drug administration or decreasing the dosage. Antiemetics can often ameliorate nausea and vomiting; however, discontinuation of ETA may be necessary. A metallic taste, likely related to the sulfur, sometimes has been noted. Postural hypotension, depression, and drowsiness have been observed. Additional side effects include convulsions, peripheral neuropathy, olfactory disturbances, diplopia, blurred vision, dizziness, paresthesias, headache, tremors, and hallucinations.

Transient elevations of serum bilirubin, AST (SGOT), and ALT (SGPT) have occurred in patients taking ETA. Hepatitis has been reported to occur and is usually reversible after ETA is discontinued. Rash, stomatitis, photosensitivity, thrombocytopenia, purpura, and goiter (with and without hypothyroidism) rarely have been associated with use of ETA. In addition, hypoglycemia, gynecomastia, menorrhagia, joint pain, and acne have been reported. ETA should be used cautiously in patients with diabetes mellitus because management of diabetes may become difficult. ETA should be avoided in patients with severe hepatic dysfunction. The safety of ETA during pregnancy has not been established.

3. Drug Interactions

Seizures associated with cycloserine use may be aggravated by concurrent use of ETA.

III. RIFAMYCINS

A. Rifampicin (Rifampin)

In the 1950s, Lepetit Laboratories in Italy recognized a new class of antimicrobials called rifamycins. One of the original compounds, rifamycin B, was isolated from an organism belonging to the genus Streptomyces, later reclassified as *Nocardia mediterranei*. Subsequent chemical modifications of the original compounds resulted in agents with increased antibacterial activity, rifamycin SV and rifamycin B diethylamide. Rifampin (RIF), 3-4 (4-methylpiperazyinyl-iminomethylidene)-rifamycin SV, was synthesized in 1965.

RIF is an important agent in the treatment of tuberculosis, leprosy, and diseases caused by the nontuberculous mycobacteria. RIF has good *in vitro* and *in vivo* activity against *M. tuberculosis*, *M. kansasii*, and *M. marinum*.[43,44] It has modest *in vitro* and *in vivo* activity against *M. avium* complex[45-47] and poor activity against the rapid growers *M. fortuitum* and *M. chelonae*.[44,48]

The mechanism of action of RIF is inhibition of the β-subunit of DNA-dependent RNA polymerase.[39,49] RIF is considered to be bactericidal and is active against both intracellular and extracellular *M. tuberculosis*. Its use in combination with isoniazid in treatment regimens for tuberculosis allowed the duration of therapy to be decreased from 18 to 24 months to 6 to 9 months. Resistance to RIF results from mutations in the β-subunit of the DNA-dependent RNA polymerase (rpoβ).[50,51] The mutations (insertions, deletions, or missence) are most frequent within an 81-base pair fragment of rpoβ. Some of these mutations result in cross-resistance to all rifamycins while other mutations yield resistance to RIF and rifapentine but not to rifabutin and KRM-1648.[52]

1. Absorption, Distribution, and Elimination

RIF is well absorbed from the gastrointestinal tract, although the presence of food decreases absorption. A single 600 mg dose in fasting patients results in peak serum concentrations between 8 and 12 μg/ml at 2 h after administration (range of 1 to 4 h).[53] Rifampin should be taken 1 h before or 2 h after eating due to reduced absorption when ingested with food. RIF penetrates tissues well and reaches effective concentrations both in tuberculous cavities and in cerebrospinal fluid in the setting of inflamed meninges. RIF crosses the placenta and infrequently has been associated with limb deformities and central nervous system defects, although not significantly so.[54] Thus, isoniazid and rifampin are first-line drugs in pregnant women with tuberculosis (see Chapter 8).

RIF is deacetylated in the liver and enters the bile where there is subsequent enterohepatic circulation. RIF induces its own hepatic metabolism over time; however, the deacetylated metabolite retains antimycobacterial activity. Both RIF and the deacetylated metabolite are excreted in the urine. The half-life does not differ in patients with renal failure at doses not exceeding 600 mg per day and, consequently, no dosage adjustment is required.

RIF is not appreciably cleared by either peritoneal dialysis or hemodialysis. Rifampin should be used cautiously when hepatic dysfunction is present with monitoring of serum transaminases.

2. Adverse Effects

Patients should be advised that RIF is widely distributed in bodily fluids and will impart an intense orange-red color to urine, sweat, saliva, and tears; soft contact lenses may be permanently

TABLE 11.3
Potential Rifamycin Interactions[a]

Anticonvulsants	Phenytoin
Antiarrhythmics	Disopyramide, quinidine, mexiletine
Antibiotics	Chloramphenicol, clarithromycin, dapsone, doxycycline fluoroquinolones
Anticoagulants	Warfarin
Antifungals	Fluconazole, itraconazole, ketoconazole
Barbituates	—
Benzodiazepines	Diazepam
Beta-blockers, calcium channel blockers	Diltiazem, nifedipine, verapamil
Corticosteroids	—
Cardiac glycosides	—
Oral or other systemic hormonal contraceptives	—
Haloperidol	—
HIV protease inhibitors	Indinavir, ritonavir, nelfinavir, saquinavir
Oral hypoglycemics	Sulfonylureas
Immunosuppressive agents	Cyclosporine, tacrolimus
Levothyroxine	—
Narcotic analgesics	Methadone
Quinine	—
Reverse transcriptase inhibitors	Efavirenz, delavirdine
Theophylline	—
Tricyclic antidepressants	Amitriptyline, nortriptyline

[a] Dosage adjustments may be necessary when these agents are used concurrently with rifamycins. In some cases, rifampin is contraindicated — see text for details.

discolored. The most common side effects are rash (seen in 1%), fever (seen in 1%), and nausea or vomiting. Transient abnormalities in liver function have been reported, but severe hepatotoxicity due to RIF is infrequent.[43] The occurrence of severe toxicity may increase with underlying liver disease and concomitant use of isoniazid. Thrombocytopenia also has been described with RIF use.

Intermittent administration of higher doses of RIF has been associated with immunologically mediated reactions, such as anemia, thrombocytopenia, leukopenia, acute renal failure, and a "flu-like" syndrome consisting of chills, fever, myalgias, arthralgias, and gastrointestinal upset. These reactions occur mostly in persons receiving a dosage of 15 mg/kg or greater and are rare at the recommended daily or twice-weekly dose.

3. Drug Interactions

RIF is a potent inducer of hepatic microsomal enzymes. Its use may result in decreased activity of warfarin derivatives, oral contraceptives, sulfonylureas, corticosteroids, digoxin, methadone, barbiturates, phenytoin, ketoconazole, fluconazole, β-adrenergic blocking agents, verapamil, cyclosporine, and theophylline (Table 11.3).[43,55,56] When RIF and methadone are used concurrently, methadone doses must be increased at least 50% over baseline doses. In addition, methadone may need to be administered in divided doses when used with RIF. Because of induced alterations in steroid metabolism, breakthrough bleeding and pregnancy have been reported with concurrent use of RIF and oral contraceptive agents. An alternative method of contraception is recommended during therapy with a RIF-containing regimen.

Rifampin markedly lowers the serum levels of HIV protease inhibitors (saquinavir, ritonavir, indinavir, and nelfinavir) and the nonnucleoside reverse transcriptase inhibitors; therefore, it should not be used in combination with these agents.[57]

B. Rifabutin

Rifabutin (ansamycin), a semisynthetic derivative of rifamycin S, belongs to the spiropiperdylrifa-mycins. Rifabutin is more active than RIF *in vitro* against *M. tuberculosis, M. kansasii, M. marinum, M. xenopi, M. haemophilum,* and *M. avium* complex.[45,47,58,59] Cross resistance to rifabutin is incom-plete for RIF-resistant isolates of *M. tuberculosis* and *M. avium* complex.[58,59] The mechanism of action of rifabutin is similar to that of RIF.

Rifabutin has been used as part of multidrug regimens for the treatment of RIF-resistant tuberculosis,[60,61] for the treatment of pulmonary *M. avium* complex disease[62] and for disseminated *M. avium* complex infections in persons with acquired immune deficiency syndrome.[63-65] The efficacy of these regimens and of rifabutin in particular is not clear. Rifabutin (300 mg/day) is approved for prevention of disseminated *M. avium* complex (MAC) infection in persons with AIDS.[66] Daily rifabutin in combination with weekly azithromycin (1200 mg) was more effective than either agent alone in a MAC preventive therapy study.[67] Rifabutin is recommended as a substitute for rifampin in HIV-infected individuals with drug-sensitive tuberculosis who are receiv-ing antiretroviral agents[57] (see Chapter 6).

1. Absorption, Distribution, and Elimination

Rifabutin is incompletely absorbed from the gastrointestinal tract, with bioavailability ranging from 12 to 20%.[68] A peak serum concentration of less than 1 µg/ml is achieved 2 to 3 h after a single 600 mg oral dose.[66] Peak plasma levels of 0.38 µg/ml were achieved 3.3 h after a 300 mg oral dose of rifabutin in healthy volunteers. Rifabutin is taken up by tissues and the level achieved in lung is approximately five- to tenfold higher than that in serum.[58] Elimination occurs through both the liver and kidney. There appear to be two major metabolites, 31-OH rifabutin and 25-deacetyl rifabutin.[69] The terminal $t_{1/2}$ ranges from 12 to 18 h, making it suitable for intermittent administration.

2. Adverse Effects

Rifabutin generally appears to be well tolerated. The most common adverse effects are rash, gastrointestinal distress, and neutropenia.[69] Uveitis (unilateral or bilateral) characterized by pain, redness, and loss of vision, occasionally occurs in patients receiving rifabutin, particularly higher dosages in combination with clarithromycin and/or fluconazole.[70] The symptoms of uveitis usually resolve after discontinuing rifabutin and therapy with topical corticosteroids and/or mydriatics. The safety of rifabutin during pregnancy has not been established.

3. Drug Interactions

Induction of hepatic microsomal enzymes and autoinduction of its own metabolism occurs with RFB,[71] but may be less than that seen with RIF. The interaction between RFB and methadone may be less than that seen with RIF. RFB reduces the area under the zidovudine concentration time curve by 20 to 30%; however, the clinical significance of this interaction is not clear. There currently is no recommendation to alter the zidovudine dose because of this reported interaction. No clinically significant interaction was observed when rifabutin is given concomitantly with didanosine. Rifabutin is contraindicated for patients taking saquinavir or delavirdine. If rifabutin is used concurrently with nelfinavir, indinavir, or amprenavir the daily dose of rifabutin should be reduced from 300 mg to 150 mg (the twice-weekly dose of rifabutin is unchanged).[57] The serum levels of rifabutin decrease when administered with efavirenz; therefore, the dose of rifabutin (both daily and twice weekly) should be increased from 300 mg to 450 mg.[57] See Chapters 6 and 13 for further details.

C. Rifapentine

Rifapentine is rifamycin-3{-[(4-cyclopentyl-l-piperazinyl)imino]methyl}. Its activity *in vitro* is superior to that of RIF against isolates of *M. tuberculosis* and *M. avium* complex.[45,59,72,73] It also has enhanced activity compared to RIF in murine models of infection due to these mycobacterial species.[46,74]

1. Absorption, Distribution, and Elimination

The relative bioavailability of rifapentine after a single 600 mg dose is 70%. The maximum concentrations occur between 5 and 6 h after administration. Unlike RIF, absorption is enhanced by approximately 40% (AUC and C_{max}) when administered with food (850 total calories). No significant auto-induction effect on steady-state pharmacokinetics has been observed. The C_{max} and $t_{1/2}$ for rifapentine and 25-desacetyl rifapentine (active metabolite) were 15 µg/ml and 13 h, and 6.3 µg/ml and 13.4 h, respectively, on day 10 following a 600 mg dose every 72 h in healthy volunteers. Both rifapentine and its active metabolite are highly protein bound ($\approx 95\%$).

Rifapentine is predominantly excreted in the feces with a small percentage recovered in the urine. Only 17% of rifapentine is excreted via the kidneys; however, the clinical significance of impaired renal function on the disposition of rifapentine and its 25-desacetyl metabolite is not known. The elimination of these agents are primarily by the liver; however, the clinical significance of impaired hepatic function on the disposition of rifapentine and its metabolite is not known.

2. Adverse Effects

The rifamycins are associated with serious hepatic events; therefore, serum transaminases should be carefully monitored when these agents are given to patients with abnormal liver tests and/or liver disease. Diarrhea secondary to *Clostridium difficile*-associated colitis has been reported after rifamycin use. Rifapentine may cause a red-orange discoloration of body fluids (urine, tears, sweat, and CSF) and contact lenses may be permanently stained. Adverse events of moderate or severe intensity (<1% of patients) include: hyperbilirubinemia, hepatitis, urticaria, thrombocytopenia, hyperkalemia, fatigue, and gout. Rifapentine should not be used during pregnancy since it is teratogenic in rats and rabbits. Patients with abnormal liver enzymes and/or liver disease should have frequent monitoring (every 2 to 4 weeks) of serum transaminases during therapy.

3. Drug Interactions

Rifapentine induces cytochromes P 4503A4 and P 4502C8/9; thus, the levels of other coadministered drugs that are metabolized by these enzymes may be decreased. Enzyme induction occurred within 4 days after the first dose with a return to baseline levels 14 days after discontinuation of the drug. Dosage adjustments of the drugs listed in Table 11.3 may be necessary when given concurrently with rifapentine. Patients using hormonal contraceptives should change to nonhormonal methods of birth control. Interactions between protease inhibitors or nonnucleoside reverse transcriptase inhibitors and rifapentine have not been adequately studied.

IV. ETHAMBUTOL

A. Description

Ethambutol hydrochloride is a synthetic agent that was developed from *N,N'*-diisopropylethylenediamine, which was found to be active against *M. tuberculosis* in a screening program.[75] The *d*-enantiomer of ethambutol is approximately 200 times more active than the *l*-enantiomer.

Ethambutol (the *d*-enantiomer) is active against *M. tuberculosis, M. kansasii, M. avium* complex, and some other nontuberculous mycobacteria. Ethambutol inhibits the introduction of D-arabinose into lipoarabinomannan and arabinogalactan.[76,77] One mechanism of resistance to ethambutol results from overexpression or mutation of embAB (arabinosyl transferase) which facilitates arabinan synthesis.[78,79] Ethambutol is active against growing organisms and is thought to be "weakly" bactericidal.

1. Absorption, Distribution, and Elimination

Ethambutol is rapidly absorbed from the gut with a bioavailability of approximately 80% of administered dose.[80] Peak serum levels 2 to 4 h after oral doses of 25 mg/kg or 12.5 mg/kg were 4 to 5 µg/ml and 2 µg/ml, respectively.[80] Lee et al. measured a mean peak serum level of 4 µg/ml after a 15 mg/kg oral dose.[81] Ethambutol can be taken with or without food.

Ethambutol appears to have a large volume of distribution which is due in part to active uptake of drug by erythrocytes. Plasma protein binding is between 20 and 30%.[82] Ethambutol crosses the placenta. It is present in breast milk at levels comparable to that in serum.

The $t_{1/2}$ is between 3 and 4 h in patients with normal renal function. Ethambutol is primarily eliminated by the kidneys in part by active tubular secretion.[80,81] Hepatic metabolism (oxidation to an aldehyde intermediate which is converted to the dicarboxylic acid) accounts for approximately 20% of the total body clearance of ethambutol. Approximately 50% of an oral dose of the drug is excreted unchanged in the urine, and 8 to 15% is excreted as inactive metabolites. Approximately 20% of the initial dose is excreted in the feces unchanged. Accumulation of drug has been observed in patients with decreased renal function. Modification of dosing is necessary in patients with severe renal insufficiency. In patients with creatinine clearances of 10 ml/min or less the dosing interval should be increased to every 48 h.

2. Adverse Effects

Ethambutol has been well tolerated at the usual daily dose of 15 mg/kg.[83] Its most important toxicity is retrobulbar neuritis which can present with decreased visual acuity, constriction of visual fields, central and peripheral scotomas, or loss of red-green color discrimination. Optic neuritis appears to be related to dose and duration of therapy, being quite unusual at 15 mg/kg/day. Visual acuity should be measured with a Snellen eye chart prior to and during therapy.

Subjective visual symptoms may occur before or concurrent with decreased visual acuity; therefore, patients should be asked periodically about blurred vision and other visual symptoms. Each eye should be tested separately since changes in visual acuity may be unilateral or bilateral. Ocular toxicity, when detected early, usually is reversible during a period of weeks to months after ethambutol is discontinued. Recovery of visual function can take a year or more. Rarely the dysfunction is not reversible. Ethambutol should be used only when visual acuity can be monitored.

Dermatitis, pruritus, headache, malaise, dizziness, fever, mental confusion, disorientation, joint pain, GI discomfort, abdominal pain, nausea, vomiting, anorexia, and rarely anaphylactoid reactions have been associated with use of ethambutol. Peripheral neuropathy infrequently has been reported. Elevated serum uric acid levels (in approximately 50% of patients) and the occurrence of acute gout occasionally have been associated with ethambutol.[84]

Although ethambutol is teratogenic in animals in high doses, it has not been reported to produce fetal abnormalities during human pregnancy.

3. Drug Interactions

There have been no significant drug interactions reported for ethambutol.

V. AMINOGLYCOSIDES (AMINOGLYCOSIDIC AMINOCYCLITOLS): STREPTOMYCIN, KANAMYCIN, AND AMIKACIN

A. DESCRIPTION

Aminoglycosides contain one or two amino sugars linked to an aminocyclitol nucleus. Streptidine is the nucleus of streptomycin, and 2-deoxystreptamine is the nucleus of kanamycin and amikacin. The aminoglycosides are bactericidal and are thought to inhibit protein synthesis by binding to the 30S ribosomal subunit. They are effective against extracellular mycobacteria. Resistance to an aminoglycoside may result from decreased cell wall permeability, mutations in the rpsl (S12 ribosomal protein) gene, the rrs (16S rRNA) coding region, or to aminoglycoside-modifying enzymes (acetylation, adenylation, or phosphorylation).[85,86] The latter mechanism (usually plasmid-mediated) frequently is present in Gram-positive and Gram-negative bacteria. Cross-resistance between kanamycin (amikacin) and streptomycin in mycobacteria has not been reported.[87] Cross-resistance occurs between kanamycin and amikacin in *M. tuberculosis* isolates; therefore, aminoglycoside-modifying enzymes are not likely to be involved in these organisms.[88]

1. Absorption, Distribution, and Elimination

The aminoglycosides are well absorbed after parenteral (intramuscular or intravenous) administration. They are poorly absorbed from the gut. These agents are usually given in divided doses for the therapy of bacterial infections; however, they should be used in a single daily dose for the treatment of infections caused by slow-growing mycobacteria. Following an intramuscular (im) dose, peak plasma levels are usually achieved within 0.5 to 2 h and measurable levels may be present for 8 to 12 h or longer.

Aminoglycosides are widely distributed into body fluids (extracellular fluids) and are minimally protein bound. They diffuse poorly and unpredictably into the CSF even in patients with meningeal inflammation, achieving levels less than 50% of the serum level. Aminoglycosides accumulate in body tissues and are slowly released after therapy is discontinued. Aminoglycosides cross the placenta and reach levels in fetal serum of 16 to 50% of that in maternal serum.

The $t_{1/2}$ of aminoglycosides are usually 2 to 4 h. The serum levels and the $t_{1/2}$ are higher and longer, respectively, in patients with decreased renal function. These agents are not metabolized and are excreted predominantly by glomerular filtration. Particular caution must be used in monitoring renal function in elderly patients who start out with age-related decreases in GFR. The majority of a single parenteral dose of an aminoglycoside is excreted within 24 h in the urine. Aminoglycosides can be removed by hemodialysis and to a lesser extent by peritoneal dialysis. It has been suggested that patients with renal insufficiency be given 1 g loading dose of streptomycin followed by 7.5 mg/kg at 24 h intervals for creatinine clearances of 50 to 80 ml/min, 24 to 72 h intervals for creatinine clearances of 10 to 50 ml/min, and 72 to 96 h intervals for creatinine clearances less than 10 ml/min. Patients undergoing hemodialysis should receive 50 to 75% of the initial loading dose at the end of each dialysis. The author's preference is to use amikacin in patients with creatinine clearances below 50 ml/min since appropriate serum peak levels can be monitored (30 to 50 μg/ml).

2. Adverse Effects

Eighth cranial nerve toxicity may occur as a result of aminoglycoside therapy. Streptomycin usually is associated with vestibular symptoms such as dizziness, ataxia, vertigo, and nystagmus. Kanamycin and amikacin usually are associated with auditory symptoms such as hearing loss (decreased high-frequency perception detectable by audiometric testing occurs prior to middle frequency impairment), tinnitus, or roaring in ears. Auditory nerve damage may be irreversible.

Aminoglycoside-induced nephropathy may be associated with elevation of BUN and serum creatinine, with decreased creatinine clearance due to tubular necrosis. Nonoliguric azotemia is the common form, with oliguria occurring rarely. Nephropathy is generally reversible after discontinuation of drugs; however, dialysis is sometimes necessary. Streptomycin is thought to be less nephrotoxic than kanamycin or amikacin at usual doses.

Headache, tremor, lethargy, paresthesia, peripheral neuropathy, arachnoiditis, encephalopathy, and acute brain syndrome rarely have been associated with aminoglycoside therapy. Optic neuritis also has been associated with use of aminoglycosides. Hypersensitivity reactions including rash, urticaria, stomatitis, pruritus, fever, generalized burning, and eosinophilia have been associated with aminoglycoside therapy. Anaphylaxis and transient agranulocytosis have occurred rarely. Cross-allergenicity occurs among the aminoglycosides.

Less frequent adverse effects such as nausea, vomiting, anemia, granulocytopenia, thrombocytopenia, tachycardia, arthralgia, hepatic necrosis, myocarditis, transient elevation of hepatic enzymes, and serum bilirubin have been associated with use of aminoglycosides.

Ototoxicity and nephrotoxicity are more likely to occur in elderly patients (due to decreased creatinine clearance), dehydrated patients, patients with preexisting renal impairment, or patients concurrently receiving other nephrotoxic and/or ototoxic agents. Aminoglycoside therapy should be accompanied by periodic assessments of renal function and eighth cranial nerve function. During antimycobacterial therapy, monitoring serum levels is more useful to assure that appropriate therapeutic levels are achieved rather than to predict nephrotoxicity. The safety of amikacin and kanamycin during pregnancy has not been established. Streptomycin has been associated with congenital deafness in children whose mothers received this drug during their pregnancy; therefore, it should be used only in situations where there are no safer alternative drugs.

3. Drug Interactions

The concurrent use of other agents with nephrotoxic potential should be avoided.

VI. CAPREOMYCIN SULFATE

A. DESCRIPTION

Capreomycin is a polypeptide derived from *Streptomyces capreolus*. It is a complex of capreomycin IA, IB, IIA, and IIB. Capreomycin is thought to be bacteriostatic and to inhibit protein synthesis. Resistance to this agent develops in a step-wise manner *in vitro*. "Partial" cross-resistance between capreomycin and kanamycin has been observed.

1. Absorption, Distribution, and Elimination

Capreomycin is given im due to poor absorption from the gut. One gram of capreomycin im yields peak serum levels between 20 to 47 μg/ml at 1 to 2 h and approximately 10 μg/ml at 6 h. It is not known how this agent is distributed in body tissue or fluids, or whether it crosses the placenta. The $t_{1/2}$ of capreomycin is 4 to 6 h. In patients with decreased renal function, the serum levels are higher and the $t_{1/2}$ is prolonged. It is excreted in the urine predominantly by glomerular filtration without metabolic transformation. Approximately 57% of a 1 g dose is excreted in the urine within 24 h.

2. Adverse Effects

Renal dysfunction associated with increased BUN and serum creatinine results from tubular necrosis. Renal dysfunction is usually reversible after discontinuation of capreomycin. Renal function should be carefully monitored particularly in those patients at increased risk (i.e., elderly patients, patients with preexisting renal dysfunction, and patients receiving other potentially nephrotoxic drugs). Hypokalemia, hypocalcemia, hypomagnesemia, and alkalosis may occur secondary to renal tubular dysfunction.

Capreomycin therapy can result in auditory and vestibular dysfunction secondary to eighth nerve injury. Hearing loss is usually reversible. Headache, tinnitus, and vertigo associated with capreomycin have been reported.

Capreomycin can cause pain, induration, and sterile abscesses at injection sites. Eosinophilia occurs frequently in patients on daily therapy and usually resolves when the frequency is reduced to less than three times per week. Leukocytosis, leukopenia, and thrombocytopenia have been associated with this agent. In addition, hypersensitivity reactions (rash, urticaria, and photosensitivity) have been reported. The safety of capreomycin during pregnancy has not been determined.

Dosage reduction based on creatinine clearance is necessary for patients with decreased renal function. Dosage adjustments are designed to achieve a mean steady-state capreomycin level of 10 μg/ml.

3. Drug Interactions

No data are available on drug interactions with capreomycin. The concurrent use of other agents with nephrotoxic potential should be avoided.

VII. CYCLOSERINE

A. DESCRIPTION

Cycloserine, an analog of D-alanine, is derived from *Streptomyces orchidaceus* and also has been synthesized. Cycloserine inhibits cell wall synthesis by blocking alanine racemase and D-alanine-D-alanine synthetase. These components are needed for synthesis of peptidoglycan which is an essential part of bacterial cell walls.[89] Primary and acquired resistance to cycloserine has been demonstrated. The mechanism of resistance to cycloserine in *M. tuberculosis* has not been determined. In *M. smegmatis,* overexpression of the alanine racemase gene due to upregulation of its promoter has been demonstrated to be a mechanism of resistance to cycloserine.[90] Streptococcus mutants selected for resistance to cycloserine had increased levels of alanine racemase and D-alanine-D-alanine synthetase.[91]

1. Absorption, Distribution, and Elimination

After oral administration of cycloserine, approximately 70 to 90% is absorbed from the gut. Peak levels of 8 to 20 μg/ml occur within 2 to 4 h after a 250-mg dose.[92]

Cycloserine is widely distributed in body fluids and tissues in concentrations approximately equal to that in the serum. The CSF level of cycloserine is reported to be 80 to 100% of the serum level in patients with inflamed meninges and 50 to 80% of the serum level in patients with uninflamed meninges. This agent is not bound to plasma proteins. Cycloserine crosses the placenta and is present in breast milk.

The serum $t_{1/2}$ is approximately 10 h in patients with normal renal function. Approximately 65% of an oral dose of cycloserine appears unchanged in the urine after glomerular filtration. Most of the remaining 35% is metabolized to unknown products. Serum levels of cycloserine are greater and the $t_{1/2}$ is longer in patients with compromised renal function.

2. Adverse Effects

Nervous system symptoms appear to be related to doses of cycloserine greater than 500 mg/day. Drowsiness, somnolence, dizziness, headache, lethargy, depression, tremor, dysarthria, hyperreflexia, anxiety, vertigo, confusion, and disorientation with loss of memory, paresis, clonic seizures, convulsions, and coma have been associated with use of this drug. Alcohol appears to increase the occurrence of seizures. Psychosis with suicidal behavior, personality changes, hyperirritability and aggression have occurred in patients treated with cycloserine. Nervous system effects are thought to be reduced when the serum levels of cycloserine are below 30 µg/ml. Many of the neurotoxic effects (convulsions, anxiety, and tremor) associated with cycloserine can be prevented or ameliorated by treatment with pyridoxine hydrochloride (100 to 300 mg daily).

Hypersensitivity reactions (rash or photosensitivity) rarely have been associated with this agent. Renal, hepatic, and hematologic parameters should be monitored while patients are receiving cycloserine. Cycloserine should not be used in patients with severe renal impairment unless serum levels can be monitored. The safety of cycloserine during pregnancy has not been established.

3. Drug Interactions

Concurrent use of ethionamide has been reported to potentiate the neurotoxicity of cycloserine.

Cycloserine inhibits hepatic metabolism of phenytoin; therefore, serum levels of phenytoin should be monitored and evidence of phenytoin intoxication should be assessed in patients treated concurrently with these agents.

VIII. p-AMINOSALICYLIC ACID

A. DESCRIPTION

p-aminosalicylic acid (PAS), a weak bacteriostatic agent, is currently available as enteric-coated granules (Paser) designed for gradual drug release. PAS is thought to competitively inhibit conversion of aminobenzoic acid to dihydrofolic acid and/or to inhibit iron uptake.[93]

1. Absorption, Distribution, and Elimination

PAS and its salt are well absorbed from the gastrointestinal tract. After 2 h in simulated gastric acid, 10% of a dose of nonenteric-coated PAS is decarboxylated to form m-aminophenol, a hepatotoxin. The enteric coating of Paser granules protects against degradation in the stomach. Peak serum PAS concentrations of 20 µg/ml (range, 9 to 35 µg/ml) are achieved after a 4 g oral dose of enteric-coated granules with food. A serum concentration of 2 µg/ml is maintained for an average of 7.9 h, and a level of 1 µg/ml was maintained for an average of 8.8 h. Higher serum concentrations of PAS can be achieved with PAS tablets or the sodium salt of PAS (neither is available in the U.S.).

PAS is distributed into peritoneal fluid, pleural fluid, and synovial fluid in concentrations similar to plasma levels. CSF concentrations of 10 to 50% of the plasma level are achieved in patients with inflamed meninges. It is not known whether PAS crosses the placenta; however, low levels of drug are present in milk and bile.

The plasma $t_{1/2}$ of PAS is approximately 1 h. Plasma PAS levels are not significantly changed by renal or hepatic insufficiency. PAS is rapidly metabolized in the liver and intestinal mucosa primarily by acetylation. The drug and its metabolites are excreted in urine by glomerular filtration and tubular secretion. Approximately 80% of PAS is excreted in the urine, with approximately 50% in the acetylated form. Patients with severe renal insufficiency will accumulate PAS and its metabolites. End-stage renal disease patients should not be treated with PAS. Paser granules should be taken with food or drink having a pH less than 5, such as apple sauce, yogurt, or fruit juices (e.g., orange, apple, grapefruit, grape, or cranberry).

2. Adverse Effects

There is a high frequency of gastrointestinal intolerance manifested by nausea, vomiting, diarrhea, and abdominal pain. Hypersensitivity reactions to PAS often include rash (including exfoliative dermatitis) followed by fever and, much less frequently, anorexia, nausea, and diarrhea. If these symptoms develop, the medication should be stopped and clinical follow-up arranged. Hepatitis has been reported in 0.5% of patients receiving rapidly absorbed PAS preparations.[43] Other rare side effects include hypoprothrombinemia, leukopenia, agranulocytosis, thrombocytopenia, Coombs' positive hemolytic anemia, goiter, and a lupus-like syndrome.[93] The safety of PAS during pregnancy has not been established.

3. Drug Interactions

PAS reduces the rate of acetylation of INH; however, the effect is not clinically significant. Vitamin B_{12} absorption has been reduced approximately 50% by PAS with significant erythrocyte abnormalities developing after depletion. Patients receiving PAS for more than 1 month should be considered for vitamin B_{12} maintenance.

IX. THIACETAZONE

A. DESCRIPTION

Thiacetazone currently is not available in the U.S.; therefore, many practitioners are not familiar with this agent. In many developing countries, thiacetazone is included in a conventional regimen in combination with INH and SM.[94] A study by Heifets et al. employed the BACTEC methodology to evaluate the activity of thiacetazone against *M. tuberculosis* and *M. avium*.[95] Although the bactericidal activity against either species was low, the inhibitory levels for *M. tuberculosis* (n = 14) and for *M. avium* (n = 68) were 0.08 to 1.2 µg/ml and 0.02 to 0.15 µg/ml, respectively.

1. Absorption, Distribution, and Elimination

Thiacetazone has not been well studied from a pharmacokinetic standpoint. It appears to be well absorbed from the gastrointestinal tract, with peak serum levels reported between 4 to 5 h after administration.[96] Peak serum levels are in the range of 1 to 4 µg/ml following a 150 mg oral dose.[53,96] Two potential metabolites have been identified, *p*-aminobenzaldehyde-thiosemicarbazone and *p*-acetylaminobenzoic acid, although the metabolic fate of thiacetazone has not been clearly delineated.[53,96] Approximately 20% of drug is excreted unchanged in the urine.

2. Adverse Effects

Minor side effects of thiacetazone include anorexia or gastrointestinal distress in up to 10%, flushing or transient rash, dizziness, headache, and drowsiness. Serious side effects include severe cutaneous reactions, agranulocytosis, hepatotoxicity, and deafness.[97] Hypersensitivity reactions may be more severe in individuals who are seropositive for the human immunodeficiency virus.[98]

3. Drug Interactions

Thiacetazone may potentiate the vestibular toxicity of streptomycin. Severe liver damage has been reported in patients receiving INH and thiacetazone concurrently, although the contribution of each individual agent is not clear.

X. FLUOROQUINOLONES

The quinolone class of antimicrobials includes several groups of heterocyclic carbonic acid derivatives. These agents are structurally related to nalidixic acid. The mechanism of action of the quinolones is inhibition of DNA gyrase, an enzyme essential for maintenance of DNA superhelical twists. The predominant mechanism of resistance to fluoroquinolones is mutation in subunit A of DNA gyrase (gyrA) which prevents interaction with these agents.[99,100]

The newer quinolones have significant advantages in pharmacokinetics and tissue penetration compared with the parent compounds, although development of clinical resistance remains a problem.

A. Ciprofloxacin

Ciprofloxacin is active *in vitro* against *M. tuberculosis* with MICs in the range of 0.125 to 2.0 µg/ml.[101,102] Activity has also been reported *in vitro* against *M. malmoense, M. fortuitum,* and *M. kansasii.* Clinical experience with ciprofloxacin therapy in patients with mycobacterial infections is limited.[48,103,104] MICs for *M. avium* complex are less favorable and range from 1 to 16 µg/ml;[101,105] however, ciprofloxacin has been included as part of multidrug regimens for the treatment of disseminated *M. avium* complex infection in persons with AIDS.[106]

1. Absorption, Distribution, and Elimination

Ciprofloxacin hydrochloride is rapidly and well absorbed from the gastrointestinal tract. The rate of absorption is slowed in the presence of food. Magnesium-, aluminum-, or calcium-containing antacids will decrease the bioavailability of ciprofloxacin. Peak serum concentrations are generally attained within 0.5 to 2 h after oral administration. Peak serum concentrations following 500 mg and 1000 mg oral doses are 1.6 to 2.9 µg/ml and 3.4 to 5.4 µg/ml, respectively. Ciprofloxacin is widely distributed into body tissues, and tissue levels typically exceed that seen in serum. The exception is penetration into the cerebrospinal fluid, where levels may only be 6 to 10% of peak serum concentrations. Ciprofloxacin crosses the placenta and is distributed into breast milk.

The elimination half-life in adults with normal renal function is 3 to 5 h. In persons with impaired renal function, serum concentrations are higher and the half-life is prolonged. Ciprofloxacin is metabolized in the liver yielding at least four metabolites, some of which retain antibacterial activity. Ciprofloxacin and its metabolites are excreted in urine and feces.

2. Adverse Effects

Ciprofloxacin generally is well tolerated but side effects include gastrointestinal distress (nausea, vomiting, diarrhea, and abdominal pain) in 2 to 10% of patients.[107] Headache, restlessness, and neuropsychiatric symptoms (phobia, depersonalization, anxiety, depression, manic reactions, and psychosis) have been reported but occur in only 1 to 2% of patients. Some of the neuropsychiatric side effects may be related to the fact that ciprofloxacin, like other fluoroquinolones, is a GABA inhibitor. Rash occurs in 1 to 4% of patients. Severe hypersensitivity reactions have been described. Crystalluria, cylinduria, hematuria, and transient liver function abnormalities are infrequent adverse effects. Arthropathy is noted in juvenile animals receiving ciprofloxacin; therefore, this agent should not be used in pregnant women, children, or adolescents.

3. Drug Interactions

Antacids containing magnesium, aluminum, or calcium can decrease absorption of ciprofloxacin. Antacids should not be administered within 4 h of ciprofloxacin dosing. Probenecid interferes with renal tubular secretion of ciprofloxacin and may result in increased serum concentration and a prolonged half-life. Concomitant administration of ciprofloxacin and theophylline derivatives may result in higher theophylline concentrations and subsequent toxicity.[108] Concomitant administration of ciprofloxacin and warfarin derivatives may result in a prolonged prothrombin time, perhaps due to displacement of warfarin from plasma proteins.[109]

B. OFLOXACIN

Ofloxacin is active against *M. tuberculosis*, with MICs in the range of 0.3 to 2.5 µg/ml.[110,111] Ofloxacin has been evaluated in a clinical study of 19 "treatment-failure" cases of cavitary pulmonary tuberculosis. The study evaluated the activity of ofloxacin (300 mg/day for 6 to 8 months) in combination with the patients' previous "ineffective" regimen; thus, the study was considered in effect to evaluate the use of ofloxacin alone.[112] Conversion of sputum to negative occurred in 5 of 19 patients, with a decline in the number of recoverable bacilli in the majority of the remaining patients. In a subsequent uncontrolled trial of ofloxacin in the treatment of multidrug-resistant tuberculosis, 10 of 17 patients responded.[60] Ofloxacin is active *in vitro* against *M. bovis* and *M. fortuitum*, but has limited activity against *M. avium* complex and *M. chelonae*.

1. Absorption, Distribution, and Elimination

Absorption of ofloxacin is rapid and nearly complete with oral bioavailability of 85 to 100%. Peak serum concentration are reached within 0.5 to 2 h. Peak serum concentrations following 200 mg and 400 mg doses are 1.5 to 2.7 µg/ml and 2.9 to 5.6 µg/ml, respectively. Ofloxacin is widely distributed into body tissues and peak concentrations in cerebrospinal fluid are 28 to 87% of serum levels. Ofloxacin crosses the placenta and is present in breast milk.

The elimination half-life in adults with normal renal function ranges from 4 to 8 h. Ofloxacin will reach higher serum levels and exhibit a prolonged half-life in patients with decreased creatinine clearance. Less than 10% of a single dose of ofloxacin is metabolized. The majority of drug is excreted unchanged in the urine; the remainder is excreted as metabolites in the urine or feces.

2. Adverse Effects

The side effect profile for ofloxacin is similar to that of ciprofloxacin. Gastrointestinal distress has been reported in 3 to 10% of patients. CNS symptoms (including drowsiness, cognitive changes, depression, and euphoria) can be seen in 1 to 3% of patients. Rash, arthropathy, and transient liver function abnormalities have been reported. Crystalluria has not been demonstrated in animal studies.

3. Drug Interactions

Ingestion of antacids, multivitamins, and mineral supplements containing divalent or trivalent cations may decrease absorption of ofloxacin. Interaction between ofloxacin and theophylline derivatives may be less than that seen with ciprofloxacin; however, plasma theophylline concentrations should be monitored if ofloxacin is used concurrently.

C. LEVOFLOXACIN

Ofloxacin is a racemic mixture of two isoenantiomers. Levofloxacin, the *l*-isoenantiomer, is 8 to 128 times as active against susceptible Gram-positive and Gram-negative organisms as the *d*-isoenantiomer and approximately twice as active as racemic ofloxacin.[113,114] Studies of levofloxacin in a murine model of tuberculosis show greater than a twofold improvement in activity compared with ofloxacin.[115] There are currently limited data regarding the activity of this agent for the treatment of human tuberculosis. It is unclear whether a significant increase in efficacy would be achieved with daily doses greater than 500 mg/day. This agent has been well tolerated at doses of 1000 mg/day; however, long-term toxicology studies have not been done. In the author's opinion, levofloxacin currently is the quinolone of choice for the treatment of human tuberculosis.

1. Absorption, Distribution, and Elimination

Levofloxacin is rapidly and essentially completely absorbed after oral dosing. It can be taken without regard to meals. Peak plasma concentrations are approximately 5.7 µg/ml after 500 mg once daily. The trough plasma levels are approximately 0.5 µg/ml.

Levofloxacin is well distributed into body tissues with lung concentrations two- to fivefold higher than plasma concentrations. This drug is primarily excreted unchanged in the urine with less than 4% recovered in the feces. The desmethyl and *N*-oxide metabolites are present in urine (<5% of an administered dose).

The $t_{1/2}$ of levofloxacin is approximately 6 to 8 h. The renal clearance exceeds the glomerular filtration rate; therefore, tubular secretion occurs. Cimetidine or probenicid administration reduces renal clearance (24 and 25%, respectively). Dosage adjustment is required in patients with impaired renal function (creatinine clearance ≤ 50 ml/min). In these patients, the levofloxacin dose should be based on the level of renal impairment as recommended in the package insert. Neither hemodialysis nor continuous ambulatory peritoneal dialysis effectively removes levofloxacin from the body. Levofloxacin dose adjustment is not necessary for patients with hepatic insufficiency.

2. Adverse Effects

The side effect profile for levofloxacin includes diarrhea, nausea, vaginitis, flatulence, pruritus, rash, abdominal pain, genital moniliasis, dizziness, dyspepsia, insomnia, taste perversion, and vomiting. Convulsions and toxic psychoses have been reported in patients receiving levofloxacin. Serious hypersensitivity and/or anaphylactic reactions also have been reported. This agent should be discontinued at the first appearance of a skin rash or other sign of hypersensitivity reaction. Pseudomembranous colitis has been associated with administration of quinolones; therefore, this diagnosis should be considered in patients with diarrhea. Shoulder, head, and Achilles tendon rupture have occurred in patients receiving quinolones. If tendinitis or tendon rupture occurs, levofloxacin should be discontinued.

3. Drug Interactions

Antacids containing magnesium or aluminum, metal cations (iron or calcium), multivitamin preparations with zinc, and sucralfate may decrease the absorption of levofloxacin leading to significantly lower plasma levels. These agents should be taken at least 2 h before or 2 h after administration of levofloxacin.

There does not appear to be a significant interaction between theophylline and levofloxacin. No significant interactions have been observed with warfarin, cyclosporine, or digoxin. Hyperglycemia and hypoglycemia have been reported in patients treated concurrently with oral antidiabetic agents.

D. Newer Quinolones

Two promising quinolones with improved activity against *M. tuberculosis* are currently in the late stages of clinical development. Moxifloxacin and gatifloxacin may become the quinolones of choice for the treatment of tuberculosis. Further study of these agents in the treatment of human tuberculosis would be helpful to determine their potential role in the treatment of tuberculosis.

XI. CLOFAZIMINE

A. Description

Clofazimine has been in use since 1962 for the treatment of leprosy. It is a substituted iminophenazine dye with the chemical name 3-(*p*-chloroanilino)-10-(*p*-chlorophenyl)-2,10-dihydro-2-(isopropylimino) phenazine. Clofazimine has activity *in vivo* in the mouse foot-pad model of *M. leprae* infection and is used in combination drug therapy for multibacillary leprosy.[116]

Clofazimine has *in vitro* activity against *M. tuberculosis*, with MICs in the range of 0.1 to 10 μg/ml, depending on the pH of the media. Clofazimine has activity in murine and guinea pig models of tuberculosis, but had neither therapeutic nor prophylactic activity in a rhesus monkey model of infection.[117] Interspecies differences in peak serum levels may help explain the observed variation in activity. Clofazimine activity in a murine model of drug-resistant tuberculosis has been reported.[4] Assessment of its activity in human disease is necessary to determine whether clofazimine has a role as an antituberculosis agent.

Clofazimine has activity *in vitro* and *in vivo* against *M. avium* complex and has been used in multidrug regimens for the treatment of *M. avium* complex infection in persons with AIDS.[64]

The mechanism of action of clofazimine is not well understood, but may involve inhibition of the template function of the DNA strand, thus resulting in growth inhibition.[116]

1. Absorption, Distribution, and Elimination

Clofazimine is slowly and incompletely absorbed from the gastrointestinal tract. Bioavailability of the commercial preparation (microcrystalline suspension in an oil-wax base) approximates 70%. The rate and extent of absorption of clofazimine appears to be increased in the presence of food. After a single 200 mg oral dose in fed subjects, peak serum concentrations average 0.41 μg/ml, with a prolonged time (8 to 12 h) to reach maximum concentrations.[118] Clofazimine distributes into fatty tissues and is taken up by macrophages. It crosses the placenta and is distributed into breast milk.

Few data are available regarding the metabolism of clofazimine. Three urinary metabolites have been identified, but the overall metabolic fate of clofazimine and its metabolites is not known.

Elimination characteristics of clofazimine are interesting and seem to correspond to a two-phase elimination. The initial elimination half-life is 7 to 10 days, followed by a much longer elimination half-life of approximately 70 days as the drug is slowly released from tissues.[118] The effects of peritoneal dialysis and hemodialysis on clofazimine levels are not known.

2. Adverse Effects

The most frequently reported side effects include discoloration of the skin and abdominal pain. Red-brown discoloration of the skin and conjunctiva occurs in the majority of patients and may last several years after discontinuation of the drug. Other bodily fluids, such as sweat, tears, sputum, and feces also may be discolored. Additional skin conditions, such as xeroderma, pruritus, and exfoliative dermatitis occur as well. Corneal discoloration and maculopathy have been reported.

Gastrointestinal side effects include abdominal pain, nausea, anorexia, diarrhea, and weight loss. Irritation of the GI tract and deposition of clofazimine crystals have been implicated in these reactions. The safety of clofazimine during pregnancy has not been established.

3. Drug Interactions

Reduction in the rate of absorption of rifampin has been described with clofazimine, although overall bioavailability of rifampin was not significantly affected.

XII. MACROLIDES

Erythromycin is produced by *Streptomyces erythraeus* and belongs to the macrolide group of antimicrobial agents. The mechanism of action of the macrolides appears to be inhibition of protein synthesis by reversible binding to the 50S ribosomal subunit. Erythromycin has limited activity against mycobacteria and is used only in infections caused by susceptible strains of *M. chelonae*.[48]

A. CLARITHROMYCIN

Clarithromycin differs structurally from erythromycin only by the methylation of a hydroxyl group at position 6 of the lactone ring. The presence of the methyl group minimizes the acid-catalyzed degradation to the inactive hemiketal and spiroketal products, which may mitigate the adverse gastrointestinal effects seen with erythromycin. Clarithromycin has activity *in vitro* and *in vivo* against *M. kansasii*, *M. fortuitum*, *M. chelonae*, *M. leprae*, and *M. avium* complex with MICs generally less than 2 μg/ml against these species.[105,119,120] It has good activity for the treatment of disseminated *M. avium* complex infection in persons with AIDS.[121-123] MICs against *M. tuberculosis* are not as favorable, and currently clarithromycin is not considered a useful agent against this species.

In *M. avium* complex, resistance to clarithromycin has been associated with mutations in the peptidyltransferase region in 23S rRNA (A-2058→G,C,orU).[124] This is consistent with the previous observation that modification of adenine 2058 by dimethylation (chromosomal or plasmid mediated constituitive or inducible methylase) is a frequent cause of macrolide resistance in bacteria. There is cross resistance between azithromycin and clarithromycin.

1. Absorption, Distribution, and Elimination

Clarithromycin is rapidly absorbed from the gastrointestinal tract; its absorption exceeds that of erythromycin. Bioavailability is on the order of 50 to 55%. Administration with food may delay the rate but not the overall extent of absorption. Peak serum concentrations of 2.1 μg/ml are achieved following a single 400 mg dose of clarithromycin,[125] but much higher tissue concentrations are reached. Concentrations of the drug and its 14-hydroxy metabolite in HIV-infected adults receiving 500 mg orally every 12 h were comparable to those achieved in similarly treated healthy individuals. The extent of penetration into CSF is not known.

Clarithromycin is eliminated by both renal and nonrenal means. Clarithromycin is metabolized in the liver primarily by oxidative *N*-demethylation and hydroxylation at the 14 position. The principal metabolite, 14-hydroxyclarithromycin, is the only one with substantial antibacterial activity. The elimination half-life following a single 250 mg dose is approximately 4 h, with approximately 38% of the dose excreted in urine and 40% excreted in feces. The serum half-life is prolonged in patients with renal failure and a dosage reduction may be required. Moderate-to-severe hepatic impairment reduces formation of the 14-hydroxy metabolite, but is accompanied by increased renal clearance of the parent drug. Dosage modification is necessary only when concurrent hepatic dysfunction and renal impairment are present. In patients with creatinine clearances less than 30 ml/min the clarithromycin dosing interval should be doubled. Clarithromycin can be taken with or without food.

2. Adverse Effects

The overall incidence of side effects with clarithromycin is similar to or lower than that with erythromycin. Diarrhea, nausea, abnormal taste, abdominal discomfort, and dyspepsia are reported in 2 to 3% of patients taking the drug. Oral candidiasis, glossitis, stomatitis, vomiting, flatulence, constipation, pancreatitis, and tongue discoloration also have been reported. Hepatomegaly and elevation of liver enzymes have been reported infrequently. Headache, increased prothrombin, and elevated BUN occur in 1 to 4% of patients receiving clarithromycin. Allergic reactions (urticaria, anaphylaxis, and Stevens-Johnson syndrome), pruritus, and rash also have been attributed to this drug. The safety of clarithromycin during pregnancy has not been established.

3. Drug Interactions

Use of clarithromycin in patients who are receiving theophylline may result in an increase in serum theophylline concentrations. Serum theophylline concentrations should be monitored closely if these agents are used concurrently. There is a two-way interaction between clarithromycin and rifabutin. The latter induces hepatic microsomal enzymes which reduce serum clarithromycin levels by approximately 50%. Clarithromycin increases serum levels of rifabutin and its desacetyl metabolite by inhibiting the cytochrome P-450 3A pathway responsible for its metabolism.[126,127]

Peak serum concentrations of zidovudine are reduced when clarithromycin is used concurrently, but the clinical significance of this finding is uncertain.

Elevated serum digoxin levels have been reported with coadministration of clarithromycin; therefore, digoxin levels should be monitored in this setting. Clarithromycin is contraindicated in patients receiving terfenadine, cisapride, or pimozide and is not recommended with astemizole due to potential for serious cardiotoxicity.

B. Azithromycin

Azithromycin is an azalide antibiotic that differs from erythromycin chemically by the addition of a methyl-substituted nitrogen in the macrolide ring. Azithromycin has *in vitro* and *in vivo* activity against *M. avium* complex and *M. kansasii*, although MICs are several-fold higher than those of clarithromycin.[128-130] Azithromycin has good activity for the treatment of disseminated *M. avium* complex infection in persons with AIDS.[131]

1. Absorption, Distribution, and Elimination

Azithromycin is rapidly but incompletely absorbed after oral administration. Bioavailability is between 34 to 52% with single doses of 500 to 1200 mg. Peak plasma concentrations following a 500 mg oral dose is 0.5 µg/ml. Azithromycin is widely distributed into most tissues and body fluids. The high and persistent tissue concentrations of this agent are thought to result from uptake of this basic compound into lysosomes.[132] The concentration within phagocytes is substantially greater than that achieved by other antimicrobial agents. Tissue concentrations of azithromycin usually exceed plasma concentrations by 10- to 100-fold following a single dose. Multiple dosing yields higher ratios. Very low levels of this agent have been found in CSF when noninflamed meninges are present. The $t_{1/2}$ of azithromycin in plasma is approximately 68 h. The tissue $t_{1/2}$ is thought to be 1 to 4 days.

Azithromycin is principally excreted intact in feces. The primary route of metabolism involves *N*-demethylation of the desoamine sugar or the 9a position on the azalide ring. A small portion of azithromycin is excreted in urine. The extent of absorption of azithromycin tablets or suspension in adults is not significantly affected by food. It is not known whether dosage adjustments are necessary for patients with renal or hepatic impairments.

2. Adverse Effects

Azithromycin usually is well tolerated. The side effect profile is similar to that of clarithromycin.[133] Nausea, vomiting, diarrhea, and abdominal pain are the most frequent therapy-limiting adverse effects. Hearing loss, deafness, or tinnitus have been reported in <1% of patients receiving 1200 mg of azithromycin weekly for prevention of disseminated MAC infections. The safety of azithromycin during pregnancy has not been established.

3. Drug Interactions

Interactions between erthryomycin or clarithromycin with digoxin, dihydroergotamine, triazolam, or agents metabolized by the cytochrome P-450 isoenzymes (carbamazepine, cyclosporine, phenytoin) have been reported. Azithromycin does not appear to affect the cytochrome P-450 enzyme system; therefore, interactions mediated by this system are not expected. Patients receiving other drugs, mentioned above, in combination with azithromycin should be monitored carefully. Azithromycin dosing should be separated from administration of aluminum- or magnesium-containing antacids. Azithromycin does not appear to affect plasma theophylline levels. Concomitant administration of rifabutin and azithromycin does not affect the average serum level of either agent.

XIII. β-LACTAMS

β-lactams have *in vitro* activity against slow growing and rapid growing mycobacteria. Amoxicillin/clavulanate and other β-lactam/β-lactamase inhibitor combinations have been reported to have activity *in vitro* against *M. tuberculosis*;[134,135] however, clinical efficacy or convincing activity in a murine infection model has not been demonstrated. Cefoxitin, cefmetazole, and imipenem have *in vitro* activity against *M. fortuitum*.[136-141] Cefoxitin was less active against *M. chelonae* subsp. *chelonae*.[139] Cefoxitin has been used for treatment of pulmonary and nonpulmonary infections caused by rapid growers.[139] Imipenem and cefmetazole were more active than cefoxitin against *M. fortuitum*, and imipenem was the only β-lactam active against *M. chelonae* subsp. *chelonae*.[138] The pharmacology of the β-lactams has been well summarized previously.[107]

XIV. SULFONAMIDES

The *in vitro* activity of sulfonamides against rapid growers has been extensively evaluated.[137] *M. fortuitum* isolates are susceptible to sulfonamides; however, *M. chelonae* isolates usually are resistant to the sulfonamides.[137,140] Trimethoprim is not active against *M. fortuitum* or *M. chelonae* isolates when used alone, nor is there enhanced activity when combined with sulfamethoxazole. Ahn et al. have reported *in vitro* activity of sulfonamides against *M. kansasii* and a good clinical response to sulfonamide-containing regimens in *M. kansasii*-infected patients.[141] The *in vitro* activity of sulfonamides against other nontuberculous mycobacteria has not been adequately evaluated; however, they have been found to have *in vitro* activity against *M. marinum* and *M. scrofulaceum* isolates.[140] Testing of *M. avium* complex isolates *in vitro* with sulfisoxazole has yielded variable results.[142,143]

XV. TETRACYCLINES

Tetracycline and its derivatives (minocycline and doxycycline) have modest *in vitro* activity against *M. fortuitum* and *M. chelonae*.[144,145] These agents have not been found to be particularly active against *M. tuberculosis* and other slow growing mycobacteria with the exception of *M. leprae*.[146,147] Tetracyclines presently do not have a role in treatment of disease caused by *M. tuberculosis*.

XVI. FUTURE PROSPECTS

The revival of interest in mycobacterial infections is due in part to the emergence of multidrug-resistant *M. tuberculosis* and the frequent occurrence of disseminated *M. avium* complex infection in patients with advanced HIV infection. New agents can be developed by modification of current agents, by screening existing chemical libraries, by evaluating natural products, and perhaps by targeting specific biochemical pathways with sophisticated molecular biological techniques. Agents that will facilitate ultra-short-course (2 or 3 month) treatment for tuberculosis and preventive therapy are desirable. Agents with efficacy against multidrug-resistant tuberculosis also are needed.

Immunomodulators are not likely to have broad clinical application for the treatment of tuberculosis. Liposome-encapsulated antimicrobial agents have been demonstrated to have enhanced activity compared to free nonencapsulated drug in macrophage culture[148] as well as in murine models of mycobacterial disease.[149] This novel drug delivery system is unlikely to be clinically practical unless the candidate product has exceptional activity and can be utilized intermittently on a once or twice a week dosing schedule.

Analogs of currently used agents with enhanced activity can be synthesized as our understanding of the common mechanisms of resistance are better understood.[31] The quinolones remain the most promising class of new antituberculosis agents. The macrolides are another fertile group for chemical manipulation, based on their existing activity against *M. avium* complex.

At the present time it is not known whether ultra-short-course regimens would be achievable with currently available agents (INH/rifapentine/PZA). Ultra-short-course therapy is a desirable goal for the mycobacterial therapeutic research and development agenda.

REFERENCES

1. Pablos-Mendez, A., Raviglione, M. C., Laszlo, A., Binkin, N., Rieder, H. L., Bustreo, F., Cohn, D. L., Lambregts-van Weezenbeck, C. S., Kim, S. J., Chaulet, P., and Nunn, P., Global surveillance for antituberculosis-drug resistance, 1994-1997. World Health Organization-International Union against Tuberculosis and Lung Disease Working Group on Anti-Tuberculosis Drug Resistance Surveillance, *N. Engl. J. Med.*, 338, 1641, 1998.
2. Fischl, M. A., Uttamchandiani, R. B., Daikos, G. L., Poblete, R. B., Moreno, J. N., Reyes, R. R., Boota, A. M., Thompson, L. M., Cleary, T. J., and Lai, S., An outbreak of tuberculosis caused by multiple-drug resistant tubercle bacilli among patients with HIV infections, *Ann. Intern. Med.*, 117, 177, 1992.
3. Centers for Disease Control, Nosocomial transmission of multi-drug resistant tuberculosis among HIV-infected persons — Florida and New York, 1988–1991, *MMWR*, 40, 585, 1991.
4. Klemens, S. P., DeStefano, M. S., and Cynamon, M. H., Therapy of multidrug resistant tuberculosis (MDR-TB): lessons from mice, *Antimicrob. Agents Chemother.*, 37, 2344, 1993.
5. Chorine, M. V., Action of nicotinamide on bacilli of the species mycobacterium, *C.R. Hebd. Seances Acad. Sci.*, 220, 150, 1945.
6. Fox, H. H., The chemical attack on tuberculosis, *Trans. N.Y. Acad. Sci.*, 15, 234, 1953.
7. Kushner, S., Dalalian, H., Sanjurjo, J. L., Bach, F. L., Safir, S. R., Smith, V. L., and Williams, J. H., Experimental chemotherapy of tuberculosis, *J. Am. Chem. Soc.*, 74, 3617, 1952.
8. Solotorovsky, M., Gregory, F. J., Ironson, E. J., Bugie, E. J., O'Neill, R. C., and Pfister, K., Pyrazinoic acid amide — An agent active against experimental murine tuberculosis, *Proc. Soc. Exp. Biol. Med.*, 79, 563, 1952.
9. World Health Organization, Antituberculosis drug resistance in the world: the WHO/IUATLD Global Project on Antituberculosis Drug Resistance Surveillance, WHO, Geneva, Switzerland, 1997.
10. Victor, T. C., Warren, R., Butt, J. L., Jordaan, A. M., Felix, J. V., Venter, A., Sirgel, F. A., Shaaf, H. S., Donald, P. R., Richardson, M., Cynamon, M. H., and Van Helden, P. D., Genome and MIC stability in *Mycobacterium tuberculosis* and indications for continuation of use of isoniazid in multidrug-resistant tuberuculosis, *J. Med. Microbiol.*, 46, 847, 1997.
11. Quemard, A., Lacave, C., and Lancelle, G., Isoniazid inhibition of mycolic acid synthesis by cell extracts of sensitive and resistant strains of *Mycobacterium aurum, Antimicrob. Agents Chemother.*, 35, 1035, 1991.
12. Davidson, L. A. and Takayama, K., Isoniazid inhibition of the synthesis of monounsaturated long-chain fatty acids in *Mycobacterium tuberculosis* H37Ra, *Antimicrob. Agents Chemother.*, 16, 104, 1979.
13. Takayama, K., Wang, L., and David, H. L., Effect of isoniazid on the *in vivo* mycolic acid synthesis, cell growth, and viability of *Mycobacterium tuberculosis, Antimicrob. Agents Chemother.*, 2, 29, 1972.
14. Winder, F. G. and Collins, P. B., Inhibition by isoniazid of synthesis of mycolic acids in *Mycobacterium tuberculosis, J. Gen. Microbiol.*, 63, 41 1970.
15. Iwainsky, H., INH-mode of action, in *Antituberculosis Drugs*, Bartmann, K., Ed., Springer-Verlag, Berlin, 1988, 476.
16. Krishna Murti, C. R., Isonicotinic acid hydrazide, in *Antibiotics*, Vol. III, Corcoran, J. W. and Hahn, F. E., Eds., Springer-Verlag, Berlin, 1975, 623.
17. Zhang, Y., Heym, B., Allen, B., Young, D., and Cole, S., The catalase-peroxidase gene and isoniazid resistance of *Mycobacterium tuberculosis, Nature*, 358, 591, 1992.

18. Banjerjee, A., Dubnau, E., Quemard, A., Balasubramanian, V., Um, K. S., Wilson, T., Collins, D., de Lisle, G., and Jacobs, W. R., Jr., Inh A, a gene encoding a target for isoniazid and ethionamide in *Mycobacterium tuberculosis*, *Science*, 263, 227, 1994.

19. Mdluli, K., Slayden, R. A., Zhu, Y., Ramaswamy, S., Pan, X., Mead, D., Crane, D. D., Musser, J. M., and Barry, C. E. III, Inhibition of a *Mycobacterium tuberculosis* β-ketoacyl ACP synthase by isoniazid, *Science*, 280, 1607, 1998.

20. Musser, J. M., Kapur, V., Williams, D. L., Kreiswirth, B. N., van Soolingen, D., and Van Emden, J. D., Characterization of the catalase-peroxidase gene (kat G) and inh A locus in isoniazid-resistant and -susceptible strains of *Mycobacterium tuberculosis* by automated DNA sequencing: restricted array of mutations associated with drug resistance, *J. Infect. Dis.*, 173, 196, 1996.

21. Heym, G., Starropoulos, E., Honore, N., Demenech, P., Saint-Toanis, B., Wilson, T. M., Collins, D. M., Colston, M. J., and Cole, S., Effects of over expression of the alkyl hydroperoxidase reductase AhpC on the virulence and isoniazid resistance of *Mycobacterium tuberculosis*, *Infect. Immun.*, 65, 1395, 1997.

22. Weber, W. W. and Hein, D. W., Clinical pharmacokinetics of isoniazid, *Clin. Pharmacokinet.*, 4, 410, 1979.

23. Bowersox, D. W., Winterbauer, R. H., Steward, G. L., Orme, B., and Barron, E., Isoniazid dosage in patients with renal failure, *N. Engl. J. Med.*, 289, 84, 1973.

24. Public Health Service, U.S. Department of Health, Education, and Welfare, Isoniazid-associated hepatitis: summary of the report of the Tuberculosis Advisory Committee and special consultants to the director, Center for Disease Control, *MMWR*, 23, 97, 1974.

25. Garibaldi, R. A., Drusin, R. E., Ferebee, S. H., and Gregg, M. B., Isoniazid-associated hepatitis, report of an outbreak, *Am. Rev. Respir. Dis.*, 106, 357, 1972.

26. Maddrey, W. C. and Boitnoit, J. K., Isoniazid hepatitis, *Ann. Intern. Med.*, 79, 1, 1973.

27. Mitchell, J. R., Zimmerman, H. J., Ishak, K. G., Thorgeirsson, U. P., Timbrell, J. A., Snodgrass, W. R., and Nelson, S. D., Isoniazid liver injury: clinical spectrum, pathology, and probable pathogenesis, *Ann. Intern. Med.*, 84, 181, 1976.

28. Konno, L., Feldmann, F. M., and McDermott, W., Pyrazinamide susceptibility and amidase activity of tubercle bacilli, *Am. Rev. Respir. Dis.*, 95, 461, 1967.

29. Scorpio, A. and Zhang, Y., Mutations in pncA, a gene encoding pyrazinamidase/nicotinamidase, cause resistance to the antituberculosis drug pyrazinamide in tubercle bacillus, *Nature Med.*, 2, 662, 1996.

30. Sreevatsan, S., Pan, X., Zhang, Y., Kreiswirth, B. N., and Musser, J. M., Mutations associated with pyrazinamide resistance in pncA of *Mycobacterium tuberculosis* complex organisms, *Antimicrob. Agents Chemother.*, 41, 636, 1997.

31. Cynamon, M. H., Klemens, S.P., Chou, T-S., Gimi, R. H., and Welch, J. T., Antimycobacterial activity of a series of pyrazinoic acid esters, *J. Med. Chem.*, 35, 1212, 1992.

32. Mitchison, D. A., The Garrod lecture: understanding the chemotherapy of tuberculosis-current problems, *J. Antimicrob. Chemother.*, 29, 477, 1992.

33. Grosset, J. H., Present status of chemotherapy for tuberculosis, *Rev. Infect. Dis.*, 11 (Suppl. 2), S347, 1989.

34. Ellard, G.A., Absorption, metabolism and excretion of pyrazinamide in man, *Tubercle*, 50, 144, 1969.

35. Weiner, I. M. and Tinker, J. P., Pharmacology of pyrazinamide: metabolic and renal function studies related to the mechanism of drug-induced urate retention, *J. Pharmacol. Exp. Ther.*, 180, 411, 1972.

36. McDermott, W., Ormond, L., Muschenheim, C., Deuschle, K., McCune, R. M., and Tompsett, R., Pyrazinamide-isoniazid in tuberculosis, *Am. Rev. Tuberc.*, 69, 319, 1954.

37. Veterans Hospital (Madison, WI): Thioisonicotinamides, *Quart. Prog. Rep. V.A. Chem. Tuberc.*, 10, 44, 1955.

38. Rist, N., Grumbach, F., and Liberman, D., Experiments on the antituberculous activity of α-ethyl-thionicotinamide, *Am. Rev. Tuberc.*, 79, 1, 1959.

39. Winder, F. G., Mode of action of the antimycobacterial agents and associated aspects of the molecular biology of the mycobacteria, in *The Biology of Mycobacteria*, Vol. 1, Ratledge, C. and Stanford, J., Eds., Academic Press, New York, 1982, 353.

40. Quemard, A., Lancelle, G., and Lacave C., Mycolic acid synthesis: a target for ethionamide in mycobacteria? *Antimicrob. Agents Chemother.*, 36, 1316, 1992.

41. Jenner, P. J., Ellard, G. A., Gruer, P. J. K., and Aber, V. R., A comparison of the blood levels and urinary excretion of ethionamide and prothionamide in man, *J. Antimicrob. Chemother.*, 13, 267, 1984.

42. Girling, D. J., Adverse effects of antituberculosis drugs, *Drugs*, 23, 56, 1982.
43. Perez-Stable, E. J. and Hopewell, P. C., Current tuberculosis treatment regimens, in *Clinics in Chest Medicine*, Vol. 10, Snider, D.E., Jr., Ed., W.B. Saunders, Philadelphia, 1989, 323.
44. Wolinsky, E., Mycobacterial diseases other than tuberculosis, *Clin. Inf. Dis.*, 15, 1, 1992.
45. Cynamon, M. H., Comparative *in vitro* activities of MDL 473, rifampin and ansamycin against *Mycobacterium intracellulare, Antimicrob. Agents Chemother.*, 28, 440, 1985.
46. Klemens, S. P. and Cynamon, M. H., Activity of rifapentine against *Mycobacterium avium* infection in beige mice, *J. Antimicrob. Chemother.*, 29, 555, 1992.
47. Saito, H., Sato, K., and Tomioka, H., Comparative *in vitro* and *in vivo* activity of rifabutin and rifampicin against *Mycobacterium avium* complex, *Tubercle*, 69, 187, 1988.
48. Wallace, R. J., Jr., The clinical presentation, diagnosis and therapy of cutaneous and pulmonary infections due to the rapid growing mycobacteria, *M. fortuitum* and *M. chelonae*, in *Clinics in Chest Medicine*, Vol. 10, Snider, D. E., Jr., Ed., W.B. Saunders, Philadelphia, 1989, 419.
49. Kono, K., Oizumi, K., and Oka, S., Mode of action of rifampin in mycobacteria. II. Biosynthetic studies on the inhibitors of ribonucleic acid polymerase of *Mycobacterium bovis* BCG by rifampin and uptake of rifampin-^{14}C by *Mycobacterium phlei, Am. Rev. Respir. Dis.*, 107, 1006, 1973.
50. Cole, S. T., Rifamycin resistance in mycobacteria, *Res. Microbiol.*, 147, 48, 1996.
51. Williams, D. L., Waquespack, C., Eisenach, K., Crawford, J. T., Portaels, F., Salfinger, M., Nolan, C. M., Abe, C., Sticht-Groh, V., and Gillis, T. P., Characterization of rifampin resistance in pathogenic mycobacteria, *Antimicrob. Agents Chemother.*, 38, 2380, 1994.
52. Williams, D. L., Spring, L., Collins, L., Miller, L. P., Heifets, L. B., Gangadharam, P. R., and Gillis, T. P., Contributions of rpoβ mutations to development of rifamycin cross-resistance in *Mycobacterium tuberculosis, Antimicrob. Agents Chemother.*, 42, 1853, 1998.
53. Peloquin, C. A., Antituberculosis drugs: pharmacokinetics, in *Drug Suspectibility in the Chemotherapy of Mycobacterial Infections*, Heifets, L. B., Ed., CRC Press LLC, Boca Raton, FL, 1991, 61.
54. Snider, D., Pregnancy and tuberculosis, *Chest*, 86 (Suppl.), 10S, 1984.
55. Van Scoy, R. E. and Wilkowske, C. J., Antituberculous agents, *Mayo Clin. Proc.*, 67, 179, 1992.
56. Borcherding, S. M., Baciewicz, A. M., and Self, T. H., Update on rifampin drug interactions II, *Arch. Intern. Med.*, 152, 711, 1992.
57. Centers for Disease Control and Prevention, Prevention and treatment of tuberculosis among patients infected with human immunodeficiency virus: principles of therapy and revised recommendations, *MMWR*, 47 (RR-20), 1, 1998.
58. Traxler, P., Vischer, W. A., and Zak, O., New rifamycins, *Drugs Future*, 13, 845, 1988.
59. Dickinson, J. M. and Mitchison, D. A., *In vitro* activity of new rifamycins against rifampicin-resistant *M. tuberculosis* and MAIS-complex mycobacteria, *Tubercle*, 68, 177, 1987.
60. Hong Kong Chest Service/British Medical Research Council, A controlled study of rifabutin and an uncontrolled study of ofloxacin in the retreatment of patients with pulmonary tuberculosis resistant to isoniazid, streptomycin and rifampicin, *Tuberc. Lung Dis.*, 73, 59, 1992.
61. Chan, S. L., Yew, W. W., Ma, W. K., Girling, D. J., Aber, V. R., Flemingham, D., Allen, B. W., and Mitchison, D. A., The early bactericidal activity of rifabutin measured by sputum viable counts in Hong Kong patients with pulmonary tuberculosis, *Tuberc. Lung Dis.*, 73, 33, 1992.
62. O'Brien, R. J., Geiter, L. J., and Lyle, M. A., Rifabutin (ansamycin LM 427) for the treatment of pulmonary *Mycobacterium avium* complex, *Am. Rev. Respir. Dis.*, 141, 841, 1990.
63. Agins, B. D., Berman, D. S., Spicehandler, D., El-Sadr, W., Simberkoff, M. S., and Rahal, J. J., Effect of combined therapy with ansamycin, clofazimine, ethambutol, and isoniazid for *Mycobacterium avium* infection in patients with AIDS, *J. Infect. Dis.*, 159, 784, 1989.
64. Dautzenberg, B., Truffot, C., Mignon, A., Rozenbaum, W., Katlama, C., Perrone, C., Parrot, R., and Grosset, J., Rifabutin in combination with clofazimine, isoniazid and ethambutol in the treatment of AIDS patients with infections due to opportunist mycobacteria, *Tubercle*, 72, 168, 1991.
65. Shafran, S., Prevention and treatment of disseminated *Mycobacterium avium* complex infection in Human Immunodeficiency Virus-infected individuals, *Int. J. Infect. Dis.*, 3, 39, 1998.
66. Nightingale, S. D., Cameron, D. W., Gordin, F. M., Sullam, P. M., Cohn, D. L., Chaisson, R. E., Eron, L. J., Sparti, P. D., Bihari, B., Kaufman, D. L., et al., Two controlled trials of rifabutin prophylaxis against *Mycobacterium avium* complex infection in AIDs, *N. Engl. J. Med.*, 329, 828, 1993.

67. Havlir, D. V., Dube, M. P., Sattler, F. R., Fortha, D. N., Kemper, C. A., Dunne, M. W., Parenti, D. M., Lavelle, J. P., White, A. C., Jr., Witt, M. D., Bozzette, S. A., and McCutchan, J. A., Prophylaxis against disseminated *Mycobacterium avium* complex with weekly azithromycin, daily rifabutin, or both, *N. Engl. J. Med.*, 335, 392, 1996.

68. Skinner, M. H., Hsieh, M., Torseth, J., Pauloin, D., Bhatia, G., Harkonen, S., Merigan, T. C., and Blaschke, T. F., Pharmacokinetics of rifabutin, *Antimicrob. Agents Chemother.*, 33, 1237, 1989.

69. Battaglia, R., Pianezzola, E., Salgarollo, G., Zini, G., and Benedetti, M. S., Absorption, disposition and preliminary metabolic pathway of ^{14}C-rifabutin in animals and man, *J. Antimicrob. Chemother.*, 26, 813, 1990.

70. Shafran, S. D., Singer, J., Zarowny, D. P., Phillips, P., Salit, I., Walmsley, S. L., Fong, I. W., Gill, M. J., Rachlis, A. R., Lalonde, R. G., Fanning, M. M., and Tsoukas, C. M., A comparison of two regimens for the treatment of *Mycobacterium avium* complex bacteremia in AIDS: rifabutin, ethambutol, and clarithromycin versus rifammpin, ethambutol, clofazimine, and ciprofloxacin, *N. Engl. J. Med.*, 335, 377, 1996.

71. Strolin Benedetti, M., Efthymiopoulos, C., Sassella, D., Moro, E., and Repetto, M., Autoinduction of rifabutin metabolism in man, *Xenobiotica*, 20, 1113, 1990.

72. Dickinson, J. M. and Mitchison, D. A., *In vitro* properties of rifapentine (MDL 473) relevant to its use in intermittent chemotherapy of tuberculosis, *Tubercle*, 68, 113, 1987.

73. Heifets, L. B., Lindholm-Levy, P. J., and Flory, M. A., Bactericidal activity *in vitro* of various rifamycins against *Mycobacterium avium* and *Mycobacterium tuberculosis, Am. Rev. Respir. Dis.*, 141, 626, 1990.

74. Dhillon, J., Dickinson, J. M., Guy, J. A., Ng, T. K., and Mitchison, D. A., Activity of two long-acting rifamycins, rifapentine and FCE 22807, in experimental murine tuberculosis, *Tuberc. Lung Dis.*, 73, 116, 1992.

75. Thomas, J. P., Baughn, C. O., Wilkinson, R. G., and Shepard, R. G., A new synthetic compound with antituberculous activity in mice: ethambutol (dextro-2-2′-(ethylenediimino)-di-1-butanol), *Am. Rev. Respir. Dis.*, 83, 891, 1961.

76. Takayama, K., Armstrong, E. L., Kunugi, K. A., and Kilburn, J. D., Inhibition by ethambutol of mycolic acid transfer into the cell wall of *Mycobacterium smegmatis, Antimicrob. Agents Chemother.*, 16, 240, 1979.

77. Mikusova, K., Slayden, R. A., Besra, G. S., and Brennan, P. J., Biogenesis of the mycobacterial cell wall and the site of action of ethambutol, *Antimicrob. Agents Chemother.*, 39, 2484, 1995.

78. Belanger, A. E., Besra, G. S., Ford, M. E., Mikusova, K., Belisle, J. T., Brennan, P. J., and Inamine, J. M., The embAB genes of *Mycobacterium avium* encode an arabinosyl transferase involved in cell wall arabinan biosynthesis that is the target for the antimycobacterial drug ethambutol, *Proc. Natl. Acad. Sci.*, 21, 1919, 1996.

79. Telenti, A., Philipp, W., Sreevatsan, S., Bernascon, C., Stockbauer, K. E., Wieles, B., Musser, J. M., and Jacobs, W. R., Jr., The emb operon: a gene cluster of *Mycobacterium tuberculosis* involved in resistance to ethambutol, *Nature Med.*, 3, 567, 1997.

80. Place, V. A., Peets, E. A., Buyske, D. A., and Little, R. R., Metabolic and special studies of ethambutol in normal volunteers and tuberculosis patients, *Ann. N.Y. Acad. Sci.*, 135, 775, 1966.

81. Lee, C. S., Brater, D. C., Gambertoglio, J. G., and Benet, L. Z., Disposition kinetics of ethambutol in man, *J. Pharmacokin. Biopharmocol.*, 8, 335, 1980.

82. Lee, C. S., Gambertoglio, J. G., Brater, D. C., and Benet, L. Z., Kinetics of oral ethambutol in the normal subject, *Clin. Pharmacol. Ther.*, 22, 615, 1977.

83. Doster, B., Murray, F. J., Newman, R., and Woolpert, S. F., Ethambutol in the initial treatment of pulmonary tuberculosis, *Am. Rev. Respir. Dis.*, 107, 177, 1973.

84. Postlethwaite, A. E., Bartel, A. G., and Kelley, W. N., Hyperuricemia due to ethambutol, *N. Engl. J. Med.*, 286, 761, 1972.

85. Finken, M., Kirschner, P., Meier, A., Wrede, A., and Bottger, E. C., Molecular basis of streptomycin resistance in *Mycobacterium tuberculosis:* alterations of the ribosomal protein S12 gene and point mutations within a functional 16S ribosomal RNA pseudoknot, *Mol. Microbiol.*, 9, 1239, 1993.

86. Honore, N. and Cole, S., Streptomycin resistance in mycobacteria, *Antimicrob. Agents Chemother.*, 38, 238, 1994.

87. Hoffner, S. E. and Kallenius, G., Susceptibility of streptomycin-resistant *Mycobacterium tuberculosis* strains to amikacin, *Eur. J. Clin. Microbiol. Infect. Dis.*, 7, 188, 1988.

88. Allen, B. W., Mitchison, D. A., Chan, Y. C., Yew, W. W., Allan, W. G., and Girling, D. J., Amikacin in the treatment of pulmonary tuberculosis, *Tubercle*, 64, 111, 1983.

89. Neuhaus, F. C., D-cycloserine and D-carbamyl-D-serine, in *Antibiotics,* Vol. I, Gottlieb, D. and Shaw, P. D., Eds., Springer-Verlag, New York, 1967, 40.

90. Caceres, N. E., Harris, N. B., Wellehan, J. F., Feng, Z., Kapur, V., and Barletta, R. G., Overexpression of the D-alanine racemase gene confers resistance to D-cycloserine in *Mycobacterium smegmatis, J. Bacteriol.*, 179, 5046, 1997.

91. Reitz, R., Slade, H. D., and Neuhaus, F. C., On the biochemical basis of D-cycloserine resistance. *Fed. Proc.*, Abstr. 25, 344, 1966.

92. Nair, K. G. S., Epstein, I. G., Baron, H., and Mulinos, M. G., Absorption, distribution, and excretion of cycloserine in man, *Antibiot. Annual*, 1955, 136.

93. Masel, M. A., A lupus-like reaction to antituberculous drugs, *Med. J. Aust.*, 2, 738, 1967.

94. Hopewell, P. C., Sanchez-Hernandez, M., Baron, R. B., and Ganter, B., Operational evaluation of treatment of tuberculosis: results of a "standard" 12-month regimen in Peru, *Am. Rev. Respir. Dis.*, 129, 439, 1984.

95. Heifets, L. B., Lindholm-Levy, P. J., and Flory, M., Thiacetazone: *in vitro* activity against *Mycobacterium avium* and *M. tuberculosis, Tubercle*, 71, 287, 1990.

96. Ellard, G. A., Dickinson, J. M., Gammon, P. T., and Mitchison, D. A., Serum concentrations and antituberculosis activity of thiacetazone, *Tubercle*, 55, 41, 1974.

97. Miller, A. B., Fox, W., and Tall, R., An international co-operative investigation into thiacetazone (thioacetazone) side effects, *Tubercle*, 47, 33, 1966.

98. Nunn, P., Kibuga, D., Gathua, S., Brindle, R., Imalingat, A., Wasunna, K., Lucas, S., Gilks, C., Omwega, M., and Were, J., Cutaneous hypersensitivity reactions due to thiacetazone in HIV-1 seropositive patients treated for tuberculosis, *Lancet*, 337, 627, 1991.

99. Cambau, E. and Jarlier, V., Resistance to quinolones in mycobacteria, *Res. Microbiol.*, 147, 52, 1996.

100. Takiff, H. E., Salazar, L., Guerrero, C., Philipp, W., Huang, W. M., Kreisworth, B., Cole, S. T., Jacobs, W. R., Jr., and Telenti, A., Cloning and nucleotide sequence of *Mycobacterium tuberculosis* gyrA and gyrB genes and detection of quinolone resistance mutations, *Antimicrob. Agents Chemother.*, 38, 773, 1994.

101. Heifets, L. B. and Lindholm-Levy, P. J., Bacteriostatic and bactericidal activity of ciprofloxacin and ofloxacin against *Mycobacterium tuberculosis* and *Mycobacterium avium* complex, *Tubercle*, 68, 267, 1987.

102. Van Caekenberghe, D., Comparative *in vitro* activities of ten fluoroquinolones and fusidic acid against *Mycobacterium* spp., *J. Antimicrob. Chemother.*, 26, 381, 1990.

103. Bergstermann, H. and Ruchardt, A., Ciprofloxacin once daily versus twice daily for the treatment of pulmonary tuberculosis, *Infection*, 25, 227, 1997.

104. Kennedy, N., Berger, L., Curram, J., Fox, R., Gutmann, J., Kisyombe, G. M., Ngowi, F. I., Ramsay, A. R., Saruni, A. O., Sam, N., Tillotson, G., Uiso, L. O., Yates, M., and Gillespie, S. H., Randomized controlled trial of a drug regimen that includes ciprofloxacin for the treatment of pulmonary tuberculosis, *Clin. Infect. Dis.*, 22, 827, 1996.

105. Gorzynski, E. A., Gutman, S. I., and Allen, W., Comparative antimycobacterial activities of difloxacin, temafloxacin, enoxacin, pefloxacin, reference fluoroquinolones, and a new macrolide, clarithromycin, *Antimicrob. Agents Chemother.*, 33, 591, 1989.

106. Chiu, J., Nussbaum, J., Bozzette, S., Tilles, J. G., Young, L. S., Leedom, J., Heseltine, P. N. R., McCutchan, J. A., and the California Collaborative Treatment Group, Treatment of disseminated *Mycobacterium avium* complex infection in AIDS with amikacin, ethambutol, rifampin and ciprofloxacin, *Ann. Intern. Med.*, 113, 358, 1990.

107. McEvoy, G. K., Ed., Anti-infective agents, in *American Hospital Formulary Service Drug Information*, American Society of Hospital Pharmacists, Inc., Bethesda, MD, 1998.

108. Janknegt, R., Drug interactions with quinolones, *J. Antimicrob. Chemother.*, 26 (Suppl. D), 7, 1990.

109. Jolson, H. M., Tanner, L. A., Green, L., and Grasela, T. H., Jr., Adverse reaction reporting of interaction between warfarin and fluoroquinolones, *Arch. Intern. Med.*, 151, 1003, 1991.

110. Truffot-Pernot, C., Ji, B., and Grosset, J., Activities of pefloxacin and ofloxacin against mycobacteria: *in vitro* and mouse experiments, *Tubercle*, 72, 57, 1991.

111. Tomioka, H., Sato, K., and Saito, H., Comparative *in vitro* and *in vivo* activity of fleroxacin and ofloxacin against various mycobacteria, *Tubercle*, 72, 176, 1991.

112. Tsukamura, M., Nakamura, E., Yoshii, S., and Amano, H., Therapeutic effect of a new antibacterial substance ofloxacin (DL 8280) on pulmonary tuberculosis, *Am. Rev. Respir. Dis.*, 131, 352, 1985.

113. Fu, K. P., Lafredo, S. C., Locodo, J., Isaacson, D., and Tobia, A. J., *In vivo* antibacterial activity of a L-isomer of ofloxacin (L-ofloxacin; DR-3355), an active isomer of racemic ofloxacin (OFL) in murine infection models, in Program Abstr. 31st Interscience Conf. Antimicrob. Agents Chemother., Abstr., 1202, 1991.

114. Kawada, Y., Aso, Y., Kamidono, S., Ohmori, H., and Kumazawa, J., Comparative study of DR-3355 and ofloxacin in complicated urinary tract infections, in *Program Abstr. 31st Interscience Conf. Antimicrob. Agents Chemother.*, Abstr., 884, 1991.

115. Klemens, S. P. and Cynamon, M. H. (unpublished data).

116. Garrelts, J. C., Clofazimine: a review of its use in leprosy and *Mycobacterium avium* complex infections, *DICP*, 25, 525, 1991.

117. Schmidt, L. H., Observations on the prophylactic and therapeutic activities of 2-(p-chloranilino)-5-(p-chlorophenyl)-3,5-dihydro-3-(isopropylimino)phenazine (B.663), *Bull. Int. Union Tuberc.*, 30, 316, 1959.

118. Holdiness, M. R., Clinical pharmacokinetics of clofazimine: a review, *Clin. Pharmacokinet.*, 16, 74, 1989.

119. Heifets, L. B., Lindholm-Levy, P. J., and Comstock, R. D., Clarithromycin minimal inhibitory and bactericidal concentrations against *Mycobacterium avium*, *Am. Rev. Respir. Dis.*, 145, 856, 1991.

120. Klemens, S. P. and Cynamon, M. H., Activity of clarithromycin against *Mycobacterium avium* complex infection in beige mice, *Antimicrob. Agents Chemother.*, 36, 2413, 1992.

121. Dautzenberg, B., Truffot, C., Legris, S., Meyohas, M-C., Berlie, H. C., Mercat, A., Chevret, S., and Grosset, J., Activity of clarithromycin against *Mycobacterium avium* infections in patients with the acquired immune deficiency syndrome, *Am. Rev. Respir. Dis.*, 144, 564, 1991.

122. Chaisson, R. E., Benson, C. A., Dube, M. P., Heifets, L. B., Korvick, J. A., Elkin, S., Smith, T., Craft, J. C., and Sattler, F. R., Clarithromycin therapy for bacteremic *Mycobacterium avium* complex disease in patients with AIDS, *Ann., Intern. Med.*, 121, 905, 1994.

123. Chaisson, R. E., Keiser, P., Pierce, M., Fessel, W. J., Ruskin, J., Lahart, C., Benson, C. A., Meek, K., Siepman, N., and Craft, J. C., Clarithromycin and ethambutol with or without clofazime for the treatment of bacteremic *Mycobacterium avium* complex disease in patients with HIV infection, *AIDS*, 11, 311, 1997.

124. Meier, A., Kirschner, P., Springer, B., Steingrube, V. A., Brown, B. A., Wallace, R. J., Jr., and Bottger, E., Identification of mutations in 23S rRNA gene of clarithromycin-resistant *Mycobacterium intracellulare*, 38, 381, 1994.

125. Kirst, H. A. and Sides, G. D., New directions for macrolide antibiotics: pharmacokinetics and clinical efficacy, *Antimicrob. Agents Chemother.*, 33, 1419, 1989.

126. Wallace, R. J., Jr., Brown, B. A., Griffith, D. E., Girard, W., and Tanaka, K., Reduced serum levels of clarithromycin in patients treated with multidrug regimens including rifampin or rifabutin for *Mycobacterium avium* — *M. intracellulare* infection, *J. Infect. Dis.*, 171, 747, 1995.

127. Hafner, R., Bethel, J., Power, M., Landry, B., Banach, M., Mole, L., Standiford, H. C., Follansbee, S., Kumar, P., Raasch, R., Cohn, D., Mushatt, D., and Drusano, G., Tolerance and pharmacokinetic interactions of rifabutin and clarithromycin in human immunodeficiency virus-infected volunteers, *Antimicrob. Agents Chemother.*, 42, 631, 1998.

128. Kirst, H. A. and Sides, G. D., New directions for macrolideantibiotics: structural modifications and *in vitro* activity, *Antimicrob. Agents Chemother.*, 33, 1413, 1989.

129. Cynamon, M. H. and Klemens, S .P., Activity of azithromycin against *Mycobacterium avium* infection in beige mice, *Antimicrob. Agents Chemother.*, 36, 1611, 1992.

130. Naik, S. and Ruk, R., *In vitro* activities of several new macrolide antibiotics against *Mycobacterium avium* complex, *Antimicrob. Agents Chemother.*, 33, 1614, 1989.

131. Young, S. L, Wiviott, L., Wu, M., Kolonoski, P., Bolan, R., and Inderlied, C. B., Azithromycin for treatment of *Mycobacterium avium-intracellulare* complex infection in patients with AIDS, *Lancet*, 388, 1107, 1991.

132. Girard, A. E., Girard, D., English, A. R., Gootz, T. D., Cimochowski, C. R., Faiella, J. A., Haskell, S. L., and Retsema, J. A., Pharmacokinetics and *in vivo* studies with azithromycin (CP-62,993), a new macrolide with an extended half-life and excellent tissue distribution, *Antimicrob. Agents Chemother.*, 31, 1948, 1987.

133. Bahal, N. and Nahata, M. C., The new macrolides: azithromycin, clarithromycin, dirithromycin, and roxithromycin, *Ann. Pharmacol.*, 26, 46, 1992.

134. Wong, C. S., Palmer, G. S., and Cynamon, M. H., *In vitro* suspectibility of *Mycobacterium tuberculosis, Mycobacterium bovis*, and *Mycobacterium kansasii* to amoxicillin and ticarcillin in combination with clavulanic acid, *J. Antimicrob. Chemother.*, 22, 863, 1988.

135. Sorg, T. B. and Cynamon, M. H., Comparison of four β-lactamase inhibitors in combination with ampicillin against *Mycobacterium tuberculosis, J. Antimicrob. Chemother.*, 19, 59, 1987.

136. Cynamon, M. H. and Palmer, G. S., *In vitro* susceptibility of *Mycobacterium fortuitum* to *N*-formimidoyl thienamycin and several cephamycins, *Antimicrob. Agents Chemother.*, 22, 1079, 1982.

137. Swenson, J. M., Wallace, R. J., Jr., Silcox, V. A., and Thornsberry, C., Antimicrobial susceptibility of five subgroups of *Mycobacterium fortuitum* and *Mycobacterium chelonae, Antimcrob. Agents Chemother.*, 28, 807, 1985.

138. Wallace, R. J., Jr., Brown, B. A., and Onyi, G. O., Susceptibilities of *Mycobacterium fortuitum* biovar. *fortuitum* and the two subgroups of *Mycobacterium chelonae* to imipenem, cefmetazole, cefoxitin and amoxicillin-clavulanic acid, *Antimicrob. Agents Chemother.*, 35, 773, 1991.

139. Wallace, R. J., Jr., Swenson, J. M., Silcox, V. A., and Bullen, M. G., Treatment of nonpulmonary infections due to *Mycobacterium fortuitum* and *Mycobacterium chelonei* on the basis of *in vitro* susceptibilities, *J. Infect. Dis.*, 152, 500, 1985.

140. Wallace, R. J., Jr., Wiss, K., Bushby, M. B., and Hollowell, D. C., *In vitro* activity of trimethoprim and sulfamethoxazole against the nontuberculous mycobacteria, *Rev. Infect. Dis.*, 4, 326, 1982.

141. Ahn, C. H., Wallace, R. J., Jr., and Steele, L. C., Sulfonamide containing regimens for disease caused by rifampin-resistant *Mycobacterium kansasii, Am. Rev. Respir. Dis.*, 135, 10, 1987.

142. Berlin, O. G. W., Clancy, M. N., and Bruckner, D. A., *In vitro* susceptibility of sulfisoxazole against *Mycobacterium avium* complex, in *Prog. Abstr. 28th Intersc. Conf. Antimicro. Agents Chemother.*, Abstr. 1227, 1988.

143. Davis, C. E., Jr., Carpenter, J. L., and Trevino, S., *In vitro* susceptibility of *Mycobacterium avium* complex to antibacterial agents, *Diagn. Microbiol. Infect. Dis.*, 8, 149, 1987.

144. Swenson, J. M., Wallace, R. J., Jr., Silcox, V. A., and Thornsberry, C., Antimicrobial susceptibility of five subgroups of *Mycobacterium fortuitum* and *Mycobacterium chelonae, Antimicrob. Agents Chemother.*, 28, 807, 1985.

145. Wallace, R. J., Jr., Dalovisio, J. R., and Pankey, G. A., Disk diffusion testing of susceptibility of *Mycobacterium fortuitum* and *Mycobacterium chelonei* to antibacterial agents, *Antimicrob. Agents Chemother.*, 16, 611, 1979.

146. Gelber, R. H., Activity of minocycline in *Mycobacterium leprae*-infected mice, *J. Infect. Dis.*, 156, 236, 1987.

147. Ji, B., Perani, E. G., and Grosset, J. H., Effectiveness of clarithromycin and minocyline alone and in combination against experimental *Mycobacterium leprae* infection in mice, *Antimicrob. Agents Chemother.*, 35, 579, 1991.

148. Majumdar, S., Flasher, D., Friend, D. S., Nassos, P., Yajko, D., Hadley, W. K., and Duzgunes, N., Efficacies of liposome-encapsulated streptomycin and ciprofloxacin against *Mycobacterium avium — M. intracellulare* complex infections in human peripheral blood monocyte/macrophages, *Antimicrob. Agents Chemother.*, 36, 2808, 1992.

149. Cynamon, M. H., Klemens, S. P., and Swenson, C. E., TLCG-65 in combination with other agents in the therapy of *Mycobacterium avium* infection in beige mice, *J. Antimicrob. Chemother.*, 29, 693, 1992.

150. Maller, R., Isaksson, B., Nilsson, L., and Soren, L., A study of amikacin given once versus twice daily in serious infection, *J. Antimicrob. Chemother.*, 22, 75, 1988.

151. Holdiness, M. R., Clinical pharmacokinetics of the antituberculosis drugs, *Clin. Pharmacokinet.*, 9, 108, 1984.

152. Heifets, L. B., Lindholm-Levy, P. J., and Flory, M., Comparison of bacteriostatic and bactericidal activity of isoniazid and ethionamide against *M. avium* and *M. tuberculosis, Am. Rev. Respir. Dis.*, 143, 268, 1991.

153. Heifets, L. B., Antituberculosis drugs: antimicrobial activity *in vitro*, in *Drug Susceptibility in the Chemotherapy of Mycobacterial Infections*, Heifets, L. B., Ed., CRC Press LLC, Boca Raton, FL, 1991, 20.

154. Salfinger, M. and Heifets, L., Determination of pyrazinamide MICs for *Mycobacterium tuberculosis* at different pHs by the radiometric method, *Antimicrob. Agents Chemother.*, 32, 1002, 1988.

155. Trnka, L., Rifampicin (RMP), in *Antituberculosis Drugs*, Bartmann, K., Ed., Springer-Verlag, Berlin, 1988, 205.

156. Heifets, L. B. and Iseman, M. D., Determination of *in vitro* susceptibility of mycobacteria to ansa-mycin, *Am. Rev. Respir. Dis.*, 132, 710, 1985.

157. Otten, H., Ethambutol (EMB), in *Antituberculosis Drugs*, Bartmann, K., Ed., Springer-Verlag, Berlin, 1988, 197.

158. Suo, J., Chang, C-E., Lin, T. P., and Heifets, L. B., Minimal inhibitory concentrations of isoniazid, rifampin, ethambutol, and streptomycin against *M. tuberculosis* strains isolated before treatment of patients in Taiwan, *Am. Rev. Respir. Dis.*, 138, 999, 1988.

159. Heifets, L. B., MIC as a quantitative measurement of the susceptibility of *M. avium* strains to seven antituberculosis drugs, *Antimicrob. Agents Chemother.*, 32, 113, 1988.

160. Otten, H., Cycloserine (CS) and Terizidone (TZ), in *Antituberculosis Drugs*, Bartmann, K., Ed., Springer-Verlag, Berlin, 1988, 158.

12 Drug Resistance

Marian Goble, M.D.

CONTENTS

0-8493-1565-4/97/$0.00+$.50
© 2000 by CRC Press LLC

I. BACKGROUND[1]

The thrust of treatment programs for tuberculosis is to avoid treatment failure and to prevent the emergence of drug-resistant strains. Nevertheless, drug-resistant tuberculosis remains a problem and appears to be increasing in prevalence and in complexity.[2]

A. HISTORICAL

Early in the antibiotic era, streptomycin, given as a single agent, was shown to be highly effective in producing clinical, roentgenographic, and bacteriologic improvement in patients with serious illness from tuberculosis. Frequently the improvement was short lived and patients relapsed with tubercle bacilli resistant to streptomycin.[3] Subsequently, with the development of new antituberculosis medications, resistance of tubercle bacilli to any effective drug could be induced if that drug was used as a single agent.[4,5] It was discovered that properly administered multiple drug therapy prevented the emergence of drug resistance.[6,7] Until it was understood that patients required prolonged multiple drug therapy for tuberculosis, inadequate regimens were prescribed commonly. Drug-resistant disease followed.

New drugs were developed. Specific regimens for drug-resistant tuberculosis were studied over the years. Earlier studies[8-14] involved the use of pyrazinamide, cycloserine, p-aminosalicylate (PAS), ethionamide, kanamycin, and viomycin (viomycin is no longer available in the U.S., but is of interest because of common cross-resistance with capreomycin). Later, as ethambutol, capreomycin, and rifampin became available, regimens including these drugs also were studied in retreatment situations.[15,16] Although some reports were not based on carefully controlled studies with uniform criteria, results suggest that in using drugs to which the bacilli were susceptible, three drugs in the regimens gave better results than two drugs.[8,12,17,18]

In several studies outside the U.S., retreatment regimens of pyrazinamide, cycloserine, and ethionamide were given to patients with tuberculosis resistant to isoniazid, PAS, and streptomycin; a successful outcome was reported in 90% of cases.[8,12,13] In a developing nation where isoniazid, streptomycin, and thiacetazone (an antituberculosis drug that never became commercially available in the U.S.) had been standard therapy for tuberculosis, patients who had experienced treatment failure were retreated with a regimen including pyrazinamide and PAS; results were acceptable.[19,20]

At National Jewish Medical and Research Center in Denver, CO,[21] prior to 1971, a regimen of kanamycin, ethionamide, and pyrazinamide was given to 108 patients with tubercle bacilli resistant to isoniazid and streptomycin; a successful outcome occurred in 92% of these patients. A similar group of 164 patients was treated with capreomycin or viomycin in place of kanamycin, with either ethambutol or rifampin replacing one of the oral drugs; similar results were achieved, provided the organisms were susceptible to the drugs chosen. For 36 patients, cycloserine or PAS were among the drugs selected; a successful outcome occurred in 78%. Because of the limited number of drugs that were effective when taken orally, one injectable medication usually was included in these regimens, along with two oral drugs.

Prior to the late 1980s, most of the patients with drug-resistant tuberculosis were isolated cases who had acquired drug resistance because of inadequate treatment or nonadherence. Only occasional clusters of drug-resistant cases were reported. [22-27] The prevalence of drug resistance in the U.S. remained stable for many years.[28-34] Sporadic cases with rifampin resistance were noted shortly after the introduction of this important drug in the U.S. in 1971. Then no new highly effective antituberculosis medications were introduced for several decades. Results of therapy for rifampin-resistant tuberculosis (almost always with concomitant resistance to isoniazid, and often with resistance to other drugs) were dire. Among 134 patients (without infection with the human immunodeficiency virus) with resistance to a median of six antituberculosis drugs and treated with individually tailored regimens at National Jewish Center between 1973 and 1983, only 65% responded favorably to medical regimens.[35] The fluoroquinolones were introduced in the mid-1980s. When one of these drugs was included in individually tailored multidrug regimens along with aggressive use of expertly performed surgical resection of major residual lesions, favorable outcome improved to 85% in a group of 109 similar patients treated at National Jewish Center.[36]

In the late 1980s the overall incidence of tuberculosis started to increase. Prior cutbacks in tuberculosis control programs had led to increasing numbers of patients receiving inadequate therapy. Some inadequately treated patients developed drug-resistant disease. Socioeconomic conditions favored overcrowding and spread of tuberculosis in poorly ventilated facilities. Persons infected with the human immunodeficiency virus, if exposed to tuberculosis, were unusually vulnerable to developing active (rather than latent) disease very soon after exposure. Thus, they were capable of transmitting the infection very soon after having become infected themselves. Frequently their tuberculosis was not recognized promptly and appropriate treatment was delayed. Infection control measures often were not implemented due to delay in suspicion of a diagnosis of tuberculosis in these immunosuppressed hosts with atypical manifestations of the disease. In some cases, adequate isolation and infection control measures were not available, further favoring nosocomial spread of infection. In the early 1990s, increasing outbreaks of drug-resistant tuberculosis were reported, with extremely high mortality. [37-53]

With the resurgence of tuberculosis and the apparent increasing incidence of drug-resistant disease, resources were mobilized to control the problem. In 1992, the U.S. Centers for Disease Control and Prevention (CDC) devised a National Action Plan to combat multidrug-resistant tuberculosis.[54] Identification of the extent of the problem was necessary. Therefore, performance of susceptibility studies on all culture-positive cases was recommended. Previously, in the U.S., routine susceptibility studies were not advocated. Surveys of the prevalence of drug-resistant tuberculosis had been conducted between 1961 and 1986, using various methods. [29-33] Between 1986 and 1990, drug resistance surveys had been discontinued.[55] Surveys for drug resistance were resumed in 1991[56] and 1992. Since 1993, data have been collected with increasing regularity and consistency.

With the implementation of the National Action Plan, along with increased efforts and allocated resources on local levels, the overall incidence of tuberculosis in the U.S. decreased from its recent peak of 26,673 in 1992 to 19,851 in 1997. The prevalence of isoniazid resistance decreased from 9.1% in 1991 to 7.8% in 1997, and of combined isoniazid and rifampin resistance from 3.4% in 1991 to 1.4% in 1997.[56,57] Notably, in New York City,[58,59] where tuberculosis and drug resistance has been a particularly bad problem, the prevalence of combined isoniazid and rifampin resistance decreased from 13.9% in 1991 to 3.8% in 1997.[56,57]

With renewed awareness of tuberculosis and of drug-resistant tuberculosis in particular, and increasing resources to control the problem, the early outcome for patients improved. In the outbreaks in the late 1980s and early 1990, 60 to 89% of the patients with drug-resistant tuberculosis, many of whom were severely immunosuppressed from coinfection with HIV, died in a median of 4 to 16 weeks.[1] When appropriate therapy was started promptly, the outcome was less bleak.[60] Median survival was 315 days in one series of patients with multidrug-resistant tuberculosis coinfected with HIV.[61] Among another series of patients with HIV-related multidrug-resistant tuberculosis, who were diagnosed early and treated appropriately, 59% survived 1 year or more.[62]

In a series of patients with multidrug-resistant tuberculosis without HIV infection, who were treated promptly and apppropriately, 96% had a favorable clinical response; bacteriological response was not documented in all cases.[63]

Along with renewed interest in the clinical and epidemiological aspects of drug-resistant tuberculosis, interest in the basic science aspects began to flourish. More scientists are studying the basic mechanisms of drug resistance[64,65] and the details of host response to infection with *M. tuberculosis*. New technologies from other fields have been applied to tuberculosis. The genome of *M. tuberculosis* has been sequenced;[66] clinical applications are to be anticipated.[67]

Although the prevalence of drug-resistant tuberculosis in the U.S. has declined and outbreaks involving large clusters of patients have been controlled, drug-resistance continues to be a serious problem.[55] Outbreaks of drug-resistant disease are being reported from other countries [68-71] and the overall prevalence of drug-resistant tuberculosis worldwide is alarmingly high. (See Chapter 16.)

B. MECHANISMS[65,72-74]

The development of drug resistance in *M. tuberculosis* occurs through random genetic mutation. Approximately 95% of strains resistant to rifampin exhibit mutation in the rpoβ gene, which involves alterations of RNA polymerase.[75] Resistance to isoniazid may be associated with mutations in any of a number of genes, including KatG,[76] involved in catalase and peroxidase production, and inhA,[77] involved in mycolic acid biosynthesis. The inhA gene also has been associated with resistance to ethionamide.[77] Genes involved in resistance to the quinolones, streptomycin, and pyrazinamide also have been identified.[65] (See also Chapter 11.)

The drug resistance conferred by genetic mutations of *M. tuberculosis* is spontaneous and not dependent on exposure to drugs. Although it is conceivable that a person could become infected with a tubercle bacillus bearing a spontaneous mutation conferring resistance to a drug, it is more likely for a person to have inhaled a fully susceptible bacillus. When this bacillus multiplies in the person's body, most of its progeny will be drug susceptible; a few will be drug-resistant mutants. In the process of multiplication of *M. tuberculosis*, mutations having resistance to any drug occur at a fairly predictable rate.[78] Mutants resistant to rifampin have a probable incidence of 1 in 10^8 bacilli; mutants resistant to isoniazid, streptomycin, ethambutol, kanamycin, or PAS have a probability of 1 in 10^6; mutants resistant to ethionamide, capreomycin, cycloserine, or thiacetazone occur at a rate of approximately 1 in 10^3 tubercle bacilli.[79] When large numbers of tubercle bacilli are present in a person who is ill with tuberculosis, the use of a single antituberculosis medication selects for drug resistance by killing or suppressing susceptible bacilli and leaving the resistant bacilli unaffected and free to multiply. Natural resistance to more than one drug (i.e., multiple drug resistance due to spontaneously occurring mutations) is very unlikely, suggesting that the mutations to various drugs are unlinked genetically. Other mechanisms of resistance have been proposed.[80-84]

1. Primary Resistance

Primary resistance refers to drug resistance of the bacilli from a patient who has never received treatment, who presumably has contracted his or her infection from an index case with drug-resistant tubercle bacilli. Initial resistance is another term used, to include drug-resistant bacilli from patients with no prior treatment, or with no known prior treatment with antituberculosis chemotherapy. The term "transferred resistance" is sometimes used to refer to drug-resistant tuberculosis acquired from contact with a drug-resistant index case.

2. Secondary Resistance

Secondary, or acquired resistance, refers to resistance of the bacilli after exposure to an antimicrobial agent, the mutant bacilli having been selected for survival. A patient with untreated cavitary tuberculosis has on the order of 1 in 10^8 tubercle bacilli in the cavity.[72,73] Since mutations to isoniazid resistance occurs at a frequency of 1 in 10^6, an infection with 10^8 bacilli would include approximately 10^2 that are resistant to isoniazid. If the patient is treated with isoniazid alone, almost all the bacilli would be killed, but those few remaining would be isoniazid resistant. At the time of the reduction in the number of the isoniazid-susceptible bacilli, the patient may improve clinically, roentgenographically, and even bacteriologically. The bacterial count may become very low, even low enough that the bacilli are no longer detectable by usual bacteriologic tests. However, if the host defenses are unable to control the resistant bacilli, they multiply and become the predominant organisms; the patient then has isoniazid-resistant tuberculosis. A decrease in the numbers of bacilli, followed by an increase associated with the emergence of drug resistance is called the "fall and rise" phenomenon.[72]

Sometimes the host defenses control the drug-resistant bacilli temporarily and these persisting, living, drug-resistant bacilli remain dormant. However, if the balance between the host's defenses and the bacilli changes, and the drug-resistant persisters[83,84] later multiply aggressively, the patient will relapse with drug-resistant tuberculosis. Inadequate therapy may result in treatment failure or relapse with secondary or acquired drug resistance. Most commonly, this inadequate therapy results from inappropriate prescription, such as the use of a single effective agent or because of the patient's nonadherence to the prescribed regimen.[85]

3. Multidrug Resistance

The occurrence of multidrug-resistant tuberculosis is favored by inappropriate management of tuberculosis. In the presence of tuberculosis already resistant to a single drug, therapy with that drug is ineffective. If one other single drug is included in the regimen, or added to the regimen, this is equivalent to monotherapy with the potentially effective second drug. Emergence of resistance to this second drug is to be anticipated, superimposed upon the previously existing resistance to the first drug;[86] thus, multiple drug resistance emerges. Infectious patients with multidrug resistance may spread their multidrug-resistant bacilli to their contacts. It has been common practice in the 1990s in the U.S. and some other industrialized nations, to limit the term "multidrug-resistant tuberculosis" or "MDR-TB" to tuberculosis exhibiting resistance to both isoniazid and rifampin, with or without resistance to additional drugs.

4. Cross Resistance[72,87]

Cross resistance between streptomycin and kanamycin or capreomycin is unusual; between kanamycin and capreomycin is fairly frequent;[88] between kanamycin and amikacin is frequent. Cross resistance between thiacetazone (a drug not available in the Untied States, but used in developing nations) and ethionamide, and between isoniazid and ethionamide has been reported.[89,90] Cross resistance between the quinolones[91] and between rifamycin derivatives[92,93] also occurs.

C. PREVALENCE OF DRUG RESISTANCE[28,33,55,56,94-96]

In 1996, in the U.S., the overall prevalence of drug resistance of *M. tuberculosis* to any drug was 13.4%, resistance to isoniazid was 8.0%, resistance to rifamin was 2.3%, and combined resistance to both isoniazid and rifampin was 1.6%. Resistance to streptomycin was 6.2%, resistance to pyrazinamide was 2.3%, and resistance to ethambutol was 2.2%.[55] In 1997, resistance to isoniazid was 7.8% and combined resistance to both isoniazid and rifampin was 1.4%. Drug resistance is distributed unevenly. In New York City in 1997, resistance to isoniazid was 10% and combined resistance to isoniazid and rifampin was 3.8%.[57,97] (See Chapter 1 for a discussion of prevalence in the U.S.)

In many countries throughout the world, data on drug resistance has been scanty and surveys for drug resistance often have not used comparable criteria.[98] Two recent publications have reviewed these surveys.[99,100] In 1997 the World Health Organization and the International Union Against Tuberculosis and Lung Disease prepared guidelines for surveillance of drug resistance in tuberculosis.[101] Reports of the results of surveys in individual countries are being published periodically. (See Chapter 16 for a discussion of international issues in tuberculosis.)

II. PREVENTION OF DRUG RESISTANCE[54,102-104]

A. APPROPRIATE THERAPEUTIC REGIMENS

There is no known way to prevent nature's mutations to resistance. However, thoughtful treatment of tuberculosis can significantly minimize the selection of these drug-resistant mutants as the predominant population in patients being treated for the first time and in patients undergoing retreatment. Applying an effective and efficient tuberculosis treatment program has been followed ultimately by a decrease in the prevalence of drug resistance.[105-107]

1. Initial Treatment

It is a well-accepted practice to employ more than one drug in therapy of disease due to *M. tuberculosis* (see Chapter 6). If two effective antimicrobial drugs are administered, the mutants resistant to drug A are controlled by drug B, and the drug-resistant mutants to drug B are controlled by drug A.[108] Two-drug therapy with agents such as isoniazid and rifampin works well *if* the bacterial population is susceptible to both drugs. However, sometimes the tubercle bacilli are resistant to one of the drugs chosen. This resistance may be unsuspected and not documented until the susceptibility studies are reported, often belatedly. Meanwhile, the patient is receiving therapy with only one effective drug. If the bacterial population is large, mutants will emerge that are resistant to the drug that has been working, in addition to the inherited resistance of these same organisms to the originally ineffective drug. These multiply resistant tubercle bacilli will become the predominant strain in the infection. This scenario of compounding the problem of drug resistance can be prevented if a sufficient number of effective antimycobacterial drugs are given from the start. Accordingly, the American Thoracic Society (ATS) and the CDC have recommended that patients being treated for the first time be started on isoniazid, rifampin, pyrazinamide, and either ethambutol or streptomycin, until the results of susceptibility tests of their bacilli are known, unless there is little possibility of primary resistance to isoniazid.[109,110] Overtreatment in the early phase of therapy is preferable to undertreatment that favors the emergence of multidrug resistance.

2. Retreatment

The patient's history, especially regarding prior antituberculosis chemotherapy, and the susceptibility of the tubercle bacilli he or she is harboring should be fully evaluated before starting treatment. After the susceptibility of the organism is known, it is important to prescribe at least three previously unused drugs to which the patient's strain of *M. tuberculosis* is susceptible. In this way the likelihood of selecting mutants resistant to the drugs in the new regimen is minimized. *A single drug should never be added to a failing regimen.*

B. ASSURANCE OF ADHERENCE[111-114]

A regimen is effective only if it is taken appropriately. If a patient takes only part of the drugs prescribed, either by taking a reduced (ineffective) dose or by omitting one or more drugs, there is danger of resistance emerging. Nonadherence is known to lead to treatment failure and to drug resistance. If a patient with a history of treatment failure associated with prior nonadherence is being considered for retreatment, it is unwise to add new drugs until the compliance issue is dealt with. If the patient does not follow the new regimen, the patient may destroy the potential effectiveness of the additional drugs and render himself or herself essentially untreatable. (For further discussion on adherence issues, please refer to Chapter 14.)

C. PREVENTION OF TUBERCULOUS DISEASE AMONG THOSE EXPOSED OR LIKELY TO BE EXPOSED TO A PATIENT WITH ACTIVE DRUG-RESISTANT TUBERCULOSIS

Early in the chemotherapy era, transmission of tuberculosis from a drug-resistant index case was questioned. More recently, evidence for such transmission of drug-resistant tuberculosis has been substantiated.[42,43,46,115-118]

1. Environmental Measures[119-121]

(See Chapter 3 for a discussion of environmental issues.)

2. BCG

Bacillus Calmette-Guérin (BCG) vaccine may be appropriate for tuberculin-negative contacts unavoidably exposed to a patient with multidrug-resistant tuberculosis. There is disagreement among experts regarding this approach.[122,123] (See Chapters 8 and 15.)

3. Preventive Chemotherapy[103,124]

(See Chapter 13 for a discussion of chemotherapeutic regimens.)

III. RECOGNITION AND EVALUATION

A. PERSONS AT RISK

Overall, in recent years the prevalence of drug resistance among patients with tuberculosis in the U.S. has been estimated at 8 to 14%.[33,54,55] Accordingly, drug resistance should be a consideration in any patient. However, drug resistance is distributed unevenly throughout the U.S. Large cities tend to have a high prevalence of drug resistance.[23,125-128] New York City[27,129-131] has an especially high prevalence. Certain groups of patients have a greater likelihood of harboring drug-resistant bacilli.

1. Previously Treated Patients[132-134]

In a survey of specimens from 30 large health departments in the U.S. (1982 to 1986), 23% of strains of *M. tuberculosis* from unselected, previously treated patients showed resistance to one or more drugs.[33] During 1993 to 1996, the overall prevalence of resistance to one or more drugs among previously treated patients was 22.4%, compared to 13% among patients with no history of prior tuberculosis. Resistance to isoniazid occurred in 17%, to rifampin in 8.6%, and to both isoniazid and rifampin in 6.9% of previously treated patients. This contrasts with resistance to isoniazid in 7.9%, to rifampin in 2.7%, and to both isoniazid and rifampin in 1.9% of those patients who had no prior history of tuberculosis.[55] Pockets with even higher prevalence of drug resistance have been reported. Drug resistance was found less frequently among those who responded to a good regimen initially and later relapsed[135] than among those who initially had a poor regimen and failed to respond.[136]

2. Patients on Therapy But Not Responding

Ordinarily, a person on a good antituberculosis regimen should have sputum smears negative for acid-fast bacilli 2 to 3 months after the initiation of therapy. If symptoms, such as fever, do not resolve in 2 weeks,[62] or if sputum conversion does not occur in 2 to 3 months, drug resistance should be suspected. (Also suspect nonadherence or poor absorption of medications.)[137,138]

3. Nonadherent Patients[139]

By taking only part of the prescribed therapy, drug-resistant bacilli can be selected for survival. However, if a patient is totally noncompliant and does not take any antituberculosis medicine, his tubercle bacilli will remain drug susceptible.

4. Patients with Conditions that Impair Delivery of Drugs to the Site of Infection

Patients who have undergone gastrectomy[140] or ileal bypass surgery may not absorb sufficient antituberculosis medications to cure their tuberculosis, but enough to select out drug-resistant mutants for survival. Patients with HIV infection may not absorb their medications well.[141]

Patients with tuberculosis involving extensively calcified pleura,[142,143] or very thick-walled cavities or heavily fibrotic areas, although absorbing their drugs properly, may have insufficient blood supply to the infected tissue site. The impaired circulation cannot deliver sufficient antimicrobial drugs to the infected tissue site to cure the tuberculosis. The extremely large number of organisms increases the likelihood of multidrug-resistant organisms. Also, variable penetration of antituberculosis medications may have the effect of monotherapy at the site of infection, thus selecting the resistant members of the bacterial population for survival.

5. Persons Likely to be in Contact with Drug-Resistant Patients

It is reasonable to infer that persons who have become infected with the tubercle bacillus during a time frame when they have been in contact with a contagious tuberculosis patient have acquired the same strain of *M. tuberculosis* as that patient. Recent studies have compared and contrasted certain features of the specific molecular structure of strains of tubercle bacilli, using techniques such as restriction fragment-length polymorphism (RFLP) analysis. These "genetic fingerprinting" techniques strongly support the inference of recent transmission of drug-resistant tuberculosis in cluster[69,144-146] and in community[53,147,148] situations.

a. Household Contacts

Household contacts who have converted to tuberculin positive while exposed to a patient with infectious drug-resistant tuberculosis can be expected to be infected with the same strain as the index case. If these contacts subsequently develop disease, it is likely to be drug resistant with a pattern comparable to that of the index case at the time of transmission of infection.

b. Homeless Persons[149] and Prisoners[42]

Homeless persons may have been present in a crowded, poorly ventilated shelter while a person with infectious drug-resistant disease was present in the facility. Prisoners similarly may have been exposed to drug-resistant tuberculosis in crowded, poorly ventilated facilities.

c. Persons in Medical Care Situations[40,42-48,121]

Persons in medical care situations may have been present when a patient with drug-resistant tuberculosis had contaminated the air. The diagnosis of tuberculosis may not have been suspected. Precautions for airborne infection may have been omitted, exposing healthcare staff and possibly other patients to viable, airborne tubercle bacilli.

6. Immunocompromised Patients[40,42-44,46-48,150,151]

See Chapters 6 and 13 for a discussion of immunocompromised patients. Patients infected with HIV, especially those with the acquired immunodeficiency syndrome (AIDS), are at very high risk of developing active tuberculous disease (rather than latent infection alone) when exposed to an infectious case of drug-susceptible or -resistant tuberculosis. Since the time course from infection to the development of active disease is short (months to a few years) in HIV-infected individuals, patterns of resistance are likely to reflect recent prevalence of drug resistance in the community where they were exposed.[152] Prevalence of drug resistance among HIV-infected individuals has been variable among reported surveys.[137,153] In one series, conducted on all cases of tuberculosis in selected communities in 1992 to 1994, the prevalence of resistance to at least one drug was 15% among HIV-infected patients in communities other than New York; 2.8% had resistance to both isoniazid and rifampin. Among HIV-infected patients in the New York City area, 37% had resistance to at least one drug; 19% had resistance to both isoniazid and rifampin. This compares to 19% single drug resistance and 6% isoniazid and rifampin resistance among persons in that area not known to be HIV infected.[152] In regions where there is a significant probability of exposure to drug-resistant tuberculosis, treatment should be started promptly using sufficient medications to cover for the possibility of both drug-susceptible and drug-resistant organisms. Drug-resistant disease requires appropriate, prompt, aggressive management in these immunosuppressed patients.[154] Drug susceptibility studies certainly should be done. When the results of the susceptibility studies are known, treatment can be modified.

Patients may have been infected with tuberculosis prior to having become infected with HIV. These individuals are at risk of developing tuberculosis disease at a rate of about 7 to 10% per year.[54] Whether the disease is drug resistant is primarily dependent upon the susceptibility of the organisms of the source case at the time of transmission of the infection. As with other patients, HIV-infected patients with active tuberculosis disease are at risk of acquiring drug resistance by taking an inadequate regimen, by failing to adhere to a good regimen, and by having inadequate tissue concentrations of all the prescribed drugs. Malabsorption has been reported to occur frequently in persons with AIDS.[141] Therapy with rifabutin to prevent *M. avium* disease in a patient with unrecognized active tuberculosis may inadvertently lead to rifampin cross resistance of the *M. tuberculosis*. For this reason and for other reasons only partially understood,[155] resistance to rifampin (without resistance to other drugs), occurs almost exclusively in patients infected with HIV. Because of severe impairment of the immune system, a patient with HIV infection is at risk of reinfection with a drug-susceptible or a drug-resistant strain of tubercle bacilli, even after having successfully completed antituberculosis chemotherapy.[69] Transmission of multidrug-resistant disease due to *Mycobacterium bovis* among HIV-infected patients also has been reported.[156,157]

7. Persons from Developing Nations or Nations with Inadequate Tuberculosis Control Programs[85,158-162]

In countries with very limited resources, it may not be possible to furnish adequate drugs on a regular, predictable basis to impoverished patients with tuberculosis. The infrastructure may be inadequate to deliver and monitor therapy. Policies for treating tuberculosis may not be based on assured administration of multiple effective drugs over a prolonged period of time. Therefore, patients may take only one drug at a time, or may receive drugs in inadequate combinations, or may receive medication irregularly. In some areas it is possible for patients to receive medicine for tuberculosis without a prescription, further promoting inadequate therapy and the emergence of drug resistance. (See Chapter 16 for discussion of international issues.)

B. History: Emphasis on Details of Prior Chemotherapy

The usual medical history should be taken. In addition, it is important to question the patient about any of the above mentioned risk factors, and to follow through on any leads by finding out more details. History should include surgical procedures and collapse therapy for tuberculosis. History of antituberculosis chemotherapy is of paramount importance. Obtaining details in complex cases may be difficult, especially if the patient has been under the care of multiple providers, in multiple localities. Frequently it is necessary to contact the previous providers in order to obtain as complete

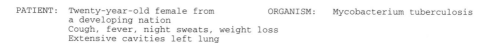

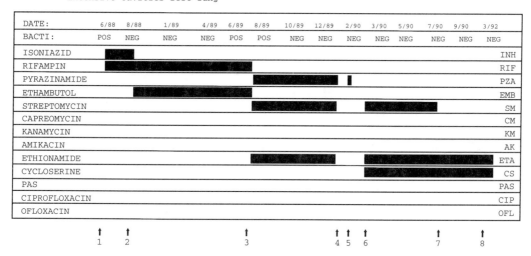

PATIENT: Twenty-year-old female from   ORGANISM: Mycobacterium tuberculosis
          a developing nation
          Cough, fever, night sweats, weight loss
          Extensive cavities left lung

DATE:	6/88	8/88	1/89	4/89	6/89	8/89	10/89	12/89	2/90	3/90	5/90	7/90	9/90	3/92	
BACTI:	POS	NEG	NEG	NEG	POS	POS	NEG	NEG	NEG	NEG	NEG	NEG	NEG	NEG	
ISONIAZID															INH
RIFAMPIN															RIF
PYRAZINAMIDE															PZA
ETHAMBUTOL															EMB
STREPTOMYCIN															SM
CAPREOMYCIN															CM
KANAMYCIN															KM
AMIKACIN															AK
ETHIONAMIDE															ETA
CYCLOSERINE															CS
PAS															PAS
CIPROFLOXACIN															CIP
OFLOXACIN															OFL

↑   ↑   ↑   ↑ ↑ ↑   ↑   ↑
1   2   3   4 5 6   7   8

1. INH and RIF started.   5. Challenge dose of PZA.
2. Pretreatment isolate reported resistant to INH;   6. SM, ETA, CS started.
   INH stopped; EMB started.   7. SM stopped.
3. Resistance to INH and RIF reported;   8. Therapy completed.
   RIF and EMB stopped; PZA, SM, ETA started.
4. Liver enzymes six times normal; all drugs stopped.

FIGURE 12.1 (Example 1) Patient with primary resistance to isoniazid was treated inappropriately with isoniazid and rifampin. Ethambutol was added as a single drug, inappropriately. Resistance to rifampin was acquired. Retreatment with pyrazinamide, streptomycin, and ethionamide was started. The bacilli were susceptible to these previously unused drugs. Liver function abnormalities developed; all drugs were stopped. Challenge with pyrazinamide was followed by liver function abnormalities. Streptomycin, ethionamide, and cycloserine were tolerated. Long-course chemotherapy was completed. (See Figure 12.3 for details of management of liver function abnormalities.) (From Friedman, L. N., Ed., *Tuberculosis: Current Concepts and Treatment,* 1st ed., CRC Press LLC, Boca Raton, FL, 1994. With permission.)

a history as possible. Patients may not be reliable in presenting their histories, possibly due to lack of information, forgetfulness, or embarrassment regarding poor adherence. A complete and accurate medication history is essential; prior use of an antituberculosis drug, especially if it was used ineffectively, can compromise its usefulness in the regimen being proposed. In retreatment of patients with multidrug-resistant tuberculosis, the use of three antituberculosis drugs that the patient had not received before was predictive of a favorable outcome.[35] Medication history should include:

1. Drugs received, with dosages and dates.
2. How the drugs were added: one at a time (favoring selection for resistance) or several simultaneously.
3. Adherence to therapy.
4. Adverse reactions to medications.
5. Response to therapy, including bacteriological response. In cases where the patient has received more than one regimen, effort should be made to determine the response to each regimen employed.
6. In complex cases, a flow sheet can organize the important aspects of the drug history into a manageable form, thus simplifying analysis and decision making. (Figures 12.1 and 12.2)

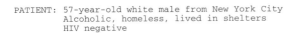

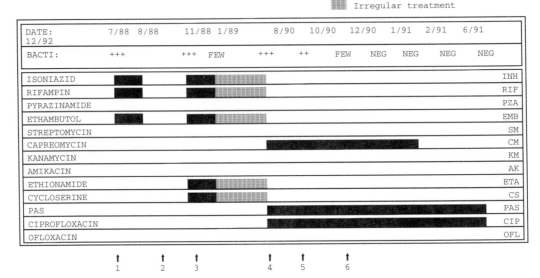

1. Cough, weight loss, RUL cavity.
2. Lost to follow-up.
3. Report on initial isolate: resistant INH, RIF, PZA, EMB, SM.
4. Cough, weight loss, RUL cavities-few nodules, resistant INH, RIF, PZA, EMB, SM, ETA, CS.
5. Cough improved, gained weight.
6. 12/19/90 right upper lobectomy.

FIGURE 12.2 (Example 2) Patient with multidrug resistance was treated with isoniazid, rifampin, and ethambutol. He was noncompliant. Retreatment with isoniazid, rifampin, ethambutol, ethionamide, and cycloserine was started; compliance was poor. Additional drug resistance was acquired. He was retreated with capreomycin, PAS, and ciprofloxacin under supervision. The bacilli in his sputum diminished. Adjunctive right upper lobectomy was followed by culture conversion to negative. Long-term supervised chemotherapy was continued for an additional 2 years. (From Friedman, L. N., Ed., *Tuberculosis: Current Concepts and Treatment,* 1st ed., CRC Press LLC, Boca Raton, FL, 1994. With permission.)

C. CLINICAL MANIFESTATIONS

Clinical manifestations of drug-resistant tuberculosis are the same as for drug-susceptible tuberculosis. However, patients with acquired drug-resistant tuberculosis may have more pulmonary parenchymal scarring because of the chronicity of their disease. This may be associated with respiratory impairment. Patients with tuberculosis not responding to therapy in the expected manner should be evaluated or reevaluated for drug resistance. As in drug-susceptible disease, extrapulmonary tuberculosis is common among patients with AIDS and drug-resistant disease.

D. SUSCEPTIBILITY STUDIES[163-165]

Susceptibility testing and history of prior chemotherapy have been cornerstones in the detection and management of drug-resistant tuberculosis (see Chapter 4). The ATS and CDC recommend that susceptibility studies be performed routinely on an isolate from every patient who has a positive culture.[109,110] Susceptibility studies should be done in a reliable laboratory. In the earlier years of the chemotherapy era, the clinical relevance of susceptibility testing and the criteria for resistance of tubercle bacilli to various antituberculosis medications were debated.[81,166] Nonuniformity of drug resistance of tubercle bacilli from patients with chronic tuberculosis has been recognized.[72,167] At the National Jewish Center, during the 1960s and 1970s, retreatment regimens for isoniazid-resistant tuberculosis were based on *in vitro* susceptibility of the organisms to the drugs in the individually tailored regimens prescribed. *In vitro* susceptibility to three drugs in a regimen was predictive of a favorable outcome.[21]

More recently, 134 previously treated cases of multidrug-resistant tuberculosis were reviewed at the National Jewish Center.[35] These patients were shedding tubercle bacilli resistant to an average of six drugs, including isoniazid and rifampin. Increasing numbers of drugs to which the bacilli were resistant was predictive of poor outcome. Surprisingly, *in vitro* susceptibility of the organisms to the drugs used in the new retreatment regimens was not necessarily predictive of outcome. The latter observation in this series of very complex cases is unexplained. This study does not negate the usefulness of *in vitro* susceptibility studies. However, it does indicate that the need persists for research in better methodology and in the application of the information obtained.

Where multidrug resistance is likely, isolates should be sent to a reference laboratory experienced in the testing of drugs that are used less commonly. Results of susceptibility studies serve as a guide for determining therapy for patients with newly diagnosed tuberculosis and for patients with long-standing disease. Methods of reporting may vary from one laboratory to another. If there is any uncertainty about the interpretation of the test results, it is essential to communicate with the laboratory performing the test or with their clinical consultants. Recently methods have been developed to identify drug resistance by genetic markers. For rifampin, mutations in the rpoβ gene correlate well with resistance to this drug.[75,168-170] The clinical usefulness of this technology for rapidly identifying rifampin-resistant strains is being explored.

IV. TREATMENT

Tuberculosis resistant to one or more drugs is treated with multiple other drugs to which the bacilli are susceptible.[21,171,172] If the patient has received prior medications for tuberculosis and the regimen has failed, the drugs employed in the failing regimen cannot be relied upon to have full efficacy.[173] The new regimen should contain at least three antituberculosis agents, especially in the early phase of therapy. Drugs and dosages are listed in Table 12.1 (see also Chapter 11). Although selection of a regimen of first-line drugs is desirable, the usefulness of these drugs in patients with drug-resistant disease is limited. They are the drugs to which the organisms are most likely to be resistant.

A. First-Line and Second-Line Drugs

The first-line drugs, also known as primary or standard drugs, are those recommended for the treatment of newly diagnosed tuberculosis. The drugs considered first line do not always remain the same and are related to the historical and geographic context. In the U.S. in the 1990s, they were the drugs applicable to short-course (6 to 9 months) chemotherapy. They include isoniazid and rifampin (the two most effective drugs), pyrazinamide, ethambutol, and streptomycin. In some developing nations, thiacetazone (an inexpensive drug not available in the U.S.) is used as a standard drug, along with isoniazid and streptomycin. The other antituberculosis medications are considered second line, secondary, or reserve drugs. They are used in cases of resistance or intolerance to the otherwise preferred first-line drugs.

In the 1960s, pyrazinamide was considered a second-line drug. It was used effectively during the entire course of therapy in patients being retreated, but was considered too hepatotoxic for routine use. Ethionamide, although effective, has always been a reserve drug because it is difficult to tolerate in therapeutic dosages. Cycloserine is another secondary drug; it is associated with frequent central nervous system toxicity and has a small window between the therapeutic and toxic dose. PAS was employed as a first-line drug in the 1950s and 1960s. Several formulations of PAS were available during that time. Because of frequent gastrointestinal side effects, and possibly lesser efficacy, PAS lost its position as a first-line drug when ethambutol and rifampin became available. Then PAS was used infrequently as a second-line drug; by 1990, any formulation of PAS became

TABLE 12.1
Drugs, Dosage, and Monitoring

Drugs[a]	Adult Dosage[b]	Monitoring/Comments[c]
Isoniazid	300–600 mg po daily	SGOT baseline and monthly; give with pyridoxine 50 mg daily if using larger dose
Rifampin[d]	600 mg po daily	SGOT and Bilirubin baseline and monthly; single dose on empty stomach (2 h before or after eating)
Ethambutol	25 mg/kg until culture negative; then 15 mg/kg po daily	Visual acuity and color vision baseline and monthly Question patient about visual symptoms
Pyrazinamide	30–40 mg/kg po daily	SGOT and uric acid baseline and monthly; may split dose initially to improve tolerance; then single daily dose
Fluoroquinolones (use one)		Antacids, sucralfate, calcium, iron, and zinc decrease absorption
Ofloxacin	400–800 mg po daily	
Ciprofloxacin	500–750 mg po daily	
Levofloxacin	500–750 mg po daily	
Sparfloxacin	400 mg po first day; then 200 mg po daily	May prolong QT-interval on ECG Photosensitivity common
Ethionamide	500–1000 mg po daily	SGOT baseline and monthly; may split dose or give at bedtime to improve tolerance
Cycloserine	500–1000 mg po daily	Serum drug levels weekly until stable; give with pyridoxine 50-200 mg daily
p-aminosalicylic acid (PAS)	6–12 g po daily	Take granules with acid juice, applesauce, or yogurt; may split dose to improve tolerance; SGOT baseline and monthly
Clofazimine	100–300 mg po daily	Efficacy unproven
Streptomycin, capreomycin, kanamycin, or amikacin[f]	15 mg/kg im[e] 5 days weekly until culture negative, then 3 days weekly	Creatinine, electrolytes, and audiometry baseline and at least monthly; observe for problems with balance; reduce dose and monitor serum drug concentrations in the elderly and in patients with impaired renal function

[a] Oral drugs are listed in the order of preference; use at least two oral drugs and one injectable drug that the patient has not received previously and to which the bacilli are susceptible.

[b] Dosages suggested for drug resistant tuberculosis may not apply to drug susceptible disease.

[c] On multidrug therapy, monitor complete blood count at baseline and every 1 to 3 months. For more complete information on side effects, see Chapter 11.

[d] Rifabutin may be substituted for rifampin if the organisms are susceptible. See Chapter 6. The usefulness of rifapentine in drug-resistant tuberculosis has yet to be investigated.

[e] Alternatively, capreomycin, kanamycin, or amikacin may be given 12 mg/kg by intravenous infusion 5 days weekly until culture negative, then 3 days weekly; check serum drug concentrations.

[f] Amikacin may be given by intravenous infusion 12 to 22 mg/kg twice weekly, with close monitoring, including serum drug concentrations.

Source: Adapted from Friedman, L. N., Ed., *Tuberculosis: Current Concepts and Treatment,* 1st ed., CRC Press LLC, Boca Raton, FL, 1994.

difficult to obtain in the U.S. More recently, a new, better tolerated formulation of PAS has become available in enteric-coated granule form and is being used as a second-line drug.

Among the drugs that must be given parenterally because of poor gastrointestinal absorption, capreomycin is approved for long-term use in tuberculosis. It has remained a second-line drug, used as a substitute for streptomycin. Kanamycin, although not officially approved for long-term use in tuberculosis, has been used effectively for several decades as a second-line drug in retreatment. Similarly, amikacin is being used as a secondary drug. One of these parenteral drugs usually is prescribed along with several oral drugs for the treatment of multidrug-resistant tuberculosis.

In the 1980s, fluoroquinolones became available. Several drugs in this group show good *in vitro* susceptibility[174] against *M. tuberculosis* as well as pharmacokinetic properties that suggest clinical usefulness in treating tuberculosis. Although no large, controlled clinical trials have been done using these drugs for treating patients with tuberculosis, uncontrolled clinical studies using ciprofloxacin or ofloxacin suggest their usefulness in multidrug regimens for drug resistant tuberculosis.[175-181] They have the advantage of being better tolerated than some of the other secondary drugs.[182] Levofloxacin, the *l*-isomer (the active component) of ofloxacin, recently has become available, and has the advantage of yielding higher serum drug concentrations than comparable doses of ofloxacin.[183] As more experience is gained using levofloxacin, it may become the quinolone of choice in treating drug-resistant tuberculosis.[179] Sparfloxacin, a long-acting new fluoroquinolone, appears highly effective *in vitro*,[184] but its use is limited by the occurrence of a prolonged QT-interval on the electrocardiogram and photosensitivity. Sparfloxacin in regimens for drug-resistant tuberculosis needs to be studied further. The quinolone antibiotics should not be used for the initial treatment of drug-susceptible tuberculosis. Rather, one of the medications from this group should be selected when designing multidrug regimens for drug-resistant tuberculosis.

Among the rifamycins, rifabutin has a profile of drug interactions different from rifampin. Rifabutin has the advantage of allowing greater bioavailability of some of the drugs given in HIV infection for conditions other than tuberculosis, but toxic levels of rifabutin may occur when used with certain antiretroviral drugs[151] (see also Chapters 6 and 11). Otherwise, rifabutin does not appear to have advantages over rifampin, except in occasional instances when rifabutin may be tolerated by patients who have had side effects to rifampin. Reports of the clinical efficacy of rifabutin have been conflicting.[185-190] Rifapentine has the advantage of long duration of action and, hence, infrequent dosing.[191] Its role in the treatment of tuberculosis has yet to be worked out. Rifabutin or rifapentine are potentially useful for drug-resistant tuberculosis that is not rifampin resistant. Unfortunately, since these drugs show significant cross resistance with rifampin, they may not be useful in rifampin-resistant disease.[92,93]

B. PROGRAM APPROACH

1. Situations Suitable for a Program Approach

In regions where the prevalence of drug resistance is high, it may be advisable to treat all newly diagnosed tuberculosis patients with a regimen designed to be effective against both drug-susceptible and drug-resistant tubercle bacilli. This presupposes knowledge of the susceptibility patterns of the tuberculosis cases in the community. It is essential to survey for drug resistance periodically. It also is important to know which regimen or regimens have been used commonly in the community, and what the treatment practices have been.[105] Resistance is likely to be directed against drugs used in the community, especially if the drugs have been employed in inadequate or unsupervised regimens.

By administering a regimen likely to be effective against both drug-susceptible and drug-resistant disease, the patient can be spared the wait for the results of susceptibility studies before starting effective therapy.[173] Immediate initiation of empirical therapy is especially important in patients with immunodeficiency and in patients who are ill with rapidly progressive tuberculosis.[154]

2. Examples

In localities where isoniazid and streptomycin resistance is prevalent, a reasonable approach is to begin all patients on a regimen of isoniazid, rifampin, ethambutol, and pyrazinamide.[192] This is excellent therapy for patients with drug-susceptible disease. If susceptibility of the patient's bacilli is documented, ethambutol is stopped; after 2 months of therapy pyrazinamide is stopped and the patient continues to receive isoniazid and rifampin to complete 6 months. The four-drug regimen also provides good therapy for patients with isoniazid- and/or streptomycin-resistant bacilli. When the laboratory studies document resistance to isoniazid (with or without resistance to streptomycin) but susceptibility to rifampin and ethambutol, isoniazid can be stopped; pyrazinamide can be stopped after 2 months of therapy. Rifampin and ethambutol should be continued to complete at least 12 months either daily or intermittently.

Short-course and intermittent regimens, using various combinations of the primary drugs, have yielded varying results.[193-200] Excellent results have been reported[198] with short-course regimens involving the use of isoniazid, rifampin, pyrazinamide, plus either ethambutol or streptomycin, for the full 6-month period. The drugs were given either daily or three times weekly for tuberculosis, including disease resistant to isoniazid and/or streptomycin. Although the latter drugs were included in the study, they probably did not contribute to the efficacy of the regimens when resistance to them was present. These short-course regimens are applicable if the patient has received no prior therapy with rifampin nor pyrazinamide nor a third drug in the regimen, and the tubercle bacilli from the patient are fully susceptible to these drugs. Other regimens for drug-resistant tuberculosis, not consisting exclusively of first-line drugs, must be given daily for longer periods (see Duration of Therapy — IV,C,3, this chapter). For dosages of drugs used in intermittent regimens, see Chapter 6.

In sections of New York City,[154] outbreaks of tuberculosis resistant to isoniazid, rifampin, ethambutol, pyrazinamide, streptomycin, and ethionamide have been reported. Initial treatment regimens employing six drugs may be appropriate, aiming to provide adequate antimicrobial coverage while awaiting the results of susceptibility studies on the patient's organisms. A regimen of isoniazid, rifampin, pyrazinamide, capreomycin, ciprofloxacin, and cycloserine has been proposed. The first three drugs give excellent coverage if the patient has a drug-susceptible strain; the latter three provide coverage for anticipated drug resistance. When the susceptibility studies have been reported, the regimen is adjusted appropriately. The potential for toxicity of such a regimen is high. However, the patient is likely to be spared the risk of acquiring resistance to additional drugs resulting from inadequate therapy during the waiting period.

C. INDIVIDUALLY TAILORED APPROACH[21,173,201-205]

A standard regimen, or "program approach," is not applicable to all situations. Many patients require a regimen tailored to their particular circumstances.

1. Selection of Drugs

Patients who already have undergone several courses of therapy and have been exposed to multiple antituberculosis medications, require individually prescribed regimens. These regimens should contain at least three[8,12,17,18] previously unused drugs to which the tubercle bacilli are susceptible. Currently, the trend is toward using four effective drugs, especially if isoniazid or rifampin are not included in the regimen. Thorough evaluation is essential (as described in the previous section). Frequently these patients are chronically ill, but generally do not have acute or urgent illness. Thus, the benefit accrued by deferring treatment to obtain the necessary information upon which to base rational therapy, (i.e., a detailed drug history and full susceptibility studies) outweighs the potential risk of waiting. There are relatively few drugs effective against *M. tuberculosis*. Drug resistance and suboptimal prior use will have rendered some drugs ineffective against the patient's bacilli, so choices are limited. If any primary drug has not been used previously and shows *in vitro* susceptibility, that drug should be included in the regimen, barring a contraindication. The newly introduced quinolone antibiotics, if not given to the patient previously, usually inhibit *M. tuberculosis*. Since these drugs are potentially effective and usually are well tolerated,[182] one of these drugs, such as ofloxacin, generally should be included in regimens for tuberculosis resistant to multiple other drugs. The oral drugs remaining may be unpleasant to take and may be less effective than the primary drugs. Frequently, selection must be made from among these. An injectable drug usually is included in the regimen. Options for effective therapy are limited. These patients cannot afford another experience of treatment failure.

Sometimes a patient will have received adequately selected medications for a brief time, the drugs having been stopped simultaneously, but prematurely, at a time when the drug regimen was working. In such cases, a short duration of prior therapy correlates with continuing *in vitro* susceptibility and continuing clinical efficacy of the drugs so used.[135] However, if previously used drugs were employed in a regimen that was failing or in which the drugs had been added in inadequate combinations, those drugs cannot be depended upon for efficacy, despite *in vitro* susceptibility.[206] Sometimes physicians have included isoniazid in a regimen where susceptibility tests have shown resistance to low concentrations, but sensitivity to higher concentrations of this drug. Impairment of efficacy is similar with low levels or high levels of resistance.[166] If any degree of resistance to isoniazid is found, isoniazid cannot be depended on as a major effective drug in the regimen.

Patient factors, such as preexisting medical conditions that may predispose to side effects, should be considered where possible in selecting specific drugs for the new retreatment regimen. For instance, patients with gastrointestinal problems are likely to have problems tolerating ethionamide; patients with prior hearing loss may develop significantly impaired hearing when treated with an aminoglycoside. Where possible, it is preferable to avoid drugs to which the patient is particularly likely to react, provided other drugs are capable of controlling the tuberculosis. The antituberculosis drugs currently available, along with their potential side effects are discussed in Chapter 11.

2. Examples

Example 1. (Figure 12.1): A 20-year-old woman from a developing nation had been treated (inappropriately) with isoniazid and rifampin for cavitary tuberculosis. (Primary) isoniazid resistance of the initial isolate was reported belatedly and ethambutol was added as a single new drug (inappropriately). After a short period of improvement, including conversion to negative cultures, positive cultures again were reported (the fall and rise phenomenon), this time with resistance to both isoniazid and rifampin. The patient was referred for retreatment. At that time, options among the oral drugs were pyrazinamide, ethionamide, cycloserine, and PAS; ethambutol was not considered a good option since it had been in use in a regimen that was ultimately failing. All of the injectable drugs were potentially effective. Streptomycin was chosen since it had not been used before, is slightly more effective, and was less expensive than the other parenteral drugs. Pyrazinamide and ethionamide were chosen because of slight superiority compared to the other available oral drugs; they were likely to be tolerated by this young patient. The regimen of streptomycin, pyrazinamide, and ethionamide was effective. The patient's sputum cultures converted to negative.

However, the patient developed liver function abnormalities during therapy (see Section V.B.1 and Figure 12.3). Either pyrazinamide or ethionamide could have caused the problem. All medications were stopped until the liver function tests stabilized at normal values. Pyrazinamide challenge resulted in elevation of liver enzymes. Another drug had to be substituted for pyrazinamide. Available options were cycloserine and PAS. Because of the potential of PAS for producing gastrointestinal side effects that might enhance the gastrointestinal side effects of ethionamide, PAS seemed undesirable. Cycloserine was chosen and was introduced with streptomycin uneventfully. The replacement of pyrazinamide with a single drug was appropriate in this case in which the patient's disease was responding to therapy. This is not the same as adding a single drug to a *failing* regimen. Small doses of ethionamide produced no abnormalities in the liver function tests. Therefore, the patient received a full dosage of ethionamide along with cycloserine and streptomycin. The oral drugs were continued for an additional 2 years. Streptomycin was stopped after 5 months on the revised regimen. The patient continued to have negative cultures.

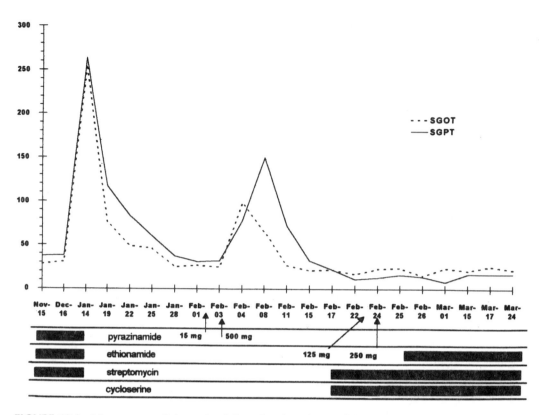

FIGURE 12.3 Management of drug-related liver function abnormalities. The patient had been receiving pyrazinamide, ethionamide, and streptomycin. After 4 months of therapy, the SGOT (AST) rose to 6 times the upper limit of normal (normal, 8 to 40). Either pyrazinamide or ethionamide could have produced the abnormality. All drugs were stopped. Liver function tests returned to normal gradually. The patient was rechallenged with pyrazinamide, 15 mg, with no change in SGOT or SGPT (ALT). The next day, she was rechallenged with pyrazinamide 500 mg, followed by elevation of the serum enzymes. Medications were withheld until the enzymes became normal. Streptomycin and cycloserine were introduced without problem. Ethionamide 125 mg; then, the next day, 250 mg was given with no increase in the enzymes. The full dosage of ethionamide was tolerated, along with streptomycin and cycloserine. (See also Figure 12.1 and Section IV.C.2.) (From Friedman, L. N., Ed., *Tuberculosis: Current Concepts and Treatment,* 1st ed., CRC Press LLC, Boca Raton, FL, 1994. With permission.)

Example 2 (Figure 12.2): A 57-year-old homeless alcoholic man from New York City had been started on what appeared to be a reasonable regimen of isoniazid, rifampin, and ethambutol for extensive cavitary tuberculosis. His initial isolate later was reported to be resistant to isoniazid, rifampin, pyrazinamide, ethambutol, and streptomycin. Two new drugs, ethionamide and cyclos-erine, were added to the regimen. This might have salvaged the situation if the bacterial count had been low and if the patient had cooperated with therapy. The patient took his treatment irregularly and developed resistance to these drugs as well. He was referred for retreatment with tubercle bacilli resistant to isoniazid, rifampin, pyrazinamide, ethambutol, streptomycin, ethionamide, and cycloserine. Among the oral drugs, the only choices for a new effective regimen were PAS and ciprofloxacin or ofloxacin. Among the injectable antibiotics, capreomycin, kanamycin, and amikacin were potentially effective. Capreomycin was chosen because of its lesser toxicity; it was given in combination with PAS and ciprofloxacin. This was believed to be a weak regimen for a patient with extensive disease, but no further medical options were available. Since the tuberculosis was fairly well localized, the option of adjunctive pulmonary resection was pursued. At the time of surgery, sputum smears were negative and few tubercle bacilli were present on sputum cultures.

The right upper lobe was resected without complications. All smears and cultures were negative postoperatively. Therapy with multiple drugs was continued for 2 years beyond culture conversion.

3. Duration of Therapy

Regimens based on drugs other than rifampin must be given for prolonged periods. In cases of rifampin resistance with isoniazid susceptibility, isoniazid and ethambutol (with streptomycin for the first 1 to 3 months) should be continued to complete 18 months. When resistance to both isoniazid and rifampin is present, at least two drugs should be continued for 2 years beyond culture conversion. The third drug, usually an injectable drug, is stopped 4 to 6 months after the first of a series of negative cultures. The date of culture conversion is suggested as a marker for timing the duration of treatment so that patients with slow responses (probably associated with more refractory disease) will be given longer courses of therapy. Patients with acquired drug resistance already have demonstrated their ability to fail to respond to treatment, or to respond and later relapse. Giving them a prolonged course of therapy seems prudent. Studies done before the availability of rifampin suggest that 18 to 24 months of chemotherapy was associated with lower relapse rates than shorter regimens.[133,207,208] Accordingly, patients who, because of drug resistance, cannot benefit from rifampin require prolonged therapy. A possible exception to this is a regimen of streptomycin, pyrazinamide, and isoniazid given daily or 3 times weekly for 9 months. Under study conditions this 9-month regimen was effective against drug-susceptible tuberculosis.[209] Since rifampin was not included in the regimen, one might infer that the regimen would be effective against tuberculosis resistant to rifampin but susceptible to the other drugs.

D. MULTIDRUG-RESISTANT TUBERCULOSIS[1,210]

At the National Jewish Center, the current practice is to tailor regimens based on a history of no prior use of a given drug, along with full *in vitro* susceptibility to that drug.[202] A recent review[35] of 134 patients who had *M. tuberculosis* resistant to a median of six drugs, including isoniazid and rifampin, and who previously had received a median of six drugs showed a favorable response in 65%. Twelve of the patients who responded subsequently relapsed, making the overall response rate 56%. These patients were treated in the era before AIDS had become a widespread problem. They received a median of four drugs in their new regimens. Many of these patients did not have an ideal regimen available to them. Employing more than three drugs when the selected drugs did not appear to have promise of maximal efficacy may have salvaged some patients; however, the results were not as good as those achieved when three optimal antituberculosis drugs were available. Some patients did not have two potentially effective oral drugs for their regimens. Two injectable medications (usually kanamycin and capreomycin) and one oral antituberculosis drug were given. Limited (unpublished) data suggests that, although toxicity was not doubled, efficacy was diminished when compared to regimens employing one injectable and two oral drugs. At another institution, medical treatment of patients resistant to multiple drugs, including isoniazid and rifampin, was effective for 34 of 102 patients.[211] In both of these series, adjunctive surgery salvaged a few additional patients. In subsequent years, one of the quinolones often was used as an additional drug in regimens, and surgical resection was used more frequently. A comparable group of 109 patients at the National Jewish Center had an overall cure rate of 85%. Among the 47 patients who had only medical treatment, 64% converted to negative. Among the 62 patients treated with medical therapy plus surgical resection, 95% became culture negative.[36] Other series of patients likewise have responded favorably to intensive medical and sometimes surgical therapy.[61,62,212]

Because of the possibility of ruining the patient's last chance for effective therapy, multiple-drug regimens containing every known drug with potential effectiveness against a patient's multi-drug-resistant bacilli sometimes are prescribed. The aggressive approach of treating tuberculosis resistant to multiple drugs with four or more effective drugs including a quinolone, although not based on controlled clinical trials, appears superior to the historical comparison with regimens based on three effective drugs. Caution is necessary in making these comparisons; however, since, in some instances, the cases being treated were very different in the extent of drug resistance, the extent and complexity of disease, and in prior exposure to antituberculosis drugs.[213,214]

E. PATIENTS INFECTED WITH HIV[151]

Patients with immune deficiency and drug-resistant disease, including those with AIDS, are treated with multiple drug therapy in a manner similar to patients with drug-resistant disease and a normal immune system. Starting therapy immediately upon suspicion of drug-resistant tuberculosis is critical. The CDC recommends the following,[151] all to be given under careful supervision and management:

- For patients with tuberculosis disease resistant to isoniazid only, a regimen of rifampin (or rifabutin), pyrazinamide, and ethambutol for the duration of treatment. These drugs can be given daily throughout, or daily for at least the first 14 doses, then twice weekly to complete therapy. Treatment should be continued for a minimum of 6 months, or 4 months after culture conversion.
- For patients with tuberculosis disease resistant to rifampin only, a 9-month regimen, with isoniazid, streptomycin, pyrazinamide, and ethambutol for the first 2 months. (These drugs should be given daily for at least 2 weeks, after which they may be given either daily or 2 to 3 times weekly.) After this intensive phase of treatment, isoniazid, strepto-mycin, and pyrazinamide should be given 2 to 3 times weekly for an additional 7 months.
- For patients with multidrug-resistant tuberculosis disease, management should be by or in consultation with physicians experienced in the management of MDR-TB. Early aggressive treatment with appropriate regimens decreases deaths associated with MDR-TB.[151] The multiple drug regimens, based on known or suspected drug-resistance patterns, usually include an aminoglycoside (e.g., streptomycin, kanamycin, or amikacin) or capreomycin, and a fluoroquinolone, along with other appropriate drugs. Monitoring of serum drug concentrations may be helpful in managing these patients. Treatment should be continued for 24 months after culture conversion, and post-treatment follow-up visits to monitor for tuberculosis relapse should be conducted every 4 months for 24 months. Directly observed therapy should always be used, plus whatever enhancements are needed to assure that these patients adhere to therapy.

F. EXTRAPULMONARY TUBERCULOSIS

Experience in managing drug-resistant extrapulmonary tuberculosis is limited. Because bacterial counts are low in most extrapulmonary sites, spontaneous mutation of bacilli to resistance and subsequent selection of these resistant bacilli for survival is unlikely. Thus, acquired resistance in extrapulmonary tuberculosis has not been a major problem. However, in recent years, primary drug resistance in extrapulmonary tuberculosis has increased, due to the fact that immunocompromised patients, including those infected with a drug-resistant strain of *M. tuberculosis*, have a high incidence of extrapulmonary disease. When the infecting bacilli are drug resistant, the bacilli in the extrapulmonary site of tuberculosis are drug resistant. Treatment is recommended with regimens selected in the same manner as for drug-resistant pulmonary tuberculosis. Specific studies on the treatment of drug-resistant extrapulmonary tuberculosis are needed. For management of problems related to site of infection, see Chapter 7.

G. OTHER MEDICATIONS[179] AND THERAPEUTIC APPROACHES

In recent years, the fluoroquinolones[180,181] (ciprofloxacin, ofloxacin, levofloxacin, and sparfloxacin) and the new rifamycins (rifabutin and rifapentine) have been added to the therapeutic armamen-tarium against tuberculosis.[179] (See also Chapter 11.)

Clofazimine,[215] a drug employed extensively in treating leprosy, has been used in the management patients with multidrug-resistant tuberculosis for whom therapeutic options were limited. Since many variables and adverse factors were present in this group of patients, the independent effect of this drug was impossible to determine. Clofazimine certainly was not outstanding in its efficacy against *M. tuberculosis* in these clinical situations despite favorable *in vitro* susceptibility. Its role in the treatment of tuberculosis has yet to be determined.

The macrolides, such as clarithromycin, generally do not show favorable *in vitro* susceptibility against *M. tuberculosis*, but appear to show *in vitro* synergy with other antituberculosis drugs;[216] the clinical significance of this is unknown. The macrolides are effective against certain other mycobacteria, such as *M. avium*. β-lactams, such as amoxacillin/clavulanate have been used anecdotally.[217] Metronidazole,[218] which is believed to affect organisms under anaerobic conditions, is being investigated with the hope of preventing tubercle bacilli in the latent phase from becoming active. "Nonantibiotics," such as phenothiazines, are being studied for synergistic antimicrobial activity with conventional antimicrobials.[219]

Better understanding of the biochemical structure of the tubercle bacillus should facilitate the design of targeted new drugs.[220] With the sequencing of the genome of *M. tuberculosis*,[66,67] it is anticipated that design of new therapies will be enhanced further. In recent years, pharmaceutical companies have shown interest in cooperating with other researchers in the development of new forms of therapy for tuberculosis.

Immunologic modulation of the host is being explored. γ-interferon has been tried in patients with a poor chance of recovery by more conventional means; preliminary results have been encouraging.[221] Interleukin-2 also has been employed with equivocal results.[222] *M. vaccae* has been used in the treatment of drug-resistant tuberculosis with some encouraging results.[223] These forms of therapy are investigational at this time and need further validation. New vaccines against tuberculosis are being investigated[224] (see Chapter 15).

Collapse therapy for cavitary disease was used in the prechemotherapy era with the hope of depriving the tubercle bacilli of oxygen by flattening cavities, and kinking the bronchi to prevent endobronchial spread of bacilli. This form of therapy included therapeutic pneumoperitoneum, which was revisited at the National Jewish Center for a brief time recently for a few patients with poor therapeutic options. It did not appear helpful in this group of patients with chronic cavitary disease. Their lesions probably were too fibrotic to permit collapse of cavities by indirect pressure from air injected into the abdominal cavity.[225] Collapse therapy by plombage (insertion of a foreign substance into the thorax, outside the parietal pleura) has been tried (unsuccessfully) in a few patients in recent decades. Historically, it has been associated with foreign body complications. Resectional surgery, however, shows promise for many selected patients with drug-resistant tuberculosis[36,226] (see Section VI: Surgery).

H. Children and Pregnant Women

See Chapter 8 for a discussion of tuberculosis in children and pregnant women.

I. Monitoring

1. Adherence to Therapy

It is basic that medication, no matter how carefully prescribed, will not work unless it is taken. Some patients do not take their medicine, and it is not always easy to determine which patients are not adherent. Therefore, supervision of medication ingestion is part of treating these patients who have so much to lose if their course of treatment fails. Even in the hospital, it is necessary for nurses to watch the patients swallow their pills, rather than leave the medications by the bedside and assume that the patient will take them. When hospitalized patients approach the time of anticipated discharge, rather than being served their pills, they can come to the nurses' station and request their medication, which is taken under observation, similar to what will be done in the outpatient setting. Also, in anticipation of hospital discharge, medications which had been given in split dosages in order to improve tolerance, may be given in a single daily dose, if possible, thus facilitating directly observed therapy as outpatients. Arrangement for assured administration of medication, both in the hospital and in the outpatient setting, is an essential ingredient in the management of patients with drug-resistant tuberculosis, many of whom will have no alternative treatment if their current regimen fails. See Chapter 14 for a full discussion of adherence issues.

2. Efficacy

A favorable response of patients, especially complex multidrug-resistant cases, to regimens for drug-resistant tuberculosis is less predictable than the response of drug-susceptible cases to appropriate therapy. Therefore, careful monitoring of response is appropriate. The antituberculosis regimen, ancillary treatments, potential and observed benefits of the therapeutic approach, vs. the risks entailed, should be reassessed carefully and frequently during the course of therapy. If a change in the antituberculosis regimen or in the therapeutic approach is considered, consultation with experts in the field is strongly advised before making such a change.

a. Reversal of Infectiousness

It is unwise to assume that a patient with drug-resistant tuberculosis is noninfectious because he or she has received a given duration of therapy, such as 2 weeks. Reversal of infectiousness must be documented by sputum smears and cultures. The consequences of exposure to a patient with drug-resistant tuberculosis must be considered (see also Chapter 3).

A suggested schedule for obtaining bacteriology is as follows:

1. Sputum smear and culture every 2 weeks until three consecutively negative cultures have been documented.
2. Sputum smear and culture every 2 months for the next 2 years.
3. Sputum smear and culture twice yearly for the following 2 years.
4. Bacteriology should be reevaluated if the patient has symptoms suggestive of active tuberculosis.

A patient with a positive sputum smear should be considered potentially infectious and kept in isolation. A patient with drug-resistant pulmonary tuberculosis is likely to represent minimal risk of contagion when he or she no longer is coughing and has two or three consecutively negative sputum smears. However, a series of two or three *cultures* with a final report of negative should be the criterion for release from restriction of contact. While awaiting documentation of culture conversion, the patient should avoid close contact with other persons in enclosed poorly ventilated places. He or she should not have any contact with infants or immunocompromised patients, who are particularly susceptible to tuberculosis and are at increased risk of developing very serious forms of tuberculosis.

Culture conversion occurs an average of 2 months[21] after the initiation of therapy when patients are on good regimens for drug-resistant tuberculosis. If a patient continues to have positive smears or cultures more than 3 months after starting a new regimen, the efficacy of the regimen should be questioned; treatment may be failing with the emergence of resistance to additional drugs. The patient should be reevaluated. Adherence with the regimen must be reassessed; drug dosages and timing, serum drug levels,[138] and possible drug interactions should be checked. Susceptibility studies should be done on a current specimen.

b. Chest X-rays

Chest X-rays, although important, are not reliable indicators of treatment failure or relapse.

c. Clinical Response

As in drug-susceptible tuberculosis, clinical response in drug-resistant tuberculosis frequently is observed long before bacteriological control of the disease has been accomplished. Symptoms such as cough, fever, and night sweats tend to respond to effective treatment for drug-resistant tuberculosis. However, side effects of the medications may prevent weight gain and an improved feeling of well being.

3. Serum Drug Concentrations[227,228]

Strict attention must be paid to accurate documentation of times of dosing and times of blood drawings. If other medications interfere with the assay, these should be omitted for a sufficient time to avoid this confounding factor. The measurement of serum drug concentrations should be performed by a laboratory with sufficient experience and quality control in the techniques. The physician should consult with the laboratory regarding the optimal time to draw blood levels, so that the results will be interpretable. Consultation regarding pharmacokinetic data can maximize the benefits of the proper study of serum drug levels. These services are most likely to be available at referral centers specializing in the management of drug-resistant tuberculosis.

Monitoring of serum drug concentrations is especially indicated in the following circumstances:

1. Patients with acquired immune deficiency, since they may not absorb their medications properly.[141]
2. Patients with gastrointestinal problems that may impair absorption, such as prior gastrectomy or ileal bypass.
3. Patients taking other medications that can affect antituberculosis drug metabolism.
4. Patients with reduced renal clearance (trough levels of drugs cleared by the kidneys are especially important).
5. Patients who have not improved on a regimen that should have been effective, despite documented adherence.
6. Cycloserine use: a drug with a narrow therapeutic window between effective and toxic doses.

4. Side Effects

Side effects (see also Chapter 11) are likely to occur from the medications used for treatment of tuberculosis that is resistant to the more commonly used drugs.[21,229-232] Therefore, clinical and laboratory monitoring should be done systematically and should include baseline tests before starting therapy and generally monthly testing during therapy. Testing should be in keeping with the anticipated adverse effects of the drugs employed (see Chapter 11 and Table 12.1 of this chapter). Frequent observation of the patient is essential.

V. MANAGEMENT OF ADVERSE DRUG EFFECTS

(See Chapter 11 for additional discussion of adverse effects of antituberculosis drugs.)

A. FACTORS TO CONSIDER

1. Type and Seriousness of the Reaction

If the reaction is life threatening, the offending drug must be discontinued. If it is unclear which drug in the regimen is responsible for the life-threatening reaction, all drugs must be stopped. Reactions that are uncomfortable or even damaging may not warrant stopping of medication when put into the context of the whole clinical situation.

2. Seriousness of the Patient's Illness

The seriousness of the patient's illness and its implications for the life and the long-term quality of life (including long-term isolation of the patient if the tuberculosis is not controlled) must be balanced against the seriousness of the adverse effects of the medications.

3. Timing

The time when the adverse effects of medications occur may influence the way the reaction is managed. Modifying therapy by stopping one or more drugs, either temporarily or permanently, is likely to have a more dire effect on the outcome if done early in the course of a regimen when the bacterial count is high.

4. Options for Replacement Therapy

In multidrug-resistant tuberculosis, few drugs are useful for a given patient. Some drugs have become ineffective due to drug resistance. If a drug is lost because of side effects, therapeutic options are limited further. Accordingly, the continuation of medications in the face of side effects that would be entirely unacceptable under more favorable circumstances may be justified where there are no reasonable, effective alternatives.

5. Remaining Regimen

When a medication must be stopped, one must look at the remaining regimen. The altered regimen may not contain sufficient drugs to control the infection and to protect against the development of further drug resistance. It may be preferable to stop all medications pending the introduction of a new regimen.

B. SPECIFIC PROBLEMS

For problems related to the first-line drugs, see Chapter 11.

1. Liver Toxicity

Liver function abnormalities are detected by performing blood tests of liver function regularly (generally monthly) and repeating these tests if symptoms of hepatitis develop. Clinically significant elevations of serum transaminase may occur with or without symptoms when the patient has been receiving either pyrazinamide or ethionamide. If the routine monthly SGOT (AST) is more than twice the upper limit of normal, weekly rather than monthly rechecks are advised. SGPT (ALT) and the bilirubin also should be tested. Other causes of liver function abnormalities should be evaluated. It may be possible to continue the potentially hepatotoxic medications, with close monitoring, if the enzyme levels in the serum stabilize at less than three times the upper limit of normal. If the serum enzymes continue to rise, all hepatotoxic medications must be stopped when the SGOT reaches five times the upper limit of normal. Usually, at this level, the bilirubin is not elevated.

Frequently, where pyrazinamide or ethionamide toxicity occurs, the SGOT and SGPT continue to rise for a week or two (sometimes more) despite removing all hepatotoxic agents from the regimen. Then the serum enzymes gradually come down over a course of weeks. The enzymes may take months to return to normal if the elevation is severe. As the serum enzymes approach normal, sometimes they vacillate for a time, before stabilizing at normal levels. If the bilirubin becomes elevated, it is likely to normalize before the enzymes. Although some physicians use alkaline phosphatase and GGT levels as a guide to toxicity, this author has found them elevated in many patients with drug-resistant tuberculosis without other signs suggestive of drug-induced liver toxicity (see also Section V,C).

When multiple potentially hepatotoxic drugs are in a regimen, the above and the following clinical observations may be helpful in sorting out which drug may have been responsible; Isoniazid-induced liver toxicity generally involves elevation of the hepatic enzymes. When isoniazid is stopped, the enzymes are likely to return to normal within a few days. Rifampin-induced liver toxicity is likely to affect the serum bilirubin before the hepatic enzymes increase to a significant degree. Return of liver function abnormalities to normal generally occurs within a few days after stopping the rifampin.

2. Renal Toxicity

Kidney function abnormalities can develop when the aminoglycosides (amikacin, kanamycin, and streptomycin) or the polypeptide antibiotic, capreomycin, are used. Renal dysfunction frequently is manifested by a gradual increase in the serum creatinine without accompanying symptoms. When a progressive decrease in renal function occurs, the potential benefit of the drug, as opposed to the risk it is presenting, must be reevaluated. Premature discontinuation of the drug may be the only reasonable option. However, the severity of the tuberculosis, the time of occurrence of the toxicity, and the absence of other therapeutic options may suggest that continuing the offending drug is in the best interest of the patient. Cautious modification of dosing and close monitoring of serum drug levels and creatinine may allow continuation of the injectable medication without posing an unacceptable risk.

3. Severe Central Nervous System Toxicity

Psychosis, severe depression, or convulsions associated with cycloserine mandates discontinuation of this drug. These side effects usually are associated with excessive serum levels of cycloserine. Blood for serum drug levels should be drawn at the time of the reaction. Generally, cycloserine should not be reintroduced after a severe reaction. Pyridoxine should always be given with cycloserine[233] to decrease the likelihood of serious side effects. Quinolones also may cause central nervous system toxicity. Concurrent use of cycloserine and a quinolone may increase the likelihood of central nervous system toxicity.

4. Severe Allergic Reactions

In cases of anaphylaxis, severe skin rashes, or suspected drug fever, the offending drug must be stopped. Because of uncertainty about which drug caused the problem, all medications may need to be stopped. The patient must be treated for the immediate problem, such as giving epinephrine for anaphylaxis or antihistamines for pruritic symptoms. Corticosteroids sometimes are necessary to save the life of the patient or to prevent undue morbidity; however, since they may exacerbate uncontrolled infection, their use should be avoided if possible. The risk-benefit ratio always must be considered with as much certainty as possible.

5. Toxicity to the Eighth Cranial Nerve

Eighth cranial nerve toxicity from amikacin, kanamycin, streptomycin, or capreomycin is not fatal but is likely to be permanent.

a. Vestibular

Damage to the vestibular branch may occur with or without damage to the auditory branch, and damage to the auditory branch may or may not be associated with vestibular damage. If a patient on aminoglycosides or capreomycin experiences slight balance disturbance or vertigo shortly after the injection, the experience may be transient and benign. However, caution is advised, since these minor symptoms may be the prodrome of a more serious and permanent vestibular abnormality.

The patient may not be willing to endure vertigo or impairment of mobility, even in the face of serious tuberculosis, thus demanding the decision to stop the offending agent, possibly prematurely. If a patient does develop significant balance disturbance, physical therapy may help the patient to compensate.

b. Auditory

Auditory damage generally comes on gradually, involves the high frequencies initially, and, with time, gradually affects the frequencies related to understanding speech. When the routine audiogram shows high frequency loss, the patient may be asymptomatic, or may have a feeling of fullness in the ears, or may experience tinnitus. If the offending medication is stopped at this point, chances are the damage will remain at that level, but slight improvement may follow. The damage is likely to progress and persist if the offending drug is continued. Worsening after stopping the offending drug has been reported, but this is unusual. Patients vary in the sensitivity of their eighth nerves to the adverse effects of medications. Occasional patients experience rapid hearing loss or rapid loss of vestibular function on minimal doses of aminoglycosides. More commonly, with the dosing schedule used in treating tuberculosis, the problem progresses gradually over the course of months.

In dealing with patients suffering hearing loss from their medication, it is important to be straightforward with the patient concerning the potential for permanent damage. Also, the patient must understand the importance of the toxic medicine in the long-term control of his or her tuberculosis. A patient may survive with hearing impairment (although with curtailment in quality of life). However, the tuberculosis may be fatal, if not brought under control, or may interfere more significantly with life quality. If continuing the aminoglycoside or polypeptide is indicated for the tuberculosis, the patient's informed input is helpful. In practice, patients generally opt for continuing the medication, realizing their predicament. If the hearing continues to deteriorate, the situation is reviewed with the patient again. Of course, if it is possible to decrease the dose or to stop the offending medicine without compromising the effectiveness of the regimen, this is done, and further toxicity may be curtailed. Sometimes it may be possible, provided efficacy is equivalent in the given case, to substitute capreomycin, which is likely to be somewhat less ototoxic, for kanamycin or amikacin and, thus, potentially slow down further hearing deterioration (see Section V,A).

6. Ocular Toxicity

Visual loss associated with ethambutol is more likely to occur at the higher doses used in drug-resistant disease. The patient may detect these changes before or concomitantly with objective visual screening changes. It is important to ask patients about visual changes routinely. If a patient has visual loss, usually manifested by decreased vision over a period of days to weeks (as opposed to presbyopia that occurs over months to years) or has color discrimination changes or visual field disturbances, ethambutol toxicity is likely. The drug must be stopped and ophthalmologic evaluation obtained. If ethambutol is causing the visual problem and the drug is continued, the loss may progress rapidly to blindness. Usually, after the drug is stopped, vision will return. It may take many months if impairment is advanced. Few cases have not had return of vision. Although a few patients have received ethambutol again after having recovered from ethambutol ocular toxicity, this practice is not recommended.

7. Minor Mental and Neurological Changes

Cycloserine administration commonly is associated with minor mental changes, including forgetfulness, sadness, euphoria, nervousness, and impairment of concentration or of coordination. If the patient has suicidal ideation or feels that he or she is not in control of his or her life, the medication should be discontinued. If the patient is having side effects but feels in control, reassurance is appropriate, along with careful monitoring of behavior and serum drug levels. Minor tremors may be benign; if progressive, the dosage may have to be reduced or the drug discontinued. The optimal dosage of cycloserine is difficult to predict. Serum drug levels should be monitored routinely, every 1 to 2 weeks, in the first month or two of therapy, until stabilized. At National Jewish Center, a 2-h level of 25 to 30 µg/ml is considered desirable. The serum drug levels should be repeated if the patient has increasing psychological or neurological symptoms. Dosage adjustment may be necessary. If symptoms continue to escalate, cycloserine must be stopped. Ordinarily, the serious side effects, such as psychoses or convulsions, do not occur unless the serum level of the drug is excessive. There are a few patients, however, who develop serious problems with subtherapeutic serum concentrations. Cycloserine cannot be used in such patients. Patients receiving cycloserine should be cautioned that the drug may interfere with their ability to operate a motor vehicle.

Administration of the quinolones also may be associated with central nervous system symptoms. When a regimen includes both cycloserine and a quinolone, the combination sometimes may cause more central nervous system side effects than either medication by itself. Caffeine-like effects from ciprofloxacin or ofloxacin can be made more tolerable by giving the drug early in the day.

8. Minor Cutaneous Reactions

Cutaneous reactions may occur in association with any of the antituberculosis medications. When a patient develops a minimal, localized rash, a few hives, or slight itching, close observation, with or without the use of an antihistamine, is a reasonable course of action. However, if the reaction is moderately severe, or if a mild reaction progresses, stopping medication is recommended. Often it is not possible to tell which medicine is responsible for the reaction; it may be necessary to stop all drugs, while waiting for the reaction to clear (see also Section V,C).

9. Gastrointestinal Problems

Anorexia, nausea, vomiting, abdominal pain or burning, bloating, loose stools, and bad taste in the mouth make a patient feel miserable but usually are not sufficient to warrant discontinuation of medication. These problems very frequently are associated with ethionamide and PAS and, with lesser frequency, with other antituberculosis medications. Sometimes these problems can be avoided by introducing ethionamide and PAS gradually, over the course of a few days. Prolonged periods on subtherapeutic doses should be avoided. When a patient experiences gastrointestinal symptoms, it is essential to check for more serious associated problems, such as hepatic dysfunction, that may be induced by these medications.

Once liver damage has been ruled out, palliative therapy may be given. The patient should be reassured that his or her symptoms, although very distressing, are not life threatening. When a patient recognizes the seriousness of the underlying disease and its threat to life or to long-term well being, he or she may be willing to endure minor discomfort from the medicines. However, liver function tests should be repeated periodically if symptoms persist. The problem of perverted sense of taste may be masked by lemon drops, mints, or licorice; however, the benefit is transient. Drugs causing nausea or other gastrointestinal distress may be tolerated with food (provided this does not significantly impair absorption of the drug), or at bedtime, allowing the patient to sleep off the noxious side effect. Sometimes the dosage may be split without reducing efficacy.

Frequently, however, the symptoms are severe enough that the patient cannot be expected to deal with them without some pharmacologic help. Antacids may be helpful. (These must not be given within 2 h of the quinolones). Antiemetics often will work, given on an as-needed basis if the nausea is occasional, but given regularly to prevent chronic nausea. Antiemetics themselves may be potentially hepatotoxic; liver function should be evaluated before starting them and during their use. Sometimes experimentation is necessary before arriving at the best antiemetic for a given patient. Persistence is important. Metoclopramide is helpful for some patients, either with or without an antiemetic. Patients with pain or burning may require ranitidine or cimetidine. The polypharmacy should be reevaluated periodically, since sometimes the original side effects will have run their course, making the extra drugs superfluous. Unfortunately, the medicines often given to relieve symptoms must be continued as long as the offending antituberculosis drugs are given in their full amounts.

10. Musculoskeletal Problems

Serum uric acid almost invariably is elevated when pyrazinamide is used in prolonged high dosage. Usually increasing hydration is the only treatment needed. For the occasional patient who develops clinical gout, pyrazinamide may be stopped temporarily and the gout treated. After the gout is under control, allopurinol may be added. The pyrazinamide then may be reintroduced.

Inflammation of the fascia with pain and restriction of motion of the hands and shoulders sometimes develops during ethionamide therapy.[234] Physical therapy may help maintain range of motion, making it feasible to delay having to stop the drug.

11. Endocrine Problems

Hypothyroidism occasionally may develop when a patient is receiving either ethionamide[235] or PAS.[236] When these two drugs are used simultaneously, hypothyroidism develops frequently. It is treated by thyroid replacement; stopping the offending drugs may not be necessary. Thyroid function and replacement therapy should be reassessed when the patient has completed antituberculosis therapy. Gynecomastia, impotence, menstrual disturbances, and hair loss sometimes occur, especially with ethionamide. Empathy and reassurance that the problems are drug-related and are unlikely to be permanent may help make these problems more tolerable.

12. Electrolyte Problems

Loss of electrolytes, especially magnesium and potassium, is frequent in patients receiving capreomycin or the aminoglycosides, but generally is not a reason to stop the drug. Potassium can be replaced orally, if tolerated. If significant hypomagnesemia is present, parenteral replacement is advised. Low serum potassium may not respond to potassium replacement in the presence of low serum magnesium until the hypomagnesemia has been corrected. The patient may not recognize symptoms of low serum electrolytes. However, weakness that may have been attributed to other factors may improve after normalization of the electrolytes. The potential for cardiac problems associated with electrolyte abnormalities should be appreciated.

13. Local Problems with Injections

Tenderness of injection sites may be alleviated by moist heat, exercise, massage, and ultrasound therapy (1.5 W/cm^2 for 5 min over each area immediately after the injection).[237] Intravenous administration of medication may be appropriate in some instances.

C. REINTRODUCING MEDICATIONS AFTER DRUG REACTIONS

1. Wait for the Reaction to Clear

Following liver toxicity, several consecutive normal results of liver function tests should be evident. In the case of allergic reactions, the skin should have cleared completely. The patient should be in stable condition before attempting to reintroduce medications.

If these reactions have not cleared completely, the target organs may be especially sensitive. Medications that may not have caused a problem previously, at a less vulnerable time, now may precipitate a reaction. Also, if a reaction has cleared only partially, it may be difficult to differentiate the ups and downs of the original reaction from the effect of the drug being introduced.

After a serious reaction, the waiting period before reintroducing medicines should be prolonged. Extreme caution should be observed when medications are reintroduced. Where an adverse reaction has been especially severe, one should avoid reintroducing the drugs that were present in the regimen at the time of the reaction, if possible. When a patient has tuberculosis in the usual chronic form, the disease is not likely to progress significantly during the waiting period. When a patient has aggressive tuberculosis, the omission of medications while awaiting resolution of a drug reaction may lead to the deterioration or the demise of the patient. However, the prompt introduction of a potentially toxic medication also could have dire consequences. Decision making in these circumstances is exceedingly difficult.

2. Plan a Strategy

Evaluate the options for an effective regimen, considering the likelihood that at least one drug from the former regimen must be excluded. All drugs likely to have efficacy should be considered, including drugs with the potential for side effects that are not apt to be immediately life threatening. With the listed principles in mind, determine the safest way an effective regimen can be introduced in the least amount of time.

3. Reintroduce One Drug at a Time

When reintroducing drugs that were present in the regimen at the time of the reaction, do so one at a time to clarify which drug is responsible if a reaction should recur. Whereas the original adverse event may have taken a long time to emerge, the same reaction is likely to recur within a day or two after the offending medication is reintroduced.

4. Prevent the Emergence of Additional Drug Resistance

Recognize that a long period of time may be needed to introduce previously used drugs safely. Plan a sequence of introduction that will provide adequate antimycobacterial coverage as promptly as possible, to prevent the emergence of additional drug resistance.[238] Sometimes medications deemed undesirable for extended use may be introduced temporarily to provide adequate coverage while gradually adding the medications planned for the longer term regimen. These "extra" drugs may be discontinued when the patient is tolerating adequate doses of the proposed long-term regimen.

5. Substitutions

Substitute one drug for the drug causing the adverse reaction if the reaction occurs within the first month of therapy or if the reaction occurs after the patient clearly is showing a favorable response to therapy. However, in order to decrease the likelihood of promoting additional drug resistance, two new drugs should be substituted for the one lost if there is a question of possible failure of the regimen the patient had been receiving. This may be the case in the interval between the end of the first month of the regimen and the time of documented culture conversion.

6. Reintroduce Drugs Cautiously

After a reaction affecting the liver, reintroduce suspected hepatotoxic drugs in a step-wise manner, starting with a low dose and increasing daily for 3 days. Check liver function tests before each dose. If stable, the drug challenge can proceed. When the patient is on the full regimen, liver function tests should be repeated at least every 1 to 2 weeks for the next month, to assure stability (see example in Figure 12.3).

A desensitizing schedule should be used if drugs in the former regimen are reintroduced after a skin reaction or drug fever. Emergency measures should be available immediately during desensitization. Suspected drugs may be reintroduced one at a time on a desensitization schedule. Varying schedules have been proposed; the essential ingredients in all of them are caution, close observation of the patient, immediate availability of emergency intervention (epinephrine and airway management), and incremental dosing, starting at very minute doses of the suspected drug. Complete blood count, serum creatinine, and liver enzymes should be monitored, along with close clinical observation. If the allergic reaction was particularly severe, it is wiser to avoid reintroducing the offending drug. However, when no reasonable substitute is available, very cautious desensitization, starting with a very tiny dose may make reintroduction of an effective regimen possible. Careful monitoring, under some circumstances, may require an intensive care unit setting. Desensitization can be done most safely under the care of an allergist in a hospital specializing in the management of difficult cases of tuberculosis.

VI. SURGERY[239]

A. HISTORICAL

Surgical resection of residual pulmonary lesions was performed frequently in the early years of the chemotherapy era when physicians were unsure of the long-term benefits of chemotherapy. Surgical therapy was largely abandoned when the efficacy of medical therapy was documented. With good multidrug regimens, the outcome of chemotherapy was at least 90% successful, and little additional benefit could be expected by subjecting the patient to the risk of surgery. In the 1970s and early 1980s, surgery for pulmonary tuberculosis was performed rarely, except for complications such as uncontrolled hemoptysis, bronchopleural fistula, or empyema. In cases of tuberculosis resistant to multiple drugs or when serious drug reactions limited the use of effective medications, poorer results of medical treatment were anticipated and the option of surgery became more attractive.[36,79,226,240-243]

In the 1980s, as the poor results (65% favorable response)[35] of medical therapy for MDR-TB became evident, increased use of adjunctive surgical therapy was explored. Whereas in 1973 to 1983 only 7 of 171 patients from the National Jewish Center underwent surgical resection as part of their treatment for pulmonary MDR-TB, in 1983 to 1993, 62 of 109 similar patients had surgical resection; 59 (95%) became culture negative. In the latter series, one patient developed a postoperative bronchopleural fistula and required repeat surgery, one patient died in the postoperative period of adult respiratory distress syndrome, and three patients died later of causes unrelated to surgery.[36] In both series, the patients operated upon had localized cavitary disease and, because of extensive drug resistance, were unlikely to respond to medical therapy alone.

B. FACTORS TO CONSIDER

1. Localization of Disease

The patient's disease must be sufficiently well localized to make resection feasible. Precise localization with computed tomography (CT) is helpful since, on routine chest radiography, some areas of disease may be obscured by overlying markings. A ventilation-perfusion scan is helpful in evaluating the functional status of various areas of the lungs. Since, in the pathogenesis of tuberculosis, blood vessels may be destroyed, nonfunctional lung tissue in the distribution of the involved vessel may be present despite a benign appearance on chest radiography. Leaving poorly vascularized tissue adjacent to the resected area may lead to poor healing. The perfusion status of the opposite lung may influence the decision on whether to operate.

2. Condition of the Patient

The patient's general condition and lung function must be such that the potential risk of the procedure is not prohibitive. The criteria for operability in high-risk pulmonary resective surgery have been reviewed recently.[244] An estimate of the residual lung function following resection should show a predicted postpneumonectomy FEV_1 value of greater than 0.8 l. However, in dire circumstances, the clinician may have to accept a slightly lower number. If the patient is malnourished, nutritional supplements should be given. Aggressive measures, such as tube feeding, may be needed in order to optimize the general condition of the patient prior to surgery.

3. Optimal Timing

Timing of the surgical procedure is critical. Complications of a complete or partial lung resection are reduced when the patient's infection is under good control and the sputum cultures are consistently negative. For patients who are on such poor regimens that culture conversion seems unlikely, surgery is best performed when the semiquantitative count of tubercle bacilli is at its anticipated nadir; that is, if the "fall and rise phenomenon" is in process, do the surgery after the "fall" and before the "rise." Judgment is necessary and experience is helpful in estimating the preferred time for surgery.

4. Experience of the Surgical Team

The problems of distorted anatomy, massive pleural adhesions, and destruction of tissue planes make surgery for tuberculosis very difficult. The patient should be given the benefit of a surgical team experienced with the problems involved.

5. Antituberculosis Chemotherapy

The patient should be on the best possible multidrug regimen preoperatively. Medications should be continued in the perioperative period and for 2 years beyond culture conversion to manage the inevitable residual bacilli. Occasionally, a second surgical procedure is necessary if there is a significant lesion in the contralateral lung and the patient can withstand bilateral resections. Where the amount of residual disease is small and no cavities are left behind, the bacillary load is likely to be small. The few remaining tubercle bacilli are likely to be controlled by medications that may not have been effective against a more massive bacterial burden.

VII. PROBLEMS IN THE MANAGEMENT OF DRUG-RESISTANT TUBERCULOSIS

A. NEED FOR RESOURCES AND EXPERIENCED PERSONNEL

The treatment of drug-resistant tuberculosis, especially multidrug-resistant disease, is time consuming, resource intensive, and fraught with risks. Adequate resources and experienced personnel are highly desirable in helping patients with drug-resistant tuberculosis toward recovery. In complex cases, it is possible to squander the last opportunity for the patient to undergo effective therapy by treating under less than ideal circumstances. It is strongly recommended that such patients be referred to a center specializing in the management of difficult drug-resistant cases before all reasonable options have been exhausted. With the availability of several Centers of Excellence in the management of MDR-TB, early referral of patients with MDR-TB is feasible, is in the best interest of the patients, is likely to be most cost-effective in the long run, and, in the opinion of this author, should be the standard of care.

Hospitalization frequently is required during the initiation of therapy, in view of the complexity of the regimens, the toxicity of the drugs, and the need for close monitoring of the patient. Hospitalization should be continued until the patient's condition is well stabilized. Isolation facilities within the hospital are essential. (See Chapter 3.)

Psychological support often is needed to help the patients cope with their chronic illness. Repeated teaching is helpful; some patients respond and become more cooperative with their treatment; some do not. Ancillary services such as physical therapy, occupational therapy, and recreational therapy are important in enhancing the quality of life of these chronically ill patients.

B. TREATMENT FAILURES

Patients with multidrug-resistant tuberculosis, although sometimes salvageable by aggressive therapy, have had high failure (35%) and relapse (14%) rates, according to a recent analysis from the National Jewish Center.[35] These patients are returned to the community with the recommendation of "home isolation." Some patients are conscientious and knowledgeable, and have homes with sufficient space and ventilation, along with means for delivery of food and other necessities. In such cases, home isolation presents minimal hazard. When these prerequisites are not met, individuals with refractory drug-resistant tuberculosis are potential problems in the community. At the time of this writing, the problem has not been solved. Reopening of sanatoria, in a limited way, may afford a place for some of these individuals.

Continuing partially effective therapy sometimes reduces symptoms, such as cough, and sometimes reduces the number of bacilli in the sputum. Until new drugs become available, the prospects for these patients are grim.

New drugs must be developed, and as they are developed, must be used appropriately, according to known principles of multidrug therapy. If a new drug is used as monotherapy, or if a new drug is used as a single effective agent added to a failing regimen, acquisition of resistance to the new drug is predictable. It is hoped that new drugs will be developed; it is hoped also that the new drugs will be used appropriately to reduce, rather than enhance, the problem of drug resistance.

C. DRUG RESISTANT TUBERCULOSIS INFECTION AND DISEASE WORLDWIDE

Since the treatment of drug resistant tuberculosis is resource intensive, such treatment generally has not been accessible to patients in developing nations. Even in countries where standardized secondary regimens are available and it salvages some patients with drug-resistant disease, other patients, whose drug resistance is such as to preclude response to a standard secondary regimen, remain without effective treatment. This problem has been largely ignored, but recently is being addressed in a limited way by the World Health Organization.[68,162,245-247] A large number of persons with drug-resistant tuberculosis has emerged in the developing world. Not only do these people suffer in their countries of origin, but some of them travel or emigrate to countries where drug resistance has been less prevalent, bringing their disease with them. They, as well as other persons with communicable drug-resistant tuberculosis,[50,68] are a potential source for spread of drug-resistant tuberculosis wherever they are.

As long as the problem of drug-resistant tuberculosis is not controlled worldwide, even countries where drug resistance is currently controlled continue to be vulnerable.[245] Also, many persons have latent infection with drug-resistant tubercle bacilli. Vigilance for drug resistance must be maintained because some of these persons will experience endogenous activation of drug-resistant tuberculosis in years to come.

REFERENCES

1. Villarino, M. E., Geiter, L. J., and Simone, P. M., The multidrug-resistant tuberculosis challenge to public health efforts to control tuberculosis, *Pub. Health Rpt.*, 107, 616, 1992.
2. Snider, D. E. and Roper, W. L., The new tuberculosis [editorial; comment], *N. Engl. J. Med.*, 326, 703, 1992.
3. Wolinsky, E., Reginster, A., and Steenken, W., Drug-resistant tubercle bacilli in patients under treatment with streptomycin, *Am. Rev. Tubercul.*, 58, 335, 1948.

4. Wallace, A. T., Stewart, S. M., Turbbull, F. A. W., and Crofton, J. W., Isoniazid resistance in patients with pulmonary tuberculosis treated on isoniazid alone, *Tubercle*, 35, 164, 1954.

5. American Thoracic Society, Ethambutol in the treatment of tuberculosis, a statement by the committee on therapy, *Am. Rev. Respir. Dis.*, 98, 320, 1968.

6. American Trudeau Society, Current status of drug therapy in tuberculosis, *Am. Rev. Tuberc.*, 61, 436, 1950.

7. Kass, I., Russell, W. F., Heaton, A., Miyamoto, T., Middlebrook, G., and Dressler, S. H., Changing concepts in the treatment of pulmonary tuberculosis, *Ann. Intern. Med.*, 47, 744, 1957.

8. Jancik, E., Zelenka, M., Tousek, J., and Makova, M., Chemotherapy for patients with cultures resistant to streptomycin, isoniazid and PAS, *Tubercle*, 44, 443, 1963.

9. Fischer, D. A., Lester, W., Dye. W. E., and Moulding, T. S., Re-treatment of patients with isoniazid-resistant tuberculosis. Analysis and follow-up of 146 cases, *Am. Rev. Respir. Dis.*, 97, 392, 1968.

10. Fischer, D. A., Kass, I., Dye, W. E., and Lester, W., Treatment of isoniazid-resistant tuberculosis, Antimicrobial Agents and Chemotherapy, *Proc. 4th Intersci. Conf. Antimicrob. Agents Chemother.*, American Society for Microbiology, New York, 1964, 699.

11. Somner, A. R. and Brace, A. A., Ethionamide, pyrazinamide and cycloserine used successfully in the treatment of chronic pulmonary tuberculosis, *Tubercle*, 43, 345, 1962.

12. Tousek, J., Jancik, E., Zelenka, M., and Jancikova-Makova, M., The results of treatment in patients with cultures resistant to streptomycin, isoniazid and PAS: a five-year follow-up, *Tubercle*, 48, 27, 1967.

13. Zierski, M., Treatment of patients with cultures resistant to the primary anti-tuberculosis drugs, *Tubercle*, 45, 96, 1964.

14. Zierski, M. and Zachara, A., Late results in re-treatment of patients with pulmonary tuberculosis, *Tubercle*, 51, 172, 1970.

15. Davidson, P. T., Goble, M., and Lester, W., The antituberculosis efficacy of rifampin in 136 patients, *Chest,* 61, 574, 1972.

16. Vall-Spinosa, A., Lester, W., Moulding, T., and Davidson, P. T., Rifampin in the treatment of drug-resistant *Mycobacterium tuberculosis* infections, *N. Engl. J. Med.*, 283, 616, 1970.

17. Fox, W., Changing concepts in the chemotherapy of pulmonary tuberculosis: the John Barnwell lecture, *Am. Rev. Respir. Dis.*, 97, 767, 1968.

18. International Union Against Tuberculosis, A comparison of regimens of ethionamide, pyrazinamide and cycloserine in re-treatment of patients with pulmonary tuberculosis, *Bull. Int. Union Tuberc.*, 42, 7, 1969.

19. East African/British Medical Research Councils, Streptomycin plus PAS plus pyrazinamide in the retreatment of pulmonary tuberculosis in East Africa, *Tubercle*, 52, 191, 1971.

20. Study by East African and British Medical Research Councils, Streptomycin plus PAS plus pyrazinamide in the retreatment of pulmonary tuberculosis in East Africa: 2nd report, *Tubercle*, 54, 283, 1973.

21. Lester, W., Treatment of drug resistant tuberculosis, *Dis. Month*, April 1, 1971.

22. Centers for Disease Control, Multi-drug-resistant tuberculosis — North Carolina, *MMWR,* 35, 785, 1987.

23. Schiffman, P. L., Ashkar, B., Bishop, M., and Cleary, M. G., Drug-resistant tuberculosis in a large southern California hospital, *Am. Rev. Respir. Dis.*, 116, 821, 1977.

24. Reves, R., Blakey, D., Snider, D. E., and Farer, L. S., Transmission of multiple drug-resistant tuberculosis: report of a school and community outbreak, *Am. Epidem.*, 113(4), 423, 1981.

25. Carpenter, J. L., Obnibene, A. J., Gorby, E. W., Neimes, R. E., Koch, J. R., and Perkins, W. L., Antituberculosis drug resistance in South Texas, *Am. Rev. Respir. Dis.*, 128, 1055, 1983.

26. Steiner, P., Rao, M., Mitchell, M., and Steiner, M., Primary drug-resistant tuberculosis in children: emergence of primary drug-resistant strains of *M. tuberculosis* to rifampin, *Am. Rev. Respir. Dis.*, 134, 446, 1986.

27. Steiner, P., Roa, M., Victoria, M. S., Hunt, J., and Steiner, M., A continuing study of primary drug-resistant tuberculosis among children observed at the Kings County Hospital Medical Center between the years 1961 and 1980, *Am. Rev. Respir. Dis.*, 128, 425, 1983.

28. Horne, N. W., Drug resistant-tuberculosis: a review of the world situation, *Tubercle,* (Suppl.), 50, 2, 1968.

29. Doster, B., Caras, G., and Snider, D. E., Jr., A continuing survey of primary drug resistance in tuberculosis, 1961 to 1968, *Am. Rev. Respir. Dis.*, 113, 419, 1976.

30. Hobby, G. L., Johnson, P. M., and Boytar-Papirnyik, V., Primary drug resistance: a continuing study of drug resistance in tuberculosis in a veteran population in the United States — September 1962 to September 1971, *Transact. 31st VA Armed Forces Pulon. Conf.*, 36, 1972.

31. Hobby, G. L., Johnson, P. M., and Boytar-Papirnyik, V., Primary drug resistance: a continuing study of drug resistance in tuberculosis in a veteran population within the United States. X. September 1970 to September 1973, *Am. Rev. Respir. Dis.*, 110, 95, 1974.

32. Kopanoff, D. E., Kilburn, J. O., Glassroth, J. L., Snider, D. E., Farer, L. S., and Good, R. C., A continuing survey of tuberculosis primary drug resistance in the United States, March 1975 to November 1977. A U.S. Public Health Service cooperative study, *Am. Rev. Respir. Dis.*, 118, 835, 1978.

33. Cauthen, G. M., Kilburn, J. O., Kelly, G. D., and Good, R. C., Resistance to antituberculosis drugs in patients with and without prior treatment: survey of 31 state and large city laboratories, 1982-1986, *Am. Rev. Respir. Dis.*, 137(Suppl.), 260, 1988.

34. Snider, D. E., Cauthen, G. M., Farer, L. S., Kelly, G. D., Kilburn, J. O., Good, R. C., and Dooley, S. W., Drug-resistant tuberculosis, *Am. Rev. Respir. Dis.*, 144, 732, 1991.

35. Goble, M., Iseman, M. D., Madsen, L. A., Waite, D., Ackerson, L., and Horsburgh, C. R., Jr., Treatment of 171 patients with pulmonary tuberculosis resistant to isoniazid and rifampin, *N. Engl. J. Med.*, 328, 527, 1993.

36. Iseman, M., Madsen, L., Iseman, M., and Ackerson, L., Impact of surgery on the management of MDR-TB, *Am. J. Respir. Crit. Care Med.*, 151S, A336, 1995.

37. Brudney, K. and Dobkin, J., Resurgent tuberculosis in New York City: human immunodeficiency virus, homelessness, and the decline of tuberculosis control programs, *Am. Rev. Respir. Dis.*, 144, 745, 1991.

38. Reichman, L. B., The U-shaped curve of concern [editorial], *Am. Rev. Respir. Dis.*, 144, 741, 1991.

39. Centers for Disease Control, Outbreak of multidrug-resistant tuberculosis in Texas, California, and Pennsylvania, *MMWR*, 39, 369, 1990.

40. Centers for Disease Control, Nosocomial transmission of multidrug-resistant tuberculosis to health-care workers and HIV-infected patients in an urban hospital — Florida, *MMWR*, 39, 718, 1990.

41. Centers for Disease Control, Transmission of multidrug-resistant tuberculosis from an HIV positive client in a residential substance-abuse facility — Michigan, *MMWR*, 40:8, 129, 1991.

42. Centers for Disease Control, Transmission of multidrug-resistant tuberculosis among immunocompromised persons in a correctional system — New York, 1991, *MMWR*, 41:28, 507, 1992.

43. Centers for Disease Control, Nosocomial transmission of multidrug-resistant tuberculosis among HIV-infected persons — Florida and New York, 1988-1991, *MMWR*, 40, 585, 1991.

44. Pitchenik, A. E., Burr, J., Laufer, M., Miller, G., Cacciatore, R., Bigler, W. J., Witte, J. J., and Cleary, T., Outbreaks of drug-resistant tuberculosis at AIDS center [letter], *Lancet*, 336, 440, 1990.

45. Calder, R. A., Duclos, P., Wilder, M. H., Pryor, V. L., and Scheel, W. J., *Mycobacterum tuberculosis* transmission in a health clinic, *Bull. Int. Union Tuberc. Lung Dis.*, 66, 103, 1991.

46. Edlin, B. R., Tokars, J. I., Grieco, M. H., Crawford, J. T., Williams, J., Sordillo, E. M., Ong, K. R., Castro, K. G., et al., An outbreak of multidrug-resistant tuberculosis among hospitalized patients with the acquired immunodeficiency syndrome, *N. Engl. J. Med.*, 326, 1514, 1992.

47. Fischl, M. A., Uttamchandani, R. B., Daikos, G. L., Poblete, R. B., Moreno, J. N., Reyes, R. R., Boota, A. M., Thompson, L. M., et al., An outbreak of tuberculosis caused by multiple-drug-resistant tubercle bacilli among patients with HIV infection, *Ann. Intern. Med.*, 117, 177, 1992.

48. Pearson, M. L., Jereb, J. A., Frieden, T. R., Crawford, J. T., Davis, B. J., Dooley, S. W., and Jarvis, W. R., Nosocomial transmission of multidrug-resistant *Mycobacterum tuberculosis*: a risk to patients and health care workers, *Ann. Intern. Med.*, 117, 191, 1992.

49. Busillo, C. P., Lessnau, K., Sanjana, V., Soumakis, S., Davidson, M., Mullen, M. P., and Talavera, W., Multidrug resistant *Mycobacterum tuberculosis* in patients with human immunodeficiency virus infection, *Chest*, 102, 797, 1992.

50. Bifani, P. J., Plikaytis, B. B., Kapur, V., Stockbauer, K., Pan, X., Lutfey, M. L., Moghazeh, S. L., Eisner, W., Daniel, T. M., Kaplan, M. H., Crawford, J. T., Musser, J. M., and Kreiswirth, B. N., Origin and interstate spread of a New York City multidrug-resistant *Mycobacterium tuberculosis* clone family, *JAMA*, 275, 452, 1996.

51. Neville, K., Bromberg, A., Bromberg, R., Bonk, S., Hanna, B. A., and Rom, W. N., The third epidemic — multidrug-resistant tuberculosis, *Chest,* 105, 45, 1994.

52. Centers for Disease Control, Multidrug-resistant tuberculosis in a hospital — Jersey City, New Jersey, 1990–1992, *MMWR,* 43, 417, 1994.

53. Frieden, T. R., Sherman, L. F., Maw, K.L., Fujiwara, P. I., Crawford, J. T., Nivin, B., Sharp, V., Hewlett, D., Jr., Brudney, K., Alland, D., and Kreisworth, B. N., A multi-institutional outbreak of highly drug-resistant tuberculosis: epidemiology and clinical outcomes, *JAMA,* 276, 1229, 1996.

54. Centers for Disease Control, National action plan to combat multidrug-resistant tuberculosis, *MMWR,* 41, 5, 1992.

55. Moore, M., Onorato, I. M., McCray, E., and Castro, K. G., Trends in drug-resistant tuberculosis in the United States, 1993–1996 (published erratum appears in *JAMA,* 1998 March 4; 279(9):656), *JAMA,* 278, 833, 1997.

56. Bloch, A. B., Cauthen, G. M., Oronato, I. M., Dansbury, K. G., Kelly, G. D., Driver, C. R., and Snider, D. E., Jr., Nationwide survey of drug-resistant tuberculosis in the United States, *JAMA,* 271, 665, 1994.

57. Centers for Disease Control and Prevention, Reported tuberculosis in the United States, 1997, Atlanta, GA, July 1998.

58. Frieden, T. R., Fujiwara, P. I., Washko, R. M., and Hamburg, M.. A., Tuberculosis in New York City — turning the tide, *N. Engl. J. Med.,* 333(4), 229, 1995.

59. Dorsinville, M. S., Case management of tuberculosis in New York City, *Int. J. Tuberc. Lung Dis.,* 2(9), S46, 1998.

60. Park, M. M., Davis, A. L., Schluger, N. W., Cohen, H., and Rom, W. N., Outcome of MDR-TB patients, 1983–1993. Prolonged survival with appropriate therapy, *Am. J. Respir. Crit. Care Med.,* 153, 317, 1996.

61. Turett, G. S., Telzak, E. E., Torian, L. V., Blum, S., Alland, D., Weisfuse, I., and Fazal, B. A., Improved outcomes for patients with multidrug-resistant tuberculosis, *Clin. Infect. Dis.,* 21, 1238, 1995.

62. Salomon, N., Perlman, D. C., Friedmann, P., Buchstein, S., Kreiswirth, B. N., and Mildvan, D., Predictors and outcome of multidrug-resistant tuberculosis, *Clin. Infect. Dis.,* 21, 1245, 1995.

63. Telzak, E. E., Sepkowitz, K., Alpert, P., Mannheimer, S., Medard, F., el-Sadr W., Blum S., Gagliardi, A., Salomon, N., and Turett, G., Multidrug-resistant tuberculosis in patients without HIV infection, *N. Engl. J. Med.,* 333, 907, 1995.

64. Telenti, A., Genetics of drug resistance in tuberculosis, in *Clinics in Chest Medicine,* 18, Iseman, M. D. and Huitt, G. A., Eds., W.B. Sanders, Philadelphia, 1997, 55.

65. Chopra, I. and Brennan, P., Molecular action of antimycobacterial agents, *Tuberc. Lung Dis., 78, 89, 1998.*

66. Cole, S. T., Brosch, R., Parkhill, J., Garnier, T., Churcher, C., Harris, D., Gordon, S. V., Eiglmeier, K., Gas, S., Barry, C. E., III, Tekaia, F., Badcock, K., Basham, D., Brown, D., Chillingworth, T., Connor, R., Davies, R., Devlin, K., Feltwell, T., Gentles, S., Hamlin, N., Holroyd, S., Hornsby, T., Jagels, K., Krogh, A., McLean, J., Moule, S., Murphy, L., Oliver, K., Osborne, J., Quail, M. A., Rajandream, M.-A., Rogers, J., Rutter, S., Seeger, K., Skelton, J., Squares, R., Squares, S., Sulston, J. E., Taylor, K., Whitehead, S., and Barrell, B. G., Deciphering the biology of *Mycobacterium tuberculosis* from the complete genome sequence, *Nature,* 393, 537, 1998.

67. Cole, S. T., Why sequence the genome of *Mycobacterium tuberculosis*, *Tuberc. Lung Dis.,* 77, 486, 1996.

68. Nolan, C. M., Nosocomial multidrug-resistant tuberculosis — global spread of the third epidemic (editorial), *J. Infect. Dis.,* 176, 748, 1997.

69. Ritacco, V., Di Lonardo, M., Reniero, A., Ambroggi, M., Barrera, L., Dambrosi, A., Lopez, B., Isola, N., and de Kantor, I. N., Nosocomial spread of human immunodeficiency virus-related multidrug-resistant tuberculosis in Buenos Aires, *J. Infect. Dis.,* 176, 637, 1997.

70. Breathnach, A. S., de Ruiter, A., Holdsworth, G. M. C., Bateman, N. T., O'Sullivan, D. G. M., Rees, P. J., Snashall, D., Milburn, H. J., Peters, B. S., Watson, J., Drobiniewski, F. A., and French, G. L., An outbreak of multi-drug-resistant tuberculosis in a London teaching hospital, *J. Hosp. Inf.,* 39, 111, 1998.

71. Centers for Disease Control, Multidrug-resistant tuberculosis outbreak on an HIV ward — Madrid, Spain, 1991–1995, *MMWR,* 45:330, 1996.

72. Canetti, G., The J. Burns Amberson lecture: present aspects of bacterial resistance in tuberculosis, *Am. Rev. Respir. Dis.,* 92, 687, 1965.

73. Canetti, G., *The Tubercle Bacillus in the Pulmonary Lesion of Man: Histobacteriology and Its Bearing on the Therapy of Pulmonary Tuberculosis*, Springer, New York, 1955.

74. Rattan, A., Kalia, A., and Ahmad, N., Multidrig-resistant *Mycobacterium tuberculosis*: molecular perspectives, *Emerg. Inf. Dis.*, 4(2), 195, 1998.

75. Telenti, A., Imboden, P., Marchesi, F., Lowrie, D., Cole, S., Colston, M. J., Matter, L., Schopfer, K., and Bodmer, T., Detection of rifampicin-resistance in *Mycobacterium tuberculosis*, *Lancet*, 341, 647, 1993.

76. Zhang, Y., Heym, B., Allen, B., Young, D., and Cole, S., The catalase-peroxidase gene and isonizid resistance of *Mycobacterium tuberculosis*, *Nature*, 358, 591, 1992.

77. Banerjee, A., Dubnau, E., Quemard, A., Balasubramanian, V., Um, K. S., Wilson, J., Collins, D., De Lisle, G., and Jacobs, W. R., Jr., *inhA*, a gene encoding a target for isoniazid and ethionamide in *Mycobacterium tuberculosis*, *Science*, 263, 227, 1994.

78. David, H. L., Probability distribution of drug-resistant mutants in unselected populations of *Mycobacterum tuberculosis*, *Appl. Microbiol.*, 20, 810, 1970.

79. Shimao, T., Drug resistance in tuberculosis control, *Tubercle*, 68(2) (Suppl.), 5, 1987.

80. Pollock, M. R., Drug resistance and mechanisms for its development, *Br. Med. Bull.*, 16, 16, 1960.

81. International Union Against Tuberculosis, The clinical significance of bacterial resistance: a symposium held in Paris on September 20, 1957, *Bull. Int. Union Tuberc.*, 27, 215, 1957.

82. Schmidt, L. H., Grover, A. A., Hoffmann, R., Rehm, J., and Sullivan, R., The emergence of isoniazid-sensitive bacilli in monkeys inoculated with isoniazid-resistant strains, *Transact. 17th VA Armed Forces Conf. Chemo.*, 264, 1958.

83. McDermott, W., Microbial persistence, (the Alpha Kappa Kappa lecture), *Yale J. Biol. Med.*, 30, 257, 1958.

84. McDermott, W., The J. Burns Amberson lecture — The chemotherapy of tuberculosis, *Am. Rev. Respir. Dis.*, 86, 323, 1962.

85. Hershfield, E. S., Drug resistance — response to Dr. Shimao, *Tubercle*, 68(Suppl.), 17, 1987.

86. Tripathy, S. P., Menon, N. K., Mitchison, D. A., Narayana, A. L. S., Somasundaram, P. A., Scott, H., and Velu, S., Response to treatment with isoniazid plus PAS of tuberculosis patients with primary isoniazid resistance, *Tubercle*, 50, 257, 1969.

87. Winder, F. G., Mode of action of the antimycobacterial agents and associated aspects of the molecular biology of mycobacteria, in *Biology of the Mycobacteria*, vol. 1, Ratledge, C. and Stanford, J., Eds., Academic Press, London, 1982, Chap. 8.

88. Tsukamura, M., Yamamoto, M., Hayashi, M., Noda, Y., and Torii, T., Further studies on cross resistance in *Mycobacterum tuberculosis*, with special reference to streptomycin, kanamycin, and viomycin resistance, *Am. Rev. Respir. Dis.*, 85, 426, 1962.

89. Tsukamura, M., Cross-resistance of tubercle bacilli, *Kekkaku*, 52, 47, 1977.

90. Lefford, M. J., The ethionamide sensitivity of East African strains of *Mycobacterum tuberculosis* resistant to thiacetazone, *Tubercle*, 50, 7, 1969.

91. Yew, W. W., Piddock, L. J. V., Li, M. S. K., Lyon, D., Chan, C. Y., and Cheng, A. F. B., *In vitro* activity of quinolones and macrolides against mycobacteria, *J. Antimicrob. Chemother.*, 34, 343, 1994.

92. Heifets, L. B., Lindholm-Levy, P. J., and Iseman, M. D., Rifabutine: minimal inhibitory and bactericidal concentrations for *Mycobacterum tuberculosis*, *Am. Rev. Respir. Dis.*, 137, 719, 1988.

93. Dickinson, J. M. and Mitchison, D. A., *In vitro* activity of new rifamycins against rifampin-resistant *M. tuberculosis* and MAIS-complex mycobacteria, *Tubercle*, 68, 177, 1987.

94. Kleeberg, H. H. and Boshoff, M. S., *World Atlas of Initial Drug Resistance*, prepared for the Scientific Committee on Bacteriology and Immunology of the International Union Against Tuberculosis, Paris, 1980.

95. Kleeberg, H. H. and Olivier, M., *World Atlas of Initial Drug Resistance*, 2nd rev. ed., S. Africa Med. Research Council, Pretoria, 1984.

96. Meissner, G., Primary drug resistance of the tubercle bacillus: bacteriology, therapeutic and epidemiological aspects, *Bull. Int. Union Tuberc.*, 32(2), 15, 1962.

97. Centers for Disease Control, Tuberculosis morbidity — United States, 1997, *MMWR*, 47, 253, 1998.

98. Sudre, P. and Cohn, D. L., *Mycobacterium tuberculosis* drug resistance: a call to action [editorial], *Int. J. Tuberc. Lung Dis.*, 2, 609, 1998.

99. Cohn, D. L., Bustreo, F., and Raviglione, M. C., Drug-resistant tuberculosis: review of the worldwide situation and the WHO/IUATLD Global Surveillance Project, International Union Against Tuberculosis and Lung Disease, *Clin. Infect. Dis.*, 24S1, 121, 1997.

100. Pablos-Mendez, A., Raviglione, M. C., Laszlo, A., Binkin, N., Rieder, H. L., Bustreo, F., Cohn, D. L., Lambregts-van Weezenbeek, C. S. B., Kim, S. J., Chaulet, P., and Nunn, P., Global surveillance for antituberculosis-drug resistance, 1994–1997, World Health Organization-International Union against Tuberculosis and Lung Disease Working Group on Anti-Tuberculosis Drug Resistance Surveillance, *N. Engl. J. Med.*, 338, 1641, 1998.

101. WHO Geneva/IUATLD Paris, Guidelines for serveillance of drug resistance in tuberculosis, *Int. J. Tuberc. Lung Dis.*, 2(1), 72, 1998.

102. Centers for Disease Control, Meeting the challenge of multidrug-resistant tuberculosis: summary of a conference, *MMWR*, 41, 51, 1992.

103. Centers for Disease Control, Management of persons exposed to multidrug-resistant tuberculosis, *MMWR*, 41, 61, 1992.

104. Grzybowski, S., Cost of tuberculosis control, *Tubercle*, 68(Suppl.), 33, 1987.

105. Boulahbal, F., Khaled, S., and Tazir, M., The interest of follow-up of resistance of the tubercle bacillus in the evaluation of a programme, *Bull. Int. Union Tuberc. Lung Dis.*, 64, 23, 1989.

106. Weyer, K., Primary and acquired drug resistance in adult black tuberculosis patients in South Africa, *Am. Rev. Respir. Dis.*, 143(4)(Suppl.), A121, 1991.

107. Kim, S. J. and Hong, Y. P., Drug resistance of *Mycobacterium tuberculosis* in Korea, *Tuberc. Lung Dis.*, 73, 219, 1992.

108. Cohn, M. L., Middlebrook, G., and Russell, W. F., Combined drug treatment of tuberculosis. I. Prevention of emergence of mutant populations of tubercle bacilli resistant to both streptomycin and isoniazid *in vitro*, *J. Clin. Invest.*, 38, 1349, 1959.

109. American Thorasic Society, Control of tuberculosis in the United States, *Am. Rev. Respir. Dis.*, 146, 1623, 1992.

110. Centers for Disease Control, Initial therapy for tuberculosis in an era of multidrug resistance, recommendations of the Advisory Council for the Elimination of Tuberculosis, *MMWR*, 42(RR7), 1, 1993.

111. Addington, W. W., Patient compliance: the most serious remaining problem in the control of tuberculosis in the United States, *Chest*, 76(Suppl.), 741, 1979.

112. Chaulet, P., Compliance with anti-tuberculosis chemotherapy in developing countries, *Tubercle*, 68(Suppl.), 19, 1987.

113. Reichman, L. B., Compliance in developed nations, *Tubercle*, 68(Suppl.), 25, 1987.

114. Sbarbaro, J. A., Compliance: inducements and enforcement, *Chest*, 76(Suppl.), 750, 1979.

115. Snider, D. E., Kelly, G. D., Thompson, N. J., Kilburn, J. O., and Good, R. C., Infectiousness and pathogenicity of drug resistant *Mycobacterum tuberculosis*, *Am. Rev. Respir. Dis.*, 123(Suppl.), 254, 1981.

116. Snider, D. E., Kelley, G. D., Cuathen, G. M., Thompson, N. J., and Kilburn, J. O., Infection and disease among contacts of tuberculosis cases with drug-resistant and drug-susceptible bacilli, *Am. Rev. Respir. Dis.*, 132, 125, 1985.

117. Dooley, S. W., Castro, K. G., Hutton, M. D., Mullan, R. J., Polder, J. A., and Snider, D. E., Jr., Guidelines for preventing the transmission of tuberculosis in health-care settings, with special focus on HIV-related issues, *MMWR*, 39, 1, 1990.

118. Dooley, S. W., Jarvis, W. R., Martone, W. J., and Snider, D. E., Jr., Multi-drug resistant tuberculosis [editorial; comment], *Ann. Intern. Med.*, 117, 257, 1992.

119. Nardell, E. A., Multidrug-resistant tuberculosis [letter], *N. Engl. J. Med.*, 327, 1174, 1992.

120. Nardell, E. A., Nosocomial tuberculosis in the AIDS era: strategies for interrupting transmission in developing countries, *Bull. Int. Union Tuberc. Lung Dis.*, 66, 107, 1991.

121. ACCP consensus statement, Institutional control measures for tuberculosis in the era of multiple drug resistance, ACCP/ATS Consensus Conference, American College of Chest Physicians and the American Thoracic Society, *Chest*, 108, 1690, 1995.

122. Centers for Disease Control and Prevention, The role of BCG vaccine in the prevention and control of tuberculosis in the United States: a joint statement by the Advisory Council for the Elimination of Tuberculosis and the Advisory Committee on Immunization Practices, *MMWR*, 45(RR-4), 1, 1996.

123. Reichman, L. B., Mangura, B. T., and Jordan, T., BCG immunization of health care workers exposed to multidrug-resistant tuberculosis [letter], *Int. J. Tuberc. Lung Dis.*, 1, 90, 1997.

124. Passannante, M. R., Gallagher, C. T., and Reichman, L. B., Preventive therapy for contacts of multidrug-resistant tuberculosis, a Delphi survey, *Chest*, 106, 431, 1994.

125. Ben-Dov, I. and Mason, G. R., Drug resistant tuberculosis in Southern California: trends 1969 to 1984, *Am. Rev. Respir. Dis.*, 135, 1307, 1987.

126. Barnes, P. F., The influence of epidemiologic factors on drug resistance rates in tuberculosis, *Am. Rev. Respir. Dis.*, 136, 325, 1987.

127. Riley, L. W., Arathoon, E., and Loverde, V. D., The epidemiologic patterns of drug-resistant *Mycobacterium tuberculosis*: a community-based study, *Am. Rev. Respir. Dis.*, 139, 1282, 1989.

128. Areas, A., Chaparala, B., Martin, H. K., Muthuswamy, P., and Serai, L., Drug resistant tuberculosis at Cook County Hospital, *Am. Rev. Respir. Dis.*, 139(Suppl.), A315, 1989.

129. Chawla, P. K., Klapper, P. J., Kamholz, S. L., Pollack, A. H., and Heurich, A. E., Drug resistant tuberculosis in an urban population including patients at risk for human immunodeficiency virus infection, *Am. Rev. Respir. Dis.*, 146, 280, 1992.

130. Jacobs, M., Hussain, E., and D'Amato, R. F., Incidence of drug resistant *Mycobacterium tuberculosis* in a New York City medical center, *Am. Rev. Respir. Dis.*, 145(Suppl.), A101, 1992.

131. Frieden, T. R., Sterling, T., Pablos-Mendez, A., Kilburn, J. O., Cauthen, G. M., and Dooley, S. W., The emergence of drug-resistant tuberculosis in New York City, *N. Engl. J. Med.*, 328, 521, 1993.

132. Kritski, A. L., Rodrigues de Jesus, L. S., Andrade, M. K., Werneck-Barroso, E., Vieira, M. A. M. S., Haffner, A., and Riley, L. W., Retreatment tuberculosis cases, factors associated with drug resistance and adverse outcomes, *Chest*, 111, 1162, 1997.

133. Crofton, J. and Douglas, A., Treatment of pulmonary tuberculosis, in *Respiratory Diseases*, F. A. Davis Co., Philadelphia, 1969, Chap. 14.

134. Harrow, E. M., Rangel, J. M., Arriega, J. M., Cohen, I., Regil Ruiz, M. I., DeRiemer, K., and Small, P. M., Epidemiology and clinical consequences of drug-resistant tuberculosis in a Guatemalan hospital, *Chest*, 113, 1452, 1998.

135. Suwanogool, S., Smith, S. M., Smith, L. G., and Eng, R., Drug-resistance encountered in the retreatment of *Mycobacterium tuberculosis* infections, *J. Chronic Dis.*, 37:12, 925, 1984.

136. Costello, H. D., Caras, G. J., and Snider, D. E., Jr., Drug resistance among previously treated tuberculosis patients, a brief report, *Am. Rev. Respir. Dis.*, 121, 313, 1980.

137. Bradford, W. Z., Martin, J. N., Reingold, A. L., Schecter, G. F., Hopewell, P. C., and Small, P. M., The changing epidemiology of acquired drug-resistant tuberculosis in San Francisco, *Lancet*, 348, 928, 1996.

138. Kimerling, M. E., Phillips, P., Patterson, P., Hall, M., Robinson, C. A., and Dunlap, N. E., Low serum antimycobacterial drug levels in non-HIV-infected tuberculosis patients, *Chest*, 113, 1178, 1998.

139. Matthews, J. I., Rajput, M. A., and Neimus, R., Drug resistant tuberculosis in south Texas, *Chest*, 92(2)(Suppl.), 145S, 1987.

140. Welsh, C. H., Drug-resistant tuberculosis after gastrectomy. Double jeopardy? *Chest*, 99, 245, 1991.

141. Peloquin, C. A., Nitta, A. T., Burman, W. J., Brudney, K. F., Miranda-Massari, J. R., McGuinness, M. E., Berning, S. E., and Gerena, G. T., Low antituberculosis drug concentrations in patients with AIDS, *Ann. Pharmacother.*, 30, 919, 1996.

142. Iseman, M. D. and Madsen, L. A., Chronic tuberculous empyema with bronchopleural fistula resulting in treatment failure and progressive drug resistance, *Chest*, 100, 124, 1991.

143. Elliott, A. M., Berning, S. E., Iseman, M. D., and Peloquin, C. A., Failure of drug penetration and acquisition of drug resistance in chronic tuberculous empyema, *Tuberc. Lung Dis.*, 76, 463, 1995.

144. Moss, A. R., Alland, D., Telzak, E., Hewlett, D., Jr., Sharp, V., Chiliade, P., LaBombardi, V., Kabus, D., Hanna, B., Palumbo, L., Brudney, K., Weltman, A., Stoeckle, K., Chirgwin, K., Simberkoff, M., Moghazeh, S., Eisner, W., Lutfey, M., and Kreiswirth, B., A city-wide outbreak of a multiple-drug-resistant strain of *Mycobacterium tuberculosis* in New York, *Int. J. Tuberc. Lung Dis.*, 1, 115, 1997.

145. Agerton, T., Valway, S., Gore, B., Pozsik, C., Plikaytis, B., Woodley, C., and Onorato, I., Transmission of a highly drug-resistant strain (strain W1) of *Mycobacterium tuberculosis*. Community outbreak and nosocomial transmission via a contaminated bronchoscope, *JAMA*, 278, 1073, 1997.

146. Jereb, J. A., Klevens, R. M., Privett, T. D., Smith, P. J., Crawford, J. T., Sharp V. L., Davis, B. J., Jarvis, W. R., and Dooley, S. W., Tuberculosis in health care workers at a hospital with an outbreak of multidrug-resistant *Mycobacterium tuberculosis*, *Arch. Intern. Med.*, 155, 854, 1995.

147. Alland, D., Kalkut, G. E., Moss, A. R., McAdam, R. A., Hahn, J. A., Bosworth, W., Drucker, E., and Bloom, B. R., Transmission of tuberculosis in New York City, an analysis by DNA fingerprinting and conventional epidemiologic methods, *N. Engl. J. Med.*, 330, 1710, 1994.

148. Friedman, C. R., Stoeckle, M. Y., Kreiswirth, B. N., Johnson, W. D., Jr., Manoach, S. M., Berger, J., Sathianathan, K., Hafner, A., and Riley, L. W., Transmission of multidrug-resistant tuberculosis in a large urban setting, *Am. J. Resp. Crit. Care Med.*, 152, 355 1995.

149. Pablos-Mendez, A., Raviglione, M. C., Battan, R., and Ramos-Zuniga, R., Drug-resistant tuberculosis among the homeless in New York City, *N. Y. State J. Med.*, 90, 351, 1990.

150. Lessnau, K., Talavera, W., Busillo, C., Sanjana, V., Soumakis, S., Davidson, M., and Mullen, M., Multi-drug resistant *Mycobacterium tuberculosis* in patients with human immunodeficiency virus infection, *Am. Rev. Respir. Dis.*, 145(Suppl.), A815, 1992.

151. Centers for Disease Control, Prevention and treatment of tuberculosis among patients infected with human immunodeficiency virus: principles of therapy and revised recommendations, *MMWR*, 47(RR20), 1, 1998.

152. Gordin, F. M., Nelson, E. T., Matts, J. P., Cohn, D. L., Ernst, J., Benator, D., Besch, C. L., Crane, L. R., Sampson, J. H., Bragg, P. S., and El-Sadr, W., The impact of human immunodeficiency virus infection on drug-resistant tuberculosis, *Am. J. Respir. Crit. Care Med.*, 154, 1478, 1996.

153. Asch, S., Knowles, L., Rai, A., Jone, B. E., Pogoda, J., and Barnes P. F., Relationship of isoniazid resistance to human immunodeficiency virus infection in patients with tuberculosis, *Am. J. Respir. Crit. Care Med.*, 153, 1708, 1996.

154. Fischl, M. A., Daikos, G. L., Uttamchandani, G. L., Poblete, R. B., Moreno, J. N., Reyes, R. R., Boota, A. M., Thompson, L. M., et al., Clinical presentation and outcome of patients with HIV infection and tuberculosis caused by multiple-drug-resistant bacilli, *Ann. Int. Med.*, 117, 184, 1992.

155. Ridzon, R., Whitney, C. G., McKenna, M. T., Taylor, J. P., Ashkar, S. H., Nitta, A. T., Harvey, S. M., Valway, S., Woodley, C., Cooksey, R., and Onorato, I. M., Risk factors for rifampin mono-resistant tuberculosis, *Am. J. Respir. Crit. Care Med.*, 157, 1881, 1998.

156. Samper, S., Martin, C., Pinedo, A., Rivero, A., Blazquez, J., Baquero, F., van Soolingen, D., and van Embden, J., Transmission between HIV-infected patients of multidrug-resistant tuberculosis caused by *Mycobacterium bovis*, *AIDS*, 11, 1237, 1997.

157. Guerrero, A., Cobo, J., Fortun, J., Navas, E., Quereda, C., Asensio, A., Canon, J., Blazquez, J., and Gomez-Mampaso, E., Nosocomial transmission of *Mycobacterium bovis* resistant to 11 drugs in people with advanced HIV-1 infection, *Lancet*, 350, 1738, 1997.

158. Byrd, R. B., Fish, D. E., Roethe, R. A., Glover, J. N., and Wooster, L. D., Tuberculosis in oriental immigrants: a study in military dependents, *Chest*, 76, 136, 1979.

159. Aitken, M. L., Sparks, R., Anderson, K., and Albert, R. K., Predictors of drug resistant *Mycobacterium tuberculosis*, *Am. Rev. Respir. Dis.*, 130, 831, 1984.

160. Nolan, C. M. and Elarth, A. M., Tuberculosis in a cohort of Southeast Asian refugees, a five-year study, *Am. Rev. Respir. Dis.*, 137, 805, 1988.

161. Centers for Disease Control, Recommendations for prevention and control of tuberculosis among foreign-born persons, report of the working group on tuberculosis among foreign-born persons, *MMWR*, 47(RR16), 1, 1998.

162. Farmer, P. and Kim, J. Y., Community-based approaches to the control of multidrug resistant tuberculosis: introducing "DOTS-plus," *BMJ*, 317, 671, 1998.

163. Heifets, L. B., Drug susceptibility in the management of chemotherapy of tuberculosis, in *Drug Susceptibility in the Chemotherapy of Mycobacterial Infections*, Heifets, L. B., Ed., CRC Press LLC, Boca Raton, FL, 1991, Chap. 3.

164. Heifets, L. B., Qualitative and quantitative drug-susceptibility tests in mycobacteriology, *Am. Rev. Respir. Dis.*, 137:5, 1217, 1988.

165. McClatchy, J. K., Antimycobacterial drugs: mechanisms of action, drug resistance, susceptibility testing, and assays of activity in biological fluids, in *Antibiotics in Laboratory Medicine* Lorian, V., Ed., Williams & Wilkins, Baltimore, 1985, 181.

166. Stewart, S. M. and Crofton, J. W., The clinical significance of low degrees drug resistance in pulmonary tuberculosis, *Am. Rev. Respir. Dis.*, 89, 811, 1964.

167. Wang, C. and Lou, Y., A study of the ununiformity of drug resistance of tubercle bacilli from patients with chronic pulmonary tuberculosis, *Am. Rev. Respir. Dis.*, 141(4)(Suppl.), A448, 1990.

168. Nachamkin, I., Kang, C., and Weinstein, M. P., Detection of resistance to isoniazid, rifampin, and streptomycin in clinical isolates of *Mycobacterium tuberculosis* by molecular methods, *Clin. Infect. Dis.*, 24, 894, 1997.

169. De Beenhouwer, H., De Lhiang, Z., Jannes, G., Mijs, W., Machtelinckx, L., Rossau, R., Traore, H., and Portaels, F., Rapid detection of rifampicin resistance in sputum and biopsy specimens from tuberculosis patients by PCR and line probe assay, *Tuberc. Lung Dis.*, 76, 425, 1995.

170. Telenti, A., Imboden, P., Marchesi, F., Schmidheini, T., and Bodmer, T., Direct, atomated detection of rifampin-resistant *Mycobacterium tuberculosis* by polymerase chain reaction and single-strand conformation polymorphism analysis, *Antimicrob. Agents Chemother.*, 37, 2054, 1993.

171. International Union Against Tuberculosis, Antituberculosis regimens of chemotherapy — recommendations from the committee on treatment of the International Union Against Tuberculosis, *Bull. Int. Union Tuberc. Lung Dis.*, 63, 60, 1988.

172. Moulding, T. S., Davidson, P. T., and Goble, M., The treatment of tuberculosis, *Sem. Respir. Med.*, 2, 215, 1981.

173. Crofton, J., The prevention and management of drug-resistant tuberculosis, *Bull. Int. Union Tuberc.*, 62, 6, 1987.

174. Chen, C., Shih, J., Lindholm-Levy, P. J., and Heifets, L. B., Minimal inhibitory concentrations of rifabutin, ciprofloxacin, and ofloxacin against tuberculosis isolated before treatment of patients in Taiwan, *Am. Rev. Respir. Dis.*, 140, 987, 1989.

175. Kahana, L. M. and Spino, O., Ciprofloxacin in patients with mycobacterial infections: experience in 15 patients, *DICP*, 25, 919, 1991.

176. Tsukamura, M., Nakamura, E., Yoshii, S., and Amano, H., Therapeutic effect of a new antibacterial substance ofloxacin (DL8280) on pulmonary tuberculosis, *Am. Rev. Respir. Dis.*, 131, 352, 1985.

177. Yew, W. W., Kwan, S. Y., Ma, W. K., Khin, M. A., and Chau, P. Y., *In vitro* activity of ofloxacin against *Mycobacterium tuberculosis* and its clinical efficacy in multiply resistant pulmonary tuberculosis, *J. Antimicrob. Chemother.*, 26, 227, 1990.

178. Stocks, J. S. and Wallace, R. J., Preliminary data on the safety and efficacy of drug regimens containing ofloxacin in the therapy of multiple drug resistant mycobacterial infections, *Am. Rev. Respir. Dis.*, 135(Suppl.), A136, 1987.

179. O'Brien, R. J. and Vernon, A. A., New tuberculosis drug development. How can we do better? [editorial], *Am. J. Respir. Crit. Care Med.*, 157, 1705, 1998.

180. Alanganden, G. J. and Lerner, S. A., The clinical use of fluoroquinolones for the treatment of mycobacterial diseases, *Clin. Infect. Dis.*, 25, 1213, 1997.

181. Gillespie, S. H. and Kennedy, N., Fluoroqinolones: a new treatment for tuberculosis? *Int. J. Tuberc. Lung Dis.*, 2(4), 265, 1998.

182. Berning, S. E., Madsen, L., Iseman, M. D., and Peloquin, C. A., Long-term safety of ofloxcin and ciprofloxacin in the treatment of mycobacterial infections, *Am. J. Respir. Crit. Care Med.*, 151, 2006, 1995.

183. Peloquin, C. A., Berning, S. E., Huitt, G. A., and Iseman, M. D., Levofloxacin for drug-resistant *Mycobacterium tuberculosis* [letter], *Ann. Pharmacother.*, 32, 268, 1998.

184. Ji, B., Truffot-Pernot, C., and Grosset, J., *In vitro* and *in vivo* activity of sparfloxacin (AT-4140) against *Mycobacterium tuberculosis, Tubercle,* 72, 181, 1991.

185. Lyle, M. A. and O'Brien, R. J., Rifabutin (ansamycin LM427) for the treatment of rifampin resistant tuberculosis, *Am. Rev. Respir. Dis.*, 139(4)(Suppl.), A316, 1989.

186. O'Brien, R. J., Lyle, M. A., and Snider, D. E., Jr., Rifabutin (ansamycin LM 427): a new rifamycin-S derivative for the treatment of mycobacterial diseases, *Rev. Infect. Dis.*, 9, 519, 1987.

187. Pretet, S., Lebeaut, A., Parrot, R., Truffot, C., Grosset, J., and Dinh-Xuan, A. T., Combined chemotherapy including rifabutin for rifampicin and isoniazid-resistant pulmonary tuberculosis, *Eur. Resp. J.*, 5, 680, 1992.

188. Grassi, C. and Peona, V., Use of rifabutin in the treatment of pulmonary tuberculosis, *Clin. Infect. Dis.*, 22, S50, 1996.

189. Madsen, L., Goble, M., and Iseman, M., Ansamycin (LM 427) in the retreatment of drug-resistant tuberculosis, *Am. Rev. Respir. Dis.*, 133(Suppl.), A206, 1986.

190. De Cian, W., Sassella, D., and Wynne, B. A., Clinical experience with rifabutin in the treatment of mycobacterial infections, *Scand. J. Infect. Dis.*, 98(Suppl), 22, 1995.

191. Dhillon, J., Dickinson, J. M., Guy, J. A., Ng, T. K., and Mitchison, D. A., Activity of two long-acting rifamycins, rifapentine and FCE 22807, in experimental murine tuberculosis, *Tubercle Lung Dis.*, 73, 116, 1992.

192. Davidson, P. T., Drug resistance and the selection of therapy for tuberculosis [editorial], *Am. Rev. Respir. Dis.*, 136, 255, 1987.

193. Hong Kong Tuberculosis Treatment Services/Brompton Hospital/British Medical Research Council, A controlled clinical trial of daily and intermittent regimens of rifampicin plus ethambutol in the retreatment of patients with pulmonary tuberculosis in Hong Kong, *Tubercle*, 55, 1, 1974.

194. Poland National Research Institute, A comparative study of daily followed by twice or once weekly regimes of ethambutol and rifampicin in the retreatment of patients with pulmonary tuberculosis: second report, *Tubercle*, 57, 105, 1976.

195. Zierski, M., Prospects of retreatment of chronic resistant pulmonary tuberculosis patients. A critical review, *Lung*, 154, 91, 1977.

196. Mitchison, D. A. and Nunn, A. J., Influence of initial drug resistance on the response to short-course chemotherapy of pulmonary tuberculosis, *Am. Rev. Respir. Dis.*, 133, 423, 1986.

197. Swai, O. B., Aluoch, J., Githui, W. A., Thiong'o, R., and Edwards, E. A., Controlled clinical trial of a regimen of two durations for the treatment of isoniazid resistant pulmonary tuberculosis, *Tubercle*, 69, 5, 1988.

198. Hong Kong Chest Service/British Medical Research Council, Controlled trial of four thrice-weekly regimens and a daily regimen all given for 6 months for pulmonary tuberculosis, *Lancet*, 1, 171, 1981.

199. Hong, Y. P., Kim, S. C., Chang, S. C., Kim, S. J., Jin, B. W., and Park, C. D., Comparison of a daily and three intermittent retreatment regimens for pulmonary tuberculosis administered under programme conditions, *Tubercle*, 69, 241, 1988.

200. Hong Kong Chest Service/British Medical Research Council, Controlled trial of 2, 4 and 6 months of pyrazinamide in 6-month, three-times-weekly regimens for smear-positive tuberculosis, including an assessment of a combined preparation of isoniazid, rifampin, and pyrazinamide. Results at 30 months, *Am. Rev. Respir. Dis.*, 143, 700, 1991.

201. Donath, J. and Chitkara, R. K., Drug-resistant tuberculosis: a tactical approach to therapy, *J. Respir. Dis.*, 9, 73, 1988.

202. Goble, M., Drug-resistant tuberculosis, *Sem. Respir. Infect.*, 1, 220, 1986.

203. Iseman, M. D. and Goble, M., Treatment of tuberculosis, *Adv. Intern. Med.*, 33, 253, 1988.

204. Iseman, M. D. and Madsen, L. A., Drug-resistant tuberculosis, *Clin. Chest Med.*, 10, 341, 1989.

205. McDonald, R. J., Memon, A. M., and Reichman, L. B., Successful supervised ambulatory management of tuberculosis treatment failures, *Ann. Inter. Med.*, 96, 297, 1982.

206. Crofton, J., Treatment of patients with drug-resistance in economically developed countries, *Tubercle*, 50, 65, 1969.

207. Medical Research Council report by their Tuberculosis Chemotherapy Trials Committee, long-term chemotherapy in the treatment of chronic pulmonary tuberculosis with cavitation, *Tubercle*, 43, 201, 1962.

208. Crofton, J., Tuberculosis undefeated, *Br. Med. J.*, 2, 679, 1960.

209. Hong Kong Chest Service/British Medical Research Council, Controlled trial of 6-month and 9-month regimens of daily and intermittent streptomycin plus isoniazid plus pyrazinamide for pulmonary tuberculosis in Hong Kong, the results up to 30 months, *Am. Rev. Respir. Dis.*, 115, 727, 1977.

210. Iseman, M. D., Treatment of multidrug-resistant tuberculosis, *N. Engl. J. Med.*, 329, 784, 1993.

211. Gonzalez-Montaner, L. J., Dambrosi, A. O., and Abbate, E. H., Treatment and results of multiple resistance pulmonary tuberculosis, *Am. Rev. Respir. Dis.*, 141:4, A450, 1990.

212. Park, S. K., Kim, C. T., and Song, S. D., Outcome of therapy in 107 patients with pulmonary tuberculosis resistant to isoniazid and rifampin, *Int. J. Tuberc. Lung Dis.*, 2, 877, 1998.

213. Drobniewski, F., Is death inevitable with multiresistant TB plus HIV infection? [published erratum appears in *Lancet*, 1997 March 15; 349(9054):810], *Lancet*, 349, 71, 1997.

214. Iseman, M. D. and Goble, M., Multidrug-resistant tuberculosis [letter, comments], *N. Engl. J. Med.*, 334, 267, 1996.

215. Donaldson, R. and Wallace, A., Drug-resistant pulmonary tuberculosis treated with ethambutol, a rifamycin and a riminophenazine (B663), *Br. J. Dis. Chest*, 64, 161, 1970.

216. Cavalieri, S. J., Biehle, J. R., and Sanders, W. E., Jr., Synergistic activities of clarithromycin and antituberculous drugs against multidrug-resistant *Mycobacterium tuberculosis, Antimicrob. Agents Chemother.*, 39, 1542, 1995.

217. Nadler, J. P., Berger, J., Nord, J. A., Cofsky, R., and Saxena, M., Amoxicillin-clavulanic acid for treating drug-resistant *Mycobacterium tuberculosis, Chest*, 99(4), 1025, 1991.

218. Wayne, L. G. and Sramek, H. A., Metronidazole is bactericidal to dormant cells of *Mycobacterium tuberculosis, Antimicrob. Agents Chemother.*, 38, 2054, 1994.

219. Kristiansen, J. E. and Amaral, L., The potential management of resistant infections with non-antibiotics, *J. Antimicrob. Chemother.*, 40, 319, 1997.

220. Barry, C. E., III, New horizons in the treatment of tuberculosis, *Biochem. Pharmacol., 54, 1165, 1997.*

221. Condos, R., Rom, W. N., and Schluger, N. W., Treatment of multidrug-resistant pulminary tuberculosis with interferon-γ via aerosol, *Lancet*, 349, 1513, 1997.

222. Johnson, B. J., Bekker, L.-G., Rickman, R., Brown, S., Lesser, M., Ress, S., Willcox, P., Steyn, L., and Kaplan, G., rhuIL-2 adjunctive therapy in multidrug resistant tuberculosis: a comparison of two treatment regimens and placebo, *Tuberc. Lung Dis.,* 78, 195, 1997.

223. Etemadi, A., Farid, R., and Stanford, J. L., Immunotherapy for drug-resistant tuberculosis, [letter], *Lancet,* 340, 1360, 1992.

224. Centers for Disease Control, Development of new vaccines for tuberculosis — recommendations of the Advisory Council for the Elimination of Tuberculosis (ACET), *MMWR,* 47, 1, 1998.

225. Nitta, A. T., Iseman, M. D., Newell, J. D., Madsen, L. A., and Goble, M., Ten-year experience with artificial pneumoperitoneum for end-stage drug-resistant pulmonary tuberculosis, *Clin. Inf. Dis.,* 16, 219, 1993.

226. van Leuven, M., De Groot, M., Shean, K. P., von Oppell, U. O., and Willcox, P. A., Pulmonary resection as an adjunct in the treatment of multiple drug-resistant tuberculosis [discussion 1372-3], *Ann. Thorac. Surg.,* 63, 1368, 1997.

227. Peloquin, C. A., Antituberculosis drugs: pharmacokinetics, in *Drug Susceptibility in the Chemotherapy of Mycobacterial Infections*, Heifets, L. B., Ed., CRC Press LLC, Boca Raton, FL, 1991, Chap. 2.

228. Peloquin, C. A., Using therapeutic drug monitoring to dose the antimycobacterial drugs, in *Clinics in Chest Medicine,* 18, Iseman, M. D. and Huitt, G. A., Eds., W.B. Sanders, Philadelphia, 1997, 79.

229. Moulding, T. and Davidson, P. T., Tuberculosis II: toxicity and intolerance to antituberculosis drugs, *Drug Ther.,* 41, Feb. 1974.

230. Gonzalez-Montaner, L. J., Dambrosi, A., Manassero, M., Dambrosi, V. M., Adverse effects of antituberculosis drugs causing changes in treatment, *Tubercle,* 63, 291, 1982.

231. Hajjaj, M., Xie, H. J., Enarson, D. A., Allen, E. A., and Grzybowski, S., Serious drug toxicity in tuberculosis treatment programs, *Am. Rev. Respir. Dis.,* 141, A441, 1990.

232. Johnston, R. F. and Hopewell, P. C., Chemotherapy of pulmonary tuberculosis, *Ann. Inter. Med.,* 70, 359, 1969.

233. Matsui, M. S. and Rozovski, S. J., Drug-nutrient interactions, *Clin. Ther.,* 4, 423, 1982.

234. Seaman, J. M., Goble, M., Madsen, L., and Steigerwald, J. C., Fasciitis and polyarthritis during antituberculosis treatment, *Arthritis Rheum.,* 28, 1179, 1985.

235. Moulding, T. and Fraser, R., Hypothyroidism related to ethionamide, *Am. Rev. Respir. Dis.,* 101, 90, 1970.

236. Huang, K. L., Beutler, S. M., and Wang, C., Hypothyroidism in a patient receiving treatment for multidrug-resistant tuberculosis, *Clin. Infect. Dis.,* 27, 910, 1998.

237. Casewitt, C., Ultrasound for relief of painful injection sites, *Clin. Manage.,* 4, 50, 1983.

238. Horne, N. W. and Grant, I. W. B., Development of drug resistance to isoniazid during desensitization: a report of two cases, *Tubercle,* 44, 180, 1963.

239. Pomerantz, M. and Brown, J. M., Surgery in the treatment of multidrug-resistant tuberculosis, in *Clinics in Chest Medicine,* 18, Iseman, M. D. and Huitt, G. A., Eds., W.B. Sanders, Philadelphia, 1997, 123.

240. Hui, K. K. L. and Mary-Aquines, Sr., Surgery for first line drug-resistant tuberculosis, *Dis. Chest,* 49, 57, 1966.

241. Iseman, M. D., Madsen, L., Goble, M., and Pomerantz, M., Surgical intervention in the treatment of pulmonary disease caused by drug-resistant *Mycobacterium tuberculosis, Am. Rev. Respir. Dis.,* 141, 623, 1990.

242. Mahmoudi, A. and Iseman, M. D., Surgical intervention in the treatment of drug-resistant tuberculosis: update and extended follow-up, *Am. Rev. Respir. Dis.,* 145(Suppl.), A816, 1992.

243. Muthuswamy, P., Chechani, V., and Baker, W., Surgical management of pulmonary tuberculosis, *Am. Rev. Respir. Dis.,* 145(Suppl.), A816, 1992.

244. Zibrak, J. D., O'Donnell, C. R., and Marton, K., Indications for pulmonary function testing, *Ann. Intern. Med.,* 112, 763, 1990.

245. Griffith, D. E., The United States and worldwide tuberculosis control: a second chance for Prince Prospero [editorial], *Chest,* 113, 1434, 1998.

246. Snider, D. E., Jr. and Castro, K. G., The global threat of drug-resistant tuberculosis [editorial], *N. Engl. J. Med.,* 338, 1689, 1998.

247. Iseman, M. D., MDR-TB and the developing world — a problem no longer to be ignored: the WHO announces 'DOTS Plus' strategy [editorial], *Int. J. Tuberc. Lung Dis.,* 2, 867, 1998.

13 Skin Testing and Chemoprophylaxis

Lloyd N. Friedman, M.D.

CONTENTS

0-8493-1565-4/97/$0.00+$.50
© 2000 by CRC Press LLC

I. PURIFIED PROTEIN DERIVATIVE (PPD)

Tuberculin PPD is a purified protein derivative prepared from culture filtrates of *Mycobacterium tuberculosis*. It is employed in skin testing to detect persons infected with *M. tuberculosis*. PPD-S, lot number 49608, prepared in 1939 by Siebert and Glenn,[1] was adopted in 1951 by the World Health Organization (WHO) Expert Committee on Biologic Standardization as the international standard for tuberculin PPD.[2] The international unit, also known as the tuberculin unit (TU), is the biologic activity represented by 0.00002 mg of PPD-S. PPD-S was used for comparison testing in the formulation of all commercially prepared PPD for use in the U.S.[3,4]

II. PREPARATION OF PPD

There are two basic methods of PPD preparation: the ammonium sulfate and the trichloroacetic acid precipitation methods. In both cases, the PPD is prepared by growing large amounts of *M. tuberculosis* in liquid culture, steaming for 3 h at 100°C to sterilize, and then filtering. The filtrate undergoes a series of precipitation, washing, buffering, and centrifugation steps until it becomes the concentrated stock solution. The ammonium sulfate precipitation method results in a PPD with a higher protein and lipopolysaccharide percentage, whereas the trichloroacetic acid precipitation method results in a PPD with higher percentage of nucleic acids.[2] The preparation of old tuberculin (OT), which rarely is used, is similar to the above preparation without the precipitation and centrifugation steps.

PPD-S was formulated by the ammonium sulfate precipitation method. The commercially available Aplisol® brand (Parkedale Pharmaceuticals) also was formulated by the ammonium sulfate method, whereas Tubersol® (Connaught) was formulated by the trichloroacetic acid method. For a given strength, the commercially available PPD brands are assumed to be equal in potency and in the ability to detect tuberculous infection, although in one study, 18% of subjects who underwent paired tuberculin testing with Aplisol® and Tubersol® showed a difference of 5 mm or more between the two preparations.[5] In a similar comparison, 14% of low-risk individuals who had a skin test reaction greater than 0 mm showed a 5 mm or more difference in test results.[6]

The standard strength of PPD for skin testing is 5 TU, which is the biologic equivalent of 0.0001 mg of PPD-S. One TU is one fifth and 250 TU is 50 times the concentration of 5 TU, but this is not reflected to the same degree in their biologic equivalencies. PPD RT-23 is a standard tuberculin in use in countries other than the U.S., and 2 TU is biologically equivalent to 5 TU of PPD-S.[7]

III. SKIN TEST PLACEMENT AND REACTIONS

A. PLACEMENT

The Mantoux test has been standardized as the intradermal placement of 0.1 ml (5 TU) of PPD into the volar, or rarely, the dorsal surface of the forearm. A 27-gauge, short, beveled needle is the favored instrument of delivery. Interpretation of the test is performed within 48 to 72 h. Induration is assessed by palpation, inspection, or both, and is measured in the transverse direction only.[3,4,8,9] Other techniques, such as the ballpoint pen method, have been used with some success.[10-12] Regardless of the technique, proficiency at skin test measurement occurs only after proper training and experience.[13-15]

The following reactions have been described after intradermal PPD administration: immediate hypersensitivity; Arthus reaction; retest phenomenon (early, altered, or accelerated reaction); cutaneous basophil hypersensitivity (i.e., Jones-Mote reactivity); and delayed-type hypersensitivity (DTH).

B. REACTIONS

1. Early Reactions

The early reactions, i.e., the Arthus reaction and immediate hypersensitivity reaction, occur to one or more of the components of tuberculin. The Arthus reaction is an IgG immune complex reaction peaking in 2 to 6 h with erythema, edema, hemorrhage, and necrosis. Immediate hypersensitivity is an IgE-mediated reaction with the rapid development of a wheal and flare that usually resolves by 24 h.[8] With 250 TU, the reaction may peak in 24 h and resolve slowly.[16] In a study by Tarlo et al., immediate hypersensitivity occurred to an injection of 5 TU of PPD in 76 (2.3%) of 3248 patients who underwent tuberculin skin tests, only 3 of whom also had a DTH response.[17] Prior exposure to tuberculin was not a prerequisite for this reaction, as 28% of those evaluated had had no previous exposure to tuberculin.

2. Retest Phenomenon

The retest phenomenon is a reproducible phenomenon described in past literature.[14,16,18-20] It is a form of local hypersensitivity that occurs when a tuberculin injection is placed at the site of a previous tuberculin test and induces a markedly accelerated reaction that begins usually within 3 h, peaks at 12 to 24 h, and resolves by 48 h. It may occur as an early and more pronounced component of the usual tuberculin reaction in a tuberculin-positive individual, and is a reproducible phenomenon.[18,20] A well-controlled study of the retest phenomenon was conducted by the WHO Tuberculosis Research Office on 216 unvaccinated PPD-positive individuals.[20] Repeat tests were applied to both arms 3 months after initial testing and, on average, the reaction at the retest site was 13 mm larger than the control site at 6 h, and reached a peak much earlier. The rate of vesiculation at 24 h was 30% vs. 5% of controls. Although the retest site consistently reached a maximum induration that was approximately 4 mm greater than the control site, the induration was equivalent at 3 days, and less at 6 days. The study found no appreciable retest phenomenon with 5 TU in 14 PPD-negative individuals, but Duboczy and Brown showed that it did occur, although to a lesser degree, with higher doses of tuberculin in PPD-negative individuals.[16,19] Persistence of the phenomenon has been reported for as long as 12 years after a test.[16] It is not thought to be related to the Arthus reaction, and is thought to be closely allied to delayed-type hypersensitivity.[21]

3. Cutaneous Basophil Hypersensitivity

Cutaneous basophil hypersensitivity or Jones-Mote reactivity is thought to be a form of delayed-type hypersensitivity with a prominent infiltrate of basophils.[22,23] The pure form is not seen in humans. In guinea pigs, the sensitivity usually is transient (2 to 4 weeks) and the reaction is less indurated and more erythematous than the typical tuberculin reaction. The onset of the reaction is within 4 to 6 h after injection and is maximal at 18 to 24 h.[22] The phenomenon is transferred by lymphocytes and probably represents a response to true infection. It has been stated that it does not play an important role in PPD interpretation,[3] but there has been only one study addressing this issue in humans, and the results showed a significant basophilic response in four (44%) of nine patients with tuberculosis biopsied after PPD administration.[24] Thus, this phenomenon is thought to be part of the delayed-type hypersensitivity response to tuberculin. It has not been described as a reaction to tuberculin in nonsensitized individuals.

4. Delayed-Type Hypersensitivity

The delayed-type hypersensitivity reaction is the classic reaction to tuberculin. Infected individuals may require 4 to 6 weeks to develop a sufficient immune response to react to tuberculin, but usually not more than 3 months. A description of the clinical features associated with primary infection may be found in Chapter 6, Section I. The typical tuberculin reaction begins within 4 to 6 h after injection, is maximal at 48 to 72 h, and subsides over a few days.[25] In some cases, especially in the elderly, the peak is delayed and may be maximal at 7 days. Slutkin et al. showed that a 7-day reading could add an additional 5% to the number of persons who reacted to tuberculin.[26] In general, the reaction is indurated with erythema and may have necrosis or vesiculation. It is dependent on cell-mediated immunity and is transferrable by T lymphocytes, but not by serum antibodies. A special fibrin gel network is the essential component that allows induration rather than edema alone to occur. It has been shown in recent studies that the etiology of induration in delayed-type hypersensitivity is not simply the accumulation of cells and fluid in the skin, which can occur with any type of insult, but is related to the deposition of a special fibrin gel network which can trap and hold significant amounts of fluid, protein, and cells, so that a relatively pronounced border is present in the skin.[25,27] Support for this concept may be found in a study of two patients with afibrinogenemia who had no induration, but had normal kinetics with regard to the intensity and diameter of erythema during delayed-type hypersensitivity responses to a variety of skin test antigens.[28]

Due to the possibility of an immediate reaction, Duboczy has recommended that, for the most accurate reading, an assessment of the reaction be made at 24 and 48 h.[16] For practical purposes, a patient should return for a reading once only, but should be questioned about the course of the reaction, e.g., did the patient notice a reaction soon after placement.

C. Multiple Puncture Tests

Tuberculosis skin tests have been administered with multiple puncture techniques employing both OT and PPD, but these techniques should not be used to guide treatment decisions, unless there is vesiculation. Vesiculation is considered to be a positive reaction, and it is the only reaction that may be interpreted. In three studies, the multiple puncture test, in comparison with the Mantoux test, did not achieve 100% sensitivity, even when the cutting point was 1 mm.[29-31] The range in these three studies was 96 to 99% sensitivity; the specificity was poor. Although, in general, a completely negative PPD-multiple puncture test without any erythema or induration usually indicates that the Mantoux will be negative, this has never been proved. The Centers for Disease Control and Prevention (CDC) has stated that multiple puncture tests should not be used to screen high-risk populations.[32] For further information on this matter in children, see Chapter 8.

D. False-Positive Tests

The greatest concern with false-positive tests centers on the incidence of cross reactivity with atypical mycobacteria. The mode for the diameter of induration in persons infected with tuberculosis appears to be at 16 to 17 mm,[3] with means in various groups ranging from 12.8 to 18.8 mm.[4] The mean induration to PPD-S after exposure to nontuberculous mycobacteria has been estimated to be 8 mm with very few reactions at 15 mm.[33] Therefore, a cutting point of 15 mm of induration will eliminate cross reactivity almost completely, but will decrease sensitivity.[34] A cutting point of 5 mm will yield much more cross reactivity, but will enhance the sensitivity markedly.[3]

Bacille Calmette-Guérin (BCG) vaccination also can cause false-positive reactions (see Section XIII, as well as Chapter 15).

E. BOOSTER PHENOMENON

Any PPD-reactive individual may lose skin test reactivity,[35] and persons over 55 years of age are particularly susceptible to this loss.[8,32,36] The booster phenomenon refers to the ability of a negative tuberculin skin test to reactivate the immune response in a previously infected person and cause a subsequent skin test to become positive.[37,38] PPD in standard doses cannot cause systemic sensitization. Thus, a boosted skin test represents true immunologic memory. The elderly in nursing homes, who require yearly skin test screening, are particularly prone to this phenomenon.[36,39] The prevalence of the booster phenomenon has been reported to be as high as 15% in elderly persons with an initially negative PPD.[26] If a second test is placed 1 year after the first in a PPD-negative individual who has a history of tuberculous infection, it might appear as if the individual is a new convertor. Therefore, all individuals undergoing repeated yearly skin tests should anticipate a two-step procedure,[8] as well as all individuals with diminished immune responses.[40] In persons in whom the first test is read negative, a second test should be performed 1 to 3 weeks after placement of the first test. The reading of the second test is the final result.[32]

A third sequential skin test also has been shown to add to the overall rate of tuberculin positivity. Gordin et al. showed that of 1726 elderly persons, 477 (28%) were positive to a first test, 158 (9%) were positive to a second test, and 67 (4%) were positive to a third test.[41] Some have even placed four tests.[42] However, at this time, tuberculin testing should be limited to two sequential tests due to problems with the reproducibility and, therefore, validity of boosted reactions that are less than 15 mm in diameter.[43]

There is some concern that a boosted response may, in certain circumstances, be due to BCG vaccination.[44-50] This will be discussed in Section XIII.

F. ANERGY IN NONIMMUNOCOMPROMISED HOSTS

False-negative tests may be due to a host of causes (Table 13.1). An addition to the usual list is clotting function abnormalities such as those found in persons with congenital afibrinogenemia, disseminated intravascular coagulation, hepatic failure, or in persons on anticoagulants, such as coumarin or heparin. The reduction or absence of induration is due to the lack of the special fibrin gel network mentioned earlier.

Even if none of these causes is present, 17.4 to 21.0% of patients with tuberculosis had less than 5 mm of induration response to 5 TU of PPD in three studies,[51-53] and 19.1 to 24.5% had less than 10 mm of induration in three studies.[51,52,54] Nash and Douglass found that 49 (24.5%) of 200 patients with active pulmonary tuberculosis had less than 10 mm of induration response to 5 TU of PPD, and 16 (8%) also were anergic to 250 TU PPD (<10 mm), with positive control antigens.[54] Rooney et al. showed that 16 (76%) of 21 tuberculosis patients with an initially negative response to PPD became reactive (induration of 5 mm or greater) after 2 weeks of treatment and nutritional support.[52] Proposed pathophysiologic mechanisms of skin test anergy in otherwise healthy hosts with tuberculosis may be found in Chapter 2.

Anergy testing may be performed with injections of candida antigen, mumps antigen, trichophyton antigen, diluted tetanus toxoid, streptokinase/streptodornase antigen, or the multiple puncture Multitest® (tetanus toxoid antigen, diphtheria toxoid antigen, streptococcus antigen, old tuberculin, candida antigen, trichophyton antigen, proteus antigen, and a glycerine control). The Multitest® does not deliver a standard amount of antigen. Furthermore, it does not contain mumps antigen. If anergy testing is performed, at least two separate injectable antigens, to which most healthy persons in the population would be sensitized, should be used. In one study that compared injections of tetanus toxoid, candida, mumps, and trichopyton in HIV-positive individuals, persons with more than 800 CD4 cells reacted most often to tetanus (88.5%), and those with 200 CD4 cells or less reacted most often to mumps (21.3%).[55] HIV-related anergy will be discussed below in Section VI,B,3,b.

TABLE 13.1
Factors Causing False-Negative Tuberculin Skin Tests

Factors related to the person being tested
    Infections
        Viral (measles, mumps, chicken pox, HIV)
        Bacterial (typhoid fever, brucellosis, typhus, leprosy, pertussis, overwhelming tuberculosis, tuberculous pleurisy)
        Fungal (South American blastomycosis)
    Live virus vaccinations (measles, mumps, polio, varicella)
    Metabolic derangements (chronic renal failure)
    Low protein states (severe protein depletion, afibrinogenemia)
    Diseases affecting lymphoid organs (Hodgkin's disease, lymphoma, chronic lymphocytic leukemia, sarcoidosis)
    Drugs (corticosteroids and many other immunosuppressive agents)
    Age (newborns, elderly patients with "waned" sensitivity)
    Stress (surgery, burns, mental illness, graft vs. host reactions)
Factors related to the tuberculin used
    Improper storage (exposure to light and heat)
    Improper dilutions
    Chemical denaturation
    Contamination
    Adsorption (partially controlled by adding Tween^R 80)
Factors related to the method of administration
    Injection of too little antigen
    Subcutaneous injection
    Delayed administration after drawing into syringe
    Injection too close to other skin tests
Factors related to reading the test and recording results
    Inexperienced reader
    Conscious or unconscious bias
    Error in recording

Source: American Thoracic Society/Centers for Disease Control and Prevention, *Am. J. Respir. Crit. Care Med.,* 161, 1376, 2000.

IV. SCREENING

The focus of tuberculosis screening has changed to target those groups most likely to benefit from treatment of latent tuberculosis infection (LTBI).[56] Targeted screening helps to concentrate resources where they are needed most, upon those persons at highest risk for recent infection and upon those persons at highest susceptibility for developing disease once infected (Table 13.2). The new statement from the American Thoracic Society (ATS) and the CDC entitled, "Targeted Tuberculin Testing and Treatment of Latent Tuberculous Infection," is a detailed document that addresses these issues.[56] In most circumstances, persons should be screened only if there is a plan to treat infected individuals. Low-risk individuals no longer are screened except upon initial entry into a high-risk setting, e.g., a new hire into a healthcare setting. In certain circumstances where there is great risk or high turnover, e.g., certain jails and homeless shelters, it is more appropriate to use chest radiography as the primary screening tool if there are signs or symptoms of pulmonary or pleural tuberculosis.[57] Although not on the list, potential organ donors also should be screened because of the risk to a recipient that a dormant infection might pose in an organ.[58-66] It is not necessary to treat such individuals, but their skin test status should be known.

    Although alcoholism has long been associated with tuberculosis,[67] it is not considered to be an indication for screening unless it is associated with another risk factor, such as homelessness.[32,56]

    Pet dogs and cats in close contact with a tuberculosis case should be screened. Although there have been no reported cases of transmission from pet to human, it certainly is possible that this might occur, as organisms have been recovered from laryngeal swabs of pet dogs, and fulminant lung lesions have been documented. Dogs react well to tuberculin and cats do not, but skin testing is not considered reliable in either and a chest radiograph should be performed. Preventive therapy

TABLE 13.2
Indications for Screening and Treatment

<5 mm Induration	≥ 5 mm Induration	≥ 10 mm Induration	≥ 15 mm Induration
Recent contacts who are HIV positive or are otherwise significantly immunocompromised (prescribe full course of therapy)	HIV-positive persons	Recent immigrants (within the last 5 years) from high-prevalence countries	Persons with no risk factors for TB[a]
Children <5 years old who are close contacts (HIV negative) — treat for 8 to 12 weeks after contact is broken, then retest[c]	Recent contacts of TB case (HIV negative)	Injection drug users	
	Fibrotic changes on chest radiograph consistent with old TB	Resident and employees[b] of high-risk congregate settings: prisons and jails, nursing homes and other long-term facilities for the elderly, hospitals and other healthcare facilities, residential facilities for AIDS patients, and homeless shelters	
	Patients with organ transplants and other immunosuppressed patients (receiving the equivalent of ≥ 15 mg/day of prednisone for ≥ 1 month)[d], or any other stronger chemotherapeutic agent for any length of time	Mycobacteriology lab personnel	
		Persons with clinical conditions that place them at high risk: silicosis, diabetes mellitus, chronic renal failure, some hematologic disorders (e.g., leukemias and lymphomas), other specific malignancies (e.g., carcinoma of the head or neck and lung), weight loss of ≥ 10% of ideal body weight, gastrectomy, jejunoileal bypass	
		Children < 4 years of age or infants, children, and adolescents exposed to adults in high-risk categories	

Note: Recent convertors, i.e., persons with an increase in induration of 10 mm or more within a 2-year period, should be treated regardless of age. Also, all individuals who meet the criteria for prophylaxis should receive a chest radiograph to evaluate for active tuberculosis before starting therapy; HIV-infected individuals should have sputum collected for AFB, even if the chest radiograph is normal.

[a] Generally not screened except upon initial entry into a high-exposure setting, such as a new prisoner who is not otherwise in a high risk group.

[b] For persons who are otherwise at low risk and are tested at entry into employment, a reaction of ≥ 15 mm induration is considered positive.

[c] Interim treatment also may be considered for other close contacts, especially for children < 15 years old.[8]

[d] Risk of TB in patients treated with corticosteroids increases with higher doses and longer duration.

Source: American Thoracic Society and Centers for Disease Control and Prevention, *Am. J. Respir. Crit. Care Med.*, 161, S221, 2000.

for these animals is recommended by some regardless of skin test status. Treatment of disease is very successful with current regimens.[68,69]

Since persons with active tuberculosis may be anergic to tuberculin even when they are otherwise healthy, it probably is not useful to place a skin test as part of the workup of active tuberculosis, especially in hospitalized patients who may have additional reasons to be transiently anergic. If a patient with a positive skin test has pneumonia, the likelihood that the patient has tuberculosis is dependent more upon the prevalence of tuberculosis in that patient's specific population than on the skin test result. Similarly, if a patient has a negative skin test with radiographic evidence and signs and symptoms of tuberculosis, he must be evaluated fully for active tuberculosis regardless of the skin test result. There may be certain circumstances where a positive skin test is helpful in diagnosing active tuberculosis, such as in children, but these should be evaluated on a case-by-case basis. Furthermore, it may be misleading to place a tuberculin test in a hospitalized patient because if that patient has latent tuberculosis, is transiently anergic to tuberculin, and tests positive later as an outpatient, it will appear as if he has converted his skin test when actually he has not.

In HIV-infected anergic individuals, one should consider retesting with tuberculin if, as a result of antiretroviral therapy, the immune system has responded sufficiently, and it is felt that there might be a response to skin tests.[70]

V. INTERPRETATION

Once these individuals have been screened, those who are considered infected, based on the cutting points listed in Table 13.2, should be questioned and examined for signs and symptoms of tuberculosis and should have a chest radiograph performed. These cutting points are based on the likelihood that the degree of induration represents true infection with tuberculosis (based on the prevalence of infection with typical and atypical mycobacteria in the region of interest), that the risk of developing tuberculosis once infected is high, and that the ability of isoniazid to prevent the development of disease outweighs the risk of isoniazid hepatitis. A reduction in active cases with treatment has been shown clearly for infected close contacts, persons with fibrotic lesions, and HIV-positive individuals (see later). However, strong data for other groups are not as secure, and many risk groups are represented by merit of their association with an increased incidence of tuberculous disease. Individuals with a high risk of exposure, such as foreign-born individuals who have entered the country within 5 years, have an increased risk of recent exposure to tuberculosis and, thus, an increased risk of developing the disease. The medical risk groups contain subsets almost surely at increased risk, and although they have not been studied in a well-controlled fashion, the data are compelling. Some of the pertinent information may be found in Section VI,B,6.

Vesiculation indicates that a test is positive regardless of the degree of induration or the method of placement (i.e., multiple puncture or intradermal). Treatment should be administered accordingly.

Other factors that may merit specific consideration at 10 mm but are not mentioned specifically in the official statements are radiation therapy to the lung[71,72] and collagen vascular diseases such as systemic lupus erythematosus,[73] although it is difficult to separate the immunosuppressive effects of treatment from the actual disease.

VI. TREATMENT OF LATENT TUBERCULOSIS INFECTION (LTBI)

Strictly speaking, the therapy we have called "chemoprophylaxis" is actually treatment of infection.[74] The burden of organisms in tuberculous infection is low and, thus, the development of resistance is not a major problem. Therefore, single-drug therapy with isoniazid represents an adequate course, and combination therapy might be even more effective. The CDC uses the term "primary prophylaxis" to refer to the initial treatment after exposure to tuberculosis.[70] It represents an attempt to prevent tuberculosis from infecting the individual, which is part of the purpose for beginning therapy immediately in exposed children and adolescents.

The current recommendations for treatment are found in Tables 13.2 and 13.3,[56] and are discussed below. The major changes since the previous recommendations published in 1994[75] are listed in Table 13.4. Isoniazid for 9 months now is a primary recommendation for all individuals. It also is possible, in special circumstances, to treat with rifampin and pyrazinamide for 2 months or rifampin for 4 months (see below).

Persons with a history of tuberculous disease, who were not treated with an adequate course of chemotherapy and do not have active disease presently, should receive treatment for LTBI. This includes persons treated with surgical techniques before the introduction of adequate chemotherapeutic regimens.

In order to truly eradicate tuberculosis worldwide, we must treat tuberculous infection aggressively because most active cases arise from the infected pool. Safer and more potent drugs, as well as shorter durations of therapy, will be crucial aspects of this attempt. If a safe and effective alternative to isoniazid (i.e., a single depot injection that results in a 90% reduction in cases) was developed and administered simultaneously to an entire at-risk population, there is a possibility that the tuberculosis incidence in that population could be reduced to one tenth its current rate within 1 year. This strategy should be a global priority.

A. MEDICATIONS (TABLE 13.5)

1. Isoniazid

Nine months of isoniazid, 5 mg/kg up to 300 mg/day, has been recommended for tuberculin-positive individuals, especially those who are HIV-positive or have fibrotic lesions. There are no controlled data to show the equivalency of 9 months and 12 months of therapy, although a study from Bethel, AK, from the late 1950s, has shown that there is little to be gained from treating for longer than 9 months.[76,77] There is limited justification for treating compliant patients with isoniazid for 6 months (see Section VI,B,2), but this regimen may be used if there are compliance or toxicity problems. For high-risk adults who are likely to be noncompliant, directly observed intermittent therapy should be considered strongly.

2. Two Months of Rifampin and Pyrazinamide

Two months of daily pyrazinamide with rifampin or rifabutin in HIV-infected, PPD-positive individuals now is an acceptable option to treat LTBI (see Tables 13.2 and 13.3).[56,70] There is a long history of reductions in the duration of therapy for infection and disease. In 1994, the ATS and CDC reduced the duration of chemoprophylaxis by suggesting the use of multidrug chemotherapy in persons with fibrotic lesions or silicosis.[75] This recommendation was based on the use of such regimens in smear-negative, culture-negative tuberculosis (see Section VI,B,2, as well as Chapter 6). In 1989, Grosset recommended the study of a course of 2 to 3 months of isoniazid, rifampin, and pyrazinamide.[78] In 1997, Whalen et al. showed a statistically significant reduction (compared to placebo) of 57 to 59% when 3 months of daily isoniazid and rifampin, with or without pyrazinamide, were used in HIV-positive, PPD-positive adults in Uganda.[79] Halsey et al. compared 2 months of twice-weekly rifampin and pyrazinamide with 6 months of twice-weekly isoniazid in HIV-positive, PPD-positive individuals, and showed no significant difference by the Kaplan-Meier estimate of risk at 36 months (i.e., 5.4% vs. 5.1%, respectively), although a significant benefit in favor of isoniazid was noted during the first 10 months (i.e., 3.7% vs. 1.0%, respectively, $p = 0.03$).[80]

Mwinga et al. also did not find a significant difference between these same two regimens in a similar study, but the number of subjects was too small to draw definite conclusions.[81] Gordin et al. compared 2 months of daily rifampin and pyrazinamide with 12 months of daily isoniazid in HIV-positive, PPD-positive individuals, and found no significant difference in tuberculosis rates, i.e., 0.8 cases per 100 person years vs. 1.1 cases per 100 person years, respectively.[82] Based on similar benefits of the two treatment regimens, the ATS/CDC has approved treatment of LTBI in

TABLE 13.3
Recommended Drug Regimens for Treatment of Latent Tuberculosis (TB) Infection in Adults

Drug	Interval and Duration	Comments	Rating[a] (Evidence)[b] HIV−	Rating[a] (Evidence)[b] HIV+
Isoniazid	Daily for 9 months[c,d]	In human immunodeficiency virus (HIV)-infected patients, isoniazid may be administered concurrently with nucleoside reverse transcriptase inhibitors (NRTIs), protease inhibitors, or nonnucleoside reverse transcriptase inhibitors (NNRTIs)	A (II)	A (II)
	Twice weekly for 9 months[c,d]	Directly observed therapy (DOT) must be used with twice-weekly dosing.	B(II)	B (II)
Isoniazid	Daily for 6 months[d]	Not indicated for HIV-infected persons, those with fibrotic lesions on chest radiographs, or children	B (I)	C (I)
	Twice weekly for 6 months[d]	DOT must be used with twice-weekly dosing	B (II)	C (I)
Rifampin plus pyrazinamide	Daily for 2 months	May also be offered to persons who are contacts of patients with isoniazid-resistant, rifampin-susceptible TB. In HIV-infected patients, protease inhibitors or NNRTIs generally should not be administered concurrently with rifampin; rifabutin can be used as an alternative for patients treated with indinavir, nelfinavir, amprenivir, ritonavir, or efavirenz, and possibly with nevirapine or soft-gel saquinavir[e]	B (II)	A (I)
	Twice weekly for 2–3 months	DOT must be used with twice-weekly dosing	C (II)	C (I)
Rifampin	Daily for 4 months	For persons who cannot tolerate pyrazinamide For persons who are contacts of patients with isoniazid-resistant, rifampin-susceptible TB who cannot tolerate pyrazinamide	B (II)	B (III)

[a] Strength of recommendation: A = preferred, B = acceptable alternative, C = offer when A and B cannot be given.

[b] Quality of evidence: I = randomized clinical trial data, II = data from clinical trials that are not randomized or were conducted in other populations, III = expert opinion.

[c] Recommended regimen for children < 18 years of age.

[d] Recommended regimens for pregnant women. Some experts would use rifampin and pyrazinamide for 2 months as an alternative regimen in HIV-infected pregnant women, although pyrazinamide should be avoided during the first trimester.

[e] Rifabutin should not be used with hard-gel saquinavir or delavirdine. When used with other protease inhibitors or NNRTIs, dose adjustment of rifabutin may be required (see Table 13.5).

Source: Adapted from American Thoracic Society/Centers for Disease Control and Prevention, *Am. J. Respir. Crit. Care Med.*, 161, S221, 2000.

TABLE 13.4
Changes from Prior Recommendations on Tuberculin Testing and Treatment of Latent Tuberculosis Infection (LTBI)

Tuberculin Testing

Emphasis on targeted tuberculin testing among persons at high risk for recent LTBI or with clinical conditions that increase the risk for tuberculosis (TB), regardless of age; testing is discouraged among persons at lower risk

For patients with organ transplants and other immunosuppressed persons (e.g., persons receiving the equivalent of ≥ 15 mg/day of prednisone for ≥ 1 month), 5-mm induration rather than 10-mm induration as a cut-off level for tuberculin positivity

A tuberculin skin test conversion is defined as an increase of ≥ 10 mm of induration within a 2-year period, regardless of age

No distinction made in any category for persons who are older or younger than 35 years old

Treatment of Latent Tuberculosis Infection

For human immunodeficiency virus (HIV)-negative persons, isoniazid given for 9 months is preferred over 6-month regimens

For HIV-positive persons and those with fibrotic lesions on chest x-ray consistent with previous TB, isoniazid should be given for 9 months instead of 12 months

For HIV-negative and HIV-positive persons, rifampin and pyrazinamide should be given for 2 months

For HIV-negative and HIV-positive persons, rifampin should be given for 4 months

Clinical and Laboratory Monitoring

Routine baseline and follow-up laboratory monitoring can be eliminated in most persons with LTBI, except for those with HIV infection, pregnant women (or those in the immediate postpartum period), and persons with chronic liver disease or those who use alcohol regularly

Emphasis on clinical monitoring for signs and symptoms of possible adverse effects, with prompt evaluation and changes in treatment, as indicated

Source: Adapted from American Thoracic Society/Centers for Disease Control and Prevention, *Am. J. Respir. Crit. Care Med.,* 161, S221, 2000.

HIV-infected, PPD-positive individuals with 2 months of daily rifampin and pyrazinamide. Intermittent therapy may be used if there is no alternative. Rifabutin may be substituted for rifampin where necessary (see the next section and Table 13.3). However, clinicians should use caution when administering this 2-month, 2-drug prophylactic regimen until more data are available.

The CDC also has stated that this 2-month, 2-drug regimen of pyrazinamide and a rifamycin is acceptable in normal hosts, although they state that there are no data to support this recommendation.[56,83] Clinicians must be aware that data from HIV-positive individuals do not necessarily translate to normal hosts. The interaction of the immune response with the organism is different in HIV-infected hosts where the organism may not be as well contained by granulomas and may be more accessible to chemotherapy. Thus, further study will be necessary in larger cohorts in all settings to confirm the safety and efficacy of this 2-month prophylactic regimen.

3. Rifamycins

Four months of daily rifampin has been recommended for patients who cannot take other regimens, such as patients with isoniazid-resistant tuberculosis who cannot tolerate pyrazinamide (see Table 13.3). This recommendation is based primarily on a study from Hong Kong in patients with silicosis where rifampin for 12 weeks, isoniazid and rifampin for 12 weeks, and isoniazid alone for 24 weeks were found to have similar efficacy and, when the groups were combined, reduced the incidence of tuberculosis by approximately 50% when compared to placebo.[84] In the 3-month rifampin group, the reduction was actually 63% at 5 years, but this was not analyzed separately. Because these

TABLE 13.5
Medications to Treat Latent Tuberculosis Infection: Doses, Toxicities, and Monitoring Requirements

Drug	Oral Dose in mg/kg (max. dose)				Adverse Reactions	Monitoring	Comments
	Daily		Twice Weekly[a]				
	Adults	Children	Adults	Children			
Isoniazid	5 (300 mg)	10–20 (300 mg)	15 (900 mg)	20–40 (900 mg)	Rash Hepatic enzyme elevation Hepatitis Peripheral neuropathy Mild central nervous system effects Drug interactions resulting in increased phenytoin (dilantin) or disulfiram (antabuse) levels	Clinical monitoring monthly Liver function tests[b] at baseline in selected cases[c] and repeat measurements if: Baseline results are abnormal Patient is pregnant, in the immediate postpartum period or at high risk for adverse reactions Patient has symptoms of adverse reactions	Hepatitis risk increases with age and alcohol consumption Pyridoxine (Vitamin B_6, 10 to 25 mg/day) might prevent peripheral neuropathy and central nervous system effects
Rifampin	10 (600 mg)	10–20 (600 mg)	10 (600mg)	—	Rash Hepatitis Fever Thrombocytopenia Flu-like symptoms Orange-colored body fluids (secretions, urine, tears)	Clinical monitoring at weeks 2, 4, and 8 when pyrazinamide given Complete blood count, platelets and liver function tests[b] at baseline in selected cases[c] and repeat measurements if: Baseline results are abnormal Patient has symptoms of adverse reactions	Rifampin is contraindicated or should be used with caution in human immunodeficiency virus (HIV)-infected patients taking protease inhibitors (PIs) or nonnucleoside reverse transcriptase inhibitors (NNRTIs). Decreases levels of many drugs (e.g., methadone, coumadin derivatives, glucocorticoids, hormonal contraceptives, estrogens, oral hypoglycemic agents, digitalis, anticonvulsants, dapsone, ketoconazole, and cyclosporin). Might permanently discolor soft contact lenses

Drug	Daily dose, mg/kg (maximum)	Intermittent dose, mg/kg (maximum)[a]	Adverse reactions	Monitoring	Comments
Rifabutin	5 (300 mg)[c]	—	Rash Hepatitis Fever Thrombocytopenia Orange-colored body fluids (secretions, urine, tears) With increased levels of rifabutin Severe arthralgias Uveitis Leukopenia	Clinical monitoring at weeks 2, 4, and 8 when pyrazinamide given Complete blood count, platelets, and liver function tests[b] at baseline in selected cases[c] and repeat measurements if: Baseline results are abnormal Patient has symptoms of adverse reactions Use adjusted daily dose of rifabutin and monitor for decreased antiretroviral activity and for rifabutin toxicity if rifabutin taken concurrently with PIs or NNRTIs[d]	Rifabutin is contraindicated for HIV-infected patients taking hard-gel saquinavir (Invirase™) or delavirdine; caution is also advised if rifabutin is administered with soft-gel saquinavir Reduces levels of many drugs (e.g., PIs, NNTRIs, methadone, dapsone, ketoconazole, coumadin derivatives, hormonal contraceptives, digitalis, sulfonylureas, diazepam, beta-blockers, anticonvulsants, and theophylline) Might permanently discolor contact lenses
Pyrazinamide	15–20 (2.0 g)	50 (4.0 g)	Gastrointestinal upset Hepatitis Rash Arthralgias Gout (rare)	Clinical monitoring at weeks 2, 4, and 8 Liver function tests[b] at baseline in selected cases[c] and repeat measurements if: Baseline results are abnormal Patient has symptoms of adverse reactions	Treat hyperuricemia only if patient has symptoms Might make glucose control more difficult in persons with diabetes Should be avoided in pregnancy but can be given after first trimester

[a] All intermittent dosing should be administered by directly observed therapy.

[b] AST or ALT and serum bilirubin.

[c] HIV infection, history of liver disease, alcoholism, and pregnancy.

[d] If nelfinavir, indinavir, amprenavir, or ritonavir is administered with rifabutin, blood concentrations of these protease inhibitors decrease. Thus, the dose of rifabutin is reduced from 300 to 150 mg per day when used with nelfinavir, indinavir, or amprenavir; and to 150 mg every other day (two or three times a week) when used with ritonavir. If efavirenz is administered with rifabutin, blood concentrations of rifabutin decrease. Thus, when rifabutin is used concurrently with efavirenz, the daily dose of rifabutin should be increased from 300 to 450 mg or 600 mg. Pharmacokinetic studies suggest that rifabutin might be given at usual doses with nevirapine. It is not currently known whether dose adjustment of rifabutin is required when used concurrently with soft-gel saquinavir. For patients receiving multiple PIs or a PI in combination with an NNRTI, drug interactions with rifabutin are likely more complex; in such situations, the use of rifabutin is not recommended until additional data are available.

Source: Adapted from American Thoracic Society/Centers for Disease Control and Prevention, *Am. J. Respir. Crit. Care Med.,* 161, S221, 2000.

individuals still had a high rate of development of tuberculosis (i.e., 4% per year for the combined group), it was thought that an extra month of treatment would be beneficial for broad application of this regimen.[56] Further proof of the effectiveness of this regimen will be necessary.

Rifampin was used as a sole agent in prophylaxis for a mean duration of 6.4 months in a study of Boston's homeless. None of 49 persons with documented conversions with isoniazid/streptomycin-resistant tuberculosis developed disease over a median of 27 months of follow-up, as opposed to 8.6% in the placebo group and 7.9% in the isoniazid group.[85] Six months of rifampin also was used effectively in a study of 157 adolescents recently exposed to isoniazid-resistant tuberculosis, of whom 134 (87%) had a tuberculin skin test reaction of at least 10 mm.[86] There were 41 (26%) persons with adverse effects, 18 who had therapy temporarily suspended, 2 permanently. There were no cases of active tuberculosis over a 2-year follow-up period. The estimated protective effect, based on the expected number of cases, was 56%.

Rifapentine is not recommended as a rifampin substitute because its safety and effectiveness have not been established in patients with HIV-related tuberculosis.[70]

The clinician should be familiar with other drug interactions with the rifamycins that might cause the need for dosage adjustments. Such drugs include antiretroviral agents (see below) methadone, barbiturates, hormonal contraceptives, dapsone, ketoconazole, fluconazole, itraconazole, narcotics, anticoagulants, corticosteroids, cardiac glycosides, hypoglycemics (sulfonylureas), diazepam, beta-blockers, anticonvulsants, and theophylline.

Uveitis has been reported in patients receiving rifabutin with clarithromycin, and may be mitigated by using reduced dosages of rifabutin (see Chapter 11).

a. Rifamycins and Antiretroviral Agents (see Table 13.5)

Unfortunately the protease inhibitors (PI) and the nonnucleoside reverse transcriptase inhibitors (NNRTI) generally cannot be administered with rifampin because of problems with drug metabolism, although the nucleoside reverse transcriptase inhibitors (NRTI) may be given with rifampin.[56,70] However, rifabutin is not as potent a P450 enzyme inducer as rifampin, and can be used, with dosage adjustments, with many protease inhibitors and NNRTIs. No dosage adjustment is necessary for the NRTIs. The dosage of rifabutin should be reduced to 150 mg for daily regimens (intermittent dosing should not be used unless there is no alternative) with the protease inhibitors nelfinavir, indinavir, and amprenavir, and it should be further reduced to 150 mg every other day or three times a week with ritonavir.[56,70,87] Experts do not know whether rifabutin dose modifications are needed where soft-gel saquinavir (Fortavase™) is used, and it may be best to avoid the use of this drug with rifabutin. Information about efavirenz also is limited, but because it reduces the concentration of rifabutin, it is recommended that the dose of rifabutin be increased to 450 mg.[56] Rifabutin is contraindicated with hard-gel saquinavir (Invirase™) and delavirdine.[56,70] Until more data are available, rifabutin should be avoided in persons receiving multiple PIs or a PI in combination with an NNRTI. Information about the interactions of these drugs with rifabutin is controversial and changing rapidly. Therefore, it is strongly recommended that an expert in the use of antiretroviral agents be consulted for dosage adjustments when a patient receiving these medications must be treated with an antituberculosis regimen.

B. Risk Factors

1. Close Contacts, Recent Convertors, and Skin Test Reversion

a. Close Contacts and Recent Convertors

It is recommended that children < 5 years old who have been close contacts of infectious persons within the past 3 months and have negative skin tests should receive isoniazid for at least 8 to 12 weeks after the last contact with the infectious source, at which time the skin test should be repeated.[56] If the repeat skin test is positive (5 mm or greater), therapy should be continued. These youngsters are at high risk for developing both infection and disease, and the opportunity to eradicate

TABLE 13.6
Risk of Tuberculosis in Close Contacts: Percentage Reduction With Isoniazid

Induration	No.	Risk of TB (1st Year/%)	Risk of TB (10 years/%)
5–9 mm			
Placebo	1616	0.5	1.9
Isoniazid	1716	0.2	1.0
Reduction (%)		65	45
≥ 10 mm			
Placebo	4992	1.2	2.9
Isoniazid	4852	0.2	1.2
Reduction (%)		80	60
< 5 mm initially and ≥ 5 mm at 1 year			
Placebo	867	2.0	3.7
Isoniazid	694	0.6	1.4
Reduction (%)		71	61

Source: Adapted from Ferebee, S. H., *Adv. Tuberc. Res.,* 17, 28, 1970.

the organism at this stage is one that should not be missed. Interim therapy also may be considered for other close contacts, especially for children < 15 years old.[8] Immunocompromised close contacts should be treated with a full course of therapy, regardless of the skin test result (see Table 13.2).

Before the acquired immunodeficiency syndrome (AIDS) crisis, the highest rate of development of disease from infection was in new-convertor, close contacts. In the U.S. Public Health Service (USPHS) trials, Ferebee found that there were 867 household contacts who were initially negative and converted to positive (5 mm or greater) within the first year.[74] Of those, 17 (2.0%) developed tuberculosis during the first year and 32 (3.7%) developed tuberculosis during the first 10 years (Table 13.6). This rate of disease was higher than in those who were initially skin-test positive at 10 mm. There is considerable evidence to support the use of immediate isoniazid after exposure to a tuberculosis case because of the possibility of eradicating the infection completely and reverting the skin test (see below).

Close contacts who already have converted their skin tests (i.e., 5 mm or greater) also are at high risk for the development of tuberculosis disease, with the highest rate in the first year. Ferebee, in a review of chemoprophylaxis trials, described the rate of development of disease in the first year to be between 0.6 and 7.5% of those infected,[74] with a 75% reduction in new cases by the second year. Data from the USPHS trials of household contacts show that the risk of disease in the U.S. appears to be less than that in other countries. This may be explained by the increased intensity and duration of exposure of persons in developing countries. In fact, Grzybowski et al. have shown that persons exposed to a high bacillary load not only are at greater risk for developing infection, but also are at greater risk for developing disease once infected.[88]

In the USPHS trials, 27,847 household contacts of persons with active tuberculosis were evaluated.[74] Subjects were randomized to isoniazid or placebo. Data for the convertors are presented in Table 13.6. As mentioned earlier, those persons who converted at 5 mm by the end of the first year of observation were at the highest risk for developing tuberculosis. Initial reactions of 10 mm or more were next highest, followed by initial reactions 5 mm or more, and less than 10 mm. Overall, the reduction of risk with isoniazid prophylaxis was 60 to 70%, but it varied widely between groups. The group of household contacts, who took at least 80% of their pills for a period of at least 10 months, enjoyed a 68% reduction in cases of tuberculosis over a 10-year period (88% during the treatment year and 60% in posttreatment years). These data show clearly the increased risk of developing tuberculosis in close contacts, even at 5 mm of induration, and support the use of isoniazid prophylaxis in close contacts at this level of induration. The protective effect of isoniazid is thought to continue even after the therapy ceases.[76]

"Recent convertors" are those persons with an increase in induration of 10 mm or more within a 2-year period.[56] They should be treated regardless of age.

b. Skin Test Reversion

Skin test reversion is the occurrence of a negative skin test in a person who was positive previously. It may occur spontaneously, but has been shown to be associated with chemoprophylaxis.

Experimental data to support the immediate use of isoniazid may be found in studies of guinea pigs inoculated intraperitoneally with high doses of tuberculous organisms and treated immediately with isoniazid to prevent skin test conversion or facilitate skin test reversion.[89] Clinical studies also have addressed reversion rates. Grzybowski and Allen showed the rate of reversion to be 22% in a young treated population (0 to 19 years).[90] Dahlstrom et al. found a 15% reversion rate in children on isoniazid for 1 year vs. a 3.6% reversion rate in controls.[91] In the USPHS trial, there were an equivalent amount of reverters in the placebo group (6.5%) and the isoniazid group (7.9%), suggesting little effect of isoniazid on the early eradication of organisms.[74] However, Houk et al., in a well-designed study, showed a dramatic 89% reversion rate in 179 naval personnel on isoniazid.[92] They showed clearly that this effect was related to the speed with which chemoprophylaxis was initiated after infection, with 100% reversion rates in persons started within 3 months; most reversions occurred after only 3 months of therapy. There were no reversions in controls that were known to be PPD-positive for at least 1 year. This study was important because the infections occurred aboard a ship with one primary source case, and allowed for relatively accurate timing of exposure and infection.

2. Fibrotic Lesions

Stable upper lobe fibrotic lesions associated with a positive PPD (i.e., 5 mm or greater) are assumed to be tubercular and are at increased risk for reactivation. Persons with such lesions have been shown to benefit from isoniazid prophylaxis. The largest study involved 27,830 persons from Eastern Europe and was performed by the International Union Against Tuberculosis.[93] The entry criteria included a PPD skin test reaction larger than 5 mm with a radiograph that showed "well delineated lesions of probable tuberculous origin, usually in the upper half of the lung, which had been stable during the year prior to entry."[94] There were four treatment groups: placebo, 12 weeks of isoniazid, 24 weeks of isoniazid, and 52 weeks of isoniazid. Lesions were categorized in 67% of persons as less than 2 cm², and in 30% of persons as 2 cm² or greater. Active tuberculosis was defined as a culture-positive case. The rate of development of tuberculosis in the placebo group during the first year was 0.4%, and during the first 5 years was 1.4%. Persons receiving 12 weeks of isoniazid showed a 21% reduction in cases, those who received 24 weeks showed a 65% reduction, and those who received 52 weeks showed a 75% reduction. However, when these data were analyzed for those who actually completed treatment, persons who received 24 weeks of treatment showed a 69% reduction and those who received 52 weeks of treatment showed a 93% reduction. Lesion size also appeared to influence outcome. Lesions 2 cm² or larger reactivated at a greater frequency and clearly benefited additionally from a full 52-week course of isoniazid. Compliant patients with lesions less than 2 cm² also benefited from a full 52-week course of therapy.

Other studies also have shown the benefit of treating fibrotic lesions. Falk and Fuchs, in a Veteran's Administration Cooperative Study, found administration of isoniazid to be beneficial for persons with fibrotic lesions who had not been treated previously, but not beneficial for those who had been treated previously.[95] Katz et al. also found isoniazid to be beneficial.[96] Grzybowski et al. had success with isoniazid prophylaxis, and even greater success with isoniazid plus PAS.[97] Prolongation of therapy beyond 1 year did not appear to improve results.

Ferebee reviewed the USPHS data on 1 year of isoniazid prophylaxis for fibrotic lesions in three groups: persons in whom inactive untreated fibrotic lesions were discovered, persons in whom previously active tuberculosis had never been treated, and persons in whom previously active tuberculosis had been treated.[74] For the first group of untreated never-active fibrotic lesions, the rate of reactivation during the first year was 1.9% and the rate over 5 years was 6.9%, with a 63% overall reduction noted with isoniazid prophylaxis. For the second group of previously active but untreated cases, the rate of reactivation during the first year was 1.4%, and the rate over 5 years was 4.9%, with a 51% reduction noted with isoniazid prophylaxis. For the third group of previously treated, previously active tuberculosis, the rate of reactivation during the first year was 1.2%, and the rate over 5 years was 3.3%, with only a 17% reduction noted with isoniazid prophylaxis.

These data show clearly the benefit of prophylaxis in inactive, untreated fibrotic lesions, as well as in old untreated tuberculosis. There is little benefit in the use of prophylactic isoniazid in persons who were treated previously.

The ATS/CDC state that inactive fibrotic lesions in persons with tuberculous infection can be treated with 9 months, instead of 12 months, of isoniazid.[56] This is based on a study of Inuits in Bethel, AK, as noted earlier (see Section VI,A,1).[76,77] It also is possible to use 2 months of daily rifampin and pyrazinamide or 4 months of daily rifampin with or without isoniazid, although there are no data to show that these shorter regimens are effective in patients with fibrotic lesions.

Sometimes it is difficult to distinguish active from inactive lesions. In those cases, it would not be unreasonable to start a patient on a multidrug regimen that included rifampin and pyrazinamide. After 2 months of therapy, if the cultures are reported negative, chemoprophylaxis would be considered complete. This regimen may have some support from a study in Hong Kong where a 2-month short-course, four-drug regimen in radiologically active, smear-negative, initially culture-negative tuberculosis was used, although the failure rate was 11%.[98a] Thus, it may be prudent to use 9 months of isoniazid alone,[56] or 4 months of isoniazid and rifampin as recommended previously.[75] This 4-month regimen in smear-negative, culture-negative, radiologically active cases was associated with a 1% failure rate.[98b] This regimen may be supplemented by pyrazinamide and ethambutol during the first 2 months.

3. HIV-Infected and Other Immunosuppressed Individuals

a. HIV-Infected, PPD-Positive

HIV infection is the greatest single risk factor for active tuberculosis. National registry matching has shown that during 1993 and 1994, 14% of AIDS cases also appeared on the tuberculosis registries.[99] The earliest confirmatory prospective study of risk, performed by Selwyn et al. on 513 intravenous drug abusers in a New York City methadone maintenance program, showed that the risk of reactivation was 7.9 cases per 100 person years in persons with skin-test induration of 10 mm or more.[100] Pape et al. studied 38 HIV-positive, PPD-positive (5 mm or greater) patients treated with isoniazid for 1 year and showed that the incidence of tuberculosis per 100 person years in the 38 isoniazid-treated patients vs. the 25 control patients was 1.7 vs. 10.0, respectively; a reduction with isoniazid of 83%.[101] Moreno et al. studied 121 HIV-positive, PPD-positive (induration ≥ 5 mm) subjects of whom 29 completed a 9 to 12 month course of isoniazid, and found that isoniazid reduced the incidence of tuberculosis by 83%, from 9.4 to 1.6 per 100 person years, $p < 0.006$.[102] Whalen et al. studied three prophylactic regimens in Ugandan adults and found a significant reduction in cases with daily isoniazid for 6 months (68% reduction), with daily isoniazid and rifampin for 3 months (59% reduction), and with daily isoniazid, rifampin, and pyrazinamide for 3 months (57% reduction).[79]

It also is clear that untested high-risk individuals who are not tested for HIV and are at high risk for exposure to tuberculosis need treatment. In a study in New York City where subjects were entered before HIV testing was available, the incidence of tuberculosis in drug abusers over the next 8 years was 1.0 per 100 person years.[103] There was no significant difference in rates between skin test-positive and skin test-negative individuals. This indicates that in the skin test-negative group, there may have been a significant number of anergic individuals or a significant number of new infections leading to disease.

The ATS/CDC recommend that HIV-positive adults with latent tuberculosis infection (induration $\geq$5 mm) receive isoniazid for 9 months, either daily or twice weekly or 2 months of daily rifampin and pyrazinamide.[56] In some studies, 6 months of isoniazid has been used,[79,81,104] but one study showed that 6 months of isoniazid is no different than placebo.[104] There have been no studies that compare the efficacy of 12 months with 6 months of isoniazid. Although 2 months of daily rifampin and pyrazinamide is an option in HIV-positive individuals,[56,70] only one study has shown the equivalence of this regimen to 12 months of isoniazid.[82] In fact, as noted earlier, Whalen et al. showed only 57% efficacy with 3 months of daily isoniazid, rifampin, and pyrazinamide.[79] Thus, the outcomes of this 2-month program of chemoprophylaxis will be monitored for further confirmation of this regimen.

Therapy also should be used in persons who, in the past, had skin test reactions of 5 mm or greater and were not candidates for treatment at that time, but developed HIV infection later.

There are no well-controlled studies to support the use of a prolonged regimen of isoniazid.

b. HIV-Infected, Anergic

Currently, treatment is not indicated for HIV-infected anergic individuals who have not been exposed to a case of active tuberculosis.[56,105] In the past, there was support for the use of isoniazid in HIV-positive anergic drug abusers[106,107] and other groups in which the prevalence of tuberculous infection was presumed to be 10% or greater. However, the reliability of anergy testing, the risk of tuberculosis in HIV-positive anergic individuals, and the efficacy of isoniazid prophylaxis in such individuals is questionable. Studies have shown that anergy testing can be unreliable.[108-110] One of these studies has shown that 30% of HIV-positive anergic individuals reacted to mumps or candida 12 months after anergy was documented. This finding was associated with a higher CD4 count. There also were 50 subjects in whom the PPD skin tests reverted to negative, 39% of whom had a positive mumps test at the time of tuberculin anergy.[109] Most of the anergy skin tests have not been standardized and cannot be considered reliable.[111]

Two recent studies have shown the rates of tuberculosis in HIV-positive anergic individuals to be relatively low, i.e., 3.1 cases per 100 person years in Uganda,[79] and 0.9 cases per 100 person years in a cohort in the U.S. with risk factors for tuberculosis exposure (predominantly drug abuse).[105] After 6 months of isoniazid vs. placebo, there was a 25% reduction in the Uganda study[79] and a 52% reduction in the U.S. study,[105] neither of which was statistically significant. In analyzing these results, one must consider that the number of tuberculosis cases was relatively small, i.e., 9 vs. 10 cases, and 3 vs. 6 cases, respectively. This may be due to the fact that the baseline rates of tuberculosis per 100 person years in the untreated groups were lower than one might have expected in these populations based on data from some, but not all, previous studies of anergic individuals, i.e., 12.4 (Moreno et al.[112]), 2.6 (Guelar et al.[113]), 5.7 (Pape et al.[101]), 3.0 (Antonucci et al.[114]), 6.6 (Selwyn et al.[115]), and 0.7 (Markowitz et al.[116]). If a larger cohort was studied, the 52% reduction seen in the U.S. study might have reached significance and would have led to a different conclusion, i.e., that isoniazid was effective. One also must consider that isoniazid was used for only 6 months instead of the 12 months recommended by the CDC at that time,[111] and compliance was not assured. A longer duration of treatment might have resulted in more of a difference between the treatment and placebo groups.

Low CD4 counts have clearly been associated with an increased risk of tuberculosis in HIV-positive anergic individuals.[114] When one considers that anergy testing is not reliable in patients with higher CD4 counts, it might have been useful to stratify patients in the studies noted above for CD4 counts in evaluating the effectiveness of isoniazid, although a study in Boston in HIV-positive anergic individuals at risk for tuberculosis exposure, half of whom had a CD4 count <200, showed that the rate of tuberculosis was only 0.2 cases per 100 person years.[117] Currently, the CDC no longer recommends anergy testing as a routine component of tuberculosis screening in HIV-positive persons in the U.S.[56,70,111] However, it is not entirely clear why this risk has decreased, and this reduced risk and the lack of response to isoniazid seems counterintuitive. Further, follow-up of these cohorts might provide more information.

The CDC states that a delayed-type hypersensitivity evaluation may assist in guiding individual decisions regarding therapy in selected situations.[111] Preventive therapy should be considered in HIV-positive individuals with a negative PPD (even if not anergic) in the following situations: recent contact with an infectious tuberculosis case; children who are born to HIV-infected women who are in close contact with a case of infectious tuberculosis; persons who work in situations with continuous tuberculosis exposure; and persons who have an ongoing high risk of exposure (e.g., prisons, jails, or homeless shelters in which the current prevalence of tuberculosis is high).[56,70,111] Persons with the latter two indications might require continuous therapy.

If a decision is made to treat an anergic individual, the clinician should weigh the risks, especially in Black and Hispanic females, and in those who are postpartum, because of a higher incidence of isoniazid fatalities.[106]

Persons who are anergic who begin antiretroviral agents and begin to reconstitute their immune systems should have a repeat skin test to reassess their tuberculosis infection status.[70]

c. Other Immunosuppressed Patients

Patients with organ transplants and other immunosuppressed patients (e.g., receiving the equivalent of ≥15 mg/day of prednisone for ≥1 month) should receive treatment for LTBI for skin-test induration ≥5 mm.[56] There are no controlled trials to show that the use of steroids alone in an infected patient can lead to active tuberculosis. There are numerous descriptive studies, but most are composed of cases where the patient's primary disease also caused immunosuppression (e.g., renal transplantation, bone marrow transplantation, systemic lupus erythematosus, rheumatoid arthritis, sarcoidosis, etc.).[118-121] Of interest in one study, 6 of the 14 cases were diagnosed 3 to 12 months after the steroids were discontinued.[120] There are two studies that show no risk, but both are limited by inadequate sample size and inadequate follow-up time.[122,123]

The best data on the timing of the immunosuppressive effect come from a study of 70 tuberculin reactors.[124] Each research subject was treated with 40 mg of prednisone per day in four divided doses and underwent a skin test every 72 hours. Sixty-eight (97%) of 70 subjects reverted to negative after an average of 14 days. Establishment of reactivity after the discontinuation of prednisone occurred, on average, in 6 days.

Schatz et al. suggested that a daily dose of 15 mg/day or greater was sufficient to cause anergy, although alternate day dosing was thought to mitigate this effect. In their study, therapy was maintained for a mean of 5 years.[122] This study was limited in that patients read their own skin tests by drawing a circle around the induration, transferring it to tape, and mailing it to the investigators on a postcard.

Millar and Horne suggested that immunosuppression was present in any person receiving more than 10 mg of prednisolone per day for a prolonged period of time.[119] In their study, immunosuppressive therapy lasted from 6 weeks to 10 years.

If a stronger immunosuppressive agent such as a cancer chemotherapeutic agent is used for any period of time, treatment for LTBI probably is indicated.

In cases where a patient is receiving a transplant, one must attempt to ascertain, where possible, the tuberculous status of the donor, as there have been reports of transfer of tuberculosis through transplanted organs that have presumably dormant infections.[58-66]

Therapy also is indicated for PPD-negative individuals, whether or not they are anergic, who are immunosuppressed, and are at high risk for infection, e.g., close contacts of infectious cases.[57,56]

4. HIV-Negative Intravenous Drug Abusers (IVDA)

Intravenous drug abusers specifically have been shown to have an increased prevalence of tuberculous infection and disease, whether or not they are known to be infected with HIV.[103,125] They have an increased risk of exposure to tuberculosis and HIV and, thus, are targeted for treatment for LTBI at 10 mm of induration.

5. Groups with High Risk of Exposure

Groups clearly at an increased risk for exposure have been delineated earlier in the section on screening, and include the foreign born, residents and employees of high-risk settings, and myco-bacteriology laboratory workers, among others (see Table 13.2). These individuals should be treated if they are tested and found to have induration ≥ 10 mm. If they are entering a high-risk setting, e.g., starting employment in a hospital, they should be treated only if they have induration ≥ 15 mm. If they are in the work force, are already known to be skin-test positive, and were not treated previously, they should not be treated now if there are no other risk factors.

There are abundant data to show that foreign-born persons,[126-129] migrant workers,[130,131] Blacks,[132-134] Hispanics,[132,135] Native Americans and Inuits,[132,136,137] persons of low socioeconomic status,[138-142] prisoners,[143,144] the elderly in nursing homes,[39,145] physicians and other hospital employees,[131,146-148] and funeral directors[131] have an increased prevalence of tuberculous disease. However, there are no controlled data to support the contention that any of these groups is at an increased risk of developing tuberculosis once infected, although there is evidence that Blacks may be more susceptible to the organism.[134] These persons at increased risk for exposure are targeted for treatment at 10 mm of induration, regardless of age, primarily because the probability of true infection with *M. tuberculosis* is higher than that of the general population, and because there is a higher likelihood that such individuals were infected recently.

Foreign-born individuals have been targeted specifically due to the fact that their proportion of new cases of tuberculosis in the U.S. has risen from 22% in 1986 to 39% in 1997.[139] In some groups, the risk was highest within 5 years of entrance into the U.S.,[126,129] but in others, the risk remained high for up to 20 years.[126] Therefore, assurance of screening and treatment programs for immigrants is a high priority.

6. Medical Risk Factors

The groups at medical risk are considered more susceptible to the development of tuberculosis once infected (i.e., skin test induration of 10 mm or greater). There are no well-designed, large-scale studies such as USPHS trials or the International Union Against Tuberculosis trial to sub-stantiate this claim or to show the benefit of isoniazid use. However, there are smaller studies to suggest that these risk factors are valid, and there is little disagreement that certain conditions predispose infected persons to disease. These data will be discussed below. The groups at medical risk include silicosis, diabetes, chronic renal failure, malignancy, weight loss, gastrectomy, and jejunoileal bypass. Immunosuppressed individuals are no longer considered in this section because they are considered positive at an induration of 5 mm or greater (see Section VI,B,3,c).

a. Silicosis

Persons with silicosis are at increased risk for the development of tuberculosis. There are numerous cross-sectional and retrospective studies that show an increased rate of tuberculosis in silicotics (as high as 43% in a past study).[149] Burke et al. have demonstrated that tuberculosis case-finding remained very effective among silicotic individuals. In their study in Oklahoma of former miners older than 50 years of age, 8 (1.1%/year) of 367 persons developed culture-positive tuberculosis over a period of 2 years. Approximately one third of the study group had silicosis.[150] Paul, in a 10-year survey in Rhodesian copper miners, showed that there was a 26-fold increase in tuberculosis in silicotic (2.89%/year) vs. nonsilicotic (0.11%/year) miners.[151] Westerholm et al. similarly have shown, in a 10-year retrospective survey of miners and foundry workers, a 33-fold increase in tuberculosis in silicotic cases (0.41%/year) vs. exposed miners without silicosis (0.012%/year).[152] There is conflict concerning the benefit of isoniazid prophylaxis, but in one unpublished study there was a 50% reduction in tuberculosis in silicotics with the use of isoniazid vs. placebo.[149] Another published study showed a 93% reduction in cases,[153] but it was seriously flawed by the inclusion of persons who already have been clearly shown to benefit from prophylaxis, i.e., new convertors, old untreated tuberculosis, and close contacts of diseased persons. There was no separation of these cases in the analysis. A study from Hong Kong has shown approximately 50% efficacy in treating silicotics with preventive therapy, but the overall rate of tuberculosis was still 4% per year (see Section VI,A,3).[84]

In view of the extent of the association of tuberculosis and silicosis, the experimental evidence that shows the potentiation of tuberculous growth by silica,[154] and the studies that suggest that isoniazid may be beneficial, treatment of LTBI is recommended in silicotics. As noted with fibrotic lesions, it may be difficult to distinguish between active and inactive disease in tuberculous-infected individuals with silicosis. Thus, a multidrug chemotherapy regimen in such individuals who are shown to be culture negative is not an unreasonable alternative. Such recommendations might include regimens containing isoniazid and rifampin for 4 months, or rifampin and pyrazinamide.[56,75] However, in view of a 3-month trial of isoniazid (400 mg), rifampin (600 mg), pyrazinamide (1200 mg), as Rifater®, which showed that treatment was not significantly different from placebo in preventing tuberculosis in silicotics,[155] it might be wise to use longer regimens.

b. Diabetes

Diabetes and tuberculosis have had a very strong historical association.[156] Various studies have shown the strength of this association, but none has evaluated the risk of developing disease once infected. Oscarsson and Silwer noted a fourfold increase in tuberculosis among diabetics in Sweden, with an added risk for younger diabetics or those with severe diabetes.[157] Root found that tuberculosis was 13 to 16 times more common in persons with diabetes who were less than 20 years old.[156] In 1946, Boucot, in a survey in Philadelphia of 3106 diabetics, estimated an overall twofold increase in the prevalence of tuberculosis in diabetics over the general population.[158] The overall incidence of active tuberculosis was 2.6%. It was higher in diabetics less than 40 years of age (5.3%), and much higher in diabetics less than 40 years of age who had had diabetes for longer than 10 years (17%).

The comparison was not as dramatic in autopsy studies. In 1934, Root summarized the data from numerous autopsy studies and found the incidence of tuberculosis in diabetics to be 28.4%, or 1.2 times that of the general population.[156] Similarly, Kessler, in 1971, analyzed mortality data in 10,066 diabetic patients seen at the Joslin Clinic from 1931 to 1959 and found that tuberculosis contributed to or was a cause of death in 26 (0.26%) patients, or 1.5 times the rate in nondiabetics.[159]

In an analysis of 145 relapses of tuberculosis in New York City in 1967, diabetes was found to be the second most important risk factor and was present in 12 (8.3%) of cases.[160]

Pablos-Mendez et al. have found that diabetes is an independent risk factor for Hispanics, but not Blacks, for reasons which are not clear.[161]

Rose et al. performed a decision analysis to assess the utility of isoniazid prophylaxis in PPD-positive diabetics.[162] They estimated the risk of disease to be 1.5 times that of the general infected population based on Kessler's data, and varied the risk from one- to fourfold in the sensitivity analysis. They found isoniazid to be beneficial for all persons, but it only added a few days to the life expectancy. The decision to use isoniazid was considered to be a "toss-up."

More data are necessary to make an informed decision about the treatment of diabetic patients. In the interim, it probably is safe to say that, of all diabetics, long-standing insulin-dependent diabetics with positive skin tests are at a higher risk for the development of tuberculosis, especially those who are controlled poorly.

c. Chronic Renal Failure/Dialysis

Dialysis centers have reported increased rates of tuberculosis,[163-171] varying from 0.12 to 3% per year. In one study, 7 (28%) of 26 patients on chronic dialysis in South Africa developed tuberculosis over a 14-month screening period.[170] The cases may involve extrapulmonary sites in as much as 95% of cases,[169,172] and often develop insidiously. However, many of the cases in these studies occurred in groups with other risk factors. In reviewing three reports from the U.S., with a total of 23 cases, there were 6 Asians, 11 Blacks, 1 Native American, 1 Hispanic, and 4 whites.[163,166,167] A study from Canada showed that all tuberculosis in persons with chronic renal failure occurred in persons who had other risks.[164] A study of 11 cases from a dialysis unit in the United Kingdom showed that all cases were derived from patients born in third world countries.[165] The results found in these studies at least partially reflect the increased exposure and risk of disease due to causes other than chronic renal failure and dialysis. In fact, Freeman et al. from Iowa stated that no cases of tuberculosis occurred in 327 dialysis patients observed for variable lengths of time after 1964.[173] He stated that a policy of antituberculous prophylaxis was not warranted in his patients. However, a study from Japan in a reportedly homogeneous population showed a 6- to 16-fold increased risk.[169] Furthermore, Andrew et al. showed that the annual case rate of 0.58% per year in their group was four times greater than that of local Filipinos, the ethnic group with the highest rate of tuberculosis in San Francisco.[163] In addition, Cuss et al. stated that the rate of tuberculosis in Afro-Caribbeans and Asians in England was 70 times that of a matched population.[165]

These findings, along with the predominance of extrapulmonary tuberculosis, the difficulty in arriving at an early diagnosis, and the high death rates in some of these studies, all support the use of isoniazid. Isoniazid is removed by dialysis. Therefore, on dialysis days, persons on chemoprophylaxis should receive their isoniazid following dialysis.

d. Malignancy

Malignancies are associated with immunosuppression, weight loss, and the use of immunosuppressive chemotherapeutic agents. Kaplan et al. reviewed 201 cases at Memorial Hospital in New York City between 1950 and 1971 and found that the cancers could be divided into three risk groups for tuberculosis. The highest rates were in lung cancer, reticulum cell sarcoma, lymphosarcoma, and Hodgkin's disease; followed closely by head and neck cancer, stomach cancer, acute lymphocytic leukemia, and acute myelocytic leukemia; and lastly by breast, colon, and genitourinary cancer.[174] Another study has shown similar risks, but has ranked some of the cancers differently, giving most weight to head and neck cancer.[175] In both studies, the exposure and infection histories were not known and the sample sizes were small. Nonetheless, there is no dispute that cancer patients who are infected with tuberculosis will be at increased risk for developing active disease when their cancer progresses and their general health deteriorates, especially if their cancers involve the immune system directly. Therefore, in patients with positive skin tests, isoniazid therapy is recommended for leukemias and lymphomas, and other cancers that affect the reticulo-endothelial system, "other malignancies," which include head and neck cancers, gastric cancers, probably lung cancer, and any cancer associated with profound weight loss and/or immunosuppression.

It also might be wise to use isoniazid in untreated PPD-positive individuals undergoing radiation therapy to the lung, although there are no data that address this issue directly.

e. Rapid Weight Loss

Substantial rapid weight loss is considered to be an indication for treatment if the individual loses 10% or more of ideal body weight. This weight loss may be due to malnutrition, malabsorption, or starvation, or may be associated with other risk factors for tuberculosis such as gastrectomy, intestinal bypass for obesity, or cancer. There is evidence of a twofold or greater increase in the risk of tuberculosis in patients who are underweight by 10% or more,[56,176] especially when compared to persons who are overweight.[177] However, reduced weight alone, in the absence of recent weight loss or other risk factors or evidence of malnutrition, is not an indication for therapy.

f. Chronic Peptic Ulcer Disease/Postgastrectomy

Thorn et al. evaluated 955 patients with peptic ulcer disease who underwent gastrectomy and were followed for an average of 4 years.[178] A preoperative radiograph was performed in 809 persons and was abnormal in 60. Eight of these 60 people with abnormal results were found to have active tuberculosis upon entry. Further analysis focused on 616 males who had normal preoperative radiographs, 14 (2.3%) of whom subsequently developed active pulmonary tuberculosis. The rate in this group was 0.57% per year, was three times more frequent in gastric ulcers than duodenal ulcers, and was five times more frequent than a comparison group selected from another study. The greatest risk factor was preoperative weight loss as a percentage of ideal body weight. Males at or above 95% of their standard weight had an annual rate of 0.12%, very near the rate of the historical control population; those between 85 and 95% had an annual rate of 0.4%; and those at or below 85% had an annual rate of 1.78%. There was no weight analysis of the patients who before surgery were discovered to have active tuberculosis. On the basis of these data, the authors concluded that the development of tuberculosis was due to severe or long-standing peptic ulcer disease with loss of weight and only secondarily to the effects of the operation. They stated that if the chest radiograph and weight were normal before surgery, there was no increased risk of developing pulmonary tuberculosis.

Hanngren and Reizenstein reviewed data on 38 patients who developed pulmonary tuberculosis after gastrectomy and found that dumping syndrome with malabsorption and malnutrition was a significant risk factor.[179] Frucht et al., in their study and review, found that weight loss was a major factor, and that active tuberculosis worsened after gastrectomy, but that there was no definite proof that gastrectomy itself led to an increased risk of developing tuberculosis.[180] Numerous other authors have noted the association of gastrectomy and tuberculosis, but Snider points out that a high proportion of those persons studied were older men, alcoholics, or had a low weight/height ratio.[181] He concluded, though, that it is reasonable to treat infected postgastrectomy patients, especially those with weight loss or a malabsorption syndrome.

g. Intestinal Bypass Surgery

Jejunoileal bypass, an operation associated with profound weight loss, also is associated with the development of tuberculosis.[182] In one study, 4 (4%) of 100 patients developed tuberculosis during the first year after surgery.[183] This was a 60-fold increase over the rate in the general population, and others have reported from 27 to 63 times the risk of comparison populations.[182] Furthermore, the rate of extrapulmonary involvement exceeded 80%. Fortunately, it is an extremely rare association and the operation has largely fallen out of favor.

7. Low-Risk Individuals

Decision analyses have addressed the issue of chemoprophylaxis in low-risk individuals at various ages with varying results.[184-188a] However, with targeted screening and treatment, these issues are bypassed and low-risk individuals are not tested or screened unless they are entering a high-risk setting. Such individuals should be treated only if their skin test is 15 mm or greater.[56]

VII. MONITORING TREATMENT OF LTBI

(See Table 13.5.) Before beginning isoniazid, baseline liver function tests are not routinely indicated unless the initial evaluation suggests a liver disorder. Leff and Leff found, in their survey of metropolitan health departments, that it was not standard practice to perform such tests routinely.[188b] However, testing (i.e., AST (SGOT), ALT (SGPT), and bilirubin) is indicated for persons at higher risk for hepatitis, e.g., patients with HIV infection, pregnant women and those in the immediate postpartum period (within 3 months of delivery), and persons with a history of chronic liver disease (e.g., hepatitis B or C, alcoholic hepatitis or cirrhosis, persons who use alcohol regularly, and others who are at risk of chronic liver disease).[56] Older individuals with chronic medical conditions may be considered on an individual basis. Active hepatitis and end-stage liver disease are relative contraindications to the use of isoniazid or pyrazinamide for treatment of LTBI. Regular monitoring of liver function tests is indicated in those persons who are at increased risk as defined above, and for those persons who are known to have abnormal baseline values. Some experts recommend that isoniazid be withheld if the transaminase level exceeds three times the upper limit of normal with symptoms, and five times normal if asymptomatic. All patients being treated should receive a clinical evaluation monthly if they are receiving isoniazid, and at 2, 4, and 8 weeks if they are receiving rifampin and pyrazinamide. Uric acid levels should be obtained in patients on pyrazinamide who develop acute arthritis.

Persons who are HIV-positive or hepatitis C virus-positive, even with normal transaminase levels, are more susceptible to antituberculous drug hepatic toxicity.[189] The clinician always should question for a history of previous isoniazid treatment and associated reactions; liver disease; other medications; alcohol abuse; evidence of, or risk factors for, peripheral neuropathy, such as might be the case in diabetics; and pregnancy. Pyridoxine at a dose of 25 to 50 mg daily, or 50 to 100 mg twice weekly, is recommended in alcoholics, persons with malnutrition from a poor diet or malabsorption, HIV-infected individuals, and other persons at risk for peripheral neuropathy. All persons receiving isoniazid should be questioned at monthly intervals about the presence of unexplained anorexia, nausea, vomiting, dark urine, icterus, rash, persistent extremity paresthesias, persistent fatigue, weakness, or fever for more than 3 days, and/or abdominal pain, especially in the right upper quadrant.[75] Isoniazid hepatitis usually is a subclinical chemical hepatitis. When symptoms appear, cessation of the drug is indicated and symptoms usually resolve. There have been idiosyncratic reactions with fulminant hepatic failure, but they are rare.

Hepatitis is an age-related phenomenon and, in a survey by Kopanoff et al., the criteria for hepatitis (usually greater than fivefold transaminase elevations) were met at the following rates: ages 20 to 35, 0.3%; ages 35 to 50, 1.2%; and ages 50 to 65, 2.3%.[190] However, one should not be too secure about persons who are less than 20 years old because of a report of eight patients who required liver transplants due to severe isoniazid-associated hepatitis, three of whom were less than 20 years old.[191] For persons older than 65 years old, the rate from the study of Kopanoff et al. (noted above) was 0.8%, but the Stead et al. rate of 4.4% is considered more accurate.[192] The death rate in the probable cases from the study by Kopanoff et al. was 7.6%, the majority occurring in Black females.[190] There has been controversy about the rates cited in this multicenter study by Kopanoff et al. because of the high incidence of isoniazid hepatitis-related fatalities in the Baltimore area.[193] Retrospectively, it was found that there was a striking increase in deaths related to cirrhosis in the city of Baltimore in 1972, although the cause was not discovered. If the Baltimore subjects had been excluded from the multicenter trial, the rate of isoniazid-related hepatitis fatalities would have been much lower. A recent study of 11,141 individuals has shown the overall rate of hepatitis to be 0.1% in persons 27 to 67 years old who were started on isoniazid.[194] The authors believe that clinicians should have greater confidence in the safety of isoniazid therapy. Furthermore, Snider and Caras[195] searched multiple data sources to compile 177 isoniazid-related deaths that occurred between the years 1972 and 1988. During this period, there were an estimated 1,084,760 persons who started therapy, 655,867 of whom completed therapy. Of those who completed therapy, 23.2 per 100,000 died. Of 21 postpartum deaths, 8 (38%) were within 1 year of delivery. Isoniazid-completer deaths peaked in 1972 and 1973 at rates of 91.6 and 83.3 per 100,000, respectively, but was much lower during the last 4 years of the study: 7.7, 5.8, 14.0, and 7.1 per 100,000 for years 1985, 1986, 1987, and 1988, respectively. This may give us some reassurance about the dangers of isoniazid prophylaxis.

Hepatitis tends to occur within the first few months of starting therapy. Minor elevations in transaminase levels may occur in 10 to 20% of persons and is not considered to be a contraindication to therapy. Slow acetylation is not thought to be a major factor in the development of hepatitis. Where there is close monitoring, most cases of hepatitis resolve with discontinuation of the drug. Alcoholics are at a higher risk for chemical hepatitis, but not necessarily for frank clinical hepatitis.[196] However, Black and Hispanic females, especially pregnant and postpartum Hispanics, may be at increased risk for fulminant hepatitis for reasons that are unknown.[190,197,198]

Additional information on isoniazid may be found in Chapter 11.

VIII. COMPLETION OF TREATMENT

Completion of treatment is based on the total number of doses ingested and not on the duration of treatment alone.[56] For the 9-month isoniazid regimen, the patient should receive a minimum of 270 doses administered within 12 months, thus allowing for minor interruptions in therapy. The 6-month regimen should comprise 180 doses administered within 9 months. The twice-weekly isoniazid regimens should comprise at least 76 doses within 12 months for the 9-month regimen, and 52 doses within 9 months for the 6-month regimen. The daily regimen of rifampin (or rifabutin) and pyrazinamide should comprise at least 60 doses within 3 months and the 4-month regimen of daily rifampin should comprise at least 120 doses within 6 months. If these criteria are not met, the clinician may have to completely renew the regimen. Whenever there are frequent or prolonged periods (>2 months) where medication is not administered, the clinician should perform a medical examination to rule out active tuberculosis.

IX. RETREATMENT

Once a person has been treated either to prevent or cure tuberculous disease, there are no data to support retreatment with isoniazid should one of the high-risk medical conditions occur, although one should closely monitor persons with old tuberculosis who are profoundly immunosuppressed.

X. EXOGENOUS REINFECTION

Exogenous reinfection may occur in persons with waning immunity to tuberculosis. It is more likely that, if immunity wanes, the patient will be reinfected endogenously by his own organisms.[199] However, if the primary infection has been eradicated or has been encapsulated with little or no contact with the immune system, and the PPD has reverted only to convert again with a new close exposure, isoniazid therapy probably is wise. Such exogenous reinfection has been documented by Nardell et al. in four cases at a Boston shelter.[200] Furthermore, Small et al. have reported 4 patients with advanced HIV infection and drug-sensitive tuberculosis who were reinfected with new resistant strains (documented by RFLP) during therapy for active tuberculosis,[201] Horn et al. have reported 3 cases,[202] and van Rie et al. have reported the identification of new drug-sensitive or resistant strains in 12 of 16 cases evaluated.[203]

XI. CONTACTS OF DRUG-RESISTANT CASES

Contacts of isoniazid-resistant cases will not benefit from isoniazid therapy. In the past, it was recommended that such persons be treated with rifampin for 6 months, with consideration given to adding ethambutol,[75] although some experts might have prescribed 12 months of therapy with rifampin and ethambutol.[204] Six months of rifampin has been used very effectively in 157 adolescents with isoniazid-resistant tuberculosis infection (see Section VI,A,3).[86] The CDC now recommends that 2 months of a rifamycin and pyrazinamide be used. For patients intolerant to pyrazinamide, a 4-month regimen of a rifamycin alone may be used;[56,70] it probably is best to treat for at least 6 months. If the source of contact is unclear and isoniazid resistance is only suspected, then isoniazid should be used.

   The management of persons exposed to multidrug-resistant (MDR) tuberculosis is more difficult.[56,70] Expert consultation should be sought. MDR tuberculosis is defined as resistance to at least isoniazid and rifampin. Guidelines have been published in the past by the CDC.[205] Close contacts, as well as casual contacts who are HIV-positive, must receive prophylaxis. Treatment should be delayed in most cases until the susceptibilities of the source case can be assessed. The following drug combinations may be considered: pyrazinamide and ethambutol; pyrazinamide and a quinolone

(such as levofloxacin, ofloxacin, or ciprofloxacin); and other drug combinations that include streptomycin, kanamycin, amikacin, and capreomycin. PAS acid, ethionamide, and cycloserine should
not be considered unless absolutely necessary because of their high toxicities. Quinolones cannot
be used in children. Treatment should ensue for at least 6 to 12 months in immunocompetent and
12 months in immunocompromised patients. All patients with suspected MDR tuberculosis infection
should be followed for at least 2 years.[56,70]

XII. PREGNANCY AND LACTATION

Women may be tested safely with tuberculin at any time during pregnancy. A reduction in cell-
mediated immunity is noted during pregnancy but is not thought to interfere with skin testing.[206]
In the past, prophylactic treatment was not recommended during pregnancy unless the patient was
a recent convertor or was significantly immunosuppressed.[207] However, currently, if a pregnant
woman is likely to have been infected recently or has a high-risk medical condition, especially
HIV infection, she should be treated as soon as the infection is documented.[75] It is important that
treatment not be delayed in these high-risk individuals.

Breast feeding during isoniazid administration is considered safe since less than 20% of an
infant's usual dose is ingested daily.[208] However, this decision must be individualized. In patients
on twice weekly therapy, the infant probably would receive much higher doses of isoniazid in the
breast milk, although this has not been studied. There are no published data on the effect of
pyrazinamide on the fetus in pregnant women,[70] but some experts suggest that it can be used in
the 2-month regimen in HIV-positive individuals in whom treatment is initiated after the first
trimester.[56] For further information on these topics, please refer to Chapter 8.

XIII. BACILLE CALMETTE-GUÉRIN (BCG) VACCINATION
AND SUBSEQUENT SKIN TESTING

The interpretation of the tuberculin skin test may be difficult in persons who have received BCG.
Comstock et al. showed that 8 to 15 years after BCG vaccination, 16% of persons had skin tests
greater than 10 mm compared to 2% of controls.[209] Sepulveda et al. showed that the mean tuberculin
skin reaction in persons vaccinated three times and tested at least 5 years after the last vaccination
correlated with the number of BCG scars: 2.3 mm for no scars, 6.7 mm for 1 scar, 10.9 mm for 2
scars, and 13.2 mm for 3 scars.[50] Menzies et al. evaluated tuberculin reactivity in 1511 school
children and young adults in Montreal in whom BCG-V was administered 10 to 25 years earlier.[210]
Among 1041 persons vaccinated once in infancy, 7.9% had significant tuberculin reactions
(≥10 mm); this wasn't different from controls when adjusted for socioeconomic factors. In young
adults vaccinated at age 6 years or older, the rate of significant skin test positivity was 25.5%, even
25 years after vaccination, whereas the rate in unvaccinated controls was 4.1%. However, because
skin test reactivity in persons vaccinated after infancy increased markedly from 11.7 to 28% as the
interval from vaccination increased from 10 to 17 or more years, a concern is raised that the study
group may have been more highly exposed to tuberculosis.

Tuberculin reactivity due to the BCG effect is unlikely to persist for more than 10 years,[211,212]
especially in persons who receive only one vaccination in infancy. However, it would be wise to
remember that BCG alone can cause a positive skin test, especially in persons recently vaccinated.
Also, there may be a significant booster effect due to BCG that may be expressed when two-step
testing is performed.[44-50]

The recent ATS statement, "Diagnostic Standards and Classification of Tuberculosis in Adults
and Children," asserts that "it is usually prudent to consider 'positive' reactions to 5 TU of PPD
tuberculin in BCG-vaccinated persons as indicating infection with *M. tuberculosis,* especially
among persons from countries with a high prevalence of tuberculosis."[8] The CDC recommends

that therapy be considered for a person who has been vaccinated with BCG who has a skin test reaction ≥10 mm, especially if the person is a close contact of an infectious case, if the person was born in or lived in a country with a high prevalence of tuberculosis, or if the person is continually exposed to a population with a high prevalence of tuberculosis (e.g., some healthcare workers, employees and volunteers at homeless shelters, and workers at drug treatment centers). Treatment of LTBI also should be used in BCG-vaccinated persons who are infected with HIV and have a tuberculin skin test reaction ≥5 mm.[212] For more information on this matter, refer to Chapter 15.

REFERENCES

1. Siebert, F. B. and Glenn, J. T., Tuberculin purified protein derivative: preparation and analysis of a large quantity for standard, *Am. Rev. Tuberc.*, 44, 9, 1941.
2. Landi, S., Production and standardization of tuberculin, in *The Mycobacteria: A Sourcebook*, Kubica, G. P. and Wayne, L. G., Eds., Marcel Dekker, New York, 1984, 505.
3. Comstock, G. W., Daniel, T. M., Snider, D. E., Edwards, P. Q., Hopewell, P. C., and Vandiveire, H. M., The tuberculin skin test, *Am. Rev. Respir. Dis.*, 124, 356, 1981.
4. Snider, D. E., The tuberculin skin test, *Am. Rev. Respir. Dis.*, 125, 108, 1982.
5. Duchin, J. S., Jereb, J. A., Nolan, C. M., Smith, P., and Onorato, I. M., Comparison of sensitivities to two commercially available tuberculin skin test reagents in persons with recent tuberculosis, *Clin. Infect. Dis.*, 25, 661, 1997.
6. Villarino, M. E., Burman, W., Wang, Y. C., Lundergan, L., Catanzaro, A., Bock, N., Jones, C., and Nolan, C., Comparable specificity of 2 commercial tuberculin reagents in persons at low risk for tuberculous infection, *JAMA*, 281, 169, 1999.
7. Guld, J., Bentzon, M. W., Bleiker, M. A., Griep, W. A., Magnusson, M., and Waaler, H., Standardization of a new batch of purified tuberculin (PPD) intended for international use, *Bull. WHO*, 19, 845, 1958.
8. American Thoracic Society/Centers for Disease Control and Prevention, Diagnostic standards and classification of tuberculosis in adults and children, *Am. J. Respir. Crit. Care Med.*, 161, 1376, 2000.
9. Reichman, L. B., Tuberculin skin testing: the state of the art, *Chest*, 76, 764, 1979.
10. Jordan, T. J., Sunderam, G., Thomas, L., and Reichman, L. B., Tuberculin reaction size measurement by the pen method compared to traditional palpation, *Chest*, 92, 234, 1987.
11. Sokal, J. E., Measurement of delayed skin-test responses, *N. Engl. J. Med.*, 293, 501, 1975.
12. Pouchot, J., Grasland, A., Collet, C., Coste, J., Esdaile, J. M., and Vinceneux, P., Reliability of tuberculin skin test measurement, *Ann. Intern. Med.*, 126, 210, 1997.
13. Bearman, J. E., Kleinman, H., Glyer, V. V., and LaCroix, O. M., A study of variability in tuberculin test reading, *Am. Rev. Respir. Dis.*, 90, 913, 1964.
14. Chaparas, S. D., Immunologically based diagnostic tests with tuberculin and other mycobacterial antigens, in *The Mycobacteria: A Sourcebook*, Kubica, G. P. and Wayne, L. G., Eds., Marcel Dekker, New York, 1984, 195.
15. Kendig, E. L., Kirkpatrick, B. V., Carter, H., Hill, F. A., Caldwell, K., and Entwistle, M., Underreading of the tuberculin skin test reaction, *Chest*, 113, 1175, 1998.
16. Duboczy, B. O., Two-reading technique for elimination of false readings in delayed type skin tests, *Am. Rev. Respir. Dis.*, 99, 961, 1969.
17. Tarlo, S. M., Day, J. H., Mann, P., and Day, M. P., Immediate hypersensitivity to tuberculin: *in vivo* and *in vitro* studies, *Chest*, 71, 33, 1977.
18. Duboczy, B. O., Repeated tuberculin tests at the same site in tuberculin-positive patients, *Am. Rev. Respir. Dis.*, 90, 77, 1964.
19. Duboczy, B. O. and Brown B. T., Local sensitization to tuberculin, *Am. Rev. Respir. Dis.*, 84, 69, 1961.
20. WHO Tuberculosis Research Office, Repeated tuberculin tests in the same site, *Bull. WHO*, 12, 197, 1955.
21. Arnason, B. G. and Waksman, B. H., The retest reaction in delayed sensitivity, *Lab. Invest.*, 12, 737, 1963.
22. Galli, S. J. and Askenase, P. W., Cutaneous basophil hypersensitivity, in *The Reticuloendothelial System*, vol. 9, Phillips, S. M. and Escobar, M. R., Eds., Plenum Publishing Company, New York, 1988, 321.

23. Lagrange, P. H., Cell-mediated immunity and delayed-type hypersensitivity, in *The Mycobacteria: A Sourcebook*, Kubica, G. P. and Wayne, L. G., Eds., Marcel Dekker, New York, 1984, 681.

24. Askenase, P. W. and Atwood, J. E., Basophils in tuberculin and "Jones-Mote" delayed reactions of humans, *J. Clin. Invest.*, 58, 1145, 1976.

25. Dvorak, H. F., Galli, S. J., and Dvorak, A. M., Cellular and vascular manifestations of cell-mediated immunity, *Hum. Pathol.*, 17, 122, 1986.

26. Slutkin, G., Perez-Stable, E. J., and Hopewell, P. C., Time course and boosting of tuberculin reactions in nursing home residents, *Am. Rev. Respir. Dis.*, 134, 1048, 1986.

27. Friedman, L. and Dvorak, H. F., The negative tuberculin skin test: tuberculin, HIV, and anergy panels [letter], *Am. J. Respir. Crit. Care Med.*, 151, 580, 1985.

28. Colvin, R. B., Mosesson, M. W., and Dvorak, H. F., Delayed-type hypersensitivity skin reactions in congenital afibrinogenemia: lack of fibrin deposition and induration, *J. Clin. Invest.*, 63, 1302, 1979.

29. Byrd, R. B., Gracey, D. R., Campbell, D. C., and Knies, A. A., The Mono-Vacc tuberculin skin test, *Dis. Chest,* 56, 447, 1969.

30. Catanzaro, A., Multiple puncture skin test and Mantoux test in southeast Asian refugees, *Chest,* 87, 346, 1985.

31. Donaldson, J.C. and Elliott, R. C., A study of copositivity of three multipuncture techniques with intradermal PPD tuberculin, *Am. Rev. Respir. Dis.,* 118, 843, 1978.

32. Centers for Disease Control and Prevention, Screening for tuberculosis and tuberculosis infection in high-risk populations: recommendations of the Advisory Council for the Elimination of Tuberculosis, *MMWR*, 44 (No. RR-11), 19, 1995.

33. Edwards, P. Q. and Edwards, L. B., Story of the tuberculin test: from an epidemiologic viewpoint, *Am. Rev. Respir. Dis.*, 81 (Suppl.), 1, 1960.

34. Bass, J. B., Sanders, R. V., and Kirkpatrick, M. B., Choosing an appropriate cutting point for conversion in annual tuberculin skin testing, *Am. Rev. Respir. Dis.*, 132, 379, 1985.

35. Sutherland, I., Recent studies in the epidemiology of tuberculosis, based on the risk of being infected with tubercle bacilli, *Adv. Tuberc. Res.*, 19, 1, 1976.

36. Finucane, T. E., The American Geriatrics Society statement on two-step PPD testing for nursing home patients on admission, *J. Am. Geriatr. Soc.*, 36, 77, 1988.

37. Thompson, N. J., Glassroth, J. L., Snider, D. E., and Farer, L. S., The booster phenomenon in serial tuberculin testing, *Am. Rev. Respir. Dis.*, 119, 587, 1979.

38. Menzies, D., Interpretation of repeated tuberculin tests: boosting, conversion, and reversion, *Am. J. Respir. Crit. Care Med.,* 159, 15, 1999.

39. Centers for Disease Control, Prevention and control of tuberculosis in facilities providing long-term care to the elderly, *MMWR*, 39 (No. RR-10), 7, 1990.

40. Hecker, M. T., Johnson, J. L., Whalen, C. C., Nyole, S., Mugerwa, R. D., and Ellner, J. J., Two-step tuberculin skin testing in HIV-infected persons in Uganda, *Am. J. Respir. Crit. Care Med.*, 155, 81, 1997.

41. Gordin, F. M., Perez-Stable, E. J., Flaherty, D., Reid, M. E., Schecter, G., Joe, L., Slutkin, G., and Hopewell, P. G., Evaluation of a third sequential tuberculin skin test in a chronic care population, *Am. Rev. Respir. Dis.*, 137, 153, 1988.

42. Van den Brande, P. and Demedts, M., Four-stage tuberculin testing in elderly subjects induces age-dependent progressive boosting, *Chest,* 101, 447, 1992.

43. Gordin, F. M., Perez-Stable, E. J., Reid, M., Schecter, G., Cosgriff, L., Flaherty, G., and Hopewell, P. G., Stability of positive tuberculin tests. Are boosted reactions valid? *Am. Rev. Respir. Dis.*, 144, 560, 1991.

44. Menzies, R., Vissandjee, B., and Amyot, D., Factors associated with tuberculin reactivity among the foreign-born in Montreal, *Am. Rev. Respir. Dis.*, 146, 752, 1992.

45. Sepulveda, R. L., Burr, C., Ferrer, X., and Sorensen, R. U., Booster effect of tuberculin testing in healthy 6-year-old school children vaccinated with bacillus Calmette-Guérin at birth in Santiago, Chile, *Pediatr. Infect. Dis. J.*, 7, 578, 1988.

46. Rosenberg, T., Manfreda, J., and Hershfield, E. S., Two-step tuberculin testing in staff and residents of a nursing home, *Am. Rev. Respir. Dis.*, 148, 1537, 1993.

47. Menzies, R., Vissandjee, B., Rocher, I., St. and Germain, Y., The booster effect in two-step tuberculin testing among young adults in Montreal, *Ann. Intern. Med.*, 120, 190, 1994.

48. Horowitz, H. W., Luciano, B. B., Kadel, J. R., and Wormser, G. P., Tuberulin skin test conversion in hospital employees vaccinated with bacille Calmette-Guérin: recent *Mycobacterium tuberculosis* infection or booster effect?, *Am. J. Infect. Cont.*, 23, 181, 1995.

49. Cauthen, G. M., Snider, D. E., and Onorato, I. M., Boosting of tuberculin sensitivity among southeast Asian refugees, *Am. J. Respir. Crit. Care Med.*, 149, 1597, 1994.

50. Sepulveda, R. L., Ferrer, X., Latrach, C., and Sorensen, R. U., The influence of Calmette-Guérin bacillus immunization on the booster effect of tuberculin testing in healthy young adults, *Am. Rev. Respir. Dis.*, 142, 24, 1990.

51. Holden, M., Dubin, M. R., and Diamond, P. H., Frequency of negative intermediate-strength tuberculin sensitivity in patients with active tuberculosis, *N. Engl. J. Med.*, 285, 1507, 1971.

52. Rooney, J. J., Crocco, J. A., Kramer, S., and Lyons, H. A., Further observations on tuberculin reactions in active tuberculosis, *Am. J. Med.*, 60, 517, 1976.

53. McMurray, D. N. and Echeverri, A., Cell-mediated immunity in anergic patients with pulmonary tuberculosis, *Am. Rev. Respir. Dis.*, 118, 827, 1978.

54. Nash, D. R. and Douglass, J. E., Anergy in active pulmonary tuberculosis, *Chest*, 77, 32, 1980.

55. Blatt, S. P., Hendrix, C. W., Butzin, C. A., and Freeman, T. M., Delayed-type hypersensitivity skin testing predicts progression to AIDS in HIV-infected patients, *Ann. Intern. Med.*, 119, 177, 1993.

56. American Thoracic Society and Centers for Disease Control and Prevention. Targeted tuberculin testing and treatment of latent tuberculosis infection, *Am. J. Respir. Crit. Care Med.*, 161, S221, 2000.

57. American Thoracic Society, American Academy of Pediatrics, Centers for Disease Control, and Infectious Disease Society of America, Control of tuberculosis in the United States, *Am. Rev. Respir. Dis.*, 146, 1623, 1992.

58. Carlsen, S. E. and Bergin, C. J., Reactivation of tuberculosis in a donor lung after transplantation, *Am. J. Radiol.*, 154, 495, 1990.

59. Lakshminarayan, S. and Sahn, S. A., Tuberculosis in a patient after renal transplantation, *Tubercle*, 54, 72, 1973.

60. Lenk, S., Oesterwitz, H., and Scholz, D., Tuberculosis in cadaveric renal allograft recipients, *Eur. Urol.*, 14, 484, 1988.

61. Lloveras, J., Peterson, P. K., Simmons, R. L., and Najarian, J. S., Mycobacterial infections in renal transplant recipients: seven cases and a review of the literature, *Arch. Intern. Med.*, 142, 888, 1982.

62. Schulman, L. L., Scully, B., McGregor, C. C., and Austin, J. H. M., Pulmonary tuberculosis after lung transplantation, *Chest*, 111, 1459, 1997.

63. Munoz, P., Palomo, J., Munoz, R., Rodriguez-Creixems, M., Pelaez, T., and Bouza, E., Tuberculosis in heart transplant recipients, *Clin. Infect. Dis.*, 21, 398, 1995.

64. Ridgeway, A. L., Warner, G. S., Phillips, P., Forshag, M. S., McGiffin, D. C., Harden, J. W., Harris, R. H., Benjamin, W. H., Zorn, G. L., and Dunlap, N. E., Transmission of *Mycobacterium tuberculosis* to recipient single lung transplants from the same donor, *Am. J. Respir. Crit. Care Med.*, 153, 1166, 1996.

65. Miller, R. A., Lanza, L. A., Kline, J. N., and Geist, L. J., *Mycobacterium tuberculosis* in lung transplant recipients, *Am. J. Respir. Crit. Care Med.*, 152, 374, 1995.

66. Korner, M. M., Hirata, N., Tenderich, G., Minami, K., Mannenbach, H., Kleesiek, K., and Korfer, R., Tuberculosis in heart transplant recepients, *Chest*, 111, 365, 1997.

67. Friedman, L. N., Diagnostic standards and classification of tuberculosis (letter), *Am. Rev. Respir. Dis.*, 143, 895, 1991.

68. Green, C. E., Mycobacterial infections: tuberculous mycobacterial infections, in *Infectious Diseases of the Dog and Cat*, Green, C. E., Ed., Saunders, Philadelphia, 1990, 558.

69. Snider, W. R., Tuberculosis in canine and feline populations: review of the literature, *Am. Rev. Respir. Dis.*, 104, 877, 1971.

70. Centers for Disease Control and Prevention, Prevention and treatment of tuberculosis among patients infected with human immunodeficiency virus: principles of therapy and revised recommendations, *MMWR*, 47 (No. RR-20), 1, 1998.

71. Fulkerson, L. L., Perlmutter, G. S., Zack, M. B., Davis, D. O., and Stein, E., Radiotherapy in chest malignant tumors associated with pulmonary tuberculosis, *Radiology*, 106, 645, 1973.

72. Bobrowitz, I. D., Elkin, M., Evans, J. C., and Lin, A., Effect of direct irradiation on the course of pulmonary tuberculosis (using cancerocidal doses), *Dis. Chest*, 40, 397, 1961.

73. Feng, P. H. and Tan, T. H., Tuberculosis in patients with systemic lupus erythematosus, *Ann. Rheum. Dis.*, 41, 11, 1982.

74. Ferebee, S. H., Controlled chemoprophylaxis trials in tuberculosis: a general review, *Adv. Tuberc. Res.*, 17, 28, 1970.

75. American Thoracic Society/Centers for Disease Control, Treatment of tuberculosis and tuberculosis infection in adults and children, *Am. Rev. Respir. Dis.*, 149, 1359, 1994.

76. Comstock, G. W., Baum, C., and Snider, D. E., Isoniazid prophylaxis among Alaskan Eskimos: a final report of the Bethel isoniazid studies, *Am. Rev. Respir. Dis.*, 119, 827, 1979.

77. Comstock, G. W., How much isoniazid is needed for prevention of tuberculosis among immunocompetent adults?, *Int. J. Tuberc. Lung Dis.*, 3, 847, 1999.

78. Grosset, J. H., Present status of chemotherapy for tuberculosis, *Rev. Infect. Dis.*, 11 (Suppl.), S347, 1989.

79. Whalen, C. C., Johnson, J. L., Okwera, A., Hom, D. L., Huebner, R., Mugyenyi, P., Mugwera, R. D., and Ellner, J. J., A trial of three regimens to prevent tuberculosis in Ugandan adults infected with the human immunodeficiency virus, *N. Engl. J. Med.*, 337, 801, 1997.

80. Halsey, N. A., Coberly, J. S., Desormeaux, J., Losikoff, P., Atkinson, J., Moulton, L. H., Contave, M., Johnson, M., Davis, H., Geiter, L., Johnson, E., Huebner, R., Boulos, R., and Chaisson, R. E., Randomized trial of isoniazid versus rifampicin and pyrazinamide for prevention of tuberculosis in HIV-1 infection, *Lancet,* 351, 786, 1998.

81. Mwinga, A., Hosp, M., Godfrey-Faussett, P., Quigley, M., Mwaba, P., Mugula, B. N., Nyirenda, O., Luo, N., Pobee, J., Elliott, A. M., McAdam, K. P. W. J., and Porter, J. D. H., Twice weekly tuberculosis preventive therapy in HIV infection in Zambia, *AIDS,* 12, 2447, 1998.

82. Gordin, F., Chaisson, R. E., Matts, J. P., Miller, C., de Lourdes Garcia, M., Hafner, R., Valdespino, J. L., Coberly, J., Schechter, M., Klukowicz, A. J., Barry, M. A., and O'Brien, R. J., Rifampin and pyrazinamide vs. isoniazid for prevention of tuberculosis in HIV-infected persons: an international randomized trial, *JAMA*, 283, 1445, 2000.

83. Centers for Disease Control and Prevention, Use of short-course tuberculosis preventive therapy regimens in HIV-seronegative persons, *MMWR,* 47, 911, 1998.

84. Hong Kong Chest Service/Tuberculosis Research Centre, Madras/British Medical Research Council, A double-blind placebo-controlled clinical trial of antituberculosis chemophophylaxis regimens in patients with silicosis in Hong Kong, *Am. Rev. Respir. Dis.*, 145, 36, 1992.

85. Polesky, A., Farber, H. W., Gottlieb, D. J., Park, H., Levinson, S., O'Connell, J. J., McInnis, B., Nieves, R. L., and Bernardo, J., Rifampin preventive therapy for tuberculosis in Boston's homeless, *Am. J. Respir. Crit. Care Med.*, 154, 1473, 1996.

86. Villarino, M. E., Ridzon, R., Weismuller, P. C., Elcock, M., Maxwell, R. M., Meador, J., Smith, P. J., Carson, M. L., and Geiter, L. J., Rifampin preventive therapy for tuberculosis infection: experience with 157 adolescents, *Am. J. Respir. Crit. Care Med.*, 155, 1735, 1997.

87. Havlir, D. V. and Barnes, P. F., Tuberculosis in patients with human immunodeficiency virus infection, *N. Engl. J. Med.,* 340, 367, 1999.

88. Grzybowski, S., Barnett, G. D., and Styblo, K., Contacts of cases of active pulmonary tuberculosis, *Bull. Int. Union Tuberc.*, 50, 90, 1975.

89. Bjerkedal, T. and Palmer, C. E., Effect of isoniazid prophylaxis in experimental tuberculosis in guinea pigs: action of isoniazid *in vivo, Am. J. Hyg.*, 76, 89, 1962.

90. Grzybowski, S. and Allen, E. A., The challenge of tuberculosis in decline: a study based on the epidemiology of tuberculosis in Ontario, Canada, *Am. Rev. Respir. Dis.*, 90, 707, 1964.

91. Dahlstrom, A. W., Wilson, J. L., and Sedlacek B. B., The immediate effectiveness of isoniazid chemoprophylaxis as determined by the tuberculin test, *Dis. Chest*, 38, 599, 1960.

92. Houk, V. N., Kent, D. C., Sorensen, K., and Baker, J. H., The eradication of tuberculosis infection by isoniazid chemoprophylaxis, *Arch. Environ. Health*, 16, 46, 1968.

93. International Union Against Tuberculosis Committee on Prophylaxis, Efficacy of various durations of isoniazid preventive therapy for tuberculosis: five years of follow-up in the IUAT trial, *Bull. WHO*, 60, 555, 1982.

94. Krebs, A., The IUAT trial on isoniazid preventive treatment in persons with fibrotic lung lesions, *Bull. Int. Union Tuberc.*, 51, 193, 1976.

95. Falk, A. and Fuchs, G. F., Prophylaxis with isoniazid in inactive tuberculosis: a Veterans Administration cooperative study XII, *Chest*, 73, 44, 1978.

96. Katz, J., Kunofsky, S., Damijonaitis, V., Lafleur, A., and Caron, T., Effect of isoniazid upon the reactivation of inactive tuberculosis, *Am. Rev. Respir. Dis.*, 91, 345, 1965.

97. Grzybowski, S., Ashley, M. J., and Pinkus, G., Chemoprophylaxis in inactive tuberculosis: long-term evaluation of a Canadian trial, *Can. Med. Assoc. J.*, 114, 607, 1976.

98a. Hong Kong Chest Service/Tuberculosis Research Centre, Madras/British Medical Research Council, A controlled trial of 2-month, 3-month, and 12-month regimens of chemotherapy for sputum-smear-negative pulmonary tuberculosis: results at 60 months, *Am. Rev. Respir. Dis.*, 130, 23, 1984.

98b. Dutt, A. K., Moers, D., and Stead, W. W., Smear- and culture-negative pulmonary tuberculosis: four-month short-course chemotherapy, *Am. Rev. Respir. Dis.*, 139, 867, 1989.

99. Moore., M., McCray, E., and Onorato, I., The proportion of U.S. TB cases with a match in the AIDS registry [Abstract], *Am. J. Respir. Crit. Care Med.*, 155, A23, 1997.

100. Selwyn, P. A., Hartel, D., Lewis, V. A., Schoenbaum, E. E., Vermund, S. H., Klein, R. S., Walker, A. T., and Friedland, G. H., A prospective study of the risk of tuberculosis among intravenous drug users with human immunodeficiency virus infection, *N. Engl. J. Med.*, 320, 545, 1989.

101. Pape, J. W., Jean, S. S., Ho, J. L., Hafner, A., and Johnson, W. D., Effect of isoniazid prophylaxis on incidence of active tuberculosis and progression of HIV infection, *Lancet*, 342, 268, 1993.

102. Moreno, S., Miralles, P., Diaz, M. D., Baraia, J., Padilla, B., Berenguer, J., and Alberdi, J. C., Isoniazid preventive therapy in human immunodeficiency virus-infected persons: long-term effect on development of tuberculosis and survival, *Arch. Intern. Med.*, 157, 1729, 1997.

103. Friedman, L. N., Williams, M. T., Singh, T. P., and Frieden, T. R., Tuberculosis, AIDS, and death among substance abusers on welfare in New York City, *N. Engl. J. Med.*, 334, 828, 1996.

104. Hawken, M. P., Meme, H. K., Elliott, L. C., Chakaya, J. M., Morris, J. S., Githue, W. A., Juma, E. S., Odhiambo, J. A., Thiong'o, L. N., Kimari, J. N., Ngugi, E. N., Bwayo, J. J., Gilks, C. F., Plummer, F. A., Porter, J. D. H., Nunn, P. P., and McAdam, K. P. W. J., Isoniazid preventive therapy for tuberculosis in HIV-1-infected adults: results of a randomized controlled trial, *AIDS*, 11, 875, 1997.

105. Gordin, F. M., Matts, J. P., Miller, C., Brown, L. S., Hafner, R., John, S. L., Klein, M., Vaughn, A., Besch, C. L., Perez, G., Szabo, S., and El-Sadr, W., A controlled trial of isoniazid in persons with anergy and human immunodeficiency virus infection who are at high risk for tuberculosis, *N. Engl. J. Med.*, 337, 315, 1997.

106. Jordan, T. J., Lewit, E. M., Montgomery, R. L., and Reichman, L. B., Isoniazid as preventive therapy in HIV-infected intravenous drug abusers: a decision analysis, *JAMA*, 265, 2987, 1991.

107. Centers for Disease Control, Purified protein derivative (PPD)-tuberculin anergy and HIV infection: guidelines for anergy testing and management of anergic persons at risk of tuberculosis, *MMWR*, 40, 27, 1991.

108. Caiaffa, W. T., Graham, N. M. H., Galai, N., Rizzo, R. T., Nelson, K. E., and Vlahov, D., Instability of delayed-type hypersensitivity skin test anergy in human immunodeficiency virus infection, *Arch. Intern. Med.*, 155, 2111, 1995.

109. Chin, D. P., Osmond, D., Page-Shafer, K., Glassroth, J., Rosen, M. J., Reichman, L. B., Kvale, P. A., Wallace, J. M., Poole, W. K., Hopewell, P. C., and the Pulmonary Complications of HIV Infection Study Group, Reliability of anergy skin testing in persons with HIV infection, *Am. J. Respir. Crit. Care Med.*, 153, 1982, 1996.

110. Johnson, J. L., Nyole, S., Okwera, A., Whalen, C. C., Nsubuga, P., Pekovic, V., Huebner, R., Wallis, R. S., Mugyenyi, P. N., Mugwera, R. D., and Ellner, J. J., Instability of tuberculin and Candida skin test reactivity in HIV-infected Ugandans, the Uganda-Case Western Reserve University Research Collaboration, *Am. J. Respir. Crit. Care Med.*, 158, 1790, 1998.

111. Centers for Disease Control and Prevention, Anergy skin testing and preventive therapy for HIV-infected persons: revised recommendations, *MMWR*, 46 (No. RR-15), 1, 1997.

112. Moreno, S., Baraia-Etxaburu, J., Bopuza, E., Parras, F., Perez-Tascon, M., Miralles, P., Vicente, T., Alberdi, J. C., Cosin, J., and Lopez-Gay, D., Risk for developing tuberculosis among anergic patients infected with HIV, *Ann. Intern. Med.*, 119, 194, 1993.

113. Guelar, A., Gatell, J. M., Verdejo, J., Podzamczer, D., Lozano, L., Aznar, E., Miro, J. M., Mallolas, J., Zamora, L., Gonzalez, J., and Soriano, E., A prospective study of the risk of tuberculosis among HIV-infected patients, *AIDS*, 7, 1345, 1993.

114. Antonucci, G., Girardi, E., Raviglione, M. C., and Ippolito, G., Risk factors for tuberculosis in HIV-infected persons: a prospective cohort study, *JAMA*, 274, 143, 1995.

115. Selwyn, P. A., Sckell, B. M., Alcabes P., Friedland, G. H., Klein, R. S., and Schoenbaum, E. E., High risk of active tuberculosis in HIV-infected drug users with cutaneous anergy, *JAMA*, 268, 504, 1992.

116. Markowitz, N., Hansen, N. I., Hopewell, P. C., Glassroth, J., Kvale, P. A., Mangura, B. T., Wilcosky, T. C., Wallace, J. M., Rosen, M. J., Reichman, L. B., and The Pulmonary Complications of HIV Infection Study Group, Incidence of tuberculosis in the United States among HIV-infected persons, *Ann. Intern. Med.,* 126, 123, 1997.

117. Gunn, J. E., Brett, D., and Barry, M. A., Progression to tuberculosis in HIV infected anergic persons from "high risk" populations [Abstract], *Am. J. Respir. Crit. Care Med.*, 155, A256, 1997.

118. Haanaes, O. C. and Bergmann, A., Tuberculosis emerging in patients treated with corticosteroids, *Eur. J. Respir. Dis.*, 64, 294, 1983.

119. Millar, J. W. and Horne, N. W., Tuberculosis in immunosuppressed patients, *Lancet*, 2, 1176, 1979.

120. Sahn, S. A. and Lakshminarayan, S., Tuberculosis after corticosteroid therapy, *Br. J. Dis. Chest*, 70, 195, 1976.

121. Ip, M. S. M., Yuen, K. Y., Woo, P. C. Y., Luk, W. K., Tsang, K. W. T., Lam, W. K., and Liang, R. H. S., Risk factors for pulmonary tuberculosis in bone marrow transplant recipients, *Am. J. Respir. Crit. Care Med.,* 158, 1173, 1998.

122. Schatz, M., Patterson, R., Kloner, R., and Falk, J., The prevalence of tuberculosis and positive tuberculin skin tests in a steroid-treated asthmatic population, *Ann. Intern. Med.*, 84, 261, 1976.

123. Smyllie, H. C. and Connolly, C. K., Incidence of serious complications of corticosteroid therapy in respiratory disease: a retrospective survey of patients in the Brompton Hospital, *Thorax*, 23, 571, 1968.

124. Bovornkitti, S., Kangsadal, P., Sathirapat, P., and Oonsombatti, P., Reversion and reconversion rate of tuberculin skin reactions in correlation with the use of prednisone, *Dis. Chest*, 38, 51, 1960.

125. Reichman, L. B., Felton, C. P., and Edsall, J. R., Drug dependence, a possible new risk factor for tuberculosis disease, *Arch. Intern. Med.*, 139, 337, 1979.

126. Centers for Disease Control and Prevention, Recommendations for prevention and control of tuberculosis in among foreign-born persons: report of the Working Group on Tuberculosis Among Foreign-Born Persons, *MMWR,* 47 (No. RR-16), 1, 1998.

127. Nolan, C. M. and Elarth, A. M., Tuberculosis in a cohort of southeast Asian refugees: a five-year surveillance study, *Am. Rev. Respir. Dis.*, 137, 805, 1988.

128. Powell, K. E., Meador, M. P., and Farer L. S., Foreign-born persons with tuberculosis in the United States, *Am. J. Public Health*, 71, 1223, 1981.

129. McKenna, M. T., McCray, E., and Onorato, I., The epidemiology of tuberculosis among foreign-born persons in the United States, 1986 to 1993, *N. Engl. J. Med.,* 332, 1071, 1995.

130. Centers for Disease Control, Prevention and control of tuberculosis in migrant farm workers, *MMWR,* 41 (No. RR-10), 1, 1992.

131. McKenna, M. T., Hutton, M., Cauthen, G., and Onorato, I. M., The association between occupation and tuberculosis: a population-based survey, *Am. J. Respir. Crit. Care Med.,* 154, 587, 1996.

132. Centers for Disease Control, Prevention and control of tuberculosis in U.S. communities with at-risk minority populations, *MMWR*, 41 (No. RR-5), 1, 1992.

133. Centers for Disease Control, Tuberculosis in Blacks — United States, *MMWR*, 36, 212, 1987.

134. Stead, W. W., Senner, J. W., Reddick, W. T., and Lofgren, J. P., Racial differences in susceptibility to infection by *Mycobacterium tuberculosis, N. Engl. J. Med.*, 322, 422, 1990.

135. Centers for Disease Control, Tuberculosis among Hispanics — United States, 1985, *MMWR*, 36, 568, 1987.

136. Centers for Disease Control, Tuberculosis among American Indians and Alaskan natives — United States, 1985, *MMWR*, 36, 493, 1987.

137. Rieder, H. L., Tuberculosis among American Indians of the contiguous United States, *Public Health Rep.*, 104, 653, 1989.

138. Centers for Disease Control, Prevention and control of tuberculosis among homeless persons, *MMWR*, 41 (No. RR- 5), 13, 1992.

139. Centers for Disease Control, Tuberculosis control among homeless population, *MMWR*, 36, 259, 1987.

140. Friedman, L. N., Sullivan, G. M., Bevilaqua, R. P., and Loscos, R., Tuberculosis screening in alcoholics and drug addicts, *Am. Rev. Respir. Dis.*, 136, 1188, 1987.

141. Reichman, L. B. and O'Day, R., Tuberculous infection in a large urban population, *Am. Rev. Respir. Dis.*, 117, 705, 1978.

142. Schieffelbein, C. W. and Snider, D. E., Tuberculosis control among homeless populations, *Arch. Intern. Med.*, 148, 1843, 1988.

143. Centers for Disease Control and Prevention, Prevention and control of tuberculosis in correctional institutions: recommendations of the Advisory Committee for the Elimination of Tuberculosis, *MMWR*, 45 (No. RR-8), 1, 1996.

144. Snider, D. E. and Hutton, M. D., Tuberculosis in correctional institutions (editorial), *JAMA*, 261, 436, 1989.

145. Stead, W. W., Lofgren, J. P., Warren, E., and Thomas, C., Tuberculosis as an endemic and nosocomial infection among the elderly in nursing homes, *N. Engl. J. Med.*, 312, 1483, 1985.

146. Malasky, C., Jordan, T., Potulski, F., and Reichman, L. B., Occupational tuberculous infections among pulmonary physicians in training, *Am. Rev. Respir. Dis.*, 142, 505, 1990.

147. Geiseler, P. J., Nelson, K. E., and Crispen, R. G., Tuberculosis in physicians: a continuing problem, *Am. Rev. Respir. Dis.*, 133, 773, 1986.

148. Haley, C. E., McDonald, R. C., Rossi, L., Jones, W. D., Haley, R. W., and Luby, J. P., Tuberculosis epidemic among hospital personnel, *Infect. Cont. Hosp. Epidemiol.*, 10, 204, 1989.

149. Snider, D. E., The relationship between tuberculosis and silicosis, *Am. Rev. Respir. Dis.*, 118, 455, 1978.

150. Burke, R. M., Schwartz, L. P., and Snider, D. E., The Ottawa county project: a report of a tuberculosis screening project in a small mining community, *Am. J. Public Health*, 69, 340, 1979.

151. Paul, R., Silicosis in northern Rhodesia copper miners, *Arch. Environ. Health*, 2, 96, 1961.

152. Westerholm, P., Ahlmark, A., Maasing, R., and Segelberg, I., Silicosis and risk of lung cancer or tuberculosis: a cohort study, *Environ. Res.*, 41, 339, 1986.

153. Monaco, A., Antituberculous chemoprophylaxis in silicotics, *Bull. Int. Union Tuberc.*, 35, 51, 1964.

154. Allison, A. C. and Hart, P. D., Potentiation by silica of the growth of *Mycobacterium tuberculosis* in macrophage cultures, *Br. J. Exp. Path.*, 49, 465, 1968.

155. Cowie, R. L., Short course chemoprophylaxis with rifampicin, isoniazid and pyrazinamide for tuberculosis evaluated in gold miners with chronic silicosis: a double-blind placebo controlled trial, *Tubercle Lung Dis.*, 77, 239, 1996.

156. Root, H. F., The association of diabetes and tuberculosis: epidemiology, pathology, treatment and prognosis, *N. Engl. J. Med.*, 210, 1, 1934.

157. Oscarsson, P. N. and Silwer, H., Incidence and coincidence of pulmonary tuberculosis among diabetics: search among diabetics in the county of Kristianstad, *Acta. Med. Scand.*, 161 (Suppl. 335), 23, 1958.

158. Boucot, K. R., Tuberculosis among diabetics: the Philadelphia survey, *Am. Rev. Tuberc.*, 65 (Suppl.), 1, 1952.

159. Kessler, I. I., Mortality experience of diabetic patients: a twenty-six year follow-up study, *Am. J. Med.*, 51, 715, 1971.

160. Edsall, J., Collins, J. G., and Gray, J. A. C., The reactivation of tuberculosis in New York City in 1967, *Am. Rev. Respir. Dis.*, 102, 725, 1970.

161. Pablos-Mendez, A., Blustein, J., and Knirsch, C. A., The role of diabetes mellitus in the higher prevalence of tuberculosis among Hispanics, *Am. J. Pub. Health*, 87, 574, 1997.

162. Rose, D. N., Silver, A. L., and Schechter, C. B., Tuberculosis chemoprophylaxis for diabetics. Are the benefits of isoniazid worth the risk? *Mt. Sinai. J. Med.*, 52, 253, 1985.

163. Andrew, O. T., Schoenfeld, P. Y., Hopewell, P. C., and Humphreys, M. H., Tuberculosis in patients with end-stage renal disease, *Am. J. Med.*, 68, 59, 1980.

164. Belcon, M. C., Smith, E. D. M., Kahana, L. M., and Shimizu, A. G., Tuberculosis in dialysis patients, *Clin. Nephrol.*, 17, 14, 1982.

165. Cuss, F. M. C., Carmichael, D. J. S., Linington, A., and Hulma, B., Tuberculosis in renal failure: a high incidence in patients born in the third world, *Clin. Nephrol.*, 25, 129, 1986.

166. Lundin, A. P., Adler, A. J., Berlyne, G. M., and Friedman, E. A., Tuberculosis in patients undergoing maintenance hemodialysis, *Am. J. Med.*, 67, 597, 1979.

167. Pradhan, R. P., Katz, L. A., Nidus, B. D., Matalon, R., and Eisenger, R. P., Tuberculosis in dialyzed patients, *JAMA*, 229, 798, 1974.

168. Rutsky, E. A. and Rostand, S. G., Mycobacteriosis in patients with chronic renal failure, *Arch. Intern. Med.*, 140, 57, 1980.

169. Sasaki, S., Takashi, A., Suenage, M., Tomura, S., Yoshiyama, N., Nakagawa, S., Shoji, T., Sasaoka, T., and Takeuchi, J., Ten years' survey of dialysis-associated tuberculosis, *Nephron*, 24, 141, 1979.

170. Mitwalli, A., Tuberculosis in patients on maintenance dialysis, *Am. J. Kidney Dis.*, 18, 579, 1991.

171. Chia, S., Karim, M., Elwood, R. K., and FitzGerald, J. M., Risk of tuberculosis in dialysis patients: a population-based study, *Int. J. Tuberc. Lung Dis.*, 2, 979, 1998.

172. Vartian, C. V., Tuberculosis in dialysis patients: an old association revisited, *Infect. Dis. Clin. Pract.*, 6, 247, 1997.

173. Freeman, R. M., Newhouse, C. E., and Lawton, R. L., Absence of tuberculosis in dialysis patients (letter), *JAMA*, 233, 1356, 1975.

174. Kaplan, M. H., Armstrong, D., and Rosen, P., Tuberculosis complicating neoplastic disease: a review of 201 cases, *Cancer*, 33, 850, 1974.

175. Feld, R. F., Bodey, G. P., and Groschel, D., Mycobacteriosis in patients with malignant disease, *Arch. Intern. Med.*, 136, 67, 1976.

176. Palmer, C. E., Jablon, S., and Edwards, P. Q., Tuberculosis morbidity of young men in relation to tuberculin sensitivity and body build, *Am. Rev. Tuberc.*, 76, 517, 1957.

177. Edwards, L. B., Livesay, V. T., Acquaviva, F. A., and Palmer, C. E., Height, weight, tuberculous infection, and tuberculous disease, *Arch. Environ. Health*, 22, 106, 1971.

178. Thorn, P. A., Brookes, V. S., and Waterhouse, J. A. H., Peptic ulcer, partial gastrectomy, and pulmonary tuberculosis, *Br. J. Med.*, 1, 603, 1956.

179. Hanngren, A. and Reizenstein, P., Studies in dumping syndrome, *Am. J. Dig. Dis.*, 14, 700, 1969.

180. Frucht, H., Kunkel, P., and Spiro, H. M., Pulmonary tuberculosis following gastric resection, *Ann. Intern. Med.*, 46, 696, 1957.

181. Snider, D. E., Tuberculosis and gastrectomy, *Chest*, 87, 414, 1985.

182. Snider, D. E., Jejunoileal bypass for obesity: a risk factor for tuberculosis, *Chest*, 81, 531, 1982.

183. Bruce, R. M. and Wise, L., Tuberculosis after jejunoileal bypass for obesity, *Ann. Intern. Med.*, 87, 574, 1977.

184. Taylor, W. C., Aronson, M. D., and Delbanco, T. L., Should young adults with a positive tuberculin test take isoniazid? *Ann. Intern. Med.*, 94, 808, 1981.

185. Tsevat, J., Taylor, W. C., Wong, J. B., and Pauker, S. G., Isoniazid for the tuberculin reactor: take it or leave it, *Am. Rev. Respir. Dis.*, 137, 215, 1988.

186. Rose, D. N., Schechter, C. B., and Silver, A. L., The age threshold for isoniazid chemoprophylaxis: a decision analysis for low-risk tuberculin reactors, *JAMA*, 256, 2709, 1986.

187. Colice, G. L., Decision analysis, public health policy, and isoniazid chemoprophylaxis for young adult tuberculin skin reactors, *Arch. Intern. Med.*, 150, 2517, 1990.

188a. Jordan, T. J., Lewit, E. M., and Reichman, L. B., Isoniazid preventive therapy for tuberculosis: decision analysis considering ethnicity and gender, *Am. Rev. Respir. Dis.*, 144, 1357, 1991.

188b. Leff, D. R. and Leff, A. R., Tuberculosis control policies in major metropolitan health departments in the United States. VI. Standard of practice in 1996, *Am. J. Respir. Crit. Care Med.*, 156, 1487, 1997.

189. Ungo, J. R., Jones, D., Ashkin, D., Hollender, E. S., Bernstein, D., Albanese, A. P., and Pitchenik, A. E., Antituberculous drug-induced hepatotoxicity: the role of hepatitis C virus and the human immunodeficiency virus, *Am. J. Respir. Crit. Care Med.*, 157, 1871, 1998.

190. Kopanoff, D. E., Snider, D. E., and Caras, G. J., Isoniazid-related hepatitis: a U.S. Public Health Service surveillance study, *Am. Rev. Respir. Dis.*, 117, 991, 1978.

191. Centers for Disease Control and Prevention, Severe isoniazid-associated hepatitis — New York, 1991-1993, *MMWR*, 42, 545, 1993.

192. Stead, W. W., To, T., Harrison, R. W., and Abraham, J. H., Benefit-risk considerations in preventive treatment for tuberculosis in elderly persons, *Ann. Intern. Med.*, 107, 843, 1987.

193. Comstock, G. W., Prevention of tuberculosis among tuberculin reactors: maximizing benefits, minimizing risks, *JAMA*, 256, 2729, 1986.

194. Nolan, C. M., Goldberg, S. V., and Buskin, S. E., Hepatotoxicity associated with isoniazid preventive therapy: a 7-year survey from a public health tuberculosis clinic, *JAMA*, 281, 1014, 1999.

195. Snider, D. E. and Caras, G. J., Isoniazid-associated hepatitis deaths: a review of available information, *Am. Rev. Respir. Dis.*, 145, 494, 1992.

196. Cross, F. S., Long, M. W., Banner, A. S., and Snider, D. E., Rifampin-isoniazid therapy of alcoholic and nonalcoholic tuberculous patients in a U.S. Public Health Service cooperative trial, *Am. Rev. Respir. Dis.*, 122, 349, 1980.

197. Franks, A. L., Binkin, N. J., Snider, D. E., and Rokaw, W. M., Isoniazid hepatitis among pregnant and postpartum Hispanic patients, *Public Health Rep.*, 104, 151, 1989.

198. Moulding, T. S., Redeker, A. G., and Kanel, G. C., Twenty isoniazid-associated deaths in one state, *Am. Rev. Respir. Dis.*, 140, 700, 1989.

199. Stead, W. W., Pathogenesis of the sporadic case of tuberculosis, *N. Engl. J. Med.*, 277, 1008, 1967.

200. Nardell, E., McInnis, B., Thomas, B., and Wiedhaas, S., Exogenous reinfection with tuberculosis in a shelter for the homeless, *N. Engl. J. Med.*, 315, 1570, 1986.

201. Small, P. M., Shafer, R. W., Hopewell, P. C., Singh, S. P., Murphy, M. J., Desmond, E., Sierra, M. F., and Schoolnik, G. K., Exogenous reinfection with multidrug-resistant Mycobacterium tuberculosis in patients with advanced HIV infection, *N. Engl. J. Med.,* 328, 1137, 1993.

202. Horn, D. L., Hewlett, D., Haas, W. H., Butler, W. R., Alfalla, C., Tan, E., Levine, A., Nayak, A., and Opal, S. M., Superinfection with rifampin-isoniazid-streptomycin-ethambutol (RISE)-resistant tuberculosis in three patients with AIDS: confirmation by polymerase chain reaction fingerprinting, *Ann. Intern. Med.,* 121, 115, 1994.

203. van Rie, A., Warren, R., Richardson, M., Victor, T. C., Gie, R. P., Enarson, D. A., Beyers, N., and van Helden, P. D., Exogenous reinfection as a cause of recurrent tuberculosis after curative treatment, *N. Engl. J. Med.*, 341, 1174, 1999.

204. Koplan, J. P. and Farer, L. S., Choice of preventive treatment for isoniazid-resistant tuberculous infection: use of decision analysis and the Delphi technique, *JAMA*, 244, 2736, 1980.

205. Centers for Disease Control, Management of persons exposed to multidrug-resistant tuberculosis, *MMWR*, 41(No. RR-11), 59, 1992.

206. Gillum, M. D. and Make, D. G., Brief report: tuberculin testing, BCG in pregnancy, *Infect. Cont. Hosp. Epid.*, 9, 119, 1988.

207. Medchill, M. T. and Gillum, M., Diagnosis and management of tuberculosis during pregnancy, *Obstet. Gynecol. Surv.*, 44, 81, 1989.

208. Snider, D., Pregnancy and tuberculosis, *Chest*, 86 (Suppl.), 10S, 1984.

209. Comstock, G. W., Edwards, L. B., and Nabangxang, H., Tuberculin sensitivity eight to fifteen years after BCG vaccination, *Am. Rev. Respir. Dis.*, 103, 572, 1971.

210. Menzies, R. and Vissandjee, B., Effect of bacille Calmette-Guérin vaccination on tuberculin reactivity, *Am. Rev. Respir. Dis.*, 145, 621, 1992.

211. Snider, D. E., Bacille Calmette-Guérin vaccinations and tuberculin skin tests, *JAMA*, 253, 3438, 1985.

212. Centers for Disease Control and Prevention, The role of BCG vaccine in the prevention and control of tuberculosis in the United States, *MMWR,* 45 (No. RR-4), 1, 1996.

14 Control of Tuberculosis

James L. Hadler, M.D., M.P.H.

CONTENTS

0-8493-1565-4/97/$0.00+$.50
© 2000 by CRC Press LLC

I. INTRODUCTION

Methods to control the spread of tuberculosis (TB) in the U.S. have been in a dynamic state for the past 15 years. On the one hand, a national tuberculosis control strategy was developed in the late 1980s in response to a call for tuberculosis elimination in the U.S. by early in the 21st century.[1] On the other hand, just as the U.S. tuberculosis elimination strategy was published, control of tuberculosis was threatened, first in the U.S. and now globally, with two related but distinct new problems: the HIV epidemic and the rapid emergence and spread of multidrug-resistant tuberculosis. Furthermore, just as these new problems begin to be successfully managed in the U.S., other challenges are emerging, including the increasing impact of the global tuberculosis problem on tuberculosis incidence in the U.S. and the need to integrate public health concerns into the managed care movement.

The HIV epidemic has had a profound effect on tuberculosis incidence and transmission in the U.S.,[2-7] Africa,[8-13] and increasingly in many other parts of the world.[11-13] The emergence and transmission of multidrug-resistant strains of *Mycobacterium tuberculosis*,[7,14-19] fueled by the HIV epidemic, resulted in the recognition that a true crisis was occurring and fueled an intensification of tuberculosis control efforts in the U.S.[14,15] As the challenges posed by these newer dynamics have generated initially successful initiatives,[20,21] the impact of the global tuberculosis problem has become increasingly evident. Imported tuberculosis infection rapidly has become a leading source of incident tuberculosis in the U.S.[20,21] and presents perhaps the greatest challenge to national efforts at tuberculosis control and elimination. Finally, the means by which to carry out tuberculosis control are changing, as managed care provides opportunities and challenges in the implementation of tuberculosis control strategies.[23]

The purpose of this chapter is to review the basic principles of tuberculosis control as they relate to these and other tuberculosis control issues in the U.S., and to outline and prioritize strategies for its control given the current epidemiology of tuberculosis in the U.S. Throughout this chapter it is recognized that the ultimate responsibility for successful tuberculosis control in the U.S. lies with local, state, and federal officials. However, tuberculosis control cannot be achieved without the systematic efforts and participation of individual practitioners, or without public interest and support.

II. PRINCIPLES OF TUBERCULOSIS CONTROL

For purposes of this discussion, tuberculosis control efforts can be broken into four major categories:

1. Surveillance
2. Decreasing transmission from, and preventing the emergence of, drug-resistant disease among persons with infectious tuberculosis (case finding and case management)

3. Prevention of development of infectious tuberculosis among persons with latent tuberculous infection (screening and preventive therapy)
4. Keeping uninfected persons from becoming infected with *M. tuberculosis*

A. Surveillance

Surveillance is the collection of information that leads to the effective control of a disease. For effective tuberculosis control, there are a number of types of data that need to be collected systematically.

Foremost for any geographic area (e.g., city, county, state) is the determination of the incidence and epidemiology of tuberculosis in that area. This information becomes the basis to determine what should be appropriate initial therapy for newly diagnosed persons with tuberculosis and which groups should be targeted for case finding and tuberculin screening, and to evaluate whether current efforts are effective in reducing group-specific incidence. Surveillance for incident disease generally is performed by a combination of physician and laboratory reports to local or state health departments with subsequent collection of additional information of concern and, in many states, collection of isolates of *M. tuberculosis* for antibiotic sensitivity testing and molecular subtyping as indicated.[15,24,25] In the current era of HIV-related and multidrug-resistant tuberculosis and imported tuberculous infection, it has become important to obtain information for each reported case on the HIV and drug-susceptibility status and a history of residence in high tuberculosis incidence countries.[14,15,22,24] For institutions and occupational settings such as hospitals, correctional facilities, drug treatment programs, homeless shelters, and long-term care facilities that can expect to manage or be confronted with persons with infectious tuberculosis, systematic periodic employee tuberculin screening programs may be the most effective surveillance tool to determine whether and where transmission is occurring.[26-30]

In addition to incidence measures of disease and infection, optimal tuberculosis control surveillance includes the collection of considerable information on the effectiveness of tuberculosis control activities. These include the effectiveness of case management (e.g., sputum conversion rates at set time intervals, treatment completion rates), the effectiveness of screening (e.g., the number and prevalence of latent tuberculous infections detected annually among target groups for screening, the percentage of persons started on and completing preventive therapy by target group), and, where appropriate, bacille Calmette-Guérin (BCG) vaccination rates.[24]

B. Case Finding and Case Management

The single most important tuberculosis control principle is the minimization of potential for sustained transmission from persons with infectious tuberculosis and the minimization of their potential to develop drug resistance. Early identification of persons with pulmonary tuberculosis and prompt isolation followed by initiation of effective antituberculosis chemotherapy are essential to render a person noninfectious. To minimize the potential for relapse and development of drug resistance, it is necessary to ensure that each person begins an effective drug treatment regimen and remains adherent to it.

Early recognition of suspect cases of tuberculosis and immediate placement in appropriate isolation until medical evaluation is complete and therapy is known to be working are critical early steps in case management. The failure of these measures was responsible for numerous extended multidrug-resistant tuberculosis outbreaks in congregate settings, especially hospitals and correctional facilities, in the past decade.[14-19,28] To promptly recognize and isolate tuberculosis suspects in institutional settings, it is critical to have a high index of suspicion and supportive medical screening and isolation policies.[24,26-30] The most effective means to initiate case finding in the community is to initiate investigation of contacts immediately upon diagnosis of infectious tuberculosis.[24,29]

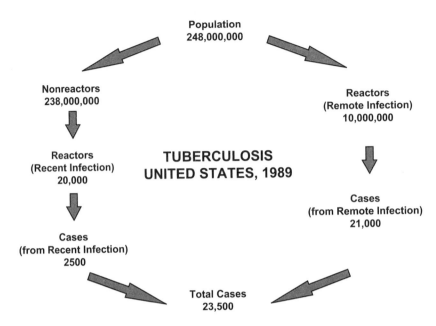

FIGURE 14.1 Epidemiology of tuberculosis and tuberculous infection, United States, 1989. (From the Centers for Disease Control and Prevention, Division of TB Elimination, Atlanta, GA.)

In the era of HIV-related and multidrug-resistant tuberculosis, the initial therapy must cover the possibility of drug resistance to both isoniazid and rifampin,[31,32] and when resistance to either is present, the duration of therapy may need to be extended. Individual physicians must report newly recognized cases of infectious tuberculosis rapidly to public health authorities so that efforts to ensure adherence can begin immediately. In the past decade, public health laws have been strengthened to give public health officials more authority and options to assure compliance, and directly observed therapy (DOT) has gradually become a standard form of therapy in the U.S.[24,31-35]

C. Screening and Preventive Therapy

The second highest priority for tuberculosis control in the U.S. is to keep latently infected persons from developing infectious tuberculosis. It has been estimated that the majority of all incident cases of infectious tuberculosis in the U.S. arise from the reservoir of 5 to 6% of the population latently infected with *M. tuberculosis*,[36] and that as few as 10% arise from recently acquired infection (Figure 14.1). To the extent that the effective reservoir of latent infection can be reduced rapidly through tuberculin screening and preventive therapy efforts, there should be a corresponding immediate impact on incident tuberculosis. Because preventive therapy is the only tuberculosis control measure that acts to reduce the major source of current and impending cases of infectious tuberculosis, its widespread use in areas with low rates of tuberculosis transmission has the potential to impact tuberculosis incidence immediately.[1,37]

HIV-related and multidrug-resistant tuberculosis and tuberculosis in persons infected in high-incidence countries play important roles in screening and preventive therapy strategies. Given that underlying HIV infection now is the strongest known predictor of infectious tuberculosis among persons with latent tuberculous infection,[2,38] screening efforts must be targeted toward the identification of persons with both HIV infection and latent tuberculosis. In addition, completion of therapy for persons with HIV-tuberculous coinfection, given their extraordinary risk of developing tuberculosis, is a major public health concern. Public health authorities must know who has tuberculous and HIV coinfection to be able to ensure the completion of preventive therapy.

The impact of multidrug-resistant tuberculosis is more problematic. Where isoniazid resistance is common among persons presenting with tuberculosis for the first time, the effectiveness of preventive therapy may be correspondingly reduced unless efficacious alternatives are readily available or can be developed.[39]

Prevention of tuberculosis in persons infected in high-incidence areas of the world requires additional strategies. Since the majority develop tuberculosis within 2 to 5 years of arrival in the U.S., they need to be identified shortly after arrival in order to derive the optimimum benefit from preventive therapy.[22] Furthermore, some come from countries where isoniazid resistance rates are high.[40] Most have had BCG in the past, complicating the interpretation of the skin test results by clinicians and by the patients themselves. Many have been educated to think that a positive tuberculin test is good — an index that BCG is conferring immunity. In addition, there may be other cultural beliefs or language problems that make the need for, and concept of, preventive treatment difficult to communicate effectively.[41]

The strategy of tuberculosis control through the widespread use of screening for latent infection and use of preventive therapy is, at most, utilized on a very limited basis in many parts of the world.[42-46] Barriers cited to its use include:

1. Limited resources and the need to focus first on case management.
2. Lack of reliability of the tuberculin skin test for diagnosis of latent infection where BCG vaccine has been in widespread use.
3. Concern that widespread use of isoniazid as preventive therapy could either directly or indirectly promote development of isoniazid-resistant *M. tuberculosis*.

While it is a common concern that widespread use of isoniazid could promote emergence of drug-resistant strains, there is little direct evidence to suggest that this is happening in the U.S., where experience with preventive therapy is the greatest. For the first 20 years of use of isoniazid in the U.S. (1966–86), no change in drug resistance patterns among persons diagnosed for the first time with tuberculosis was observed.[47-49] Anecdotal experience suggests that when active tuberculosis has been systematically ruled out before starting preventive therapy, subsequent emergence of drug-resistant disease is rare. Although all of the factors behind the emergence of multidrug-resistant *M. tuberculosis* nearly 10 years ago in the U.S. are not known yet, it appears that the use of isoniazid preventive therapy was not a factor.

Investigation of outbreaks suggests that the main contributing factors have been inadequate case management of persons with drug-susceptible tuberculosis leading to acquired drug resistance, followed by transmission to persons with underlying immune deficiency who then rapidly develop initially drug-resistant disease and continue the cycle.[7,18,50-53] In parts of the world where primary isoniazid resistance is much more common than in the U.S. (e.g., in southeast Asia), inadequate case management of initially drug-susceptible disease and widespread availability of isoniazid without prescription, permitting isoniazid monotherapy of disease, appear to underlie the problem. Preventive therapy is not used. Thus, the inability to ensure an adequate initial course of therapy (case management) in persons with drug-susceptible disease and transmission to persons without preexisting tuberculous infection appear to be the main sources of drug-resistant tuberculosis, not initial drug resistance in persons previously started on isoniazid preventive therapy.

Given limited resources, the need for better case finding and case management in many parts of the world, and the unfortunate high potential for some persons with tuberculosis to find isoniazid and begin self-medication, it is unlikely that there will be a practical role for the extensive use of preventive therapy as a major tuberculosis control strategy in those areas. However, as the HIV epidemic progresses and HIV-related tuberculosis becomes a major contributor to tuberculosis incidence, selective use of preventive therapy in persons with tuberculous and HIV coinfection may become an important adjunctive tuberculosis control strategy.[45,46] Studies in Haiti and several

African countries have shown that preventive therapy in coinfected persons is beneficial,[54-56] but questions remain about its feasibility on a programmatic basis.[57-59]

D. PREVENTION OF INFECTION

To a large extent, keeping persons without tuberculous infection from becoming infected is dependent on controlling the emission of tubercle bacilli at their source: persons with active infectious tuberculosis. However, to the extent that the potential for exposure is high (e.g., in some U.S. hospitals, in some countries) and the source is not always readily identified, strategies to directly reduce personal or group risk of exposure or to reduce risk of infection with exposure take on more importance. In particular, in the era of multidrug-resistant tuberculosis in which the potential to successfully treat latent tuberculous infection is uncertain, strategies for personal protection take on further importance.

Reduction of risk of exposure to tuberculosis can be achieved through the use of means to reduce the number of suspended infectious droplet nuclei in any given closed space (e.g., dilution by frequent air exchange, ultraviolet light) or through the use of individual protection devices that filter out droplet nuclei from inhaled air. These strategies are covered in detail in Chapter 3. Reduction of the number of suspended droplet nuclei is part of the isolation strategy to protect healthcare workers and patients wherever there is a potentially infectious suspected tuberculosis case.[28] Its more general application to situations in which there may be unrecognized infectious tuberculosis is only practical in selected institutional settings in which there is a predictably high potential for individual or group exposure to persons with infectious tuberculosis, e.g., hospitals continuously treating persons with tuberculosis or AIDS, bronchoscopy suites, some correctional institutions, and some homeless shelters.

Similarly, the use of high-quality individual protective devices needed to prevent infection is only practical when the probability that exposure to an infectious individual is high and cumulative exposure to that person is apt to total at least several hours.

Reduction of the risk of development of active tuberculosis after an exposure to tubercle bacilli also may be reduced by the use of BCG vaccination. In spite of the questionable efficacy of the currently approved strains of BCG, the World Health Organization (WHO) continues to recommend, and many countries in the world have depended on, BCG as a major component of their tuberculosis control strategy.[60] BCG is only expected to benefit persons who have not already been infected with *M. tuberculosis* and who are likely to be exposed in the future. There is no evidence that it affects subsequent disease incidence in persons who already are infected. Its potential role in an overall tuberculosis control strategy is long range. It will only result in a significant long-term decrease in tuberculosis if the new tuberculous infection rate is high, vaccine coverage is high among groups likely to be exposed, and the strain used has high and long-term efficacy. In addition, widespread BCG use makes accurate interpretation of the tuberculin skin test more difficult. For these reasons, BCG vaccination has not been part of the U.S. tuberculosis control strategy.[61] (See Chapter 15 for more information on this matter.)

The emergence of multidrug-resistant tuberculosis in the U.S. has caused experts to revisit the potential role of BCG vaccination in tuberculosis control efforts.[61] It now is recommended that BCG vaccination be considered for healthcare workers in settings where a high percentage of tuberculosis patients have multidrug-resistant strains, and where ongoing exposure is likely and comprehensive TB infection control precautions have been implemented and have not been successful. In addition, BCG vaccination of individual children should be considered if the child is continually exposed to an ineffectively treated patient with infectious tuberculosis, especially if the patient has multidrug resistance.[61] Given the recent success in curbing the resurgence of tuberculosis in the U.S. and halting the rise of multidrug resistance,[40,62,63] there no longer appear to be geographic pockets of tuberculosis in the U.S. in which community-based tuberculosis control efforts are failing and for which BCG vaccination could be considered.

Because BCG vaccines do not play a major role in the U.S. approach to tuberculosis control, they will not be discussed further in this chapter, but in more detail in Chapter 15.

III. CURRENT STRATEGIES AND METHODS FOR TUBERCULOSIS CONTROL IN THE U.S.

The preceding section outlined basic tuberculosis control principles. In this section the strategies, methods, and roles of both public health and individual healthcare providers to achieve these principles are described. In addition, tuberculosis control strategies and needs in special settings and situations are reviewed.

A. SURVEILLANCE

1. Measuring Disease Incidence

Since 1953, the Centers for Disease Control and Prevention (CDC) has been monitoring the occurrence of tuberculosis in the U.S. as a whole and in demographic subgroups through collection of standardized disease reporting from states. State and local health departments in turn have collected information in follow-up of reports of suspected tuberculosis cases from laboratories and healthcare providers. This reporting system has been the primary source of epidemiologic information on tuberculosis in the U.S., as presented in Chapter 1. This information has been supplemented periodically by special time-limited data collection efforts of state and local health departments to gather additional information of interest through individual provider or patient contact.

In response to the need to address both the increase in tuberculosis incidence in the U.S. from the mid-1980s through the early 1990s and the emergence of multidrug-resistant tuberculosis, it had been recommended by several national advisory groups that routine surveillance for tuberculosis in the U.S. include information on drug susceptibility, HIV status when known, and the occupation of each reported case of tuberculosis.[14,15] Beginning in 1993, these new variables were added to the national tuberculosis case surveillance system for all states.[25] Table 14.1 lists variables for new tuberculosis cases that currently are reported to the CDC.

2. Measuring Prevalence of Drug Resistance

In the past, surveillance for drug resistance in the U.S. was done largely through special surveillance efforts by selected state and hospital-based laboratories.[47-49] This approach was limited by the facts that only a limited number of laboratories participated and that surveillance was focused on the incidence of primary drug resistance rather than on all potentially infectious cases of tuberculosis. This system, which had been useful for determining nationwide trends in primary drug resistance, was discontinued in 1986 due to lack of funding.[49]

In the wake of recognition of the outbreaks of multidrug-resistant tuberculosis, a survey of drug susceptibility results collected by state health departments during January to March 1991 was performed by the CDC. This showed an overall prevalence of resistance to both isoniazid and rifampicin of 3.1% in new cases nationally, a marked increase from the 0.5% level from 1982 to 1986.[31] In a separate survey, 19% of 1991 cases in New York City were dually resistant.[64]

Given the magnitude of the prevalence of drug-resistant tuberculosis in some parts of the U.S. and the demonstrated potential for rapid amplification, several new surveillance efforts were recommended and have been implemented. First, it was recommended that initial isolates from all cases of tuberculosis be tested for susceptibility to first-line antituberculosis drugs.[15] Second, the results of susceptibility testing from isolates tested at each state laboratory now are collected by electronic communication at the CDC. The latter system allows for real-time estimation of the current prevalence of drug resistance. However, it does not guarantee population representation,

TABLE 14.1

Epidemiologic and Case Management Data Elements:

State and National Tuberculosis Case Reporting, 1990s

Epidemiologic Elements

Sex	HIV status[a,b]
Race	Homeless status[a]
Ethnic origin	Institutional residence at time of diagnosis[a]
City of residence	Correctional
County of residence	Long-term care
Country of origin	Drug use in past year[a]
Date of arrival in U.S.	Injecting
Date of report	Noninjecting
Date counted	Excess alcohol
	Occupation[a]

Case Management Elements

Previous diagnosis	Date therapy started
Site(s) of disease	Initial drug regimen
Smear/culture status	Sputum conversion date[a]
Drug susceptibility[a]	Date therapy stopped[a]
Initial	Reason therapy stopped[a]
Final	Means of administration[a]
Type of healthcare provider[a,c]	Directly observed
	Self-administered

[a] Added to individual case reports beginning 1993.

[b] Options include negative, positive, indeterminate, refused not offered, test done but results unknown, unknown.

[c] Options include health department, private/other, both.

Source: Adapted from Friedman, L. N., Ed., *Tuberculosis: Current Concepts and Treatment,* 1st ed., CRC Press LLC, Boca Raton, FL, 1994. With permission.

since only isolates tested by state health laboratories are included. Finally, no matter where susceptibility testing is performed, each state health department now collects such information on each new incident and recurrent case of tuberculosis and submits the information as part of a complete case report.[15] This system has enabled detailed population-based evaluations of the epidemiology of drug resistance at selected points in time, and in an ongoing fashion.[40] It has been shown, using this system, that multidrug resistance has decreased to 2.2% since 1991, that isoniazid resistance is widespread, exceeding 4% in 82% of states and that the foreign-born, persons with HIV infection, and persons with prior tuberculosis have higher rates of drug resistance.[40]

3. Measuring Incidence of New Infection

There has been no systematic population-level surveillance for the incidence of new tuberculous infections in the U.S. This is due in part to the fact that the periodic serial tuberculin testing such surveillance would require is impractical and logistically difficult to perform at the population level. Nonetheless, there is a plan to incorporate systematic serial tuberculin testing into the National Health and Nutrition Examination Survey (NHANES) beginning in 1999 in order to establish a baseline for future comparisons.

Surveillance for new infection has been an important tuberculosis control strategy and evaluation tool in institutional settings where there is substantial potential for tuberculosis exposure. It has been a long-standing and continuing recommendation to screen employees periodically with tuberculin to determine institutional exposure potential, infection rates, and preventive therapy needs.[26-30,65]

In the current era in which tuberculosis exposure among the HIV-infected can trigger outbreaks of disease with short incubation periods, determination of the incidence of infection takes on new importance. To prevent exposure of workers and patients to tuberculosis, especially HIV-infected healthcare workers and patients to multidrug-resistant tuberculosis, hospitals now are required to have effective isolation facilities and procedures.[28,66] The only outcome measure that is readily obtainable to monitor the effectiveness of these costly changes is the incidence of new tuberculous infection among employees or, where possible, long-term residents. In hospitals where testing is systematic, important program information has been obtained, i.e., information to help recognize new areas of risk and information to help confirm that current risk is low.[67-69] Employee skin testing also has been used to evaluate the effectiveness of the control measures implemented following recognition of multidrug-resistant tuberculosis outbreaks in several hospitals.[70-72]

4. Detection of Outbreaks

In the past there was no strategy to systematically detect outbreaks of tuberculosis. Given the recent recognition of many drug-sensitive and drug-resistant outbreaks of tuberculosis among HIV-infected persons, an increasing need has developed for systematic surveillance to allow early recognition of such outbreaks.

There are at least several possible strategies for outbreak detection. One is recognition of high tuberculous infection rates among employees in institutions caring for substantial numbers of HIV-infected persons, and follow-up to determine the presence of infection or disease among HIV-infected individuals who may have been exposed at the same time. This method depends on effective and systematic employee screening programs.

A second strategy for outbreak detection depends on taking advantage of the relatively short incubation period between exposure and development of tuberculosis in persons with advanced HIV infection. To the extent that local and state health officials can get HIV-related information on new tuberculosis cases and interview them for recent potential institutional exposure (in hospitals, correctional settings, drug treatment programs, and AIDS residences), outbreaks may be detected early. As yet, this method largely is untried, but it has been recommended.[15]

A third possible strategy is an application of the restriction-fragment-length polymorphism (RFLP) typing technique. This and related techniques have been used to confirm the commonality of sources in some of the multidrug-resistant tuberculosis outbreaks,[18,50] and are commonly used to assess the relationships among clusters of cases or isolates in place and time.[19,73-76] When used either prospectively or retrospectively to evaluate isolates from the same geographic area, neighborhood clusters among persons who were otherwise unrelated have been identified.[77-79] The recognition that neighborhood tuberculosis clusters of common RFLP types in urban areas occur and may account for as much as 40% of all incident TB cases has led to a call for a reexamination of how tuberculosis contact investigations are performed.[77,78,80]

5. Measuring the Effectiveness of Case Management

For several decades, tuberculosis control strategies in the U.S. have included the collection of information on the success of case management and selected screening and preventive therapy activities. The measures used have provided guidance for program review and funding, and have shown that the state of tuberculosis control in the U.S. was not good during the recent tuberculosis resurgence. In the wake of the changes in the national tuberculosis surveillance system in 1993 and the adoption of directly observed therapy as a major strategy to improve case management, the indicators now used also have changed.

Case management measures in the U.S. for decades emphasized documentation of sputum conversion rates by 3 months as an initial outcome measure of continuity and efficacy of initial therapy, and the therapy continuity rate at 6 months and eventual completion rate as major intermediate and final outcome measures. Since 1993, with the expansion of surveillance activities, case management information has been collected on each individual and reported in line-list format together with demographic and risk information by state tuberculosis control programs to the CDC (Table 14.1).[25,81] This expanded system should allow for more flexibility of analysis by population demographic characteristics, by whether or not a patient is placed on directly observed therapy, by initial treatment regimen, and by initial drug susceptibility results. Since this system was implemented, there has been an emphasis on different measures. The percentage of patients placed on directly observed therapy, the therapy completion rate at 12 months among those whose initial drug susceptibility findings indicated that therapy could be completed within 12 months, and the completion rate 2 years after diagnosis have replaced the previous measures. In addition, patients who move or are "lost" now count in the denominator of the latter two rates. Prior to the implementation of the new system, they could be excluded. Thus, current measures force tuberculosis programs to take full responsibility for monitoring the outcome of all cases initially reported to them.

For U.S. cases diagnosed in 1995, the following case management indices were documented: 57% received some directly observed therapy, 72% of those eligible completed therapy within 12 months, and 89% completed therapy by 1998.[81] The national goal in each of these areas is 90%. Although sputum conversion data still is collected for each individual, the sputum conversion rate no longer is used as a major program management index because many patients do not get systematic sputum monitoring once spontaneous cough and sputum production end.[82] Thus, many individuals cannot be counted as sputum converters, even though they may be asymptomatic and continuously taking therapy.

There have been no published analyses of what "threshold" case management indices correlate with subsequent emergence of significant problems. However, during the recent era of national TB resurgence (1985 to 1992), substantial and important differences were seen in some of these program management measures between different areas of the country, in particular for those areas with sustained increases in tuberculosis incidence and/or higher levels of drug resistance. In addition, the subsequent decrease in TB in many areas has been preceded or accompanied by a marked improvement in case management indices.[63,83] In New York City, which had the largest percentage increase in tuberculosis incidence in the U.S. and the highest percentage of cases with multidrug resistance, case management measures were among the lowest in the country. Only 56% of the cases started on therapy in 1990 in New York City were documented to have been continuously on therapy for 6 months, and 34% of all cases were declared lost to follow-up within this time period.[84] By contrast, more than 50% of states had a 6-month continuity-of-therapy index of 90% or greater and none had rates as low as in New York City. Outside of New York City, only 4% of cases were declared "lost" during the first 6 months. In addition to New York, many large urban areas of the country had relatively low continuity-of-therapy indices. For example, in 1990, the 6-month continuity-of-therapy index was only 61% for Newark, 64% for Chicago, and 66% for Houston. In each, the increase in tuberculosis incidence from 1987 to 1991 (42.3, 5.7, and 11.1 cases per 100,000 population, respectively) exceeded the overall national increase of 1.1 cases per 100,000 population.[85,86]

Since 1993, the annual TB incidence has decreased progressively.[81] By 1997, a 26% overall decrease in reported cases occurred when compared to 1992, the peak year of resurgence. The drop in incidence was associated directly in time with national and local investment in TB control and improvement in case management indices, particularly therapy completion rates.[34,35,63,83]

Cities with low therapy completion rates and high TB incidences have had striking changes in both. Between 1992 and 1997, the TB incidence in New York City had decreased by 28 cases per 100,000. Its documented therapy completion rate for 1995 cases was 93%, compared to <50% in

1990. For Newark, Chicago, and Houston, the TB incidence decreased similarly by 28, 7, and 9 cases per 100,000, respectively, while therapy completion rates rose from 60% or lower to levels above 80%. The rate of DOT use among the 1995 reported cases in New York City was 56%. It had been as low as 5% prior to "turning the tide."[83]

6. Measuring the Effectiveness of Screening and Prevention

National measures of the effectiveness of screening and prevention have focused largely on case-contact investigations. These measures have been both outcome and process oriented. One major outcome has been the number of cases of tuberculosis disease found among contacts. Process measures have included the number of latently infected contacts found and the percentages of those who are offered and complete a course of preventive therapy. From this information, it is possible to estimate the number of cases of tuberculosis that were prevented as a result of contact investigation. Contacts have been a concern because, except for persons with tuberculous-HIV coinfection, tuberculin-positive contacts of infectious tuberculosis cases have the highest predictable risk of developing infectious disease of any sizable, readily identifiable category of persons with latent tuberculous infection. Furthermore, some already have developed tuberculosis by the time they are identified. Their investigation remains a major tuberculosis control priority.[24]

In 1996, nearly 120,000 persons were tuberculin tested as a result of contact investigation in the U.S. Of these, 995 cases of active tuberculosis were found and 14,785 infected contacts began preventive therapy. Embedded in these sizable numbers are several mixed trends. Between 1987 and 1991, progressively fewer tuberculosis cases had had contacts identified. In 1987, the percentage of cases with contacts identified was 84%. By 1991, it decreased to 74%, but in 1996 it increased to 82%. During the same 3 years, the percentage of infected contacts younger than 15 years old who were started on preventive therapy had gone from 88% to 82% to 86%, respectively. Of concern, though, is that of those younger than 15 years old who were started on preventive therapy, the percentage completing it has fallen from 82% to 76% to 75%, respectively.[84,87]

Beginning in the late 1980s, federal funding supported systematic efforts to identify persons with HIV and latent tuberculous coinfection in drug treatment programs, correctional facilities, HIV counseling and testing sites, and sexually transmitted disease clinics. While recommendations have been made by a number of groups to monitor the success of such efforts,[2,24,88-90] the few reports of their efficacy and potential impact on tuberculosis prevention are limited largely to conference abstracts.[91-93] Based on the limited information in these reports, it appears that prison systems may be the most productive sites to identify and treat persons with tuberculous-HIV coinfection. In the one state in which tuberculous-HIV coinfection is systematically monitored, screening and preventive therapy programs in prisons account for more than 50% of all coinfections identified and more than 50% of all those who completed preventive therapy.[92,94]

7. Measuring Transmission

There are no systematic, population-based, surveillance efforts to measure transmission of tuberculosis in the U.S. Transmission in the community is difficult to measure accurately because the transmission rates in the U.S. generally are low and often are highly focal.[74,76-79] In general, the incidence of smear-positive tuberculosis per 100,000 population is a reasonable index of the potential for transmission in the population. In developing countries, a 1% annual rate of new tuberculosis infection correlates with an incidence of 50 smear-positive tuberculosis cases per 100,000 population.[95]

In institutional settings that can expect to take care of persons with infectious tuberculosis and which need to monitor the need for and effectiveness of environmental control and early diagnosis and isolation policies, surveillance for transmission is a priority. Thus, systematic tuberculin skin testing surveillance of workers is required in acute healthcare settings,[28,96] and is recommended strongly for correctional, drug treatment, and homeless shelter personnel.[26,27,30] In these settings, the annual tuberculin conversion rate in the absence of transmission should reflect that of the community — generally less than 5 per 1000 person-years (0.5% per year).

8. Respective Roles of Healthcare Providers and Public Health Agencies in Surveillance

Surveillance for tuberculosis cannot work effectively without substantial interaction between individual care providers and public health agencies.

To have an efficient surveillance system, individual care providers must:

- Rapidly report to local and state public health authorities new and suspected cases of tuberculosis within 24 to 72 h of starting therapy
- Assess the HIV and drug susceptibility status of each case[2,15]
- When requested, provide to public health authorities more detailed information on each reported case as outlined in Table 14.1
- Regularly obtain follow-up sputum specimens to document conversion from positive to negative culture status on each case
- Immediately report to local public health authorities any person not on directly observed therapy who is suspected of nonadherence[1]

Public health agencies must in turn:

- Promptly investigate each case of newly reported tuberculosis to establish a relationship with the patient, to assess whether some form of supervised therapy is necessary, to make a joint treatment plan with the healthcare provider, and to ensure that a thorough contact investigation is performed
- Maintain comprehensive data collection and analysis systems to ensure that complete surveillance information is collected on each newly reported case, and that the resulting data is analyzed
- Establish and maintain the capacity to ensure that at least one isolate of *M. tuberculosis* on each newly active pulmonary case is tested for susceptibility to first-line antituberculosis drugs
- Disseminate the results of tuberculosis surveillance to providers and the public on a regular basis[1,24]

B. Case Finding and Case Management

Case finding and case management are at the core of tuberculosis control in the U.S. and worldwide. The main goals of case finding and case management are to identify all infectious cases of tuberculosis, to render them noninfectious rapidly through immediate isolation and appropriate initial therapy, and to keep them on therapy until cured so that they will not relapse and become infectious again or develop drug resistance. Of these goals, the one that has been the focus of most public health attention, particularly in the U.S., has been to maintain patients on therapy until they are cured. Correspondingly, a major focus of this section is adherence to therapy.

1. Case Finding

Case finding historically has been an important tuberculosis control strategy in groups with a high tuberculosis prevalence. Methods have included population-based chest radiographic screening, initial symptom examination followed by sputum smears and/or chest radiography,[42,44] and

---

TABLE 14.2
Recommended Tuberculosis Case-Finding: Candidate Groups,
Methods, and Frequency

Group	Initial Screening Method	Frequency[a]
Contacts	Skin test and symptoms	Initial; 12 weeks
Jail[b] entrants	Symptoms or chest radiograph	Entry
Prison[c] entrants	Skin test and symptoms	Entry and Annually
Long-term care entrants	Skin test and symptoms	Entry
Homeless	Symptoms and/or chest radiograph	As possible[d]
Migrant workers	Symptoms	As possible[d]
Immigrants and refugees	Chest radiograph and skin test	See note[e]
Admissions to hospitals	Skin test and symptoms	Entry

[a] Tuberculin and symptom screening should be repeated in all groups following exposure to a potentially infectious case.

[b] "Jail" refers to a holding institution for the detention of persons accused of criminal behavior, prior to the posting of bond and/or trial.

[c] "Prison" refers to an institution for the detention of persons who are sentenced.

[d] Should be initiated by local health agencies and repeated periodically as indicated by its productivity.

[e] All refugees and legal immigrants ≥15 years are required to have a chest radiographic screening before entry into the U.S. Some children <15 years old are required to have tuberculin screening. All persons with abnormal chest radiographs should be tuberculin-tested as soon after entry as possible. All immigrants seeking adjustment of visitor status to immigrant status after arrival in the U.S. are required to have a tuberculin skin test.

Source: Adapted from Friedman, L. N., Ed., *Tuberculosis: Current Concepts and Treatment,* 1st ed., CRC Press LLC, Boca Raton, FL, 1994.

---

tuberculin skin testing followed by symptom and chest radiographic examination of all persons with significant reactions.

In the U.S., the large population-based case finding strategy of the preantibiotic era largely has been abandoned. It is logistically difficult and not cost effective in most situations. However, there still are population subgroups, other than symptomatic patients seeking medical care, for which proactive case finding is potentially cost effective and is recommended.[26-28,30,96-98] In the U.S., these groups include:

1. Persons entering institutional settings in which persons at high risk of having tuberculosis are living, the environmental characteristics are conducive to transmission, and large numbers of susceptible persons are located (e.g., prisons and jails, healthcare facilities, and nursing homes).
2. Contacts of infectious cases of tuberculosis.
3. Homeless persons living in shelters.
4. Migrant farm workers.
5. Persons entering the country with immigrant or refugee status.

The methods and frequency of attempts at case finding vary by group (Table 14.2). Where continued access to the groups is questionable and/or risk of active disease is high (jail entrants, homeless persons, migrant farm workers), screening methods should utilize initial symptom or radiographic evaluation. In groups in which the prevalence of disease is likely to be lower (e.g.,

<1%), especially if continued access for repeated screening and preventive therapy is likely (contacts, prison entrants, long-term care residents), initial tuberculin skin testing together with symptom evaluation should be performed.

The efficacy of case finding can be remarkably high in some subgroups. Based on screening at selected clinics and shelters, the prevalence of clinically active disease among the homeless has ranged as high as 1.6 to 6.8%, and the prevalence of latent infection from 18 to 57%.[26,99-102] Among migrant workers screened in 1988 in North Carolina, the prevalence of active tuberculosis was 0.5% in Hispanics and 3.5% in American Blacks.[103] Among tuberculin-positive contacts of active tuberculosis cases in 1996, 3.8% were found to have active disease.[87] Among Class B1 (chest radiograph compatible with active tuberculosis but smear negative) and Class B2 (chest radiograph compatible with inactive tuberculosis) immigrants screened overseas, 3 to 14% and 0.4 to 4%, respectively, were found to have active tuberculosis after arrival in the U.S.[22,97] Nonetheless, not all screening for active disease is so productive. Each geographic area needs to identify its own high-risk groups and assess whether active case finding is indicated.

2. Isolation

A critical component in the series of steps that need to be followed for optimal case management to stop transmission of tuberculosis is initiation of isolation as soon as tuberculosis is suspected.[24,28] Isolation must be continued until it is clear the patient is on appropriate therapy, is improving, and no longer is a risk to others. Lack of immediate isolation, of effective isolation, and of isolation of sufficient duration in hospitals and in correctional facilities were major factors in the spread of multidrug-resistant tuberculosis in New York.[83] In the wake of this recognition, the CDC guidelines for control of tuberculosis in healthcare settings were revised,[28] and OSHA established requirements for all acute healthcare facilities to have policies, procedures, and the capacity to isolate all tuberculosis suspects immediately until they are demonstrated to be not infectious.[66]

3. Choice of Therapy

Three main factors dictate the choice of antituberculosis therapy:

1. The need to cover the potential for drug resistance.
2. The need to have a regimen that is of the shortest possible duration.
3. Cost.

In principle, it is recommended that a patient be started on a regimen that contains at least two drugs to which the organism is likely to be susceptible. For most first-time cases, this has meant a two- or three-drug regimen, the latter being a necessary initiation phase for the short-course, 6- to 8-month regimens in general use in the U.S. and recommended by the USPHS and WHO.[32,36,104] However, given the emergence of multidrug-resistant tuberculosis in the U.S., it now is nationally recommended that unless there is virtual certainty that a person has fully sensitive organisms, all first-time tuberculosis cases should be started on a four-drug regimen to include isoniazid, rifampicin, pyrazinamide, and either ethambutol or streptomycin until the results of susceptibility tests are known.[31,32] This represents a major departure from pre-1992 recommendations and is intended in part to decrease the potential for institutional transmission from persons with organisms initially resistant to one or two drugs.

Shortening the course of antituberculosis treatment to make it easier to ensure that a person completes treatment has been a major practical tuberculosis control research issue for decades. Highly efficacious regimens now exist that can be completed in as little as 6 months with as few as 62 doses of antituberculosis drugs.[105,106] The shortest course regimens generally require initiation of therapy with four drugs, including isoniazid, rifampicin, and pyrazinamide with either ethambutol or streptomycin as the fourth drug. The same regimen that makes short-course treatment a possibility also covers the potential for single or even two-drug resistance. Thus, the best tuberculosis control strategy for the 1990s dictates initiation of four antituberculosis drugs in nearly all cases. Implementation of this treatment strategy combined with improvement in isolation and adherence to therapy has resulted not only in a decrease in tuberculosis incidence in the U.S. in the past 5 years, but also in a decrease in the incidence of multidrug-resistance, particularly in New York City.[81,83]

In some parts of the world, the cost of drugs has been a major concern. In particular, a standard WHO-recommended regimen previously in widespread use for either treatment from the outset or the continuation phase of an 8-month, short-course regimen had been isoniazid and thiacetazone.[44] However, in the HIV era, use of thiacetazone has proved to be problematic. Not only do regimens using thiacetazone require a longer time to complete, but among HIV-infected cases, severe reactions, including death, have been observed with unacceptable frequency, and higher relapse rates have been observed than with the use of other regimens.[107,108] In one study of children, 13% had fatal Stevens-Johnson syndrome-like reactions. In the same study, only 24% of HIV-positive children had a satisfactory response to treatment compared to 98% of those who were HIV negative.[108] Given its limitations, the role of thiacetazone in tuberculosis control worldwide has diminished. The WHO-recommended strategy of choice has become similar to that in the U.S.: directly observed therapy as often as possible accompanied by the most effective short-course regimens, which include isoniazid and rifampin.[109]

4. Adherence to Therapy

a. Background

Achieving high rates of patient adherence to therapy has been identified repeatedly as a major obstacle to tuberculosis control in the U.S.[110-116] Failure to achieve high adherence rates was a major factor underlying both the striking increase in tuberculosis in New York City[116] and in the emergence of drug resistance in the U.S.[14]

In the absence of any systematic effort to ensure that patients with infectious tuberculosis will take antituberculosis medicines for at least 6 months, it can be expected that completion rates will be low, often less than 50%. For example, only 11% of tuberculosis patients, where therapy was initiated as inpatients in Harlem Hospital Center in 1988, were shown to have completed therapy.[116] Even with active follow-up systems in place, a number of U.S. cities were able to demonstrate only 50 to 70% completion rates during the recent tuberculosis resurgence.[84] Such low completion rates were inadequate and were major contributors to the resurgence and to the emergence of drug resistance. It has been estimated that therapy completion rates of at least 70 to 85% are necessary to ensure a decline in tuberculosis incidence.[117]

Although the problem of emergence and spread of multidrug-resistant tuberculosis was most prominent in areas of the country with less than 80% completion rates, initiation of a local problem requires only a single nonadherent case with the opportunity to expose many others. Correspondingly, it is critical that public health authorities and tuberculosis control programs take an aggressive role to ensure that each infectious case of tuberculosis receives a full and continuous course of treatment.[14,15]

There is substantial medical literature dating back at least 20 years concerning factors that affect a person's healthcare-seeking behavior and adherence to recommendations to take therapy for a prolonged period.[118-122] There also has been a number of tuberculosis-specific studies of behavioral factors that influence whether a person with tuberculosis will complete a course of therapy.[123-134] The major conclusion to be drawn from a social and behavioral perspective is that adherence to antituberculosis therapy appears to be a complex interaction of a number of factors. These include the nature of the patient and his understanding and beliefs regarding the importance of therapy, the individual healthcare provider and his commitment to meaningful involvement with the patient, and the nature of the healthcare delivery system (Table 14.3).[123,132]

TABLE 14.3
Factors Affecting Adherence to Therapy

Patient Factors

1. Belief that treatment and its completion are important
2. Understanding of what is necessary to complete therapy
3. Degree to which taking medicines can be easily assimilated into daily lifestyle
4. Degree of support from community and healthcare provider for taking medicine
5. Extent of perceived benefits of completing therapy
6. Belief that there must be a degree of control over therapy
7. Duration of therapy
8. Number of pills that must be taken daily
9. Personal cost
10. Side effects
11. Stability of life style

Individual Provider Factors

1. Assumption of responsibility for completion of therapy
2. Assumption of responsibility to "educate" the patient
3. Assumption of responsibility for monitoring adherence
4. Extent of recognition of signs and symptoms of nonadherence
5. Extent to which the provider can prescribe simpler and shorter durations of therapy
6. Extent of the ability to reduce the time between the last appointment reminder and any scheduled appointment

Clinic Factors

1. Accessibility of the clinic:
   Distance from patient
   Cost of travel
   Cost of visit
   Convenient hours of operation
2. Ambience of healthcare
   Waiting times
   Cultural appropriateness including translating
   Staff attitudes
   Clinical setting
   Use of incentives (child care, free snacks)

Source: Friedman, L. N., Ed., *Tuberculosis: Current Concepts and Treatment,* 1st ed., CRC Press LLC, Boca Raton, FL, 1994. With permission.

The extent to which each of these factors can be influenced to improve treatment outcome has been less well studied.[123] However, it has been demonstrated that passive tuberculosis clinic models in which the physician and healthcare delivery system expect the patient to conform to their orders or configuration and in which little responsibility is taken for the patient's adherence to therapy do poorly when compared to more active models.[135-139] A comprehensive approach to the clinical aspects of tuberculosis control can be highly successful, even with a challenging clinic population, when individual clinicians are aware of their responsibility for each patient's adherence, and the healthcare delivery system is shaped, in part, around the needs of the tuberculosis patient.[135-137]

The rest of this section describes the specific case-management options that need to be considered to maximize the potential for continuous adherence to therapy.

TABLE 14.4
Strategies to Ensure Adherence to Therapy

1. Directly observed therapy
     The maximum benefits of DOT will occur when:
          The supervisor is acceptable to patient
          Flexibility is used in selecting the place to give therapy (e.g., home, work, street)
          Twice-weekly therapy is used
          Inducements and incentives are used to ensure meetings
2. Self-administered therapy
     Patients started on self-administered therapy will do best when:
          They are reported to local and state health departments
          They have a supportive family and physician
          They have periodic home visits
          Their pill-taking regimen is simple and associated with a daily activity
          Clinic visits and medicines are free or low-cost
          Pills are given out in small quantities (≤30-day supply)
          Clinic and/or home visits are scheduled at least monthly
          Preappointment reminders are used
3. Promptly identify potential nonadherence
     Clinicians need to use the following methods to promptly identify nonadherence so that it can be
     reported to public health agencies for immediate follow-up:
          Use DOT wherever possible or dispense medicines in small quantities and closely monitor refills
          Count pills frequently: home visits, medication monitors
          Measure INH metabolites in urine
     Assess response to therapy:
          Frequent symptom evaluation
          Frequent sputum smears and culture

Source: Adapted from Friedman, L. N., Ed., *Tuberculosis: Current Concepts and Treatment,* 1st ed., Boca
Raton, FL, 1994.

b. Directly Observed/Supervised Therapy

A wide range of methods have been used in an attempt to ensure high levels of adherence to therapy.
These methods generally can be categorized into two groups: (1) those in which therapy is
supervised or directly observed by a healthcare worker or other observer, and (2) those that are
intended to enhance adherence where the patient is self-administering medicines (Table 14.4).

Directly observed therapy has long been recognized as a highly effective way to achieve
adherence.[140] However, until recently, it usually was used only with demonstratedly difficult to
manage patients. With the recognition of the failure of passive tuberculosis control efforts in New
York City and the rapid emergence of multidrug-resistant tuberculosis, DOT has quickly become
the treatment adjunct of choice for most tuberculosis patients in the U.S. and the world.[31,32,83,109]
Because of the increasing concern that even a single case of drug resistance could be amplified
rapidly if many HIV-infected persons were exposed, the U.S. Public Health Service (USPHS) has
recommended since 1993 that most persons on antituberculosis therapy be on DOT.[31] New York
City, the epicenter of drug-resistant tuberculosis in the U.S., also has made this a programmatic
goal.[83] These recommendations are based on the facts that:

- DOT provides immediate feedback on whether a patient is receiving prescribed therapy
- Very high adherence rates have been achieved with DOT[83,138,141-144]
- DOT has proved to be highly cost effective when compared with hospitalization for
  retreatment and/or the consequences of acquired drug resistance[145-146]

High adherence rates have been achieved repeatedly by DOT in therapeutic trials of twice-weekly therapy. In public health practice, the success of DOT also has been demonstrated.[83,141-146] Since the 1993 recommendation that DOT be used as part of the initial treatment plan wherever possible, and the commitment of fiscal resources to enable its widespread implementation, the use of DOT has increased rapidly. Of tuberculosis cases reported in the U.S. in 1995, DOT was used in 58% at some time during drug therapy and in 37% as the sole form of therapy.[81] In 15 states including New York, more than 50% of cases were started on DOT. In Mississippi, which routinely has used DOT since 1984 after having an outbreak of multidrug-resistant tuberculosis generated by a nonadherent case,[147,148] 99% of all patients were started on DOT in 1995. The rapid implementation of DOT in New York City is considered to be the primary reason for the rapid improvement in therapy completion rates and the drop in tuberculosis incidence that followed.[83]

DOT is cost effective when compared to self-administered alternatives.[141,145,146] While the cost for outreach personnel to deliver therapy is not inconsequential and it has taken considerable national and local investment to make the current levels of DOT possible,[83] the cost is more than offset by savings in shorter initial hospital stays, and lower relapse, retreatment, rehospitalization, and drug-resistance rates. Furthermore, the cost of outreach can be minimized by the use of twice-weekly regimens. Using twice-weekly regimens, as few as 62 meetings for DOT are necessary to complete a full course of treatment.[105]

DOT can be given in a variety of settings and by a variety of personnel. No single rigid model is necessary other than having a responsible person who is acceptable to the patient administer medicines and observe their ingestion on a daily, twice- or thrice-weekly basis at a site mutually agreed upon by both patient and observer. DOT has been given in clinic settings, in correctional institutions, in methadone and other drug treatment modalities, in the workplace, in schools, in homeless shelters, in the home, and on the street. Although DOT usually is provided by public health personnel such as outreach workers or clinic nurses, it also can be given by other trusted persons with regular predictable contact with the patient; e.g., nurses in drug treatment or occupational settings, teachers, social workers, and relatives.

Compliance with DOT sometimes can be a problem in settings in which the patient is not "captive," especially when the patient is homeless and/or is a substance abuser, may not predictably be in the same location at a given time, or may not agree on the importance of completing therapy. To maximize the potential for the person supervising the therapy and the patient to interact, incentives[132,133,149,150] or legal inducements[34,140] have been used successfully. Such incentives include free bus tokens, returnable cans and bottles, free meals, arrangements for housing and other social services, and small but meaningful gifts of use to the patient.[132,133,149,150] Legal inducements are discussed further in the Section III,B,4,e. Although DOT by itself can result in high adherence rates, the best rates of therapy completion are achieved by DOT combined with enhancements and enablers.[141]

c. Self-Administered Therapy

Traditionally, most patients have been managed initially with daily self-administered therapeutic regimens. Such regimens, if successful, are cheaper to administer than DOT and some physicians and patients prefer the implication of trust associated with them. However, as experience has shown, they are less reliable and more cumbersome when it comes to ensuring adherence to therapy.

Many of the factors that determine whether or not a patient will complete therapy (Table 14.3) can be influenced by the healthcare provider and local public health authorities (Table 14.4). Of particular importance is that local health authorities know of each patient's diagnosis as soon as therapy is started. Reporting will enable them to become part of the "team" that lends educational and outreach support to the patient from the outset.[1,24]

Multiple studies have shown that in the majority of tuberculosis cases there is no single factor that determines full adherence to therapy. An individual but comprehensive approach is needed for each patient.[123,132] Among the factors to be considered are patient education, provider and family support, and the establishment of simple and inexpensive pill-taking regimens. Patients need to know and understand why, what, how, and for how long they should take their antituberculosis therapy. This information may need to be reinforced repeatedly, in a culturally sensitive way, and with audiovisual aids.[123] Some patients may need guided practice and demonstration in pill ingestion.[132]

Supportive family, friends, and healthcare providers are important to increase patient motivation.[123,132] Where support is lacking, some patients may need motivational incentives similar to those used with DOT.[128,132,149,150] Frequently scheduled clinic visits and/or home visits provide an opportunity for healthcare providers to demonstrate interest as well as to monitor adherence to therapy. Minimizing clinic waits, providing bus tokens, scheduling appointments at the patient's convenience, assisting with the patient's other medical and social problems can help to provide a supportive environment. Preappointment reminders, especially telephone calls, avoid potential embarrassment about missing or forgetting appointments and provide an opportunity to address remediable obstacles to keeping an appointment.

Cost should not be a barrier to therapy for tuberculosis. Most public health departments provide antituberculosis therapy and clinic support free of charge to the patient. Patients should be aware of this option. Pill-taking regimens should be as simple as possible and designed to minimize side effects. Combined drug preparations, where available, mean fewer pills. Regimens can be most easily remembered if associated with a daily activity (e.g., tooth brushing, eating). Medication side effects may be minimized by taking all pills at one time in the evening.[132]

For the patient for whom adherence to self-administration of antituberculosis drugs is a recognized problem, therapy should be switched to DOT immediately.

d. Monitoring for Adherence

Methods to monitor adherence to therapy are listed in Table 14.4. The use of directly observed therapy is the optimal way to obtain prompt information on whether a patient is adhering to therapy. When an appointment is missed or a patient refuses to ingest pills, nonadherence is apparent immediately. Even with DOT, however, the potential exists for a patient to have unsuspected drug resistance or, rarely, to fake ingestion of therapy. Thus, it also is important to monitor the patient's response to therapy with follow-up sputum cultures and symptom evaluation, and if the response to therapy is poor, to consider testing for the presence of isoniazid metabolites in the urine.[151-155]

Urine testing is the most practical direct measure of drug ingestion. At least two companies market such test products.[132] Nonetheless, urine testing for isoniazid metabolites has some qualifications. The normal rate of isoniazid metabolism varies in different populations and the average time for its clearance from the urine can be as short as 4 h.[132,151-155] Thus, testing must be performed at an appropriate time interval following ingestion. In addition, some patients may not cooperate with urine testing.

For persons who are responsible for maintaining and ingesting their own antituberculosis drugs, two additional techniques have been used to monitor and reinforce adherence. These include: (1) giving pills out in small amounts (≤30-day supply) and having the patient return frequently for refills, and (2) attempting to determine periodically whether pills are consumed at the expected rate (home visits and pills counts, pill dispensers that record when pills are removed).[156-158] Dispensing isoniazid and other antituberculosis drugs in less than 30-day quantities has been a standard recommendation of the American Thoracic Society (ATS) and the CDC to enable earlier recognition of side effects and nonadherence.[32,36] Monitoring adherence by noting a high frequency of clinic visits may not be adequate. Prediction of adherence to antituberculosis therapy based on patient reports of adherence, subjective assessment of behavior and personality traits, or by having patients bring back empty pill bottles has been shown to be less than completely reliable.[32,110,111,132,156] Thus, spot home visits for pill counts often have been used to supplement clinic observations. In addition, the widespread use of pill-dispensing devices that can automatically record when pills have been removed ("medication monitors") has been recommended.[158,159] Whether "medication monitors" will further enhance the early ability to predict which patients on self-administered therapy should be on directly observed therapy has not been evaluated yet.

Overall, there is no currently proved single, easy way to recognize nonadherent behavior other than by beginning all persons on DOT from the outset. Given that acceptance of DOT as the standard for administration of antituberculosis therapy is not yet universal, many patients will still be started on self-administered therapy and will be monitored individually via a variety of currently available methods.

e. Confinement/Quarantine

The emergence and rapid spread of multidrug-resistant tuberculosis in some urban areas caused many to reexamine the potential role of the legal system to encourage adherence to therapy and/or minimize the potential of spread to others from persons who remain infectious for prolonged time periods.[33,34,160,161] Unfortunately, there will be some patients for whom voluntary compliance with directly observed therapy will be a chronic problem, and some who will develop multidrug resistance and will not be expected to respond well to therapy. For these persons, a progressive course of legal alternatives should be available to minimize their potential to infect others and/or develop multidrug resistance.

Most states have laws that enable the courts to order directly observed therapy for persons who are not on therapy and who are suspected of being infectious, or who have stopped therapy before completing the recommended course. Such laws have been very useful in ensuring adherence to DOT and avoiding the potential expense of institutional confinement.[34,140,162]

For those few patients for whom institutional confinement may be necessary to remove them from situations where the potential for transmission is high (e.g., homeless persons who do not cooperate with court-ordered directly observed therapy, persons with chronic multidrug-resistant tuberculosis who cannot be successfully managed or confined to their homes), suitable institutional settings in many states no longer exist and may need to be identified.[163-165] Acute care hospitals are expensive and may not be equipped to successfully isolate for prolonged periods persons who are chronically infectious. Many chronic disease hospitals do not have staff with sufficient training to manage patients with multidrug-resistant tuberculosis, especially those who also may be HIV infected and have substance abuse or mental health problems. Neither setting may have appropriate security to protect against patients who are determined to leave. At least two states have identified appropriate institutional settings and have demonstrated that, in some cases at least, institutional treatment of selected patients may be cost effective.[34,165]

f. Respective Roles of Healthcare Providers, Public Health Agencies, and Managed Care Organizations

To ensure appropriate therapeutic strategies and high completion rates, it is essential that clinicians and public health authorities collaborate on the management of each case from the outset, and that managed care organizations enable the clinician to manage each case according to nationally recommended standards.[1,24,36,166] To initiate collaboration, clinicians and institutions should report suspected and confirmed cases of tuberculosis within 24 to 72 h of starting therapy, as required by law in every state. In addition, they need to update health departments regularly on the current treatment and clinical status of each patient and promptly notify them when patients under their care do not take therapy as prescribed or do not return for scheduled follow-ups.

Public health authorities are responsible for ensuring that each patient is started and maintained throughout the treatment period on an appropriate and continuous course of therapy. To do this in settings where health departments are not directly responsible for the patient's care, it has been recommended that a specific health department employee be assigned to each tuberculosis case. This person should interview the patient and help develop the initial specific treatment and monitoring plan, including methods to be used to assess and ensure adherence (e.g., directly observed therapy).[1] This person also should be responsible for ensuring the education of the patient and the continuity of therapy. Other health department responsibilities for case finding and management include: provision of outreach services, maintenance of a record system to evaluate area-wide success with case management, provision of drugs and support of clinic services so that cost is not a barrier to administering appropriate therapy, and institution of legal measures, should they become necessary, to ensure that all persons complete therapy in a timely manner.[1,24]

Nearly 50% of tuberculosis cases in the U.S. now are treated by nonhealth department-based clinicians.[81,166] Most of these providers work for managed care organizations. Their ability to fully diagnose and treat persons with tuberculosis according to public health standards can be constrained by cost-managing policies of the managed care organizations. For example, managed care organizations may contract with laboratories that do not provide timely, complete, or quality tuberculosis diagnostic services. They may limit the number of cultures, antibiotic sensitivity tests, or clinical monitoring visits that will be reimbursed, or the length of time they will pay for a person to be hospitalized. Thus, it is incumbent upon both public health agencies and providers to assure that the climate exists in which optimal tuberculosis case management can be achieved.[166]

As part of their respective roles, public health agencies must work with providers to determine whether managed care organizations' policies are constraining optimal care and, if they are, meet with the managed care organizations and the state Medicaid program to try to modify their policies accordingly. Model contract specifications have been developed that can be used as a foundation for future managed care policy development.[166]

C. SCREENING AND PREVENTIVE THERAPY

Efforts to reduce the reservoir of latently infected persons who give rise to as much as 90% of incident tuberculosis cases annually in the U.S. is second only to case management and case finding in importance as a tuberculosis control strategy.[1,36] To make best use of limited resources, it is essential to target screening to persons who are potential candidates for preventive therapy, and who have a reasonable probability of completing it.[29,37] Currently, screening and preventive therapy are underutilized.[29,167-169] In one study to determine why tuberculosis is not prevented, it was found that although three quarters of the tuberculosis patients surveyed had contact with a healthcare provider within 5 years before the diagnosis of tuberculosis, less than one third had been tuberculin tested, even though many had risk factors for tuberculosis.[167] Of those who had positive skin tests and other factors placing them at increased risk of disease, only 5% had been offered preventive therapy.

1. On Whom and Where to Perform Tuberculin Screening

In any given geographical area it is essential to know the epidemiology of incident tuberculosis cases to effectively plan screening programs. There are some groups at particularly high risk, regardless of geographic area, toward which screening programs should be directed. Table 14.5 lists these groups and sites where screening programs should optimally be placed. In Chapter 13, the rationale behind screening these groups and indications for preventive therapy are presented in detail.

a. HIV-Infected Persons and Intravenous Drug Users (IVDUs)

Given their extraordinarily high risk of disease once infected, intensive efforts are needed to identify persons with, or at risk for, tuberculous and HIV coinfection and ensure a complete course of therapy. Federal funding has been available since 1989 to support screening efforts in methadone maintenance drug treatment programs and in correctional settings where many IVDUs are incarcerated. In both, the opportunity exists to use directly observed preventive therapy (DOPT) given by staff with regular client contact to ensure adherence to therapy.[170-172] Early results from multiple states involved in the federally supported screening initiative suggest that it is highly successful in identifying persons with coinfection and achieving completion of therapy.[91-93] Overall, 17% of those

TABLE 14.5
Potential Sites and Groups for Tuberculin Screening Programs by Risk Group

Risk Group	Possible Screening Sites, Groups
HIV-infected and IVDUs	Correctional facilities: all admissions
	Drug treatment program admissions
	HIV specialty clinics: all clients
	HIV counseling and testing sites: all high-risk clients
	Hospitals: all at-risk admissions
	Jails: all admissions
Case contacts	Household: all
	Workplace: all close contacts
	"Recreational"[a]: all close contacts
	Institutional[b]: all close or high-risk contacts
Abnormal chest radiograph[c]	Radiology reading rooms: all chest radiographs
Medical risk factors	Hospitals: all admissions
	Physicians' offices: patients with risk factors
	Dialysis units: all clients
	Transplant units: all clients
	Oncology clinics: all clients
	Clinics specializing in autoimmune or rheumatoid diseases: all on chronic immunosuppressive therapy
Foreign-born	After arrival in the U.S.: all refugees and immigrants
	School and colleges: all entrants
	Selected occupational settings: all workers
High-risk urban residents and minorities	Selected hospitals: all admissions
	Physicians' offices
	Schools, entry and each mandated health assessment
	Selected occupational settings
Institutionalized	Correctional facilities: all admissions
	Long-term care facilities: all admissions
High-risk healthcare workers	Acute care hospitals: all workers[d]
	Tuberculosis clinics: all workers
	HIV specialty clinics: all workers
	Correctional facilities: all workers
	Drug treatment programs: all workers
	Long-term care facilities: all workers
	Homeless shelters: all workers

[a] Includes contacts such as those in crack houses, bars (see text).

[b] Includes outpatient clinics specializing in the care of the HIV-infected or drug addicted, as well as hospital wards, residential correctional, long-term care, and drug treatment programs.

[c] Screening in this case is for chest radiographs suggestive of old tuberculous scarring, not tuberculin screening.

[d] Some workers will need more frequent screening than others, e.g., those working with HIV-infected patients, in bronchoscopy rooms, with patients who have undiagnosed pulmonary symptoms.

Source: Friedman, L. N., Ed., *Tuberculosis: Current Concepts and Treatment,* 1st ed., CRC Press LLC, Boca Raton, FL, 1994. With permission.

tested were found to be tuberculin positive, and 84% completed preventive therapy.[91] In addition, a recent analysis suggests that such initiatives are highly cost-effective.[172]

Other sites where HIV-infected persons can be expected to be found in higher than background prevalence include HIV counseling and testing sites, hospitals, other drug treatment modalities, and jails. Even if systematic skin testing programs were implemented in all, most only provide an opportunity for screening, not follow-up or DOPT. It may be difficult to ensure continuity of therapy once persons with coinfection have been identified, especially for those who may have a history of drug abuse and who are not in the captive settings of either drug treatment or prison.[173-176] At least one state has attempted to address this concern. HIV-tuberculous coinfection has become a reportable condition in Connecticut. Reported persons are monitored similarly to tuberculosis cases and DOPT is offered to patients who are likely or have been proved to be nonadherent.[92] While rates of completion of preventive therapy have been high (>75%), persons identified by correctional setting screening, who then are discharged, have been difficult to locate.[94] Use of a 2-month preventive therapy regimen should make it possible to achieve even higher completion rates in this otherwise difficult-to-reach population.[2]

Anergy screening panels were once used routinely to help interpret the tuberculin skin test in persons with HIV infection.[177] Recent data showing their low predictive value and the relatively low efficacy of preventive therapy in persons with anergy, however, has diminished enthusiasm for anergy testing.[178] Only one group of HIV-infected persons who are found to be anergic are potential candidates for a full course of preventive therapy: contacts of known potentially infectious cases of pulmonary tuberculosis. In addition, anergy testing may be helpful to decide whether ongoing preventive therapy is needed in tuberculin-negative, HIV-positive persons with continuous periodic exposure to tuberculosis, such as may occur in an occupational setting where satisfactory control of tuberculosis transmission cannot be achieved.[178] Anergy testing currently does not play an important role in tuberculosis control.

b. Contacts of Infectious Cases

Screening of close contacts of infectious cases has long been an effective tuberculosis control strategy. In 1996, in the U.S., more than 26,000 infected contacts of cases of tuberculosis were identified, most starting and completing a course of preventive therapy. Tuberculous infection prevalence among identified contacts was higher than 20%. In addition, nearly 1000 cases of tuberculosis were identified and started on treatment before they otherwise would have been diagnosed.[87]

Several factors are critical in initiating a contact investigation.[36] These include the timing of the investigation, the potential infectiousness of the case, and the places where the case has had the potential to transmit. In the HIV era, rapid initiation of contact investigation is crucial. Among immunosuppressed HIV-infected contacts, incubation periods as short as 20 days from exposure to overt disease have been observed. Initiation of investigation should take place as soon as there is a positive smear or other strong evidence that a patient has infectious tuberculosis. Correspondingly, as contacts are identified, appropriate counseling and HIV testing of contacts should occur if their HIV status is not known.

Any patient with pulmonary tuberculosis should be considered potentially infectious. Patient factors that increase the likelihood of transmission to the community and workplace include smear positivity, positive sputum culture, presence of cavitation on chest radiograph, presence of cough, long duration of respiratory symptoms, and laryngeal involvement.[179,180] In hospital and healthcare settings, additional factors include the possibility that the patient has been hospitalized for a period of time without appropriate isolation before being rendered noninfectious by therapy,[17,18,50-52] and the possibility that cough-inducing (e.g., bronchoscopy) or other aerosol-generating procedures may have been performed.[181,182]

The sites where the patient has had indoor contact with others also are important to consider. In addition to household and workplace contacts, "recreational" contacts may have had sufficient exposure for transmission to occur. Transmission of tuberculosis among crack house contacts has been described,[183,184] transmission to HIV-infected persons in a gay bar has been recognized,[185] and transmission has occurred in a "floating card game."[74] "Home" increasingly includes homeless shelters, prison, and AIDS residences or other chronic-care facilities. Many patients have been in a variety of healthcare settings for prolonged periods during which they were symptomatic before diagnosis.[186] In some of these settings, significant numbers of persons with HIV infection may have been exposed.

Given that there may be many persons identified as contacts to any given case, it is critical to establish priorities for starting and ending a contact investigation. During the interview, a hierarchy of exposure among the identified contacts should be established. Those contacts with the greatest potential exposure to the index should be screened first. The investigation should end when there appears to be no evidence of transmission of tuberculous infection to contacts with progressively lesser levels of exposure. Although most persons with infectious tuberculosis infect few contacts, there are occasional individuals who are superdisseminators and can infect hundreds.[74-76]

Because conversion of the tuberculin skin test can take as long as 12 weeks after the infecting exposure occurs, it is essential, in those who were initially negative, to perform repeat testing at 10 to 12 weeks after contact with the source has been broken. As discussed in Chapter 13, it is recommended that close contacts with an initial tuberculin skin test reaction of less than 5 mm of induration be evaluated further by chest radiography and be considered for interim preventive therapy if: (1) circumstances suggest a high probability of infection, or (2) the contact is a child, adolescent, or is immunosuppressed (e.g., infected with HIV).[36]

c. Persons with Medical Conditions that Increase Tuberculosis Risk

Persons with medical conditions that increase tuberculosis risk, including those with abnormal chest radiographs, represent a diverse group. However, they all are candidates for preventive therapy if found to have tuberculous infection. Their common points of identification usually are clinical medical settings, such as specialty clinics, hospitals, or individual clinicians. Correspondingly, tuberculin screening efforts should occur where they receive medical care for their underlying medical conditions.

Baseline and periodic repeat tuberculin screening should be routine in transplant, renal dialysis, and oncology units. Clinics specializing in the management of autoimmune conditions for which steroid therapy is used commonly, and clinics specializing in the management of silicosis, diabetes, and cancer, particularly hematologic cancers, also should have routine tuberculin screening protocols. Radiologists should be taught to provide chest radiographic readings that specifically note upper lobe fibrotic changes consistent with past tuberculosis and, thus, alert the clinician that the patient may be a candidate for preventive therapy.

Routine tuberculin screening of all admissions to hospitals also may be relatively productive in identifying latently infected persons with medical conditions that predispose to the development of tuberculosis. In a study of two urban Connecticut hospitals, more than 60% of admissions to general medical and surgical wards had conditions that would have prompted preventive therapy if the patients had been infected. Few persons in either hospital had been screened, including those with HIV infection.[187]

d. Persons Born in High-Incidence Countries

Persons born in high-incidence countries are responsible for almost 40% of all incident tuberculosis cases in the U.S.[22] Most tuberculosis in foreign-born persons is thought to arise from tuberculous infection acquired before arrival in the U.S. Thus, a critical tuberculosis control strategy for this group is identification and treatment of persons with latent infection who are candidates for preventive therapy.[22] Overall, in 1998, there were an estimated 7 million tuberculosis-infected foreign-born persons in the U.S., i.e., approximately half of all tuberculosis-infected persons in the country. Approximately 2 to 3% of them are expected to develop tuberculosis in the absence of effective screening and preventive therapy programs.[22]

Tuberculin screening of persons born in high tuberculosis-incidence countries, particularly those born in Asia, Africa, Latin America, and Oceania, may be highly productive. The incidence of tuberculosis among this group in the U.S. is 5 to 20 times higher than that of the U.S. population as a whole,[22] and the prevalence of tuberculous infection is as high as 50%. Given that the risk of development of tuberculosis is highest during the first 5 years after arrival (i.e., nearly half of all foreign-born tuberculosis cases in the U.S. develop tuberculosis within 5 years of arrival), screening should be targeted at recent arrivals. Further, since the risk of tuberculosis is considerably higher for persons from some countries than others,[22,188] special efforts should focus on arrivals from these very high-risk countries.

There is only one systematic national effort targeted at preventing tuberculosis in the foreign-born. Screening and preventive therapy programs have been supported for refugees entering the U.S. since the early 1980s. All states receive lists of all refugees entering the U.S. who reside in their state, and have the opportunity to ensure that a health assessment that includes tuberculin screening is performed. Similar initiatives have been recommended for immigrants, a group nearly 10 times the size of refugees.[189] Currently, immigrant screening overseas includes chest radiography.[190] States receive lists of all Class B1 and B2 immigrants (those with abnormal chest radiographs) and are expected to screen them for active tuberculosis. In the process, tuberculin testing can be done and preventive therapy considered. In one study, nearly 50% of Class B1 and 25% of Class B2 immigrants were considered candidates for preventive therapy.[191] In immigrants who adjust their immigrant status after arrival in the U.S., a physical examination including a tuberculin skin test is required and must be performed by designated "civil surgeons." These requirements provide public health departments with an opportunity to reach a substantial number of new immigrants with preventive therapy initiatives.[192]

Given the emphasis on finding foreign-born persons shortly after arrival and on screening those who are clear candidates for preventive therapy, it has been recommended that programs be established throughout the U.S. to require tuberculin test screening at all school levels, including college, for foreign-born students from high-incidence countries entering school for the first time.[22,189,193,194] In addition, screening programs in occupational settings employing a high percentage of recent immigrants may be productive in identifying persons who are candidates for preventive therapy. Other opportunities for systematic screening and preventive therapy initiatives may be identified by working with community groups and/or physicians who are focal points for social concerns and medical care for immigrant groups from high-risk countries.[22] Prior BCG vaccination is not a contraindication to tuberculin screening and the use of preventive therapy.[36]

Screening programs in schools and stable occupational settings offer the opportunity to use DOPT to ensure adherence to a complete course of therapy. Where possible, culturally sensitive outreach workers who speak the same language as new arrivals should be hired and trained to work with the persons responsible for giving DOPT.[189] Such an approach in the refugee program has ensured higher preventive therapy completion rates than for the U.S. as a whole.

e. High-Risk Persons Who are Medically Underserved

High-risk persons who are medically underserved tend to be characterized by poverty, but otherwise are a diverse group. In general they consist of geographically or race/ethnicity-defined population subgroups with a relatively high tuberculosis incidence. This high incidence is due in part to varying combinations of adverse social and economic factors, the HIV epidemic, and the immigration of persons with tuberculous infection. There also may be a contribution from physician nonadherence to tuberculosis control recommendations and patient nonadherence in following prescribed recommended treatment regimens.[116,195,196] Correspondingly, each state or town needs to look at its tuberculosis epidemiology to identify who, if any, are the local high-risk groups.

Recommended sites for targeted screening programs also will be dependent upon those targeted. It is recommended that broadly constituted local tuberculosis coalitions be built to review the underlying epidemiologic data. Planning, developing, and implementing screening programs should be a joint effort among the local health departments, public and private community organizations, and healthcare providers.[195] At a minimum, screening and preventive therapy programs should be considered in local correctional facilities, drug treatment centers, long-term care facilities and school settings. In all of these, directly observed preventive therapy is possible. With proper coordination of services, tuberculin screening also may be highly effective in hospitals, outpatient facilities, and homeless shelters, particularly if the latter have relatively stable populations.

f. Institutionalized Persons

A number of studies have shown that persons living in correctional facilities and in long-term care facilities, particularly nursing homes, are at considerably increased risk for tuberculosis compared to their noninstitutionalized counterparts,[27,30,197,198] and that preventive therapy can reduce that risk.[199,200] In both settings, the purpose of tuberculin screening is multifold: to help detect persons with active disease at the time of entry, to identify candidates for preventive therapy to lower the risk of disease occurrence within the institution, and to establish baseline skin-test reactivity for future potential contact investigations and/or evaluation of in-facility tuberculosis transmission. In addition, as discussed above, screening and preventive therapy efforts in correctional settings may contribute to community tuberculosis control, given that many come from high tuberculosis incidence communities and groups, that there is a high rate of turnover in the prison population, and that these otherwise difficult-to-reach persons can be screened easily and treated while incarcerated.[30,201-203] Rates of tuberculin positivity in prisons have been found to be as high as 25% in Philadelphia and have averaged 18% in New York State.[204,205]

Tuberculin screening in these settings should be done at entry to the institution and again following exposure to a potentially infectious case of tuberculosis. In correctional settings with a high or increasing incidence of tuberculosis and a substantial percentage of HIV-infected inmates, annual screening programs for inmates may be productive. In addition to tuberculin screening, symptom and/or radiographic screening also may be warranted to rule out active disease at the time of admission. All preventive therapy should be given as DOPT, which can be given in a twice- or thrice-weekly regimen.[30]

While screening in the prison setting may contribute markedly to reduced tuberculosis prevalence in the community, screening for latent tuberculous infection in many jail settings has less potential unless the average length of stay is long enough to complete a course of preventive therapy. Once an inmate has been discharged from jail, it has been difficult to ensure completion of a course of preventive therapy.[173-175]

g. High-Risk Healthcare Workers

Persons working in hospital settings in recent years have been shown to be at increased risk of acquiring tuberculous infection independent of the outbreaks associated with multidrug-resistant tuberculosis.[69,181,182,206-211] Workers in areas of hospitals where tuberculosis patients are apt to be seen before diagnosis (clinic waiting areas, emergency rooms), where HIV patients congregate, and where sputum or abscess material may be aerosolized (bronchoscopy suites, sputum induction and aerosol treatment areas, autopsy rooms) probably are at the highest risk.[28] While specific ongoing risks cannot generally be quantified, as many as a third of healthcare workers in high-risk areas have been known to convert their tuberculin test in a 1- to 2-year time period.[18,50,51] Because of this, systematic employee skin-testing programs have been recommended and now are required by OSHA in acute medical care facilities in the U.S.[28]

Skin testing should be performed by the facility employee health service with testing done at initiation of employment and at least annually thereafter.[28,36] Persons working in areas with particularly high risk should be tested more often. In addition to periodic screening, healthcare workers should be evaluated again if they have been exposed to a potentially infectious tuberculosis patient for whom recommended precautions were not taken.

Because of their risk for rapid progression from infection to disease, HIV-infected healthcare workers pose an additional concern, especially when they are exposed to multidrug-resistant tuberculosis. Management of exposure and infection is no different for them than for other healthcare workers, other than recommending a different and longer course of preventive therapy.[28,39] Preventive therapy for workers infected with multidrug-resistant tuberculosis is discussed in Chapter 13.

2. Frequency of Screening

At a minimum, individuals for whom tuberculin screening is recommended should have at least one tuberculin test and have it recorded in a prominent place in an ongoing medical record. The frequency of repeat testing should be determined by the likelihood of exposure to infectious tuberculosis. This may require review or generation of local data and assistance of local public health officials in its interpretation.

Because the likelihood or consequences of continued exposure to tuberculosis is high for some high-risk persons, annual screening, at a minimum, is recommended for the following groups:

- Persons with HIV infection and the staffs of TB clinics
- Healthcare facilities caring for HIV-infected patients
- Mycobacteriology laboratories
- Shelters for the homeless
- Substance abuse treatment centers
- Dialysis units
- Correctional institutions
- Nursing homes[36]

Depending on the local incidence and infection rates, annual testing also may be indicated for prisoners.[30] All persons should be retested if exposure to an infectious case occurs.

3. Adherence to Preventive Therapy

The primary methods to maximize the potential for adherence to preventive therapy are the same as those used to ensure adherence to therapy.

DOPT should be used wherever possible. Given their extraordinary risk for development of tuberculosis, it is cost effective to place most persons with HIV-tuberculous coinfection on DOPT.[172] Where required by state law, persons with coinfection should be reported to local and state public health departments so that close monitoring of patients can be performed and outreach provided, including provision of DOPT. Persons receiving preventive therapy in "captive" settings also should be receiving DOPT wherever possible.[2,30,36,37] Such settings include correctional institutions, drug treatment programs that require at least twice-weekly interaction with the patient, schools, and occupational settings in which screening programs or contact investigations have been performed. Where resources are particularly scarce and the need for DOPT exists, twice-weekly therapy should be used.[30,37]

For patients on self-administered therapy, dispensing a supply of medicines to last 30 days or less assures that there will be at least monthly monitoring and reinforcement of the importance of completing therapy.[36] Dispensing medicines in 3-month supplies no longer is acceptable practice. Where possible, home visits for patient education and pill counts are helpful. Use of "medication monitors"[156-158] and testing of urine for isoniazid metabolites[151-155] may be helpful to determine whether particularly high-risk persons should be switched to directly observed preventive therapy.

Achieving high levels of patient motivation is particularly important when using preventive therapy. Patient education should address cultural concerns about taking preventive therapy and often can be performed by trained workers of the same cultural background as the patient.[22] Clinic visits should not be cumbersome or unpleasant to the patient. Waiting time should be minimized, hours of operation convenient, and costs kept to a minimum. Enablers, such as bus tokens and babysitting services, may ensure that a patient gets to the clinic. Incentives such as food, clothes, and small rewards help some patients complete therapy.[36,123,132]

For patients who are found to be nonadherent, DOPT should be considered if the resources exist and other motivational methods have failed. The highest priority group for DOPT are those who are coinfected with HIV.

4. Role of Healthcare Providers, Institutions, Public Health Agencies, and Managed Care

The responsibility for the success of screening and preventive therapy is more diffuse than for case finding and case management. However, it requires equal amounts of collaboration at the community level.

A substantial portion of the responsibility for success of tuberculin screening and preventive therapy efforts in the U.S. lies with individual healthcare providers. Many persons in high-risk groups are only readily identifiable to the individual provider, particularly those with medical factors that increase the risk of development of disease once a person has latent infection. Providers must be aware of the indications for screening and preventive therapy and must implement them aggressively. Lack of general application of preventive therapy will continue to slow efforts toward tuberculosis elimination.[1,196]

Institutions also have a substantial role in tuberculin screening and preventive therapy efforts, particularly correctional institutions, drug treatment programs, hospitals, long-term care facilities, and schools. In each setting there is an opportunity not only to detect and control transmission within institutional confines, but to contribute to shrinking the effective reservoir of latent infection in the surrounding community. Each needs to have enforced policies and procedures to ensure that both high-risk staff and clients are screened and, as indicated, are started on preventive therapy. In addition, policies should encourage the administration of directly observed preventive therapy within the institution wherever feasible.

Public health agencies have a broad responsibility to oversee screening and preventive therapy efforts in the community.[22,24,29,37] They need to review surveillance data and provide guidelines for those who are at high-risk and require screening. They must identify and work with institutions and healthcare providers who provide services to high-risk populations and help them develop and institute appropriate screening programs. They should provide clinical and outreach support to help monitor persons started on preventive therapy and to ensure adherence. They are responsible for overseeing the investigation of contacts of infectious tuberculosis cases. They should collect surveillance information to determine how well screening and preventive therapy efforts are working in each setting in which they have been initiated and to adjust screening recommendations where necessary.[24] Finally, they need to assess whether any cost-containment initiatives by managed care companies interfere with recommended provider-based screening and preventive therapy efforts. In particular, together with state Medicaid programs, they need to assure that recommended standards for screening, evaluation, and follow-up can be readily implemented by Medicaid managed care providers.[166]

Conversely, managed care organizations need to collaborate with public health departments to be sure that they are aware of effective prevention practices and have policies in place which enable providers to practice them.

D. Special Settings

Tuberculosis transmission has been a threat in indoor settings where large numbers of persons at risk for infectious tuberculosis may reside. With the emergence of HIV-related tuberculosis and multidrug-resistant tuberculosis, three settings in particular have come to the fore: hospitals, correctional institutions, and homeless shelters. In each of these settings, environmental as well as human source control measures must be considered, and special surveillance efforts are necessary to determine the ongoing risk of transmission.

1. Hospitals

Hospitals to which persons with tuberculosis may be admitted now are required to have their own systematic tuberculosis control programs.[28] These programs are based on a broad approach to tuberculosis control with attention paid to: (1) prevention of the generation of infectious airborne particles by early identification and effective treatment of persons with tuberculous infection and active tuberculosis, (2) prevention of the spread of infectious droplet nuclei into the general air circulation by applying effective isolation methods, (3) reduction of the number of infectious droplet nuclei in air by application of environmental control methods, and (4) systematic surveillance of personnel for tuberculous infection and evidence of continued risk of transmission.[28] Investigation of outbreaks of both sensitive and multidrug-resistant tuberculosis in recent years has shown that where inadequate attention is given to any of these approaches, the risk of tuberculosis transmission is increased.[16-19,28,50-53]

Specific elements of hospital control programs include:

- Screening patients for active tuberculosis and tuberculous infection on admission
- Provision of rapid diagnostic services (e.g., AFB smear reading time in 24 h or less)
- Prescription of appropriate therapy for prevention and disease
- Provision and use of isolation rooms for persons with, or suspected of having, infectious tuberculosis
- Maintenance of physical measures to reduce microbial contamination in the air, particularly in areas where procedures are performed in which respiratory aerosols are generated
- Enforced systematic screening of healthcare facility personnel for tuberculous infection and tuberculosis
- Prompt investigation and control of outbreaks
- Continued assessment of the extent to which these elements are in place and are effective[28]

Further detailed information on isolation and physical measures to reduce transmission may be found in Chapter 3. The CDC initially published detailed guidelines for preventing transmission in healthcare settings in 1990[212] and updated them in 1994.[28]

2. Correctional Institutions

Correctional facilities, like acute care hospitals, have had particular problems with transmission of tuberculosis, including multidrug-resistant strains.[16,213] Crowding and poor ventilation, combined with a particularly high-risk population (HIV-infected), make it necessary to implement a systematic approach to institutional tuberculosis control. Guidelines for such programs were published originally in 1989 and recently have been updated.[30,214] These call for:

- Having a designated person or group be responsible for tuberculosis infection control oversight
- Rapid and aggressive identification and initiation of isolation and DOT of persons with infectious tuberculosis
- Appropriate isolation facilities for persons suspected of being infectious
- Routine, systematic tuberculin screening and preventive therapy programs with DOPT for all prison inmates and staff, beginning at admission
- Centralized recordkeeping to ensure continuity of therapy on transfer or discharge
- Periodic assessment of tuberculous infection and disease rates and continuity of therapy and preventive therapy, particularly among those who are transferred from institution to institution.

In addition, HIV counseling and testing expertise should be readily available so that HIV-antibody testing can be offered to all inmates found to be tuberculin positive.

3. Homeless Shelters

Homeless shelters have long been recognized as places where high-risk groups for tuberculosis reside and where tuberculosis transmission is common.[78,215-221] Nonetheless, tuberculosis control in homeless shelters continues to be problematic, in part because staff with medical expertise often are not available and shelter users often are transient.

Recently, guidelines have been published that consider these facts and advocate collaboration among healthcare providers, health departments, shelter operators, and social service agencies to achieve certain basic tuberculosis control elements.[26] These include: (1) detection, evaluation, and reporting of homeless persons who have current symptoms of active tuberculosis; (2) ensuring completion of an appropriate course of therapy in those diagnosed with active tuberculosis; (3) maintenance of high levels of ventilation, possibly supplemented by appropriately installed ultra-violet light;[222] and (4) routine tuberculin skin testing for staff and regular volunteers. Tuberculin screening and preventive therapy initiatives among homeless persons generally have been unproductive because of poor patient adherence to follow-up visits and treatment regimens.[26] Screening should be undertaken only if there is a reasonable possibility that most infected persons will complete preventive treatment. Priority groups for screening initiatives include those with HIV infection and recent contacts of persons with infectious tuberculosis.[26]

E. MATHEMATICAL MODELING TO SELECT TUBERCULOSIS CONTROL STRATEGIES

Mathematical modeling can be used to assess the relative importance of different disease control strategies and to assist in related policy development. Recently, mathematical models of population-based tuberculosis transmission and control have been developed[223-227] and have been applied to selected issues in tuberculosis control. Among the questions the models have attempted to address are: what is necessary for tuberculosis elimination;[223,224] what is the relative importance of case finding, case treatment, preventive treatment and vaccination;[223-226] and what levels of treatment success are necessary to keep drug-resistant tuberculosis under control?[223,228]

The models developed vary in the type of outcomes they measure and in the parameters they examine. One theoretical model has been constructed to examine predictors of the average number of secondary infectious cases, "R," that result from each new infectious case that occurs in an otherwise disease-free population.[223,228] When R is less than 1, the tuberculosis incidence will decrease; when it exceeds 1, the tuberculosis incidence will increase. R is dependent on three independent variables: the average number of susceptible persons that one case infects per unit time (modified by changes in degree of crowding, case finding, treatment and vaccination); the average duration of infectiousness of a case (modified by treatment); and the probability that an infected individual will become an infectious case (modified by preventive treatment and by vaccination). With a simple modification, this model also can be used to examine the transmission and changing importance of acquired drug resistance resulting from unsuccessful initial treatment of drug-sensitive cases.[223,228]

Examination of the dynamics of tuberculosis control using this type of theoretical model results in several important findings. First, it is possible to eradicate tuberculosis by high levels of successful treatment alone or with a combination of treatment and preventive therapy, but not by preventive therapy alone.[223] Second, if drug-resistant tuberculosis is not treated as a problem in its own right, drug-resistant tuberculosis will emerge as a separate tuberculosis epidemic. In particular, any of the following scenarios could cause the rapid emergence and persistence of a drug-resistant tuberculosis problem: significant treatment failure rates of drug-sensitive tuberculosis (>10% in countries with a high tuberculosis incidence); failure to adequately treat a high percentage (at least 70%) of drug-resistant cases; or high rates of case-finding of drug-sensitive tuberculosis that are not accompanied by high success rates of treatment.[228]

Application of the previous theoretical model to real populations and inclusion of a subpopulation that is HIV-infected also has been accomplished.[225] In this case, the outcomes examined were the expected numbers of new tuberculosis cases and deaths worldwide over a 30-year time period and the extent to which they might be modified by different mass tuberculosis control strategies. The most successful strategies for reducing the number of deaths over 30 years were: implementation of a continuously active radiographic case-finding initiative accompanied by highly successful treatment; achievement of high rates of implementation and success of the WHO Directly Observed Therapy, Short Course (DOTS) strategy[109] (see also Chapter 16) in all areas of the world (resulting in 80 to 98% smear-positive cure rates); and mass population vaccination with a vaccine that has 50% long-term efficacy. In the short term, a single 12-year effort at mass tuberculin screening with successful preventive therapy in 33% of those identified would be at least equally effective for the 12-year period.[225] Limitations of this analysis are that no consideration was given to drug-resistant tuberculosis and the model was "run" for only 30 years. In a separate analysis, if the adequate treatment of drug-resistant cases was not achieved, drug-resistant tuberculosis could emerge in 50 to 100 years to fully offset the success in controlling drug-sensitive tuberculosis.[228]

A different type of model was developed to study treatment options in France.[226] In this model, the outcome was annual risk of infection (ARI), a measure used in many parts of the world and which correlates with prevalence of smear positivity.[95] Among the parameters examined were the prevalence of "open" cases of tuberculosis, the prevalence of "closed" cases, the number of susceptible persons infected by each open case, the case detection rate, the cure rate, and the percentage vaccinated with a BCG vaccine that provides time-limited protection. The potential effect of preventive therapy was not considered. When applied to the current epidemiology in France and projected over 20 years, the most important determinants of ARI were the cure rate and the open-case detection rate. The model predicted that in France, at least, BCG vaccination of infants could be discontinued with little adverse impact on the ARI.

Finally, a model was developed to fit U.S. epidemiologic data and to examine the impact of a modest 10% improvement in different tuberculosis control strategies on the elimination of tuberculosis in the U.S.[224] The outcome of this model was the prevalence of tuberculosis cases and of tuberculosis deaths each year over a 10-year period following a change in tuberculosis control parameters. The U.S. population was categorized by age and HIV-infection status into a number of different tuberculosis-related clinical states (e.g., uninfected, infected and at high or low risk of tuberculosis, and drug-resistant tuberculosis or drug-sensitive tuberculosis). Over the 10-year period, persons moved from one tuberculosis clinical state to another based on the current understanding of the risk of acquiring infection or developing tuberculosis as modified by vaccination, being identified and treated with chemoprophylaxis or being identified and treated for disease. The changes in current tuberculosis control practices studied were a 10% increase in the percentage of persons identified and receiving chemoprophylaxis or treatment and a 10% increase in the efficacy of chemoprophylaxis or treatment. Of these four strategies, those resulting in improvement of tuberculosis treatment (improving successful therapy rate and case finding) had more effect on tuberculosis incidence over 10 years than those that improved tuberculosis preventive treatment by a similar percentage. A second important understanding from this model is that even if all tuberculosis treatment and preventive therapy control measures improved by 10% and the theoretical impact of a highly effective BCG vaccine were added in, we could expect only a 48% reduction in tuberculosis incidence after 10 years. The implication is that to achieve the stated U.S. tuberculosis elimination goals by 2010,[1] we will need new tuberculosis control tools.[229]

Overall, the results of the initial modeling work done over the past few years confirm the more empirically derived tuberculosis control emphasis that has been the focus of national guidelines, has been presented in this chapter, and has been confirmed by recent experience in the U.S. The highest priority for tuberculosis control in all parts of the world should be to achieve high-quality case management and cure rates of both drug-sensitive and drug-resistant tuberculosis. Case-finding activities also are very important, but only if the cases found can be well managed. While preventive therapy activities at current levels do not have the same impact as case management, they contribute substantially to tuberculosis elimination and, when intensively applied, will greatly hasten tuberculosis elimination. Additional probing and development of these models to account for immigration and the stochastic nature of tuberculosis in the U.S., should provide better insight into how intensive an application of existing tools is needed to achieve tuberculosis control and elimination in the varied communities in the U.S. in which tuberculosis remains a problem.

IV. TUBERCULOSIS ELIMINATION

In 1987, an Advisory Committee for Elimination of Tuberculosis was established to provide recommendations to the U.S. Department of Health and Human Services for developing new technology, applying prevention and control methods, and managing state and local tuberculosis programs targeted at eliminating tuberculosis as a public health problem. In 1989, a strategic plan was published.[1] At that time the committee urged the nation to establish a goal of tuberculosis elimination (less than one case per million population) by the year 2010.

The basis for creating a strategic plan was threefold. First, tuberculosis incidence had been steadily declining and remained a significant problem in fewer and fewer geographic areas and in limited demographically defined pockets. In the remaining pockets, however, it continued to be a significant problem. It was felt that existing methods of tuberculosis control were often underapplied, particularly the use of screening and preventive therapy. Second, the biotechnical revolution had yet to be applied to tuberculosis research; there was substantial potential for generating better diagnostic, treatment, and preventive modalities with which to hasten the decline of tuberculosis. Finally, computer, telecommunications, and other technologies had the potential to allow rapid dissemination and application of new information and new methods for tuberculosis control.

The plan called for a three-step effort: (1) more effective and intensive use of existing prevention and control methods, especially prevention in high-risk populations; (2) research, both basic science and applied, that will lead to the development and evaluation of new technologies for treatment, diagnosis, and prevention; and (3) rapid assessment and transfer of any newly developed technologies into clinical and public health practice. The plan notes that all three steps are essential to eliminate tuberculosis in the near future, and significant delays in the accomplishment of any of them are likely to be detrimental to that goal. In the published plan, it also was recognized that the effect of present tuberculosis control efforts is fragile. It was stated that tuberculosis had the potential for spreading more widely in the community.[1] Indeed, that statement was borne out while the plan was being developed and for several years after its publication.

Although the development of the plan and the initial resurgence of tuberculosis stimulated some of the necessary public investment, it took the crisis of the emergence and spread of multidrug-resistant tuberculosis and the development of an action plan to generate the infrastructure needed to progress with tuberculosis elimination. With that investment, the steady decline in tuberculosis incidence that led to the concept of tuberculosis elimination has resumed.

Whether tuberculosis can be eliminated in the U.S. in the next 20 years without major scientific breakthroughs in vaccination against tuberculosis or in the diagnosis and treatment of latent infection remain matters for conjecture and modeling. It has become increasingly evident, however, based on the increasing importance of tuberculosis in the foreign-born in the U.S., that elimination of endemic tuberculosis in the U.S. will not be possible without successful efforts to control tuberculosis globally. Global tuberculosis control faces some of the same challenges that U.S. tuberculosis control now has faced successfully: the HIV epidemic, the focal deterioration of the public health infrastructure needed to keep tuberculosis in check, and the spread of multidrug-resistant strains.

While tuberculosis elimination will not be easy, it is clear that the existence of the U.S. plan, the recent real-life demonstration in New York that its principles work where there are resources and the determination to apply them, and the affirmation of these principles by mathematical modeling, all offer hope that continued progress toward elimination will be possible. The Strategic Plan for the Elimination of Tuberculosis[1] as supplemented by the National Action Plan to Combat Multidrug-Resistant Tuberculosis[15] and the series of recommendations for implementation of various aspects of the plan[2,22,24-32,36,37,61,98,178,195] provide a blueprint for action. The achievement of elimination will be dependent largely upon our collective will.[88,230]

REFERENCES

1. Centers for Disease Control, A strategic plan for the elimination of tuberculosis in United States, *MMWR*, 38 (No. S-3), 1, 1989.
2. Centers for Disease Control, Prevention and treatment of tuberculosis among patients infected with human immunodeficiency virus: principles of therapy and revised recommendations, *MMWR*, 47 (No. RR-20), 4, 1998.
3. Cantwell, M. F., Snider, D. E., Cauthen, G. M., and Onorato, I. M., Epidemiology of tuberculosis in the United States, 1985-1992, *JAMA*, 272, 535, 1994.
4. Burwen, D. R., Bloch, A. B., Griffin, L. D., Ciesielski, C. A., Stern, H. A., and Onorato, I. M., National trends in the concurrence of tuberculosis and acquired immunodeficiency syndrome, *Arch. Intern. Med.*, 155, 1281, 1995.
5. Markowitz, N., Hansen, N. I., Hopewell, P. C., Glassroth, J., Kvale, P. A., Mangura, B. T., Wilcosky, T. C., Wallace, J. M., Rosen, M. J., Reichman, L. B., and the Pulmonary Complications Study Group, Incidence of tuberculosis in the United States among HIV-infected persons, *Ann. Intern. Med.*, 126, 123, 1997.
6. Daley, C. L., Small, P. M., Schechter, G. F., Schoolnik, G. K., McAdam, R. A., Jacobs, W. R., Jr., and Hopewell, P. C., An outbreak of tuberculosis with accelerated progression among persons infected with the human immunodeficiency virus: an analysis using restriction-fragment-length-polymorphisms, *N. Engl. J. Med.*, 326, 231, 1992.
7. Centers for Disease Control, Nosocomial transmission of multidrug-resistant tuberculosis among HIV-infected persons — Florida and New York, 1988-1991, *MMWR*, 40, 585, 1991.
8. Perriens, J. H., Colebunders, R. L., Karahunga, C., Willame, J., Jeugmans, J., Kaboto, M., Mukadi, Y., Pauwels, P., Ryder, R. W., Prignot, J., and Piot, P., Increased mortality and tuberculosis treatment failure rate among human immunodeficiency virus (HIV) seropositive compared with HIV seronegative patients with pulmonary tuberculosis treated with "standard" chemotherapy in Kinshasa, Zaire, *Am. Rev. Respir. Dis.*, 144, 750, 1991.
9. Nunn, P., Brindle, R., Carpenter, L., Odhiambo, J., Wasunna, K., Newnham, R., Githui, W., Gathua, S., Omwega, M., and McAdam, K., *Am. Rev. Respir. Dis.*,146, 849, 1992.
10. Cantwell, M. F. and Binkin, N. J., Impact of HIV on tuberculosis in sub-Saharan Africa: a regional perspective, *Int. J. Tuberc. Lung Dis.*, 1, 205, 1997.
11. Raviglione, M. C., Snider, D. E., Jr., and Kochi, A., Global epidemiology of tuberculosis: morbidity and mortality of a worldwide epidemic, *JAMA*, 273, 220, 1995.
12. Dolin, P. J., Raviglione, and Kochi, A., Global tuberculosis incidence and mortality during 1990–2000, *Bull. WHO*, 72, 213, 1994.
13. DeCock, K. M., Binkin, N. J., Zuber, P. L. F., Tappero, J. W., and Castro, K. G., Research issues involving HIV-associated tuberculosis in resource-poor countries, *JAMA, 276, 1502, 1996.*
14. Centers for Disease Control, Meeting the challenge of multidrug-resistant tuberculosis: summary of a conference, *MMWR*, 41(No. RR-11), 51, 1992.
15. Centers for Disease Control, National action plan to combat multidrug-resistant tuberculosis, *MMWR*, 41(No. R-11), 1, 1992.
16. Centers for Disease Control, Transmission of MDR-TB among persons in a correctional system — New York, 1991, *MMWR*, 41, 507, 1991.
17. Dooley, S. W., Villarino, M. E., Mercedes, L., Salinas, L., Amil, S., Rullan, J. V., Jarvis, W. R., Bloch, A. B., and Cauthen, G. M., Nosocomial transmission of tuberculosis in a hospital unit for HIV-infected patients, *JAMA*, 267, 2632, 1992.

18. Edlin, B. R., Tokars, J. I., Grieco, M. H., Crawford, J. T., Williams, J., Sordillo, E. M., Ong, K. R., Kilburn, J. O., Dooley, S. W., Castro, K. G., Jarvis, W. R., and Holmberg, S. D., An outbreak of multidrug-resistant tuberculosis among hospitalized patients with the acquired immunodeficiency syndrome, *N. Engl. J. Med.*, 326, 1514, 1992.

19. Frieden, T. R., Sherman, L. F., Maw, K. L., Fujiwara, P. I., Crawford, J. T., Nivin, B., Sharp, V., Hewlett, D., Jr., Brudney, K., Alland, D., and Kreiswirth, B. N., A multi-institutional outbreak of highly drug-resistant tuberculosis. Epidemiology and infection outcomes, *JAMA*, 276, 1229, 1996.

20. Leff, D. R. and Leff, A. R., Tuberculosis control policies in major metropolitan health departments in the United States, *Am. J. Respir. Crit. Care Med.*, 156, 1487, 1997.

21. Centers for Disease Control, Reported tuberculosis in the United States, 1996, USDHHS, PHS, Atlanta, 1997, 5.

22. Centers for Disease Control, Recommendations for prevention and control of tuberculosis among foreign-born persons: report of a working group on tuberculosis among foreign-born persons, *MMWR*, 47 (No. RR-16), 1, 1998.

23. Goldberg, B. W., Managed care and public health departments: who is responsible for the health of the population?, *Annu. Rev. Public Health*, 19, 527, 1998.

24. Centers for Disease Control, Essential components of a tuberculosis prevention and control program, *MMWR*, 44 (No. RR-11), 1, 1995.

25. Centers for Disease Control, Expanded tuberculosis surveillance and tuberculosis morbidity — United States — 1993, *MMWR*, 43, 361, 1994.

26. Centers for Disease Control, Prevention and control of tuberculosis among homeless persons: recommendations of the Advisory Council for the Elimination of Tuberculosis, *MMWR*, 41(No. RR-5), 13, 1992.

27. Centers for Disease Control, Prevention and control of tuberculosis in facilities providing long-term care to the elderly, *MMWR*, 39(No. RR-10), 7, 1990.

28. Centers for Disease Control, Guidelines for preventing the transmission of tuberculosis in health-care settings, with special focus on HIV-related issues, *MMWR*, 39(No. RR-17), 1, 1990.

29. Centers for Disease Control, Screening for tuberculosis and tuberculous infection in high-risk populations: recommendations of the Advisory Committee for the Elimination of Tuberculosis, *MMWR*, 39(No. RR-8), 1, 1990.

30. Centers for Disease Control, Prevention and control of tuberculosis in correctional institutions: recommendations of the Advisory Committee for the Elimination of Tuberculosis, *MMWR*, 38, 313, 1989.

31. Centers for Disease Control, Initial therapy for tuberculosis in the era of multidrug resistance: recommendations of the Advisory Council for the Elimination of Tuberculosis, *MMWR*, 42 (No. RR-7), 1, 1993.

32. American Thoracic Society/Centers for Disease Control, Treatment of tuberculosis and tuberculosis infection in adults and children, *Am. J. Respir. Crit. Care Med.*, 149, 1359, 1994.

33. Gostin, L. O., Controlling the resurgent tuberculosis epidemic: a 50-state survey of tuberculosis statutes and proposals for reform, *JAMA*, 269, 255, 1993.

34. Gasner, M. R., Khin, L. M., Feldman, G. E., Fujiwara, P. I., and Frieden, T. R., The use of legal action New York City to ensure treatment of tuberculosis, *N. Engl. J. Med.*, 340, 359, 1999.

35. Fujiwara, P. I., Larkin, C., and Frieden, T. R., Directly observed therapy in New York City: history, implementation, results, and challenges, *Clin. Chest Med.*, 18, 135, 1997.

36. American Thoracic Society/Centers for Disease Control, Control of tuberculosis in the United States, *Am. Rev. Respir. Dis.*, 146, 1623, 1992.

37. Centers for Disease Control, The use of preventive therapy for tuberculous infection in the United States: recommendations of the Advisory Committee for the Elimination of Tuberculosis, *MMWR*, 39(No. RR-8), 9, 1990.

38. Selwyn, P. A., Hartel, D., Lewis, V. A., Schoenbaum, E. E., Vermund, S. H., Klein, R. S., Walker, A. T., and Friedland, G. H., A prospective study of the risk of tuberculosis among intravenous drug users with human immunodeficiency virus infection, *N. Engl. J. Med.*, 320, 545, 1989.

39. Villarino, M. E., Dooley, S. W., Geiter, L. J., Castro, K. G., and Snider, D. E., Jr., Management of persons exposed to multidrug-resistant tuberculosis, *MMWR*, 41(No. RR-11), 61, 1992.

40. Moore, M., Onorato, I. M., McCray, E., and Castro, K. G., Trends in drug-resistant tuberculosis in the United States, 1993-1996, *JAMA*, 278, 833, 1997.

41. Carey, J. W., Oxtoby, M. J., Nguyen, L. P., Huynh, V., Morgan, M., and Jeffrey, M., Tuberculosis beliefs among recent Vietnamese refugees in New York state, *Pub. Health Rep.*, 112, 66, 1997.

42. World Health Organization, *World Health Organization Expert Committee on Tuberculosis,* 9th report, Technical Report Service, WHO, 552, 1974.

43. Horne, N. W., Eradication of tuberculosis in Europe — so near and yet so far, *Bull. Int. Union Against Tuberc.*, 59, 107, 1985.

44. World Health Organization, *Managing Tuberculosis at the District Level,* World Health Organization, Geneva, 1992.

45. DeCock, K. M., Grant, A., and Porter, J. D. H., Preventive therapy for tuberculosis in HIV-infected persons: international recommendations, research and practice, *Lancet*, 345, 833, 1995.

46. World Health Organization, Tuberculosis preventive therapy in HIV-infected individuals, *Wkly. Epidemiol. Rec.*, 68, 361, 1993.

47. Kopanoff, D. E., Kilburn, J. O., Glassroth, J. L., Snider, D. E., Jr., Farer, L. S., and Good, R. C., A continuing survey of tuberculosis primary drug resistance in the United States: March 1975 to November 1977, a United States Public Health Service cooperative study, *Am. Rev. Respir. Dis.*, 118, 835, 1978.

48. Centers for Disease Control, Primary resistance to antituberculosis drugs — United States, *MMWR*, 32, 521, 1983.

49. Snider, D. E.m Jr., Cauthen, G. M., Farer, L. S., Kelly, G. D., Kilburn, J. O., Good, R. C., and Dooley, S. W., Drug-resistant tuberculosis (letter to editor), *Am. Rev. Respir. Dis.*, 144, 732, 1991.

50. Beck-Sague, C., Dooley, S. W., Hutton, M. D., Otten, J., Breeden, A., Crawford, J. T., Pitchenik, A. E., Woodley, C., Cauthen, G., and Jarvis, W. R., Hospital outbreak of multidrug-resistant *Mycobacterium tuberculosis* infections: factors in transmission to staff and HIV-infected patients, *JAMA*, 268, 1280, 1992.

51. Pearson, M. L., Jereb, J. A., Frieden, T. R., Crawford, J. T., Davis, B. J., Dooley, S. W., and Jarvis, W. R., Nosocomial transmission of multidrug-resistant *Mycobacterium tuberculosis*: a risk to patients and health care workers, *Ann. Intern. Med.*, 117, 191, 1992.

52. Fischl, M. A., Uttamchandani, M. D., Daikos, G. L., Poblete, R. B., Moreno, J. N., Reyes, R. R., Boota, A. M., Thompson, L. M., Cleary, T. J., and Lai, S., An outbreak of tuberculosis caused by multiple-drug-resistant tubercle bacilli among patients with HIV-infection, *Ann. Intern. Med.*, 117, 177, 1992.

53. Dooley, S. W., Jarvis, W. R., Martone, W. J., and Snider, D. E., Jr., Multidrug-resistant tuberculosis, *Ann. Intern. Med.*, 117, 257, 1992.

54. Pape, J. W., Jean, S. S., Ho, J. L., Hafner, A., and Johnson, W. D., Effect of isoniazid prophylaxis on incidence of active tuberculosis and progression of HIV infection, *Lancet*, 342, 268, 1993.

55. Whalen, C. C., Johnson, J. L., Okwera, A., Ham, D. L., Huebner, R., Mugyenyi, P., Mugerwa, R. D., and Ellner, J. J., A trial of three regimens to prevent tuberculosis in Ugandan adults infected with the human immunodeficiency virus, *N. Engl. J. Med.*, 337, 801, 1997.

56. Mwinga, A. G., Hosp, M., Godfrey-Faussett, P., Quigley, M., Mwaba, P., Mugala, B. N., Nyirenda, O., Luo, J. N., Pobee, J., Elliot, A. M., McAdam, K. P. W. J., and Porter, J. D. H., Twice-weekly tuberculosis preventive therapy in HIV infection in Zambia, *AIDS*, 12, 2447, 1998.

57. Aisu, T., Raviglione, M. C., Von Praag, E., Eriki, P., Narain, J. P., Barugahere, L., Tembo, G., McFarland, D., and Engwau, F. A., Preventive chemotherapy for HIV-associated tuberculosis in Uganda: an operational assessment at a voluntary counseling and testing center, *AIDS*, 9, 267, 1995.

58. Ngamvithayapong, J., Uthaivoravit, W., Yanai, H., Akarasewi, P., and Sawanpanyalert, P., Adherence to tuberculosis preventive therapy among HIV-infected persons in Chiang Rai, Thailand, *AIDS*, 11, 107, 1997.

59. Foster, S., Godfrey-Faussett, P., and Porter, J., Modelling the economic benefits of tuberculosis preventive therapy for people with HIV: the example of Zambia, *AIDS*, 11, 919, 1997.

60. World Health Organization, *BCG Vaccination of the Newborn: Rationale and Guidelines for Country Programmes,* World Health Organization, Geneva, 1986.

61. Centers for Disease Control, The role of BCG vaccines in the prevention and control of tuberculosis in the United States: a joint statement by the Advisory Council for Elimination of Tuberculosis and the Advisory Committee on Immunization Practices, *MMWR*, 45 (No. RR-4), 1, 1996.

62. Centers for Disease Control, Tuberculosis morbidity — United States, 1997, *MMWR*, 47, 253, 1998.

63. McKenna, M. T., McCray, E., Jones, J. L., Onorato, I. M., and Castro, K. G., The fall after the rise: tuberculosis in the United States, 1991 to 1994, *Am. J. Pub. Health*, 88, 1059, 1998.

64. Frieden, T. R., Sterling, T., Pablos-Mendez, A., Kilburn, J. O., Cauthen,, G. M., and Dooley, S. W., The emergence of drug-resistant tuberculosis in New York City, *N. Engl. J. Med.*, 328, 521, 1993.

65. American Thoracic Society, Control of tuberculosis, *Am. Rev. Respir. Dis.*, 128, 336, 1983.

66. National Institute of Occupational Safety and Health, NIOSH recommended guidelines for personal respiratory protection of workers in health-care facilities potentially exposed to tuberculosis, United States Department of Health and Human Services, Public Health Service, Centers for Disease Control, September 14, 1992.

67. Christie, C. D., Constantinou, P., Marx, M. L., Wilke, M. J., Marot, K., Mendez, F. L., Donovan, J., and Thole, J., Low risk for tuberculosis in a regional pediatric hospital: nine-year study of community rates and the mandatory employee tuberculin skin-test program, *Infect. Cont. Hosp. Epidemiol.*, 19, 168, 1998.

68. LoBue, P. A. and Catanzaro, A., Effectiveness of a nosocomial tuberculosis control program, *Chest*, 113, 1184, 1998.

69. Behrman, A. J. and Shofer, F. S., Tuberculosis exposure and control in an urban emergency department, *Ann. Emerg. Med.*, 31, 370, 1998.

70. Maloney, S. A., Pearon, M., Gordon, M., Del Castillo, R., Boyle, J., and Jarvis, W., The efficacy of recommended infection control measures in preventing nosocomial transmission of multidrug-resistant tuberculosis (abstract No.15-10), in *World Congress on Tuberculosis, Program and Abstracts*, Bethesda, MD, November 16–19, 1992, 51.

71. Otten, J., Chan, J., and Cleary, T., Successful control of an outbreak of multidrug-resistant tuberculosis in an urban teaching hospital (abstract No.15-11), in *World Congress on Tuberculosis, Program and Abstracts*, Bethesda, MD, November 16–19, 1992, 51.

72. Wenger, P., Beck-Sague, C., Otten, J., Breeden, A., Orfas, D., and Jarvis, W., Efficacy of control measures in preventing nosocomial transmission of multidrug-resistant *Mycobacterium tuberculosis* among patients and health-care workers (abstract No.15-16), in *World Congress on Tuberculosis, Program and Abstracts*, Bethesda, MD, November 16–19, 1992, 53.

73. Centers for Disease Control, Tuberculosis outbreaks in prison housing units for HIV-infected inmates — California, 1995-1996, *MMWR*, 48, 69, 1999.

74. Bock, N. N., Mallory, J. P., Mobley, N., DeVoe, B., and Taylor, B. B., Outbreak of tuberculosis associated with a floating card game in the rural south: lessons for tuberculosis contact investigations, *Clin. Infect. Dis.*, 27, 1221, 1998.

75. McIntyre, C. R., Plant, A. J., Hulls, J., Streeton, J. A., Graham, N. M. H., and Rouch, G. J., High rate of transmission of tuberculosis in an office: impact of delayed diagnosis, *Clin. Infect. Dis.*, 21, 1170, 1995.

76. Allos, B. M., Gensheimer, K. F., Bloch, A. B., Parrottee, D., Horan, J. M., Lewis, V., and Schaffner, W., Management of an outbreak of tuberculosis in a small community, *Ann. Intern. Med.*, 125, 114, 1996.

77. Small, P. M., Hopewell, P. C., Singh, S. P., Paz, A., Parsonnet, J., Ruston, D. C., Schechter, G. F., Daley, C. L., and Schoolnik, G. K., The epidemiology of tuberculosis in San Francisco: a population-based study using conventional and molecular methods, *N. Engl. J. Med.*, 330, 1703, 1994.

78. Barnes, P. F., Yang, Z. H., Preston-Martin, S., Pogoda, J. M., Jones, B. E., Otaya, M., Eisenach, K. D., Knowles, L., Harvey, S., and Cave, D., Patterns of tuberculosis transmission in central Los Angeles, *JAMA*, 278, 1159, 1997.

79. Alland, D., Kalkut, G. E., Moss, A. R., McAdam, R. A., Hahn, J. A., Bosworth, W., Drucker, E., and Bloom, B. R., Transmission of tuberculosis in New York City: an analysis by DNA fingerprinting and conventional epidemiologic methods, *N. Engl. J. Med.*, 330, 1710, 1994.

80. Behr, M. A., Hopewell P. C., Paz, A., Kawamura, L. M., Schechter, G. F., and Small, P. M., Predictive value of contact investigation for identifying recent transmission of *Mycobacterium tuberculosis, Am. J. Respir. Crit. Care Med.*, 158, 465, 1998.

81. Centers for Disease Control and Prevention, Reported Tuberculosis Cases in the United States, 1997, USDHHS, PHS, Atlanta, 1, July 1998.

82. Jereb, J., Centers for Disease Control, personal communication, 1999.

83. Frieden, T. R., Fujiwara, P. I., Washko, R. M., and Hamburg, M. A., Tuberculosis in New York City — turning the tide, *N. Engl. J. Med.*, 333, 229, 1995.

84. Centers for Disease Control, Division of Tuberculosis Elimination, 1990 and 1991 Case Management Reports, unpublished data, 1992.

85. U.S. Department of Health and Human Services, 1987 Tuberculosis Statistics in the United States, HHS Publication No.(CDC) 89-8322, 1989.

86. Centers for Disease Control and Prevention, 1992 Tuberculosis Statistics in the United States, Atlanta, 1, 1994.

87. Centers for Disease Control, Division of Tuberculosis Elimination, 1995 and 1996 Tuberculosis Program Management Report, unpublished data, 1998.

88. American Lung Association, Conference report: the American Lung Association conference on re-establishing control of tuberculosis in the United States, March 11–13, Washington D.C., *Am. J. Respir. Crit. Care Med.*, 154, 251, 1996.

89. Council of State and Territorial Epidemiologists, Position statement number 90-13, TB/HIV surveillance and control, Council of State and Territorial Epidemiologists, Atlanta, GA, April 1990.

90. Bloch, A. B., Onorato, I. M., Ihle, W. W., Hadler, J. L., Hayden, C. H., and Snider, D. E., Jr., The need for epidemic intelligence, *Pub. Health Rep.*, 111, 26, 1996.

91. Hayden, C. R., HIV-related tuberculosis prevention in drug treatment centers and correctional facilities (abstract No.11-02), in *World Congress on Tuberculosis, Program and Abstracts*, Bethesda, MD, November 16–19, 1992, 38.

92. Marino, J., Progress of mandatory HIV positivity reporting for TB cases and TB infections in Connecticut, 1992–1994, in Summary of Presentations, Conclusions, and Recommendations, Workshop Attenders and "Learning Experience" Abstracts, National TB Controllers Workshop, USDHHS, PHS, CDC, Atlanta, January 8–10, 1995.

93. Centers for Disease Control, Tuberculosis prevention in drug-treatment centers and correctional facilities — selected U.S. sites, *MMWR*, 42, 210, 1993.

94. Winquist A., Hadler, J. L., and Marino, J., unpublished data, 1999.

95. Styblo, K., The relationship between the risk of tuberculous infection and the risk of developing infectious tuberculosis, *Bull. Int. Union Against Tuberc. Lung Dis.*, 60, 117, 1986.

96. Occupational Safety and Health Administration, Enforcement procedures and scheduling for occupational exposure to tuberculosis, CPL. 2. 106, February 9, 1996.

97. Binkin, N. J., Zuber, P. L. F., Wells, C. D., Tipple, M. A., and Castro, K. G., Overseas screening for tuberculosis in immigrants and refugees to the United States: current status, *Clin. Infect. Dis.*, 23, 1226, 1996.

98. Centers for Disease Control, Prevention and control of tuberculosis in migrant farm workers: recommendations of the Advisory Council for the Elimination of Tuberculosis, *MMWR*, 41(No. RR-10), 1, 1992.

99. Centers for Disease Control, Drug-resistant tuberculosis among the homeless — Boston, *MMWR*, 34, 429, 1985.

100. Barry, M. A., Wall, C., Shirley, L., Bernardo, J., Schwingl, P., Brigandi, E., and Lamb, G. A., Tuberculosis screening in Boston's homeless shelters, *Pub. Health Rep.*, 101, 487, 1986.

101. Slutkin, G., Management of tuberculosis in urban homeless indigents, *Pub. Health Rep.*, 101, 481, 1986.

102. McAdam, J., Brickner, P. W., Glicksman, R., Edwards, D., Fallon, B., and Yanowitch P., Tuberculosis in the SRO/homeless population, in *Health Care of Homeless People*, Brickner, P. W., Scharer, L. K., Conanan, B., Elvy, A., and Savarese, M., Eds., Springer, New York, 1985, 155.

103. Cielsielski, S. D., Seed, J. R., Esposito, P. H., and Hunter, N., The epidemiology of TB among North Carolina migrant farm workers, *JAMA*, 265, 1715, 1991.

104. American Thoracic Society, Treatment of tuberculosis and tuberculous infection in adult and children, *Am. Rev. Respir. Dis.*, 134, 355, 1986.

105. Cohn, D. L., Catlin, B. J., Peterson, K. L., Judson, F. N., and Sbarbaro, J. A., A 62-dose, 6-month therapy for pulmonary and extra-pulmonary tuberculosis: a twice-weekly, directly observed and cost-effective regimen, *Ann. Intern. Med.*, 112, 407, 1990.

106. Combs, D. L., O'Brien, R. J., and Geiter, L. J., United States Public Health Service tuberculosis short course chemotherapy trial 21: effectiveness, toxicity and acceptability, *Ann. Intern. Med.*, 112, 397, 1990.

107. Mugerwa, R., Okwera, A., Viecha, M., Aisu, T., Huebner, R., Ellner, J., and Morrissey, A., Drug toxicity and mortality in HIV-infected Ugandan patients treated for pulmonary tuberculosis (abstract No. 13-11), in *World Congress on Tuberculosis, Program and Abstracts*, Bethesda, MD, November 16–19, 1992, 43.

108. Chintu, C., Bhat, G. T., Luo, C., Kabika, M., Raviglione, M. C., and O'Brien, R. J., HIV seroprevalence and fatal skin reactions in children treated for tuberculosis in Lusaka, Zambia (abstract No.13-13), in *World Congress on Tuberculosis, Program and Abstracts*, Bethesda, MD, November 16–19, 1992, 44.

109. Kochi, A., Tuberculosis control — is DOTS the health breakthrough of the 1990s? *World Health Forum*, 18, 225, 1997.

110. Ireland, H. D., Outpatient chemotherapy for tuberculosis, *Am. Rev. Respir. Dis.*, 82, 378, 1960.

111. Preston, D. F. and Miller, F. L., The tuberculosis outpatient's defection from therapy, *Am. J. Med. Sci.*, 247, 55, 1964.

112. Moulding, T., New responsibilities for health departments and public health nurses in tuberculosis — keeping outpatients on therapy, *Am. J. Pub. Health*, 56, 416, 1966.

113. Addington, W. W., Patient compliance: the most serious remaining problem in the control of tuberculosis in the United States, *Chest*, 76, 741, 1979.

114. Sbarbaro, J. A., Public health aspects of tuberculosis: supervision of therapy, *Clin. Chest Med.*, 1, 253, 1980.

115. Reichman, L., Compliance in developed nations, *Tuberculosis*, 68 (Suppl.), 25, 1987.

116. Brudney, K. and Dobkin, J., Resurgent tuberculosis in New York City: human immunodeficiency virus, homelessness, and the decline of tuberculosis control programs, *Am. Rev. Respir. Dis.*, 144, 745, 1991.

117. Styblo, K., How should a tuberculosis control program be evaluated? Unpublished talk at the World Congress on Tuberculosis, Bethesda, MD, November 17, 1992.

118. Meichembaum, D. and Turk, D. C., *Facilitating Treatment Adherence: A Practitioner's Guidebook*, Plenum Press, New York, 1987.

119. Gerber, K. E. and Nehemkis, A. M., Eds., *Compliance: The Dilemma of the Chronically Ill*, Springer, New York, 1986.

120. DiMatteo, M. R. and DiNicola, D. D., *Achieving Patient Compliance: The Psychology of the Medical Practitioner's Role*, Pergamon Press, New York, 1982.

121. Haynes, R. B., Taylor, D. W., and Sackett, D. L., Eds., *Compliance in Health Care*, The Johns Hopkins University Press, Baltimore, 1979.

122. Kirscht, J. P. and Rosenstock, I. M., Patients' problems in following recommendations of health experts, in *Health Psychology: A Handbook*, Stone, G. C., Cohen, F., and Adler, N. E., Eds., Jossey-Bass, San Francisco, 1979, 189.

123. Sumartojo, E., When tuberculosis treatment fails: a social behavioral account of patient adherence, *Am. Rev. Respir. Dis.*, 147, 1311, 1993.

124. Alcabes, P., Vossenas, P., Cohen, R., Braslow, C., Micheals, D., and Zoloth, S., Compliance with isoniazid prophylaxis in jail, *Am. Rev. Respir. Dis.*, 140, 1194, 1989.

125. Corcoran, R., Compliance with chemotherapy for tuberculosis, *Irish Med. J.*, 79, 87, 1986.

126. Barnhoorn, F. and Adriaanse, H., In search of factors responsible for noncompliance among tuberculosis patients in Wardha District, India, *Soc. Sci. Med.*, 34, 291, 1992.

127. Shears, P., Tuberculosis control in Somali refugee camps, *Tubercle*, 65, 111, 1984.

128. Morisky D. E., Malotte, C. K., Choi, P., Davidson, P., Rigler, S., Sugland, B., and Langer, M., A patient education program to improve adherence rates with antituberculosis drug regimens, *Health Educ. Q.*, 17, 253, 1990.

129. Wurtele, S. K., Galanos, A. N., and Roberts, M. C., Increasing return compliance in a tuberculosis detection drive, *J. Behav. Med.*, 3, 311, 1980.

130. Seetha, M. A., Srikantaramu, N., Aneja, K. S., and Singh, H., Influence of motivation of patients and their family members on the drug collection by patients, *Indian J. Tuberc.*, 28, 182, 1981.

131. Wobeser, W., To, T., and Hoeppner, V. H., The outcome of chemoprophylaxis on tuberculosis prevention in the Canadian Plains Indian, *Clin. Invest. Med.*, 12, 149, 1989.

132. Centers for Disease Control and Prevention, Improving Patient Adherence in Tuberculosis Treatment, revised, USPHS, Atlanta, Georgia, 1, 1994.

133. Centers for Disease Control, Approaches to improving adherence to antituberculosis therapy — South Carolina and New York — 1986–1992, *MMWR*, 42, 74, 1993.

134. Volmink, J. and Garner, P., Systematic review of randomised controlled trials of strategies to promote adherence to tuberculosis treatment, *Br. Med. J.*, 315, 1403, 1997.

135. Curry, F. J., Neighborhood clinics for more effective outpatient treatment of tuberculosis, *N. Engl. J. Med.*, 279, 1262, 1968.

136. McAdam, J. M., Brickner, P. W., Scharer, L. L., Crocco, J. A., and Duff, A. E., The spectrum of tuberculosis in a New York City men's shelter clinic (1982–1988), *Chest*, 97, 798, 1990.

137. McDonald, R. J., Memon, A. M., and Reichman, L. B., Successful supervised ambulatory management of tuberculosis treatment failures, *Ann. Intern. Med.*, 96, 297, 1982.

138. Werhane, M. J., Snukst-Torbeck, G., and Schraufnagel, D. E., The tuberculosis clinic, *Chest*, 96, 815, 1989.

139. Adler J. J., Ruggiero, D., Langhorne, W., Heetderks, A., and Nivin, B., Residential facility for homeless tuberculosis patients (abstract), *Am. Rev. Respir. Dis.*, 141, A458, 1990.

140. Sbarbaro, J. A., Compliance: inducements and enforcements, *Chest*, 76 (Suppl.), 750, 1979.

141. Chaulk, C. P. and Kazankjian, V. A., Directly observed therapy for treatment completion of pulmonary tuberculosis: consensus statement of the Public Health Tuberculosis Guidelines Panel, *JAMA*, 279, 943, 1998.

142. Schluger, N., Ciotoli, C., Cohen, D., Johnson, H., and Rom, W. N., Comprehensive tuberculosis control for patients at high risk for noncompliance, *Am. J. Respir. Crit. Care Med.*, 151, 1486, 1995.

143. El-Sadr, W., Medard, F., and Barthaud, V., Directly observed therapy for tuberculosis: the Harlem Hospital experience, 1993, *Am. J. Pub. Health*, 86, 1146, 1996.

144. Chaulk, C. P., Moore-Rice, K., Rizzo, R., and Chaisson, R. E., Eleven years of community-based directly observed therapy for tuberculosis, *JAMA*, 274, 975, 1995.

145. Moore, R. D., Chaulk, C. P., Griffiths, R., Cavalcante, S., and Chaisson, R. E., Cost-effectiveness of directly observed versus self-administered therapy for tuberculosis, *Am. J. Respir. Crit. Care Med.*, 154, 1013, 1996.

146. Burman, W. J., Dalton, C. B., Cohn, D. L., Butler, J. R. G., and Reves, R. R., A cost-effectiveness analysis of directly observed therapy vs. self-administered therapy for treatment of tuberculosis, *Chest*, 112, 63, 1997.

147. Centers for Disease Control, Drug-resistant tuberculosis — Mississippi, *MMWR*, 26, 417, 1977.

148. Centers for Disease Control, Follow-up on drug-resistant tuberculosis — Mississippi, *MMWR*, 27, 355, 1978.

149. Division of Tuberculosis Control, South Carolina Department of Health and Environmental Control, *Enablers and Incentives*, American Lung Association of South Carolina, 1989.

150. Snider, D. E., Jr., Anders, H. M., and Pozsik, C. J., Incentives to take up health services (letter), *Lancet*, 2, 812, 1986.

151. Burkhardt, K. R. and Nel, E. E., Monitoring regularity of drug intake in tuberculous patients by means of simple urine tests, *S. African Med. J.*, 57, 981, 1980.

152. Ellard, G. A. and Greenfield, C., A sensitive urine-test method for monitoring the ingestion of isoniazid, *J. Clin. Pathol.*, 30, 84, 1977.

153. Kilburn, J. O., Beam, R. E., David, H. L., Sanches, E., Corpe, R. F., and Dunn, W., Reagent-impregnated paper strip for detection of metabolic products of isoniazid in urine, *Am. Rev. Respir. Dis.*, 106, 923, 1972.

154. Henderson, W. T., The development and use of the Potts-Cozart tube test for the detection of isoniazid metabolites in urine, *J. Ark. Med. Soc.*, 82, 445, 1986.

155. Schraufnagel, D. E., Stoner, R., Whiting, E., Snukst-Torbeck, G., and Werhane, M. J., Testing for isoniazid: an evaluation of the Arkansas method, *Chest*, 98, 314, 1990.

156. Moulding, T., Onstad, G. D., and Sbarbaro, J. A., Supervision of outpatient drug treatment with the medication monitor, *Ann. Intern. Med.*, 73, 559, 1970.

157. Cheung, R., Dickins, J., Nicholson, P. W., Thomas, A. S. C., Smith, H. H., Larson, H. E., Desmukh, A. A., Dobbs, R. J., and Dobbs, S. M., Compliance with anti-tuberculous therapy: a field trial of a pill-box with a concealed electronic recording device, *Eur. J. Clin. Pharmacol.*, 35, 401, 1988.

158. Moulding, T., Medication monitors for selecting tuberculosis patients who need directly observed therapy (abstract 8-01), in *World Congress on Tuberculosis, Program and Abstracts*, Bethesda, MD, November 16–19, 1992, 35.

159. Fallab-Stubi, C. L., Zellweger, J. P., Sauty, A., Uldry, C., Iorillo, D., and Burnier, M., Electronic monitoring of adherence to treatment in the preventive chemotherapy of tuberculosis, *Int. J. Tuberc. Lung Dis.*, 2, 525, 1998.

160. Annas, G. J., Control of tuberculosis — the law and the public's health, *N. Engl. J. Med.*, 328, 585, 1993.

161. Burman, W. J., Cohn, D. L., Rietmeijer, C. A., Judson, F. N., Sbarbaro, J. A., and Reves, R. R., Short-term incarceration for the management of noncompliance with tuberculosis treatment, *Chest*, 112, 57, 1997.

162. Etkind, S., Boutotte, J., Ford, J., Singleton, L., and Nardell, E. A., Tracking hard-to-treat tuberculosis patients in Massachusetts, *Sem. Respir. Infect.*, 6, 273, 1991.

163. Yeager, H. and Medinger, A., Tuberculosis long-term care beds: have we thrown out the baby with the bath water? *Chest*, 90, 752, 1986.

164. Campion, E. W., Liberty and control of tuberculosis (editorial), *N. Engl. J. Med.*, 340, 385, 1999.

165. Singleton, L., Turner, M., Haskal, R., Etkind, S., Tricarico, M., and Nardell, E., Long-term hospitalization for tuberculosis control: experience with a medical-psychosocial inpatient unit, *JAMA*, 278, 838, 1997.

166. Miller, B., Rosenbaum, S., Stange, P., Solomon, S. L., and Castro, K. G., Tuberculosis control in a changing health care system: model contract specifications for managed care organizations, *Clin. Infect. Dis.*, 27, 677, 1998.

167. Glassroth, J., Bailey, W. C., and Hopewell, P. C., Why tuberculosis is not prevented, *Am. Rev. Respir. Dis.*, 141, 1236, 1990.

168. Mehta, J. B., Dutt, A. K., Harvill, L., and Henry, W., Isoniazid preventive therapy for tuberculosis. Are we losing our enthusiasm? *Chest*, 94, 138, 1988.

169. MacIntyre, C. R., Plant, A. J., Yung, A., and Streeton, J. A., Missed opportunities for prevention of tuberculosis in Victoria, Australia, *Int. J. Tuberc. Lung Dis.*, 1, 135, 1997.

170. Centers for Disease Control, Tuberculosis and human immunodeficiency virus infection: recommendations of the advisory committee for the elimination of tuberculosis, *MMWR*, 38, 236, 1989.

171. Centers for Disease Control, Prevention and control of tuberculosis in correctional institutions: recommendations of the Advisory Committee for the Elimination of Tuberculosis, *MMWR*, 38, 313, 1989.

172. Gourevitch, M. N., Alcabes, P., Wasserman, W. C., and Arno, P. S., Cost-effectiveness of directly observed chemoprophylaxis of tuberculosis among drug users at high risk of tuberculosis, *Int. J. Tuberc. Lung Dis.*, 2, 531, 1998.

173. White, M. C., Tulsky, J. P., Reilly, P., McIntosh, H. W., Hoynes, T. M., and Goldenson, J., A clinical trial of a financial incentive to go to the tuberculosis clinic for isoniazid after release from jail, *Int. J. Tuberc. Lung Dis.*, 2, 506, 1998.

174. Tulsky, J. P., White, M. C., Dawson, C., Hoynes, T. M., Goldenson, J., and Schecter, G., Screening for tuberculosis in jail and clinic follow-up after release, *Am. J. Pub. Health*, 88, 223, 1998.

175. Nolan, C. M., Roll, L., Goldberg, S. V., and Elarth, A. M., Directly observed isoniazid preventive therapy for released jail inmates, *Am. J. Respir. Crit. Care Med.*, 155, 583, 1997.

176. Nazar-Steward, V. and Nolan, C. M., Results of a directly- observed intermittent isoniazid preventive therapy program in a shelter for homeless men, *Am. Rev. Respir. Dis.*, 146, 57, 1992.

177. Centers for Disease Control, Purified protein derivative (PPD)-tuberculin anergy and HIV infection: guidelines for anergy testing and management of anergic persons at risk of tuberculosis, *MMWR*, 40 (No. RR-5), 27, 1991.

178. Centers for Disease Control, Anergy skin testing and preventive therapy for HIV-infected persons: revised recommendations, *MMWR*, 46 (No. RR-15), 1, 1997.

179. Shaw, J. B. and Wynn-Williams, N., Infectivity of pulmonary tuberculosis in relation to sputum status, *Am. Rev. Tuberc.*, 69, 724, 1954.

180. Loudon, R. G. and Spohn, S. K., Cough frequency and infectivity in patients with pulmonary tuberculosis, *Am. Rev. Respir. Dis.*, 99, 109, 1969.

181. Hutton, M. D., Stead, W. W., Cauthen, G. M., Bloch, A. B., and Ewing, W. M., Nosocomial transmission of tuberculosis associated with a draining abscess, *J. Infect. Dis.*, 161, 286, 1990.

182. Cantanzaro, A., Nosocomial transmission of tuberculosis, *Am. Rev. Respir. Dis.*, 125, 559, 1982.

183. Centers for Disease Control, Crack cocaine use among persons with tuberculosis — Contra Costa County, California, 1987–1990, *MMWR*, 40, 485, 1991.

184. Leonhardt, K. K., Gentile, F., Gilbert, B. P., and Aiken, M. A., A cluster of tuberculosis among crack house contacts in San Mateo County, California, *Am. J. Pub. Health*, 84, 1834, 1994.

185. Nolan, C. M., unpublished data, 1992.

186. Centers for Disease Control, Transmission of multidrug-resistant tuberculosis from an HIV-positive client in a residential substance-abuse treatment facility — Michigan, *MMWR*, 40, 129, 1991.

187. Fine, L. B., Rwambuya, D. S., Siegel, P. L., and Hadler, J. L., Tuberculosis screening policy and practices in urban Connecticut hospitals, April, 1992, unpublished, 1992.

188. Zuber, P. L. F., McKenna, M. T., Binkin, N. J., Onorato, I. M., and Castro, K. G., Long-term risk of tuberculosis among foreign-born persons in the United States, *JAMA*, 278, 304, 1997.

189. Centers for Disease Control, Tuberculosis among foreign-born persons entering the United States: recommendations of the Advisory Committee for Elimination of Tuberculosis, *MMWR*, 39 (No. RR-18), 1, 1990.

190. Binkin, N. J., Zuber, P. L. F., Wells, C. D., Tipple, M. A., and Castro, K. G., Overseas screening for tuberculosis in immigrants and refugees to the United States: current status, *Clin. Infect. Dis.*, 23, 1226, 1996.

191. Wells, C. D., Zuber, P. L. F., Nolan, C. M., Binkin, N. J., and Goldberg, S. V., Tuberculosis prevention among foreign-born persons in Seattle — King County, Washington, *Am. J. Respir. Crit. Care Med.*, 156, 573, 1997.

192. Blum, R. N., Polish, L. B., Tapy, J. M., Catlin, B. J., and Cohn, D. L., Results of screening for tuberculosis in foreign-born persons applying for adjustment of immigration status, *Chest*, 103, 1670, 1993.

193. Vaccine-Preventable Diseases Task Force, American College Health Association, ACHA guidelines: tuberculosis screening on campus, *Am. Coll. Health Assoc.*, 1, 1996.

194. American Academy of Pediatrics, Tuberculosis, in Peter, G., Ed., *1997 Redbook: Report of the Committee on Infectious Diseases*, 24th ed., Elk Grove Village, IL, American College of Pediatrics, 1997, 548.

195. Centers for Diseease Control, Prevention and control of tuberculosis in U.S. communities with at-risk minority populations: recommendations of the Advisory Council for the Elimination of Tuberculosis, *MMWR*, 41 (No. RR-5), 1, 1992.

196. Reichman, L. B., Tuberculosis elimination — what's to stop us? *Int. J. Tuberc. Lung Dis.*, 1, 3, 1997.

197. Braun, M. M., Truman, B. I., and Maguire, B., Increasing incidence of tuberculosis in a prison inmate population, *JAMA*, 261, 393, 1989.

198. Stead, W. W., Lofgren, J. P., Warren, E., and Thomas, C., Tuberculosis as an endemic and nosocomial infection among the elderly in nursing homes, *N. Engl. J. Med.*, 312, 1483, 1985.

199. Stead, W. W. and To, T., The significance of the tuberculin skin test in elderly persons, *Ann. Intern. Med.*, 107, 833, 1987.

200. Stead, W. W., To, T., Harrison, R. W., and Abraham, J. H., III, Benefit risk considerations in preventive therapy for tuberculosis in elderly persons, *Ann. Intern. Med.*, 107, 843, 1987.

201. Stead, W. W., Undetected tuberculosis in prison: source of infection for community at large, *JAMA*, 240, 2544, 1978.

202. Hutton, M. D., Cauthen, G. M., and Bloch, A. B., Results of a 29-state survey of tuberculosis in nursing homes and correctional facilities, *Pub. Health Rep.*, 108, 305, 1993.

203. Glaser, J. B. and Greifinger, R. B., Correctional health care: a public health opportunity, *Ann. Intern. Med.*, 118, 139, 1993.

204. City of Philadelphia Health Department, unpublished data, 1992.

205. Truman, B. I., Morse, D., Mikl, J., Lehman, S., Forte, A., Broaddus, R., and Stevens, R., HIV seroprevalence and risk factors among prison inmates entering New York State prisons (abstract No.4207), in Book I, 4th International Conference on AIDS, Stockholm, June 12–16, 1988, 311.

206. Barrett-Conner, E., The epidemiology of tuberculosis in physicians, *JAMA*, 241, 33, 1979.

207. Brennen, C., Muder, R. R., and Muraca, P. W., Occult endemic tuberculosis in a chronic care facility, *Infect. Cont. Hosp. Epidemiol.*, 9, 548, 1988.

208. Goldman, K. P., Tuberculosis in hospital doctors, *Tubercle*, 69, 237, 1988.

209. Ehrenkranz, N. J. and Kicklighter, J. L., Tuberculosis outbreak in a general hospital: evidence of airborne spread of infection, *Ann. Intern. Med.*, 77, 377, 1972.

210. Kantor, H. S., Poblete, R., and Pusateri S. L., Nosocomial transmission of tuberculosis from unsuspected disease, *Am. J. Med.*, 84, 833, 1988.

211. Lundgren, R., Norrman, E., and Asberg, I., Tuberculous infection transmitted at autopsy, *Tubercle*, 68, 147, 1987.

212. Centers for Disease Control, Guidelines for preventing the transmission of tuberculosis in health-care settings, with special focus on HIV-related issues, *MMWR*, 39 (No. RR- 17), 1, 1990.

213. Centers for Disease Control, Tuberculosis outbreaks in prison housing units for HIV-infected inmates — California, 1995–1996, *MMWR*, 48, 79, 1999.

214. Centers for Disease Control, Prevention and control of tuberculosis in correctional institutions: recommendations of the Advisory Committee for the Elimination of Tuberculosis, *MMWR*, 38, 313, 1989.

215. Marsh, K., Tuberculosis among the residents of hostels and lodging houses in London, *Lancet*, 1, 1136, 1957.

216. Elmwood, P. C., Tuberculosis in a common lodging house, *Br. J. Prev. Soc. Med.*, 15, 89, 1961.

217. Hurford, J. V., The "homeless" male with pulmonary tuberculosis, *Tubercle*, 43, 192, 1962.

218. Patel, K. R., Pulmonary tuberculosis in residents of lodging houses, night shelters and common hostels in Glasgow: a 5-year prospective survey, *Br. J. Dis. Chest*, 79, 60, 1985.

219. Centers for Disease Control, Drug-resistant tuberculosis among the homeless — Boston, *MMWR*, 34, 429, 1985.

220. Nardell, E., McInnis, B., Thomas, B., and Weidhaas, S., Exogenous reinfection with tuberculosis in a shelter for the homeless, *N. Engl. J. Med.*, 315, 1570, 1986.

221. Nolan, C. M., Elarth, A. M., Barr, H., Saeed, A. M., and Risser, D. R., An outbreak of tuberculosis in a shelter for homeless men, *Am. Rev. Respir. Dis.*, 143, 257, 1991.

222. Riley R. L. and Nardell, E. A., Clearing the air: the theory and application of ultraviolet air disinfection, *Am. Rev. Respir. Dis.*, 139, 1286, 1989.

223. Blower, S. M., Small, P. M., and Hopewell, P. C., Control strategies for tuberculosis epidemics: new models for old problems, *Science*, 273, 497, 1996.

224. Brewer, T. F., Heymann, S. J., Colditz, G. A., Wilson, M. E., Auerbach, K., Kane, D., and Fineberg, H. V., Evaluation of tuberculosis control policies using computer simulation, *JAMA*, 276, 1898, 1996.

225. Murray, J. L. and Salomon, J. A., Modeling the impact of global tuberculosis control strategies, *Proc. Natl. Acad. Sci.*, 95, 13881, 1998.

226. Garcia, A., Maccario, J., and Richardson, S., Modelling the annual risk of tuberculosis infection, *Int. J. Epidemiol.*, 26, 190, 1997.

227. Salpeter, E. E. and Salpeter, S. R., Mathematical model for the epidemiology of tuberculosis, with estimates of the reproductive number and infection-delay function, *Am. J. Epidemiol.*, 142, 398, 1998.

228. Blower, S. M. and Gerberding, J. L., Understanding, predicting and controlling the emergence of drug-resistant tuberculosis: a theoretical framework, *J. Mol. Med.*, 76, 624, 1998.

229. Miller, B. and Castro, K. G., Sharpen available tools for tuberculosis control, but new tools needed for elimination, *JAMA*, 276, 1916, 1996.

230. Reichman, L., The U-shaped curve of concern, *Am. Rev. Respir. Dis.*, 144, 741, 1991.

15 BCG Vaccine

Robin E. Huebner, Ph.D., M.P.H. and
George W. Comstock, M.D., Dr.P.H., F.A.C.E.

CONTENTS

I. THE HISTORY OF BCG

The discovery of *Mycobacterium tuberculosis* by Robert Koch in 1882 laid the foundation for a rational search for effective means to treat and prevent tuberculosis, a disease which at that time was the leading cause of death in much of the western world. Much research focused on the development of a vaccine; the approaches included the use of sterilized tuberculous tissue, the vaccination of cattle with human *M. tuberculosis* strains to which they were believed to be resistant, as well as the search for low virulence strains of mycobacteria.[1] In 1891 Edward Trudeau successfully attenuated a strain of *M. tuberculosis* isolated from a patient who had fatal miliary disease by inoculating the strain into a rabbit and then repeatedly subculturing the reisolated organisms on solid media.[2] While the use of these attenuated bacilli as a potential vaccine was never explored, the technique of subculturing eventually proved successful for Albert Calmette and Camille Guérin.

The history of what is known today as the bacillus of Calmette and Guérin (BCG) begins in 1908 when Calmette and Guérin began their work with "lait Nocard," a virulent bovine strain of *M. tuberculosis* isolated by Nocard from a cow that had tuberculous mastitis. The French investigators observed that the addition of bile, a natural detergent, to the laboratory media to prevent clumping of the organisms appeared also to result in attenuation in virulence. Calmette and Guérin began subculturing the organism every 3 weeks on a glycerinated beef-bile-potato medium. In 1921, after 13 years and 230 subcultures, BCG had lost its virulence for animals. Skepticism prompted attempts to restore the virulence of the now predominantly rough colony types by selecting the smooth colony types that were indicative of the original, virulent strain. These attempts proved unsuccessful.[1-3]

The original strain of BCG maintained at the Pasteur Institute in Lille, France, produced hundreds of "daughter" strains and is the progenitor of the most commonly used vaccines, the Copenhagen strain, originating in 1931 as the 423rd transfer; the Tokyo strain, sent from France as a seed culture in 1925; and the Glaxo strain, derived from the 1077th transfer of the Copenhagen strain.[4]

II. VACCINE PRODUCTION AND STANDARDIZATION

Early BCG strains, maintained as freshly prepared cultures, were propagated in hundreds of laboratories using culture methods routine to the particular laboratory. Most laboratories maintained the organisms through serial passage on potato-bile or potato-Sauton media. This method of cultivation continued into the 1960s, when such repeated subculturing was discovered to have resulted in BCG strains that differed markedly from each other. Heterogeneous *in vitro* characteristics such as colony morphology (spreading vs. nonspreading), viability on culture medium,[5] biochemical composition and activity,[6-8] drug resistance,[9] immunogenicity in animals and humans[5,10,11] and virulence in animals[12] have been found among currently available vaccines. In 1950, the World Health Organization (WHO), in an effort to limit the genetic variability among strains of BCG, issued the first in a series of recommendations for BCG production. Since 1960 the availability of lyophilized vaccine has allowed laboratories worldwide to produce seed lots, or quantities of bacteria that are processed together and are of uniform composition, to inoculate working vaccine cultures. The homogeneity of the vaccine strain can be maintained by the use of organisms that are no more than four generations from the primary seed lot.[13,14] In 1982 the responsibility for the international quality control of BCG vaccines was given to the Statens Seruminstitut in Copenhagen, Denmark. The Statens Seruminstitut provides training in vaccine production, distributes reference and seed lots, and oversees the standardization of BCG strains. Three parent strains (Glaxo, Tokyo, and Pasteur) now account for more than 90% of the vaccines used worldwide. The Pasteur strain of BCG currently serves as the international reference strain of vaccine.[15]

While no *in vitro* test has been found to correlate with protection in humans, factors such as the dose of BCG and the proportion of viable bacilli to nonviable bacilli in the preparation are thought to be important factors in the efficacy of the vaccine.[13] The WHO recommends that in addition to ensuring the absence of viable virulent mycobacteria in the preparation, quality control tests for BCG strains include measurements of the total bacterial content (dry weight), the number of viable organisms in the vaccine, the heat stability of the vaccine after incubation for 28 days at 37°C, and the ability of the vaccine to produce tuberculin sensitivity in guinea pigs.[14,15]

In the U.S., production standards for BCG vaccines set by the Food and Drug Administration, specify that they be freeze-dried preparations of live bacilli from a primary or secondary seed lot of a BCG strain identified by complete historical records. The manufacturer must provide estimates of the total bacillary mass by opacity and dry weight, viability as determined by oxygen uptake, germination rate or colony counts, and heat stability. Production lots must be incapable of producing progressive tuberculosis in guinea pigs and must be tested for potency by determination of the number of colony-forming units and by placement of the intradermal guinea pig test (Jensen's test). In addition, the vaccine must induce tuberculin reactivity in guinea pigs and in 90% of previously tuberculin-nonreactive persons.[16]

III. MECHANISM OF PROTECTIVE IMMUNITY

Immunity to tuberculosis and the mechanism of action of BCG have been investigated in different animal models using different species of animals, as well as varying routes of vaccination and challenge. An estimated 19,683 vaccine test systems are available for evaluating BCG and the events leading to protective immunity.[17] Early work examining the role of humoral immunity showed that although rabbits immunized with BCG were protected against challenge with virulent

M. bovis, the passive transfer of sera from such animals did not confer protection to *M. bovis*-naive rabbits.[17] That the induction of cell-mediated immunity results in protection against tuberculosis was demonstrated by experiments in which decreased numbers of mycobacteria were recovered from the lungs and spleens of *M. tuberculosis*-challenged mice given T-lymphocytes from BCG-vaccinated animals.[18]

Thus, BCG may be useful as a vaccine because it is able to elicit protective cell-mediated immune responses in the absence of progressive disease. Where in the chain of events following exposure to *M. tuberculosis* does BCG interfere? Levy et al.[19] demonstrated that the BCG vaccination of mice did not prevent infection or the establishment of primary foci. These findings were confirmed by Smith et al. who found that the number of organisms recovered from the lungs, spleens, and lymph nodes of vaccinated guinea pigs was not significantly different from those isolated from unvaccinated animals until 14 days post challenge.[20] Vaccinated animals showed fewer organisms in the spleen and no evidence of dissemination of bacilli to lobes of the lungs not infected at the time of challenge. These data suggest that vaccination with BCG does not protect against infection itself, but rather against uncontrolled replication and dissemination of *M. tuberculosis* from the primary foci to other parts of the lung and body.

IV. ROUTES AND METHODS OF VACCINE ADMINISTRATION

The first child immunized with BCG in July 1921 was a newborn whose grandmother had tuberculosis. Since then more than 1 billion children in more than 182 countries throughout the world have been vaccinated with BCG. The original BCG strain was given as an oral vaccine to newborns within the first 10 days of life. The oral route of vaccine administration was soon abandoned, however, as most of the infants failed to show tuberculin skin test conversions, which were thought to correlate with the development of protective immunity. The misconception that the bacilli could not penetrate the intestinal mucosa in older children and adults limited vaccination to infants. In addition, higher doses of the vaccine were required for oral immunization, causing an unacceptably high incidence of cervical lymphadenitis and damaging middle ear infections. Administration of the vaccine by the subcutaneous method produced large abscesses; therefore, the intradermal method was chosen as the best technique for BCG vaccination as it resulted in only superficial abscesses.[21] Currently, the vaccine is most commonly administered by the intradermal method with 0.1 ml of the vaccine delivered into the upper layers of the skin through a 27-gauge syringe.

A second method used to administer BCG is percutaneous scarification or multiple puncture. This technique involves placing several drops of the vaccine on the arm and then introducing the vaccine into the skin through multiple small needles on the puncture device. Though simpler and faster than the intradermal method, this procedure requires a stronger concentration of vaccine. Furthermore, because of the nature of the technique, it is impossible to determine the actual dose of the vaccine administered.[21]

Regardless of the method of administration, vaccination causes a host immune response and eventual scar formation. With the intradermal method, an indurated papule forms within 2 to 3 weeks of BCG administration. A pustule develops by 6 to 8 weeks and heals in 3 months, leaving a scar at the vaccination site.[22] With the multiple puncture technique, 2- to 3-mm papules develop within 2 weeks and begin to subside by 6 weeks after vaccination. After 3 to 4 months the lesions disappear, leaving only discoloration of the skin or slight pitting.[21]

V. TUBERCULIN REACTIVITY AFTER VACCINATION

Tuberculin reactivity develops after vaccination with BCG. Sensitivity appears as early as 10 days after vaccination; maximal responses develop after 6 to 12 weeks.[23] The size of the reaction depends on a number of factors related both to the vaccine and the host. Edwards and Gelting found that a progressive decrease in the number of viable bacilli in the vaccine resulted in a quantitative decrease in the postvaccination allergy.[24] A 1:2 dilution of vaccine reduced the average tuberculin reaction size by approximately 1 mm[25] while higher concentrations of vaccine increased the number of tuberculin reactors following vaccination.[26] One study using the Copenhagen 1331 strain found that a 10-fold increase in the dose of the vaccine reduced by 75% the number of children with negligible tuberculin reactivity 12 weeks after vaccination.[27]

Host factors also influence tuberculin reactivity after vaccination with BCG. Familial similarities influence the degree of postvaccination sensitivity in children.[28] Age at vaccination may be important in determining subsequent tuberculin reactivity. In some studies, infants who weighed less than the third percentile for their gestational age showed poor tuberculin conversions if vaccinated at birth,[29] while in other studies rates of conversion were similar for preterm infants and infants whose weight was appropriate for their gestational age.[30] Of Canadian infants vaccinated at 3 months of age, 33% developed sensitivity to tuberculin after vaccination. Only 14% of those vaccinated at birth developed tuberculin sensitivity.[31] These results agree with *in vitro* lymphocyte studies in Cree Indian children, which showed greater responses in lymphocytes from children vaccinated after 9 months of age than in those from children vaccinated at an earlier age.[32] Malnutrition also has been found to influence tuberculin reactivity after vaccination.[33]

Postvaccination sensitivity in BCG-vaccinated children ranges in size from 3 to 19 mm; this reactivity wanes with time. One study of Danish schoolchildren found that initially small postvaccination tuberculin reactions decreased by 1 to 2 mm after 5 years. In contrast, initial reaction sizes of 10 mm or greater remained unchanged over the same time period.[34] In Sri Lanka, BCG-induced sensitivity waned after 5 to 7 years.[35] Sixty-five percent of Navy recruits in the U.S. showed decreases in tuberculin reactivity within 8 to 15 years after vaccination.[36] Finally, in a study in Chicago, more than 90% of vaccinated infants were tuberculin reactive by 3 months after vaccination; the prevalence of tuberculin reactivity declined rapidly by 18 months after vaccination.[37]

Repeated tuberculin skin testing may prolong sensitivity in BCG-vaccinated persons. BCG-vaccinated children in Denmark who were tuberculin skin tested within 5 years of vaccination had significantly larger tuberculin reactions than those BCG-vaccinated children who had never been skin tested during the 5-year interval.[38] Young and Mirdad found the prevalence of 5 mm or greater induration in Canadian Indian children aged 1 to 15 years to increase with the number of documented Mantoux tests.[39] Repeated tuberculin testing also can increase the reaction size of skin tests in vaccinated persons (the booster effect, see also Chapter 13). After repeated skin testing, an increase of 6 mm or greater induration was noted in 13% of children attending day-care centers in South Africa.[40] Finally, revaccination with BCG also can increase the size of tuberculin reactions.[41]

After BCG vaccination, it is not possible on an individual basis to distinguish between a tuberculin skin test reaction caused by virulent mycobacterial infection or by vaccination itself. When interpreting skin tests, several factors increase the probability that a reaction was caused by virulent mycobacterial infection: large reaction size, a history of close contact with a person with active tuberculosis, residence in an area with a high prevalence of tuberculosis, and a long-time interval since vaccination.[42] For more information on this matter, refer to Chapter 13.

Although tuberculin sensitivity occurs after BCG vaccination, there is poor correlation between tuberculin reactivity and protection against active tuberculosis.[43] Some studies have shown that high tuberculin conversion rates correlate with little protective efficacy, while other studies with low conversion rates have found good protection after vaccination.[43,44] Nevertheless, in most developed countries where BCG is used, children are revaccinated if their tuberculin skin test reactions fail to convert to positive within 2 to 3 months of vaccination.

VI. SAFETY OF BCG VACCINE

The safety of early BCG vaccines was questioned in 1930 when active tuberculosis developed in 72 of 251 children given oral vaccination during a mass vaccination program in Lubeck, Germany.

All 72 children died.[45] Investigations into the tragedy later showed that a culture of virulent *M. tuberculosis* had been mistaken for the BCG strain, which had been kept in the same incubator. The directors and others in the laboratory were subsequently tried and convicted of negligence and malpractice.

Today, BCG is considered to be one of the safer vaccines available. The most frequent side effects after BCG vaccination are regional suppurative adenitis and osteitis.

A. REGIONAL LYMPHADENITIS

In a review of literature published between 1921 and 1982, Lotte et al.[46] found 6000 reported cases of regional lymphadenitis. The majority occurred within the first 5 months after vaccination. *M. bovis* BCG was cultured from 7% of the lesions. For those vaccinated, the risk of lymphadenitis ranged from 0.0006 per 1000 to 38 per 1000. In 1983, a prospective survey of 2 million infants vaccinated between 1979 and 1981 in six European countries (Denmark, German Democratic Republic, Hungary, Romania, and four areas within Croatia and the Federal Republic of Germany) found the risk of lymphadenitis to be 0.025 per 1000.[47]

Several factors contribute to the occurrence of regional lymphadenitis: the vaccine strain, the total number of viable and nonviable bacilli in the vaccine preparation, and the dose of BCG given. The age of the persons vaccinated also is important; for newborns the risk of lymphadenitis is 5 to 10 times greater than for preschool and school-age children.[47] Outbreaks of lymphadenitis associated with the use of the Pasteur vaccine in Africa and the Caribbean prompted the 1988 revision of the recommended dosages to be used in newborns and older children. Newborns and infants younger than 1 year old should receive 0.05 ml of vaccine; 0.1 ml is recommended for older children. The technical skill of the personnel who gave the intradermal vaccinations also was implicated in one outbreak in Zimbabwe.[48]

Opinions differ on the treatment of BCG adenitis; options range from administering no treatment to providing antibiotic chemotherapy to surgically excising the nodes. Data on the efficacy of treatment are not available from statistically proven and controlled studies; however, one prospective study compared antibiotic treatment to no active treatment.[49] No significant differences in the incidence of spontaneous drainage and suppuration were found between any of the groups. In those individuals receiving no treatment, the early onset of lymphadenitis was more likely to cause drainage and suppuration than were lesions that developed more slowly; these differences were not seen in the group receiving antibiotic treatment. While the authors concluded that medical therapy may have some beneficial effect if given to those in whom lymphadenitis develops rapidly after vaccination, there is no consensus in the medical community about what treatment is appropriate.

B. OSTEITIS

As with regional lymphadenitis, the risk of developing osteitis after BCG vaccination varies from country to country. Between 1948 and 1974, 291 cases of disseminated BCG involving lesions of the musculoskeletal system were reported from 13 countries.[47] Japan showed the lowest risk (0.1 per 100,000); Sweden and Finland showed the highest risks (325 and 434 per 100,000, respectively). A more recent review of medical records covering the years 1976 to 1995 in metropolitan Santiago, Chile, where BCG coverage is 97%, found 10 children with either culture- or histologically confirmed osteitis, for an estimated incidence of 3.2 per 100,000.[50]

The problem of BCG osteitis has been extensively investigated in Sweden where the incidence increased significantly from 1 per 100,000 to 2.5 per 100,000 in the years 1950 to 1969 to an annual rate of 25 per 100,000 to 33 per 100,000 between 1972 and 1975.[51] Osteitis developed within 4 to 144 months of vaccination; most cases occurred within 7 to 24 months. The most frequent site affected was the epiphysis of the long bones, particularly in the legs. Similar results were seen in Finland.[52] Explanations for the increases in BCG osteitis in both countries remain unclear, although cases appeared to coincide with a change in vaccine production. The Gothenburg strain, prepared in Sweden, had been used in both countries; in 1971, vaccine production was transferred to the Statens Seruminstitut in Copenhagen. Other countries also have experienced increases in BCG osteitis after changes in either the vaccine strain or the method of production.[15] In addition to the change in the vaccine manufacturer, the compulsory notification of BCG reactions to the Swedish Adverse Drug Reaction Committee, mandated in 1972, and the dissemination of information concerning the untoward reactions most likely prompted the expanded surveillance and reporting of cases of osteitis in both countries. As a result of these findings, Sweden discontinued the routine vaccination of neonates in 1975. Finland continued immunization using the Glaxo strain of vaccine.

Antituberculosis therapy, coupled in some cases with surgical curettage and debridement, usually results in healing of the skeletal lesions.

C. Disseminated Fatal BCG Disease

The most serious complication of BCG vaccination is disseminated BCG disease. Although rare, "BCGitis" can be fatal. Hematogenous dissemination of the bacilli after vaccination has been demonstrated. In most persons, the spread of the organisms is relatively benign and does not cause overt disease; however, at least 35 fatalities were reported between 1948 and 1972. BCGitis is seen most frequently in children with concomitant immunodeficiencies, such as severe combined immunodeficiency syndrome or chronic granulomatous disease. In only a few cases does disease develop in the presence of an intact immune system. Recently Tardieu et al. reported two cases of culture-confirmed BCG meningitis in immunocompetent children immunized 1.5 to 5 years previously.[53]

Although most cases of BCGitis occur within the first 6 months after vaccination, longer latent periods have been noted. In one instance, culture-confirmed BCG disease with widespread lymph node, liver, bone, and lung involvement developed in an 18-year-old boy 6 years after vaccination.[54] The patient was subsequently found to have several immunological defects, including abnormal macrophage and T-lymphocyte functions. The patient died despite prolonged antimycobacterial treatment.

Treatment for disseminated BCG disease is similar to the treatment for active tuberculosis with one exception; pyrazinamide is not used to treat BCGitis because all BCG strains are resistant to this antibiotic. Even when treated with potentially effective chemotherapeutic agents, many cases of disseminated BCG are fatal, particularly if the patient has underlying immunosuppression (for BCG vaccination in HIV-positive individuals, refer to Section X).

VII. VACCINE EFFICACY

We will consider 17 controlled trials of the efficacy of BCG vaccine in humans and one controlled trial of revaccination.[55-71,80] These trials are summarized in Table 15.1; the eight major trials are described in detail.

The first large-field trial of BCG efficacy began in 1935 among eight Native American Indian tribes.[59] The efficacy of a vaccine prepared by the Henry Phipps Institute of Philadelphia was evaluated in tuberculin-negative children and adolescents aged 0 to 20 years. The duration of follow-up was 9 to 11 years for the development of active tuberculosis; tuberculosis mortality was assessed after 20 years. Roentgenographic evidence of pulmonary tuberculosis was found in 238 of the 1457 unvaccinated persons; 64 of the 1551 given BCG vaccination developed active tuberculosis. The protective efficacy against active tuberculosis was 75%. There was an 82% reduction in deaths resulting from tuberculosis.

In their study of high-risk infants in Chicago, Rosenthal and colleagues[60] also found that BCG conferred a high degree of protection. Between 1937 and 1948, 3381 children born at Cook County Hospital were randomly assigned to receive either the Tice strain of BCG or to remain unvaccinated.

TABLE 15.1
Controlled Trials of BCG Efficacy Against Tuberculosis

Population	Vaccine	Year	Years of Follow-up	Percent Reduction		
				Cases	Deaths	Ref.
237 infants — Philadelphia	King	1927	3–4	—	83	55
1092 infant contacts — New York	IC	1933	5–11	—	8	56
609 newborns — Saskatchewan	Frappier	1933	15	81	80	57
41,301 newborns — Algiers	Oral	1935	1–11	—	11	58
3008 Native American children — U.S.	Phipps	1936	9–11	75	82	59
3381 newborns — Chicago	Tice	1937	12–23	75	83	60
262 Native American newborns — U.S.	Phipps	1938	6–8	59	100	61
451 newborn contacts — Chicago	Tice	1941	19	74	100	62
4839 children — Georgia	Tice	1947	20	–57	—	63
1025 children — Illinois	Tice	1947	13	–40	–88	64
77,972 children — Puerto Rico	Birkhaug	1949	18–20	29	38	65
34,767 adults — Georgia, Alabama	Tice	1950	20	6	—	66
21,000 villagers — Madanapalle	Danish	1950	16–21	20	—	67
27,400 adolescents — England	Danish	1950	18–20	77	—	68
16,314 miners — South Africa	Glaxo	1965	3	38	—	69
2,174 villagers — Haiti	Frappier	1965	3	67	—	70
260,000 villagers — Chingleput	Danish French	1968	15	–2	—	71
54,865 villagers — Malawi	Glaxo	1986	5–9	–4	—	80

Source: Revised from Friedman, L. N., Ed., *Tuberculosis: Current Concepts and Treatment,* 1st ed., CRC Press LLC, Boca Raton, FL, 1994.

The length of follow-up ranged from 12 to 23 years; during this time, 59 cases of tuberculosis occurred in the 1665 unvaccinated persons while only 16 of 1716 vaccinated individuals developed evidence of active disease (efficacy = 75%).

The Medical Research Council of Great Britain (MRC) conducted a large controlled trial of the Copenhagen strain of vaccine.[68] Between 1950 and 1952, a total of 14,100 tuberculin-negative schoolchildren between the ages of 14 and 16 were vaccinated; 13,300 children were randomized to the unvaccinated control group. The protective efficacy of the vaccine was 84% during the first 5 years of the study. By 15 years after vaccination, 243 cases of tuberculosis had developed in the unvaccinated group, compared with only 56 cases in those who had received BCG (efficacy = 77%). The prevalence and incidence of tuberculosis in Great Britain decreased significantly during the study period. The number of cases in the unvaccinated control group was so small during the 15 through 19 year follow-up that the trial was discontinued.

The growing support for BCG vaccination by WHO and the belief that preventive measures could significantly contribute to the control of tuberculosis prompted the U.S. Public Health Service to sponsor a series of controlled trials examining the efficacy of BCG. The first study began in 1947. A total of 2948 tuberculin-negative schoolchildren in Muscogee County, GA, were vaccinated with the Tice strain of vaccine; 2341 tuberculin-negative children were left unvaccinated.[63] Allocation to vaccine group was done by even or odd year of birth. Eight cases of tuberculosis developed during the 20-year study period; three cases occurred in unvaccinated persons and five occurred in those given BCG. No protective efficacy was detected in this study.

When it became clear that the incidence of tuberculosis in schoolchildren in Muscogee County was not as high as originally expected, a second study was begun in adults in the county as well as in the neighboring Russell County, AL.[66] The 20-year evaluation, published in 1976, again found no protection after vaccination with BCG; equal numbers of cases were found in the vaccinated and control groups.

A 29% reduction in tuberculosis incidence was observed in another U.S Public Health Service-sponsored study of Puerto Rican children aged 1 to 18 years who were given a vaccine prepared by the New York State Department of Health (Birkhaug strain).[65]

Finally, a study in a rural population in southern India found a 60% reduction in the incidence of tuberculosis in the vaccinated group as compared with the unvaccinated group 7 years after vaccination.[67] By 20 years after vaccination, the vaccine efficacy had declined to 20%.

The variable results of the published trials of BCG efficacy and the concern that the vaccines used in previous studies were so heterogeneous that they might not be of uniform potency prompted what became the largest controlled community trial ever designed to examine the efficacy of BCG vaccine. The trial, cosponsored by the Indian Council of Medical Research, WHO, and the U.S. Public Health Service, began in 1968. During the course of 3 years, 265,172 villagers older than 1 month of age and living in the Chingleput district near Madras were enrolled in the study.[71] Participants were randomized to receive either a low or high dose of the French or Danish vaccine or dextran placebo without regard to tuberculin sensitivity or radiographic findings. These two vaccines were selected for the study as they had demonstrated the best test activity in animal models and were available as freeze-dried preparations. Follow-up data were analyzed according to the degree of initial skin test sensitivity. During the 15-year follow-up period, 533 cases of pulmonary tuberculosis developed in those persons with less than 7 mm induration to tuberculin at enrollment; the number of cases was divided evenly among those receiving the placebo or the low or high doses of vaccine. Vaccination did provide some protection (17%) against pulmonary tuberculosis in children aged 0 to 14 years; adult vaccinees had more tuberculosis than the unvaccinated controls.

An additional finding of the Chingleput trial has gone unnoticed. For several decades, it had been standard practice to vaccinate without a prior tuberculin test; the purpose of the tuberculin test would have been to exclude persons already infected with *M. tuberculosis*. However, the safety of this procedure was established largely by casual and anecdotal evidence that vaccination reactions among positive tuberculin reactors did not seem sufficiently severe to contraindicate direct vaccination. The follow-up of the Chingleput trial established for the first time that BCG vaccine could be given to positively reacting children, to adults with abnormal chest radiographs, and even to persons with sputum positive for *M. tuberculosis* without demonstrable harm.[72]

Rather than resolving the issue of the efficacy of BCG, the Chingleput study brought forward even more questions about the usefulness of vaccination. The lack of protective efficacy observed in the study disappointed the public health community and forced a reevaluation of the WHO policy on the use of BCG in developing countries. Other than the two southern India trials,[67,71] none of the controlled studies were conducted in Africa or Asia, areas of the world where the incidence and prevalence of tuberculosis are highest and where BCG vaccination might be of greatest value. Another randomized, placebo-controlled trial of the efficacy of BCG would not be economically or logistically feasible and would require many years of follow-up to reach a statistically valid endpoint. In an effort to gain information on the impact of BCG on the tuberculosis burden in developing countries, WHO sponsored several case-control studies of BCG vaccination. The studies, conducted in Brazil, Burma, Sri Lanka, and Argentina, concentrated on childhood tuberculosis and used a variety of control populations, such as patients hospitalized for diseases other than tuberculosis and neighbors or siblings of tuberculosis patients.[73] As in the previous controlled prospective trials, the results varied widely: the effectiveness of the vaccination programs ranged from 2 to 84%. Protection conferred by vaccination was highest against disseminated forms of tuberculosis, such as meningitis. In recent years, numerous other case-control investigations have found similarly variable results.[74-77] Again, the majority of studies have focused on vaccine effectiveness in children and have found protection ranging from 16 to 80%. A small number of cohort studies of children who were contacts of persons with newly diagnosed, culture-confirmed tuberculosis had been funded through WHO. In these studies, the incidence of tuberculosis decreased by 53 to 66% in children who were given BCG prior to exposure to tuberculosis, compared to those who were not vaccinated with BCG.[78,79]

A more recent study conducted in northern Malawi involved revaccination of 54,865 individuals with BCG scars.[80] While repeated vaccination decreased the incidence of leprosy by 50%, no protection was seen against pulmonary tuberculosis.

In 1992, Colditz and colleagues reviewed the available published literature and databases and performed a quantitative meta-analysis of the efficacy of BCG vaccines in preventing tuberculosis.[81] Studies were included if there was a vaccinated and a concurrent control group. A total of 15 trials were included. The relative risks of developing or dying from tuberculosis associated with vaccination varied from a low of 0.16 to a high of 1.56. The overall average risk of developing tuberculosis was 0.49 among the vaccinated groups compared to the reference value of 1.00 among the controls. Although stricter methods of allocation to the two groups (as judged by the reviewers), young age at vaccination, and higher incidence of active tuberculosis, all were associated with greater protection from vaccination, these characteristics also were related to the distance of the study areas from the equator. There is evidence that the association with geographic location is due to the frequency of nontuberculous mycobacterial infections which have been found to preempt some of the protection afforded by BCG.[82a] A thorough review of the problems of the various controlled trials and how these relate to the interpretation of the conflicting findings also has been published recently.[82b]

The trend in efficacy of vaccination with time after vaccination also has been reviewed in 10 controlled trials.[83] The average annual efficacy decreased in seven trials by an average of 8% per year. Only one trial continued to show good efficacy throughout a period of 18 years after vaccination.[59]

Compilation of global data on BCG using meta-analyses can provide insight into the true efficacy of the vaccine; however, application of population-based data to individuals may be problematic. For example, while the vaccine may protect 50% of a group of vaccinated persons from developing tuberculosis, vaccination may not reduce an individual's risk of developing the disease by 50%. Caution should, therefore, be taken when applying the results of meta-analyses to public health practice.

VIII. EXPLANATIONS FOR VARIABILITY IN EFFICACY

Several hypotheses have been put forward to explain the variability in results of field trials with BCG. These hypotheses have been reviewed by Fine.[84] One hypothesis is that prior infection with nontuberculous mycobacteria could confer some protection against active tuberculosis. Natural infection with these mycobacteria could mask the effects of BCG vaccination by decreasing the susceptibility of the unvaccinated control group, thereby diluting the protective effects in the vaccinated groups. Indeed, studies in both animals and humans have found that infection with environmental mycobacteria can increase immunity to tuberculosis.[82] This hypothesis is supported by the fact that the trials showing the lowest BCG efficacy were in areas such as the southeastern U.S. where infection with the nontuberculous mycobacteria is common. However, data from studies in Puerto Rico showed no difference in protection after vaccination of persons who reacted only to a large dose (10 tuberculin units) of tuberculin, indicative of infection with nontuberculous mycobacteria.[65] In addition, two trials in the U.S. that excluded reactors to the large dose of tuberculin, showed the worst efficacy estimates of all of the trials.

There have been continued suggestions that the efficacy of BCG vaccination may be either enhanced or opposed by previous infection with environmental mycobacteria. Two types of cell-mediated immune responses may occur as a result of mycobacterial infection.[85] The first is the so-called "Koch phenomenon" which, in animals, develops 4 to 6 weeks after infection with *M. tuberculosis* and causes necrosis at the site of tuberculin skin testing. The second, described by Mackaness as a listeria-type response, occurs within days of infection, correlates with the appearance of macrophage-activating T-lymphocytes, and does not produce necrosis upon skin testing. Different species of mycobacteria have been demonstrated in animal models to produce varying levels of these two immune responses. Rook and his colleagues[85] have postulated that prior infection with *M. vaccae* or any of the nontuberculous mycobacteria that produce the listeria-type response may enhance the protective effect of subsequent vaccination with BCG. In contrast, infection with *M. scrofulaceum* or those organisms that induce the Koch phenomenon may not only inhibit the development of protective immunity following BCG but actually increase susceptibility to disease from *M. tuberculosis*. It is unlikely, however, that exposure to nontuberculous mycobacteria accounts for all of the observed variability in the efficacy of BCG.

Differences in the potency and immunogenicity of individual vaccine strains also may contribute to the variability in the efficacy of BCG. No animal model has been found to predict the efficacy of vaccination in humans; therefore, protection can only be assessed in field trials in humans. While microbiological differences between the vaccine strains do exist, studies using the same vaccines in different settings have shown both similar and varying efficacies, as have studies using different vaccines in the same setting.[84] Brewer and Colditz, in a review of the BCG efficacy data for different BCG strains, also found little evidence to suggest that the strain used for vaccination was a significant factor in the overall protective effect against tuberculosis.[86]

The efficacy of BCG is believed by some to be influenced by differences in the risk of infection of the study populations, differences in the virulence of *M. tuberculosis* isolates, or differences in the pathogenesis of disease. Some *M. tuberculosis* isolates from the Chingleput area have been found to be of low virulence for guinea pigs. One hypothesis is that BCG may not be able to protect against these "South Indian variants." This hypothesis has not been supported by laboratory data, which show that protection may be influenced by the virulence of the challenge strain of *M. tuberculosis*, but do not show evidence of poor protection against low-virulence South Indian variants.[87]

Host genetics also may play a role in the efficacy of BCG. The immune response to BCG in mice has been found to be regulated by a gene on chromosome 1; this gene also has been found on chromosome 2 in man.[88] However, no statistically significant differences in the efficacy of BCG have been found between racial groups in field trials to suggest that genetic variability is an important factor in protection following vaccination.

Although chronic moderate dietary protein deficiency has been shown to impair the ability of BCG vaccine to protect guinea pigs against challenge with virulent *M. tuberculosis*,[89] data from human trials have failed to support nutrition as a cause of variability in BCG efficacy.

BCG has been shown in animal models to protect against dissemination of organisms from the primary site of infection. Therefore, the efficacy of BCG may depend on whether disease is due to endogenous reactivation or exogenous reinfection. In the latter, the progression to disease would depend on the new primary infection. Thus, in areas where the probability of reinfection is high, such as in southern India, the efficacy of BCG may be lower than in areas where reactivation disease predominates. This hypothesis is supported by data from the Chingleput trial, which showed a high risk of infection in the study area, but a low incidence of tuberculosis in the uninfected, a high incidence of tuberculosis in the infected population, and a long interval between tuberculin conversion and evidence of disease.[90] Data from the earlier trial in Puerto Rico would appear to contradict this hypothesis. The infection rate in Puerto Rico among children initially 1 to 3 years of age was approximately 2.5% per year. At the time of study recruitment, the area also had a high tuberculosis rate, and, in the study population, the uninfected had a relatively low tuberculosis rate, and those found infected had a relatively high rate. During the 20-year follow-up, the rate of infection decreased, yet the efficacy of BCG remained constant.[91]

Finally, the different study methodologies used in the controlled studies have been blamed for the variable study results. Differences in susceptibility to tuberculosis, follow-up surveillance, diagnostic testing and interpretation, and detection of active disease in the eight major controlled trials have been reviewed by Clemens and colleagues.[92]

It is likely that a combination of some or all of the above hypotheses have influenced the observed variation in the efficacy of BCG. As Fine says, "There is no simple global answer to the problem of BCG's efficacy."[84] Current technologies may provide the tools to unravel the mysteries of protective immunity to *M. tuberculosis* and the role of BCG vaccination.

IX. RECOMMENDATIONS FOR USE OF BCG IN THE CONTROL OF TUBERCULOSIS

Given the high incidence of tuberculosis in many developing countries and the inability to control the spread of infection through chemoprophylaxis and the prompt diagnosis and effective treatment of infectious cases, WHO continues to recommend the use of BCG vaccine on a worldwide basis. BCG vaccine is given as part of the WHO Expanded Programme on Immunization; the vaccine is administered to infants as soon as possible after birth.[93]

In the U.S., the general population is at low risk for acquiring tuberculous infection. In most population groups, prevention of tuberculosis is most reliably accomplished by periodic Mantoux testing with tuberculin for high-risk children and adults and with administration of preventive therapy to selected persons with positive tuberculin tests. Therefore, a BCG vaccination policy for the entire population is not indicated. The Advisory Council for the Elimination of Tuberculosis (ACET) and the Advisory Committee on Immunization Practices have recommended that BCG vaccination be considered only for children with negative tuberculin skin tests who cannot be placed on isoniazid-preventive therapy, but who have continuous exposure to persons with active tuberculosis, particularly isoniazid and rifampin-resistant disease.[94]

The nosocomial outbreaks of multidrug-resistant tuberculosis (MDR-TB) has prompted debate on the use of BCG vaccination for healthcare workers potentially exposed to infectious tuberculosis patients. The uncertain efficacy of BCG has made policy decisions concerning the immunization of groups at increased risk, such as healthcare workers, problematic. The acceptance of a vaccine that often causes chronic ulceration also is problematic. A total of eight studies on the efficacy of BCG vaccination in healthcare workers were reviewed for the meta-analysis by Colditz; however, methodological weaknesses in the studies prevented their inclusion in the analysis.[81] Although a quantitative measurement of efficacy was not possible, published studies suggest that BCG vaccine may reduce the incidence of tuberculosis in initially tuberculin-negative healthcare workers.[95]

Unlike chemoprophylaxis with isoniazid, multidrug preventive therapy regimens for infection with MDR-TB strains are of unproven efficacy, making the choice between vaccination with BCG and chemoprophylaxis even more unclear. A decision analysis using published data from North America and New York City compared the utility of BCG vaccination with chemoprophylaxis with ciprofloxacin and pyrazinamide, the recommended preventive therapy following infection with MDR-TB.[96] Vaccination was favored by a small margin over postinfection chemoprophylaxis for nonimmunocompromised healthcare workers as long as the efficacy of BCG was greater than 26%.

An additional concern over the widespread use of BCG for healthcare workers was the recognition that the vaccine would make the tuberculin test uninterpretable and would undermine public health surveillance measures to ascertain new infections with *M. tuberculosis* and to identify ongoing epidemics. While the controversy over BCG continued, implementation of infection control practices to reduce the transmission of tuberculosis in institutional settings, such as hospitals and jails, and the strengthening of basic tuberculosis control strategies to increase patient compliance and treatment completion resulted in a decline in MDR-TB cases in New York City from 12.6% in 1991 to 1992 to 8.6% in the following 2-year period.[97]

In 1997, new guidelines for the use of BCG vaccine in healthcare workers were published and recommended consideration of BCG vaccination of healthcare workers on an individual basis in situations where MDR-TB is prevalent and likely to be transmitted to healthcare staff in spite of the implementation of comprehensive tuberculosis infection control precautions.[98] Counseling of healthcare workers on the risks and benefits of both BCG vaccination and preventive therapy should be conducted prior to vaccination. The use of the BCG vaccine is not recommended for HIV-infected or otherwise immunocompromised persons; reassignment to work areas and activities with the lowest risk for infection with *M. tuberculosis* is preferable.

X. BCG AND THE HUMAN IMMUNODEFICIENCY VIRUS (HIV)

Infection with HIV is known to be the greatest risk factor for the development of active tuberculosis. In developing countries, tuberculosis is one of the most frequent opportunistic infections in HIV-infected persons.[99] WHO has recommended BCG vaccination as part of the Expanded Programme on Immunization; however, there now is concern that many children in developing countries may be infected with HIV. For example, more than 6% of AIDS cases and more than 3% of HIV infections in Uganda occurred in children.[100] These children may face an increased risk of disseminated BCG disease after vaccination. Initial reports from Africa suggested that a higher risk of regional lymphadenitis and local abscesses occurred in HIV-infected children after BCG administration. In Zaire an outbreak of local abscesses occurred in 19 children; however, all of the children were found to be HIV seronegative, and the outbreak was attributed later to a change in the manufacturer of the vaccine.[101] Another study in Zaire found that lymphadenitis was 1.8 times as common and fistulas 2 times as common in HIV-infected children as in uninfected children.[102] A relatively high rate (10%) of post-BCG adenopathies was seen among 105 HIV-infected children, although in this study no uninfected children were included as controls.[103]

Two prospective studies of infants at risk for perinatal HIV infection found no increase in untoward reactions to BCG vaccination. Lallemant-La Coeur et al. observed 64 children born to HIV-infected mothers and 130 control children born to HIV-seronegative mothers, looking for local and regional complications of vaccination during the first month of life.[104] After 40 months of follow-up, no significant differences in the risk of lymphadenitis were seen between the HIV-infected and uninfected children (24% vs. 18%, respectively). All the cases resolved spontaneously and there were no cases of disseminated BCG.

Another prospective study in Rwanda found 6 cases of suppuration at the injection site among 377 children vaccinated during the first week of life; 1 child was HIV-infected, 1 was born to an HIV-infected mother but was seronegative at 15 months of age, and 4 were born to HIV-uninfected mothers. No other untoward reactions were reported.[105]

Dissemination of BCG and subsequent disease have been seen in HIV-infected persons. *M. bovis* BCG was cultured from the lymph node and cerebrospinal fluid of an HIV-infected child presenting with fever, adenitis, and diarrhea 4 months after vaccination.[106] The symptoms improved after antituberculosis treatment.

Culture-proven dissemination also occurred in a native American child vaccinated at 3 months of age. Organisms were isolated from blood, gastric and tracheal aspirates, and the lung.[107] The vaccination site was crusted and oozing and the child had symptoms of AIDS.

Complications of BCG vaccination also have been reported in adults who had either prior or subsequent HIV infection. Ulceration at the injection site and regional lymphadenopathy developed 4 months after vaccination of one AIDS patient; *M. bovis*, BCG strain, was identified in lesion and blood samples from this patient.[108] BCG adenitis and disseminated disease can occur from months to years after vaccination;[109-111] cases were reported to have occurred in two persons 30 years after they were vaccinated with BCG.[112,113]

To date, there have been no controlled studies of the safety of BCG vaccination in adults infected with HIV nor of the efficacy of BCG in either HIV-infected adults or children. However, given the lack of data suggesting a harmful effect of BCG vaccination in HIV-infected children and the high risk this population faces of being infected with *M. tuberculosis* and developing disease, WHO recommends BCG vaccination for asymptomatic HIV-infected children who are at increased risk of tuberculous infection. The WHO does not recommend BCG vaccination for children or adults with symptomatic HIV infection, or for persons known or suspected to be infected with HIV, who have minimal risk of infection with *M. tuberculosis*.[114] The latter recommendation would apply to most populations in the U.S. for whom BCG might be considered.[94]

XI. DEVELOPMENT OF NEW VACCINES FOR TUBERCULOSIS

The explosion of new tuberculosis cases due to concomitant infection with HIV and the emergence of MDR-TB, have led to the implementation of new control strategies, such as directly observed treatment short-course (DOTS), and better application of already existing strategies for case finding, case management, and prevention of infection. In areas of the world hardest hit by this dual HIV-TB epidemic, adequate tuberculosis control programs are not in place due in large part to financial constraints. Nor has the continuing vaccination of millions of children had a measurable effect on the spreading epidemic. A new vaccine, as inexpensive as the current BCG vaccines, and more effective and long lasting, has the potential for great benefit.

The Advisory Council for the Elimination of Tuberculosis has identifed steps that are critical to the development and implementation of a new vaccine for tuberculosis.[115] First, a consensus must be reached among vaccine manufacturers that a new tuberculosis vaccine is an urgent public health priority, warranting long-term allocation of public and private sector funding. A comprehensive strategic plan for vaccine development, as well as collaboration between the U.S. government and international funding and licensing agencies, could then ensure the appropriate use of resources and the timely evaluation of candidate vaccines in clinical trials. Finally, basic research is needed to identify *in vivo* factors related to the host immune response to tuberculous infection and the development of disease so that correlates of protection can be identified to evaluate new vaccines. Such vaccines should be well-tolerated and safe for immunocompromised persons, should protect against new infection and reactivation of existing infection, and should not confer hypersensitivity to tuberculin, thus allowing identification of new infection in vaccinated persons.

Recent technological advances have led to new approaches for the development of vaccines against tuberculosis, and at least 56 new vaccine candidates and/or strategies already have been tested in guinea pig and mouse models.[116] These include DNA vaccines, immunogenic culture filtrate proteins, subunit vaccines, mutant BCG or *M. tuberculosis* vaccines, and avirulent nontuberculous mycobacteria.[117]

DNA vaccines can protect the host after insertion of the gene for a mycobacterial antigen into a plasmid, which, when injected into the host, causes RNA transcription and production of the foreign protein. Long-lasting and protective cellular and humoral immunity can be produced with relatively few side effects.[118] Mycobacterial genes for secreted proteins Ag85A and B, ESAT6, MPT64, and PstS have shown promising results in stimulating T cell production and reducing the bacterial load in the lungs of animals challenged with virulent *M. tuberculosis*.[117-122]

Culture filtrate proteins also are being examined. Guinea pigs develop tuberculin sensitivity when immunized subcutaneously with extracellular proteins that are released when *M. tuberculosis* replicates. They also show fewer viable bacilli in their lungs following aerosol challenge with *M. tuberculosis,* and can survive a normally lethal dose of *M. tuberculosis*.[123]

Identification of the proteins capable of inducing protection might lead to the development of a subunit vaccine. This idea is supported by data demonstrating the successful insertion of a sequence that encodes *M. tuberculosis* proteins into the vaccinia virus genome. Lyons et al.[124] found that vaccinia recombinants expressing *M. tuberculosis* proteins were able to induce antibody production when injected into mice. Immunodominant T cell antigens and the secreted protein antigen ESAT6 now are being screened for their ability to stimulate IFN-γ production in T cell lines as a surrogate for protective immunity.[125,126] Data evaluating these vaccines in animal models are forthcoming.

Auxotrophic BCG mutants, deficient in leucine production, are incapable of growing in macrophages, yet appear to persist long enough to stimulate some protective immunity in mice.[117] *M.*

tuberculosis H37Rv mutants unable to synthesize the Ag85A also show attenuated virulence but no corresponding lack of immunogenicity in mice.[127]

Lastly, a vaccine incorporating *M. vaccae*, the vole bacillus, has been evaluated as a replacement for BCG, particularly in persons infected with HIV.[128] A five-dose series of inactivated bacteria was found to be safe and well-tolerated in 22 HIV-positive Zambians, and it induced *in vitro* lymphocyte proliferation in response to *M. vaccae* sonicate.

Before a new vaccine can be recommended, it must be evaluated in human trials. Unfortunately, in the past, most prospective studies have been very large, very expensive, and have required long observational periods. The infrastructure needed to conduct a randomized, placebo-controlled vaccine efficacy trial in HIV-seronegative, PPD-negative persons would require 11,200 to 81,000 participants in developed countries that have an annual incidence greater than 100 cases per 100,000 population.[129] A total of 3800 to 29,100 persons would be necessary in developing countries with an incidence greater than 400 cases per 100,000 population. Observational studies, whether case-control or cohort, also will require huge numbers or long observation periods. There are, however, ways in which large numbers of persons can be followed at little expense. It has been suggested that children be randomly allocated at birth to receive either standard BCG or a new vaccine.[130] As new tuberculosis cases are detected, household contacts could be traced and vaccinated children evaluated for active disease. This study design would require vaccination of 240,000 children over a 5-year period and evaluation of 1360 pediatric contacts of active adult TB cases (680 per group). A limitation of this design is that it could only be used in countries with high vaccine coverage rates and a TB control program with the infrastructure for vaccine delivery and TB surveillance.

The simplest and least expensive comparative study could be performed at the present time in any country with a high case rate of tuberculosis and a reasonably complete system for reporting cases. One vaccine would be administered in odd years and another in even years to newborns. The comparison could be between a new vaccine and the one in previous use. However, even before a new vaccine is ready for general administration, a comparison of two existing vaccines would be helpful. If a difference in case rates among children born in even and odd years was found, these two strains could then be tested in various animal systems to ascertain which test system correlated best with efficacy in humans.[82a]

Correlates of immunity are essential when evaluating new vaccine candidates. Potentially protective antigens should be identified and the dose, administration, scheduling of immunization, and efficacy estimates of potential vaccines should be determined prior to testing in clinical trials.[131] Production of IFN-γ by *M. tuberculosis*-stimulated whole blood cells has been proposed as a surrogate for protective immunity.[131-133] Symptomatic pulmonary tuberculosis patients, however, produce high levels of IFN-γ, suggesting that IFN-γ production alone may not correlate with protection. Further work is necessary, such as assays that mimic cytotoxic T cell activity against *M. tuberculosis*.

REFERENCES

1. Grange, J. M., Gibson, J., and Osborn, T. W., What is BCG? *Tubercle*, 64, 129, 1983.
2. Gardner, L. V., The history of the R1 strain of tubercle bacillus, *Am. Rev. Tuberc.*, 25, 577, 1932.
3. Crispen, R., History of BCG and its substrains, in *BCG in Superficial Bladder Cancer*, EORTC Genitourinary Group Monograph 6, 35, 1989.
4. Osborn, T. W., Changes in BCG strains, *Tubercle*, 64, 1, 1983.
5. Gheorghiu, M. and LaGrange, P. H., Viability, heat stability and immunogenicity of four BCG vaccines prepared from four different BCG strains, *Ann. Immunol.*, 134C, 125, 1983.
6. Minnikin, D. E., Parlett, J. H., Magnusson, M., Ridell, M., and Lind, A., Mycolic acid patterns of representatives of *Mycobacterium bovis* BCG, *J. Gen. Microbiol.*, 130, 2733, 1984.

7. Abou-Zeid, C., Smith, I., Grange, J., Steele, J., and Rook, G., Subdivision of daughter strains of Bacille Calmette-Guérin (BCG) according to secreted protein patterns, *J. Gen. Microbiol.*, 132, 3047, 1986.

8. International Union Against Tuberculosis, Phenotypes of BCG-vaccines seed lot strains: results of an International Cooperative Study, *Tubercle*, 59, 139, 1978.

9. Hesselberg, I., Drug resistance in the Swedish/Norwegian BCG strain, *Bull. World Health. Org.*, 46, 503, 1972.

10. Grange, J. M. and Gibson, J. A., Strain to strain variation in the immunogenicity of BCG, *Develop. Biol. Stand.*, 58, 37, 1986.

11. Nyboe, J. and Bunch-Christensen, K., Assay in man of different BCG products, *Bull. World Health Org.*, 35, 645, 1966.

12. Jespersen, A., The Potency of BCG Vaccines Determined on Animals, Ph.D. thesis, University of Copenhagen, 1971.

13. WHO Technical Report Series No. 8, *WHO-Sponsored International Quality Control of BCG Vaccine*, 1977.

14. WHO Expert Committee on Biological Standardization, *Requirements for dried BCG vaccine* (requirements for biological substances No. 11), 1985.

15. Milstien, J. B. and Gibson, J. J., Quality control of BCG vaccine by WHO: a review of factors that may influence vaccine effectiveness and safety, *Bull. World Health Org.*, 68, 93, 1990.

16. Federal Register, 50, 50159, 1985.

17. Smith, D. W., Protective effect of BCG in experimental tuberculosis, *Adv. Tuberc. Res.*, 22, 66, 1985.

18. Lefford, M.J., Induction and expression of immunity after BCG immunization, *Infect. Immun.*, 18, 646, 1977.

19. Levy, F. M., Conge, G. A., Pasquier, J. F., Mauss, H., Dubos, R., and Schaedler, R., The effect of BCG vaccination on the fate of virulent tubercle bacilli in mice, *Am. Rev. Respir. Dis.*, 84, 28, 1961.

20. Smith, D. W., McMurray, D. N., Wiegeshaus, E. H., Grover, A. A., and Harding, G. E., Host-parasite relationships in experimental tuberculosis. IV. Early events in the course of infection in vaccinated and nonvaccinated guinea pigs, *Am. Rev. Respir. Dis.*, 102, 937, 1970.

21. Rosenthal, S. R., Routes and methods of administration, in *BCG Vaccine: Tuberculosis — Cancer*, PSG Publishing Co., Littleton, MA, 1980, Chap. 11.

22. Myint, T. T., Yin, Y., Yi, M. M., and Aye, H. H., BCG test reaction in previously BCG vaccinated children, *Ann. Trop. Pediatr.*, 5, 29, 1985.

23. Tolderlund, K., Bunch-Christensen, K., Horwitz, O., and Kirk, L., Development of tuberculin sensitivity in children vaccinated with low doses of Danish BCG vaccine, *Acta Tub. et Pnemol. Scand.*, Suppl. LVI (56).

24. Edwards, L. B. and Gelting, A. S., BCG-vaccine studies, *Bull. World Health Org.*, 3, 279, 1950.

25. Bunch-Christensen, K., Evaluation of BCG vaccines in children, the effect of strain and dose, *J. Biol. Stand.*, 5, 159, 1977.

26. Ashley, M. J. and Siebenman, C. O., Tuberculin skin sensitivity following BCG vaccination with vaccines of high and low viable counts, *Can. Med. Assoc. J.*, 97, 1335, 1967.

27. Lehmann, H. G., Engelhardt, H., Freudenstein, H., Hennessen, W., and Widmark, R., BCG vaccination of neonates, infants, schoolchildren and adolescents. Part I: Dose finding studies with BCG strain 1331 Copenhagen, *Develop. Biol. Stand.*, 43, 127, 1979.

28. Palmer, C. and Meyer, S. N., Research contributions of BCG vaccination programs. I. Tuberculin allergy as a family trait, *Pub. Health Rep.*, 66, 259, 1951.

29. Manerikar, S. S., Malaviya, A. N., Singh, M. B., Rajgopalan, P., and Kumar, R., Immune status and BCG vaccination in newborns with intrauterine growth retardation, *Clin. Exp. Immunol.*, 26, 173, 1976.

30. Dawodu, A. H., Tuberculin conversion following BCG vaccination in preterm infants, *Acta Paediatr. Scand.*, 74, 564, 1985.

31. Kathipari, K., Seth, V., Sinclair, S., Arora, N. K., and Kukreja, N., Cell mediated immune response after BCG as a determinant of optimum age of vaccination, *Indian J. Med. Res.*, 76, 508, 1982.

32. Pabst, H. F., Gobel, J. C., Spandy, D. W., McKechnie, J., and Grace, M., Prospective trial of timing of Bacillus Calmette-Guérin vaccination in Canadian Cree infants, *Am. Rev. Respir. Dis.*, 140, 1007, 1989.

33. Heyworth, B., Delayed hypersensitivity to PPD-S following BCG vaccination in African children — an 18-month field study, *Trans. R. Soc. Trop. Med. Hyg.*, 71, 3, 251, 1977.

34. Horwitz, O. and Bunch-Christensen, K., Correlation between tuberculin sensitivity after 2 months and 5 years among BCG vaccinated subjects, *Bull. World Health Org.*, 47, 49, 1972.

35. Karalliedde, S., Katugaha, L. P., and Uragoda, C. G., Tuberculin response of Sri Lankan children after BCG vaccination at birth, *Tubercle*, 68, 33, 1987.

36. Comstock, G. W., Edwards, L. B., and Nabangxang, H., Tuberculin sensitivity eight to fifteen years after BCG vaccination, *Am. Rev. Respir. Dis.*, 103, 572, 1971.

37. Rosenthal, S. R., Routes and methods of administration, in *BCG Vaccine: Tuberculosis — Cancer*, PSG Publishing Co., Littleton, MA, 1980, Chap. 12.

38. Guld, J., Waaler, H., Sundaresan, T. K., Kaufmann, P. C., and Ten Dam, H. G., The duration of BCG-induced tuberculin sensitivity in children, and its irrelevance for revaccination, *Bull. World Health Org.*, 39, 829, 1968.

39. Young, T. K. and Mirdad, S., Determinants of tuberculin sensitivity in a child population covered by mass BCG vaccination, *Tuberc. Lung Dis.*, 73, 94, 1992.

40. Friedland, I. R., The booster effect with repeat tuberculin testing in children and its relationship to BCG vaccination, *S. Afr. Med. J.*, 77, 387, 1990.

41. Shaaban, M. A., Ati, A. M., Bahr, G. M., Stanford, J. L., Lockwood, D. N. J., and McManus, I. C., Revaccination with BCG: its effects on skin tests in Kuwaiti senior school children, *Eur. Respir. J.*, 3, 187, 1990.

42. Snider, D. E., Bacille Calmette-Guérin vaccinations and tuberculin skin tests, *JAMA*, 253, 3438, 1985.

43. Comstock, G. W., Identification of an effective vaccine against tuberculosis, *Am. Rev. Respir. Dis.*, 138, 479–480, 1988.

44. Hart, P.D'A., Sutherland, I., and Thomas, J., The immunity conferred by effective BCG and vole bacillus vaccines in relation to individual variations in tuberculin sensitivity and to technical variations in the vaccines, *Tubercle*, 48, 201, 1967.

45. Wilson, G. S., *The Hazards of Immunization*, Athlone, London, 1967.

46. Lotte, A., Wasz-Hockert, O., Poisson, N., Dumitrescu, N., Verron, M., and Couvet, E., BCG complications, *Adv. Tuberc. Res.*, 21, 107, 1984.

47. Lotte, A., Wasz-Hockert, O., Poisson, N., Engbaek, H., Landmann, H., Quast, U., Andrasofszky, B., Lugosi, L., Vadasz, I., Mihailescu, P., Pal, D., and Sudic, D., Second IUATLD study on complications induced by intradermal BCG-vaccination, *Bull. Int. Union Tuberc. Lung Dis.*, 63, 47, 1988.

48. Ray, C. S., Pringle, D., Legg, W., and Mbengeranwa, O. L., Lymphadenitis associated with BCG vaccination: a report of an outbreak in Harare, Zimbabwe, *Cent. Afr. J. Med.*, 34, 281, 1988.

49. Caglayan, S., Yegin, O., Kayran, K., Timocin, N., Kasirga, E., and Gun, M., Is medical therapy effective for regional lymphadenitis following BCG vaccination? *Am. J. Dis. Child.*, 141, 1213, 1987.

50. Castro-Rodriguez, J. A., Gonzalez, R., and Girardi, G., Osteitis caused by Bacille Calmette-Guérin vaccination: an emergent problem in Chile? *Int. J. Tuberc. Lung Dis.*, 1, 417, 1997.

51. Bottiger, M., Romanus, V., de Verdier, C., and Boman, G., Osteitis and other complications caused by generalized BCG-itis, *Acta Paediatr. Scand.*, 71, 471, 1982.

52. Peltola, H., Salmi, I., Vahvanen, V., and Ahlqvist, J., BCG vaccination as a cause of osteomyelitis and subcutaneous abscess, *Arch. Dis. Child.*, 59, 157, 1984.

53. Tardieu, M., Carriere, J. P., Truffot-Pernot, C., and Dupic, Y., Tuberculous meningitis due to BCG in two previously healthy children, *Lancet*, 440, 1988.

54. MacKay, A., Alcorn, M. J., Macleod, I. M., Stack, B. H. R., Macleod, T., Laidlaw, M., Millar, J. S., and White, R. G., Fatal disseminated BCG infection in an 18-year-old boy, *Lancet*, 1332, 1980.

55. Aronson, J. D. and Dannenberg, A. M., Effect of vaccination with BCG on tuberculosis in infancy and in childhood, *Am. J. Dis. Child.*, 50, 1117, 1935.

56. Levine, M. I. and Sackett, M. F., Results of BCG immunization in New York City, *Am. Rev. Tuberc.*, 53, 517, 1946.

57. Ferguson, R. S. and Simes, A. B., BCG vaccination of Indian infants in Saskatchewan, *Tubercle*, 30, 5, 1949.

58. Sergent, E., Catanei, A., and Ducros-Rougebief, H., Premunition anti-tuberculeuse par le BCG. Campagne controlee poursuivie a Alger depuis 1935, Troisieme note, *Arch. Inst. Pasteur d'algerile*, 38, 131, 1960.

59. Aronson, J. D., Aronson, C. F., and Taylor, H. C., A twenty-year appraisal of BCG vaccination in the control of tuberculosis, *Arch. Int. Med.*, 101, 881, 1958.

60. Rosenthal, S. R., Loewinsohn, E., Graham, M., Liveright, D., Thorne, M., and Johnson, V., BCG vaccination against tuberculosis in Chicago. A twenty-year study statistically analyzed, *Pediatrics*, 28, 622, 1961.

61. Aronson, J. D., Protective vaccination against tuberculosis with social references to BCG vaccination, *Am. Rev. Tuberc.*, 58, 275, 1948.

62. Rosenthal, S. R., Loewinsohn, E., Graham, M., Liveright, D., Thorne, M., and Johnson, V., BCG vaccination in tuberculous households, *Am. Rev. Respir. Dis.*, 84, 690, 1961.

63. Comstock, G. W. and Webster, R. G., Tuberculosis studies in Muscogee County, Georgia. VII. A twenty-year evaluation of BCG vaccination in a school population, *Am. Rev. Respir. Dis.*, 100, 839, 1969.

64. Bettag, O. L., Kaluzny, A. A., Morse, D., and Radner, D. B., BCG study at a state school for mentally retarded, *Dis. Chest*, 45, 503, 1964.

65. Comstock, G. W., Livesay, V. T., and Woolpert, S. F., Evaluation of BCG vaccination among Puerto Rican children, *Am. J. Pub. Health*, 64, 283, 1974.

66. Comstock, G. W., Woolpert, S. F., and Livesay, V. T., Tuberculosis studies in Muscogee County, Georgia. Twenty-year evaluation of a community trial of BCG vaccination, *Pub. Health Rep.*, 91, 276, 1976.

67. Frimodt-Moller, J., Acharyulu, G. S., and Kesava Pillai, K., Observations on the protective effect of BCG vaccination in a south Indian rural population: fourth report, *Bull. Int. Union Tuberc.*, 48, 40, 1973.

68. Hart, P. D. and Sutherland, I., BCG and vole bacillus vaccines in the prevention of tuberculosis in adolescence and early adult life, *Br. Med. J.*, 2, 293, 1977.

69. Coetzee, A. M. and Berjak, J., BCG in the prevention of tuberculosis in an adult population, *Proc. Mine. Med. Off. Assoc.*, 48, 41, 1968.

70. Vandiviere, H. M., Dworski, M., Melvin, I., Watson, K., and Begley, J., Efficacy of bacillus Calmette-Guérin and isoniazid-resistant bacillus Calmette-Guérin with and without isoniazid chemoprophylaxis from day of vaccination, *Am. Rev. Respir. Dis.*, 108, 301, 1973.

71. Tripathy, S. P., Fifteen-year follow-up of the Indian BCG prevention trial, *Bull. Int. Union Tuberc.*, 62, 69, 1987.

72. Narain, R. and Vallishayee, R. S., BCG vaccination of tuberculous patients and of strong reactors to tuberculin, *Bull. Int. Union Tuberc.*, 51, 243, 1976.

73. Smith, P. G., Case-control studies of the efficacy of BCG against tuberculosis, *Bull. Int. Union Tuberc.*, 62, 73, 1987.

74. Shapiro, C., Cook, N., Evans, D., Willett, W., Fajardo, I., Koch-Weser, D., Bergonzoli, G., Bolanos, O., Guerroero, R., and Hennekens, C., A case-control study of BCG and childhood tuberculosis in Cali, Colombia, *Int. J. Epidemiol.*, 14, 3, 1985.

75. Young, T. K. and Hershfield, E. S., A case-control study to evaluate the effectiveness of mass neonatal BCG vaccination among Canadian Indians, *Am. J. Pub. Health*, 76, 7, 783, 1986.

76. Houston, S., Fanning, A., and Soskolne C. L., The effectiveness of bacillus Calmette-Guérin (BCG) vaccination against tuberculosis: a case-control study in Treaty Indians, Alberta, Canada, *Am. J. Epidemiol.*, 340, 1990.

77. Blin, P., Delolme, H. G., Heyraud, J. D., Charpak, Y., and Sentilhes, L., Evaluation of the protective effect of BCG vaccination by a case-control study in Yaounde, Cameroon, *Tubercle*, 67, 283, 1986.

78. Padungchan, S., Konjanart S., and Kasiratta, S., The effectiveness of BCG vaccination of the newborn against childhood tuberculosis in Bangkok, *Bull. World Health Org.*, 64, 247, 1986.

79. Tidjani, O., Amedome, A., and Ten Dam, H. G., The protective effect of BCG vaccination of the newborn against childhood tuberculosis in an African community, *Tubercle*, 67, 269, 1986.

80. Karonga Prevention Trial Group, Randomised controlled trial of single BCG, repeated BCG, or combined BCG and killed *Mycobacterium leprae* vaccine for prevention of leprosy and tuberculosis in Malawi, *Lancet*, 348, 17, 1996.

81. Colditz, G. A., Brewer, T. F., Berkey, C. S., Wilson, M. E., Burdick, E., Fineberg, H. V., and Mosteller, F., Efficacy of BCG vaccine in the prevention of tuberculosis. Meta-analysis of the published literature, *JAMA*, 271, 698, 1994.

82a. Palmer, C. E. and Long, M. W., Effect of infection with atypical mycobacteria on BCG vaccination and tuberculosis, *Am. Rev. Respir. Dis.*, 94, 553, 1966.

82b. Comstock, G. W., Field trials of tuberculosis vaccines: how could we have done them better? *Cont. Clin. Trials*, 14, 247, 1994.

83. Sterne, J. A. C., Rodrigues, L. C., and Guedes, I. N., Does the efficacy of BCG decline with time since vaccination? *Int. J. Tuberc. Lung Dis.*, 2, 200, 1998.

84. Fine, P. E. M., BCG vaccination against tuberculosis and leprosy, *Br. Med. Bull.*, 44, 691, 1988.

85. Rook, G. A. W., Bahr, G. M., and Stanford, J. L., The effect of two distinct forms of cell-mediated response to mycobacteria on the protective efficacy of BCG, *Tubercle*, 62, 63, 1981.

86. Brewer, T. F. and Colditz, G. A., Relationship between Bacille Calmette-Guérin (BCG) strains and the efficacy of BCG vaccine in the prevention of tuberculosis, *Clin. Infect. Dis.*, 20, 126, 1995.

87. Hank, J. A., Chan, J. K., Edwards, M. L., Muller, D., and Smith, D. W., Influence of the virulence of *Mycobacterium tuberculosis* on protection induced by Bacille-Calmette-Guérin in guinea pigs, *J. Infect. Dis.*, 143, 734, 1981.

88. Blackwell, J. M., Bacterial infections, in *Genetics of Resistance to Bacterial and Parasitic Infections*, Wakelin D. and Blackwell, J. M., Eds., Taylor and Francis, London, 1988.

89. McMurray, D. N., Carlomagno, M. A., Mintzer, C. L., and Tetzlaff, C. L., *Mycobacterium bovis* BCG vaccine fails to protect protein-deficient guinea pigs against respiratory challenge with virulent *Mycobacterium tuberculosis, Infect. Immun.*, 50, 555, 1985.

90. Ten Dam, H. G. and Pio, A., Pathogenesis of tuberculosis and effectiveness of vaccination, *Tubercle*, 63, 223, 1982.

91. Comstock, G. W. and Edwards, P. Q., An American view of BCG vaccination, illustrated by results of a controlled trial in Puerto Rico, *Scand. J. Respir. Dis.*, 53, 207, 1972.

92. Clemens, J. B., Chuong, J. J. H., and Feinstein, A. R., The BCG controversy: a methodological and statistical reappraisal, *JAMA*, 249, 236, 1983.

93. WHO Study Group, BCG vaccination policies, *WHO Tech. Rep. Ser.*, 652, 1980.

94. Centers for Disease Control, The role of BCG vaccine in the prevention and control of tuberculosis in the United States. A joint statement by the Advisory Council for the Elimination of Tuberculosis and the Advisory Committee on Immunization Practices, *MMWR*, 45, 1, 1996.

95. Brewer, T. A. and Colditz, G. A., Bacille Calmette-Guérin vaccination for the prevention of tuberculosis in health care workers, *Clin. Infect. Dis.*, 20, 136, 1995.

96. Stevens, J. P. and Daniel, T. M., Bacille Calmette Guérin immunization of health care workers exposed to multidrug-resistant tuberculosis: a decision analysis, *Tuberc. Lung Dis.*, 77, 315, 1996.

97. Frieden, T. R., Fujiwara, P. I., Washko, R. M., and Hamburg, M. A., Tuberculosis in New York City — turning the tide, *N. Engl. J. Med.*, 333, 229, 1995.

98. Centers for Disease Control and Prevention, Immunization of health-care workers. Recommendations of the Advisory Committee on Immunization Practices (ACIP) and the Hospital Infection Control Practices Advisory Committee (HICPAC), *MMWR*, 46, 26, 1997.

99. Colebunders, R., Mann, J. M., Francis, H., Bila, K., Izaley, L., Kakonde, N., Kabasele, K., Ifoto, L., Nzilambi, N., Quinn, T. C., Van der Groen, G., Curran, J., Vercauteren, G., and Piot, P., Evaluation of a clinical case-definition of acquired immunodeficiency syndrome in Africa, *Lancet*, 1, 492, 1987.

100. Ten Dam, H. G., BCG vaccination and HIV infection, *Bull. Int. Union Tuberc. Lung Dis.*, 65, 38, 1990.

101. Colebunders, R. L., Izaley, L., Musampu, M., Pauwels, P., Francis, H., and Ryder, R., BCG vaccine abscesses are unrelated to HIV infection, *JAMA*, 259, 3521, 1988.

102. Mvula, M., Ryder, R. W., and Manzila, T., Response to childhood vaccinations in African children with HIV infection, *4th Int. Conf. AIDS*, Stockholm, Abstract 5112, June, 1988.

103. Bregere, P., BCG vaccination and AIDS, *Bull. Int. Union Tuberc. Lung Dis.*, 63, 40, 1988.

104. Lallemant-Le Coeur, S., Lallemant, M., Cheynier, D., Nzingoula, S., Drucker, J., and Larouze, B., Bacillus Calmette-Guérin immunization in infants born to HIV-1-seropositive mothers, *AIDS*, 5:195, 1991.

105. Centers for Disease Control, BCG vaccination and pediatric HIV infection — Rwanda, 1988–1990, *MMWR*, 40, 833, 1991.

106. Ninane, J., Grymonprez, A., Burtonboy, G., Francois, A., and Cornu, G., Disseminated BCG in HIV infection, *Arch. Dis. Child.*, 63, 1268, 1988.

107. Houde, C. and Dery, P., *Mycobacterium bovis* sepsis in an infant with human immunodeficiency virus infection, *Ped. Infect. Dis. J.*, 7, 810, 1988.

108. Centers for Disease Control, Disseminated *Mycobacterium bovis* infection from BCG vaccination of a patient with acquired immunodeficiency syndrome, *MMWR*, 34, 227, 1985.
109. Lumb, R. and Shaw, D., *Mycobacterium bovis* (BCG) vaccination. Progressive disease in a patient symptomatically infected with the human immunodeficiency virus, *Med. J. Aust.*, 156, 286, 1992.
110. Smith, E., Thybo, S., and Bennedsen, J., Infection with *Mycobacterium bovis* in a patient with AIDS: a late complication of BCG vaccination, *Scand. J. Infect. Dis.*, 24, 109, 1992.
111. Blondon, H., Guez, T., Paul, G., Truffot-Pernot, C., and Sicard, D., Adenite a BCG 6 ans apres la vaccination au cours d'un SIDA, *La Presse Medicale*, 20, 1091, 1991.
112. Reynes, J., Perez, C., Lamaury, I., Janbon, F., and Bertrand, A., Bacille Calmette-Guérin adenitis 30 years after immunization in a patient with AIDS, *J. Infect. Dis.*, 160, 727, 1989.
113. Armbruster, C., Junker, W., Vetter, N., and Jaksch, G., Disseminated Bacille Calmette-Guérin infection in an AIDS patient 30 years after BCG vaccination, *J. Infect. Dis.*, 162, 1216, 1990.
114. WHO/IUATLD, Tuberculosis and AIDS. Statement on AIDS and tuberculosis, *Bull. Int. Union Tuberc. Lung Dis.*, 64, 8, 1989.
115. Centers for Disease Control and Prevention, Development of new vaccines for tuberculosis. Recommendations of the Advisory Council for the Elimination of Tuberculosis (ACET), *MMWR*, 47, 1, 1998.
116. Orme, I., Animal model testing of new tuberculosis vaccines, Final Program of the Tuberculosis Vaccine Development and Evaluation Symposium, San Francisco, 1998.
117. Orme, I., Progress in the development of new vaccines against tuberculosis, *Int. J. Tuberc. Lung Dis.*, 1, 95, 1997.
118. Huygen, K., DNA vaccines: application to tuberculosis, *Int. J. Tuberc. Lung Dis.*, 2, 971, 1998.
119. Bean, A. G. D., Kamath, A. T., Feng, C. G., Briscoe, H., and Britton, W. J., Differential protective efficacy of DNA vaccines expressing secreted proteins of *Mycobacterium tuberculosis*, Final Program of the Tuberculosis Vaccine Development and Evaluation Symposium, San Francisco, 1998.
120. Huygen, K, D'Souza, S., and Denis, O., Immunogenicity and protective efficacy of a DNA vaccine encoding Ag85A from *M. tuberculosis* in β2-microglobulin knock-out mice, Final Program of the Tuberculosis Vaccine Development and Evaluation Symposium, San Francisco, 1998.
121. Morris, S., Li, Z., Kelley, C., Howard, A., and Collins, F., Immunogenicity and protective effectiveness of DNA vaccines against tuberculosis, Final Program of the Tuberculosis Vaccine Development and Evaluation Symposium, San Francisco, 1998.
122. Tanghe, A., Lefevre, P., Denis, O., D'Souza, S., Braibant, M., Lozes, E., Content, J., Huygen, K., Singh, M., and Montgomery, D., Immunogenicity and protective efficacy of tuberculosis DNA vaccines encoding putative phosphate transport receptors, Final Program of the Tuberculosis Vaccine Development and Evaluation Symposium, San Francisco, 1998.
123. Pal, P. G. and Horwitz, M. A., Immunization with extracellular proteins of *Mycobacterium tuberculosis* induces cell-mediated immune responses and substantial protective immunity in a guinea pig model of pulmonary tuberculosis, *Infect. Imm.*, 60, 4781, 1992.
124. Lyons, J., Sinos, C., Destree, A, Caiazzo, T., Havican, K., McKenzie, S., Panicali, D., and Mahr, A., Expression of *Mycobacterium tuberculosis* and *Mycobacterium leprae* proteins by vaccinia virus, *Infect. Imm.*, 58, 4098, 1990.
125. Alderson, M., Skeiky, Y., Durie, F., Dillon, D., Reed, S., Lewinsohn, D., and Campos-Neto, A., Towards the development of a subunit vaccine for *Mycobacterium tuberculosis*, Final Program of the Tuberculosis Vaccine Development and Evaluation Symposium, San Francisco, 1998.
126. Mustafa, A. S., Amoudy, H., Shaban, F., Oftung, F., Ravn, P., and Andersen, P., IFN-γ secreting T cell lines from pulmonary tuberculosis patients expressing a spectrum of HLA-DR molecules recognize synthetic peptides spanning the entire sequence of the *M. tuberculosis* ESAT6 antigen, Final Program of the Tuberculosis Vaccine Development and Evaluation Symposium, San Francisco, 1998.
127. Jagannath, C., Armitige, L., Pai, S., Wanger, A., Norris, S., Actor, J. K., and Hunter, R. L., Altered growth characteristics and vaccinogenic effects of a *Mycobacterium tuberculosis* H37Rv mutant deficient in antigen 85A expression, Final Program of the Tuberculosis Vaccine Development and Evaluation Symposium, San Francisco, 1998.
128. von Reyn, C. F., Waddell, R. D., Chintu, C., Lein, A. D., Arbeit, R. D., Mwinga, A., and Zumla, A., Safety and immunogenicity of a five-dose series of inactivated *Mycobacterium vaccae* vaccine for the prevention of HIV-associated tuberculosis, Final Program of the Tuberculosis Vaccine Development and Evaluation Symposium, San Francisco, 1998.

129. Horsburgh, C. R., Jr., Large simple trials of tuberculosis vaccine efficacy: preparing the foundations, Final Program of the Tuberculosis Vaccine Development and Evaluation Symposium, San Francisco, 1998.
130. Whalen, C. C., Evaluating tuberculosis vaccine efficacy in household contacts, Final Program of the Tuberculosis Vaccine Development and Evaluation Symposium, San Francisco, 1998.
131. Ellner, J. J., Correlates of immunity, Final Program of the Tuberculosis Vaccine Development and Evaluation Symposium, San Francisco, 1998.
132. Bean, A. G. D., Yow, T. T., Feng, C. G., Corte, P., and Britton, W. J., Quantifying human T cell IFN-γ responses as a correlate of protection for new vaccines against *Mycobacterium tuberculosis*, Final Program of the Tuberculosis Vaccine Development and Evaluation Symposium, San Francisco, 1998.
133. Worku, S. and Hoft, D. F., *In vitro* measurement of protective mycobacterial immunity: antigen specific expansion of T cells capable of inhibiting growth of BCG, Final Program of the Tuberculosis Vaccine Development and Evaluation Symposium, San Francisco, 1998.

16 International Tuberculosis Control in the 21st Century

Paul E. Farmer, M.D., Ph.D., David A. Walton, and Mercedes C. Becerra, Sc.D.

CONTENTS

I. INTRODUCTION

At the close of the 20th century, tuberculosis (TB) remains the world's leading infectious cause of adult mortality. In 1997, there were 3.81 million TB cases reported to the World Health Organization (WHO). With an estimated current case-detection rate of 39%, this would suggest that there are as many as 10 million incident cases of TB each year.[1] Estimates of mortality due to TB vary widely, but reliable sources report between 2 and 3 million deaths per year.[2] Active TB is common, and it stands to reason that infection with *Mycobacterium tuberculosis* is even more so. Projections based on skin-test surveys suggest that up to a third of the world's population (some 2 billion people) are currently infected with quiescent but viable tubercle bacilli.[3]

The burden of both TB infection and disease is overwhelmingly borne by those living in the Third World. Over 95% of all incident cases and over 98.6% of all TB deaths occur in countries in which TB is endemic and medical services scarce or substandard.[4] In some regions, the advent of HIV has worsened an already dire situation, doubling and even trebling TB case rates.[5,6] Finally, an increasing proportion of all cases of TB reported in low-prevalence regions in Europe and North America are diagnosed among patients born in high-prevalence countries. In the U.S., for example, almost 40% of all culture-positive cases of tuberculosis are diagnosed in the foreign-born.[7-9] In regions characterized by high rates of immigration, an even greater proportion of all TB cases are diagnosed among the foreign-born. In Massachusetts, for example, this figure now stands at 70% of all cases.[10,11] In much of Western Europe, the proportion of all cases diagnosed in the foreign-born also exceeds 60%.[12]

The last decade has seen renewed attention to TB by international bodies; major advances have been achieved. But improving TB control in the developing world represents a major challenge — likely *the* major challenge — for global TB control in the coming years. Whether one's primary approach to TB control is clinical or in terms of health policy, unnecessary TB deaths and unopposed transmission of *M. tuberculosis* in endemic regions will determine the contours of tomorrow's global pandemic. By the same logic, the emergence of drug resistance in resource-poor endemic regions will eventually pose problems for countries in which TB resources are plentiful, while TB itself is rare.[13]

This chapter will review briefly the global epidemiology of TB today, noting likely future trends. We also will review recent advances in international TB control, with a particular focus on DOTS — directly observed treatment, short-course; the strengths and weaknesses of this and other strategies currently advocated will be considered. We will then discuss the diagnosis and treatment of TB disease and infection in developing countries before turning to the emerging problem of resistance to antituberculous medications. Finally, we close by highlighting a number of new challenges and opportunities in international TB control.

II. EPIDEMIOLOGY

A. BURDEN OF DISEASE

Population-based surveys of both TB infection and TB disease reveal that the greatest burden of disease and the highest annual risk of infection are borne by those living in developing countries.[1] Within these regions, morbidity and mortality due to TB are also strikingly patterned. The World Health Organization (WHO) divides the world into six regions: Africa, the Americas, the Eastern Mediterranean, Southeast Asia, Europe, and the Western Pacific. Figure 16.1 shows the number of cases reported in each of those regions in 1997.

As is clear from Figure 16.1, fully 54% of all cases reported are diagnosed in Asia and Africa; the case-fatality rate is also highest in sub-Saharan Africa, where HIV has caused serious setbacks in TB control efforts.[14,15] Recent data also suggest a major recrudescence of TB in the former Soviet Union. In Russia, where socioeconomic decline has led to a weakening of TB surveillance and control, a steady increase in incidence has been reported. Although steady declines in incidence were registered throughout the latter half of the century, with a marked drop in case notification rates in the 1980s, incidence began to climb steadily in 1992: whereas 50,407 cases were notified in 1991, the number rose steadily to reach 121,491 in 1997.[1] Even in small and relatively affluent nations in this region, TB is on the rise. In Lithuania, for example, TB incidence increased from 39.5 per 100,000 in 1990 to 70.3 per 100,000 in 1996.[16] Similar trends have been registered in other Baltic countries, in Kazakhstan, Kyrgystan, and Georgia.[1] Although these epidemics pale in

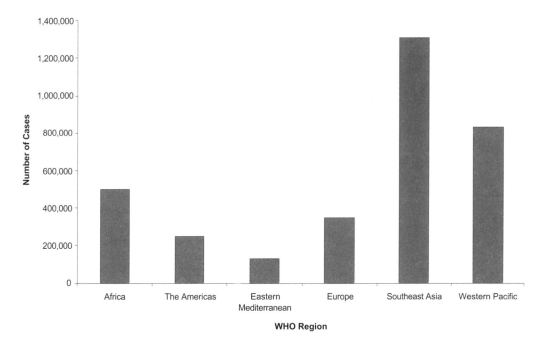

FIGURE 16.1 Incidence of Tuberculosis, 1997. (From the World Health Organization, *Global Tuberculosis Control,* WHO Report 1999, Geneva, 1999. With permission.)

comparison to those in Africa and Asia, it is important to note the relative increases in a short period, and also that death rates are climbing.[17] Most soberingly, drug-resistant TB plays a central role in these Eastern European and Central Asian setbacks.[18]

B. FUTURE TRENDS

The past 30 years have seen several attempts to model TB epidemics, including projections of likely future scenarios; we have reviewed some of these exercises elsewhere.[17] Available projections for the global pandemic and its regional subepidemics have not yet incorporated fully the effect of three developments, each with profound impact on the trends of TB in populations. First, the advent of HIV has radically altered the dynamics of TB, since reactivation of quiescent infection with *M. tuberculosis* is up to 10 times higher among patients coinfected with HIV.[19-21] It has been estimated that a third of the increase in TB incidence can be attributed to HIV in regions such as sub-Saharan Africa.[22] Second, social and economic disruption in areas of high endemicity have led to massive urbanization and also to increased traffic between far-flung locales; accordingly, microbial traffic has sped up as well.[23] Finally, resistance to antituberculous medications is now widespread, even though it was virtually unknown a mere 5 decades ago.[24] Each of these three developments will need to be considered in order to obtain more robust projections.

Even without further refining available models, it is clear that TB will not be eradicated any time soon. Recent estimates indicate that TB will remain one of the world's top 10 causes of adult mortality in the year 2020; HIV is the only other infectious pathogen slated to remain on this list.[25] It is unclear, at this writing, to what extent current control strategies are likely to inflect TB trends. The widespread adoption of DOTS could have a significant impact on the pandemic, but WHO estimates that, as of 1998, only 12% of all people sick with TB are being treated within DOTS-based programs (Figure 16.2).[26] Even optimistic scenarios are grim. If DOTS continues to be adopted widely, the numbers of projected deaths between 1998 and 2030 are still staggering: "Globally, we expect 171 million new cases and 60 million deaths in the best-case DOTS scenario

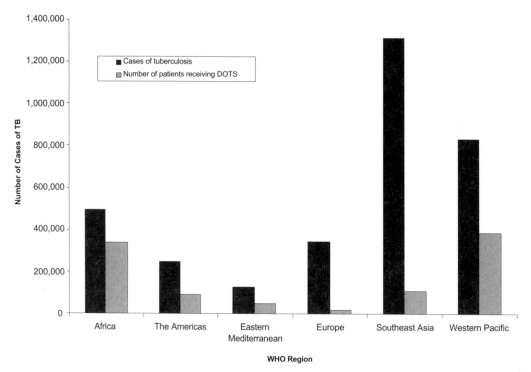

FIGURE 16.2   Implementation of DOTS, 1997. (From the World Health Organization, *Global Tuberculosis Control,* WHO Report 1999, Geneva, 1999. With permission.)

and 249 million new cases and 90 million deaths in the worse-case DOTS scenario," according to Murray and Salomon.[27]

Available modeling exercises remind us that the intrinsic dynamics of TB epidemics are slow, and that even the best control efforts based on chemotherapy will take decades to alter incidence in regions in which TB is endemic.[28,29] The impact of substandard control efforts, however, may be felt more quickly. One of the most feared consequences of inadequate therapy is acquired resistance, or the selection of organisms resistant to first-line antituberculous medications. Although the *cause* of high rates of acquired drug resistance is usually poor TB control programs,[30] the *effect* (decreased cure rates and ongoing transmission of drug-resistant strains) can subsequently weaken even the best control programs. That is, once a poor TB control program turns on the spigot of acquired drug resistance, it shortly thereafter opens a second valve, that of primary resistance. In order to interrupt this cycle, TB control measures must curb both the generation of drug-resistant TB and the transmission of drug-resistant strains of *M. tuberculosis*. Both spigots must be closed if TB control efforts are to succeed.[31]

Experience in the urban U.S. has shown that outbreaks of drug-resistant TB are only briefly local.[32] As molecular epidemiology brings into relief the transregional — often, transnational — nature of multidrug resistant TB (MDR-TB) epidemics, we are again reminded of the importance of transnational cooperation in TB control.[33] This may be especially true in efforts to curb drug-resistant tuberculosis, which is difficult and costly to treat. But future trends in the global TB pandemic will be determined by today's control activities, which we consider in the next section.

III. DOTS: THE CORNERSTONE OF INTERNATIONAL TB CONTROL

Many of the principles of modern TB control have been laid down in the last 2 decades. The key components of effective control efforts have been case finding, chemotherapy, chemoprophylaxis,

---

TABLE 16.1
Common Reasons for Patient Nonadherence to
Antituberculous Therapy in Resource-Poor Settings

- Economic barriers (including "hidden costs" of transportation, etc.)
- Drug stock-outs
- Inconvenient clinic hours or locations
- Errors in prescribing or dispensing (provider misconceptions)
- Discontinuation of therapy due to perceived adverse effects
- Patient misconceptions

---

and vaccination.[34] One of the most dynamic forces in international TB control has been the WHO's Global TB Programme, or GTB. According to the WHO-GTB, "the overall objective of TB control is to reduce mortality, morbidity, and transmission of the disease until it no longer poses a threat to public health."[35] Pioneered in East Africa and Asia in the 1960s, the DOTS strategy has been central to the WHO-recommended TB-control package since 1991.[36-40] In 1994, the World Health Assembly endorsed targets for DOTS-based global TB control to detect, by the year 2000, 70% of all existing TB cases and to cure 85% of all detected new smear-positive TB cases.[35]

When backed by the requisite political will and implemented carefully, DOTS has been shown to be highly effective, leading to greater than 90% cure rates in highly disparate settings.[41-43] This is to be compared to a worldwide average, among all cases registered in 1994, of only 43% cured.[44] Furthermore, short-course chemotherapy (SCC) regimens based on isoniazid (INH) and rifampin (RIF) are inexpensive.[42] In China, for example, a 6-month supply of drugs can cost as little as U.S. $13.[26] Accordingly, the WHO has marketed the development of strategies to extend DOTS coverage as one of the "best buys for research on major microbial diseases."[45]

Directly observed treatment is, along with SCC, the primary therapeutic innovation of DOTS.[46-51] Although there are many discrepant claims regarding the cause of patient noncompliance,[52-56] DOT serves to reduce the degree to which structural, cultural, and linguistic barriers or prior personal experience might lead to nonadherence with antituberculous therapy. The success of DOTS thus serves as a reminder that noncompliance as a cause of treatment failure should remain a diagnosis of exclusion wherever DOT is not used. This is especially true of resource-poor regions in which TB treatment has been substandard.[57] In the absence of sound DOTS-based TB programs (and 88% of all incident cases are thought to occur in regions without such programs)[1] the development of drug resistance is highly contingent on patient adherence to therapy. There are several reasons that patients may not adhere to the prescribed drug regimens. Some of these are listed in Table 16.1.

It is often noted, however, that there is more to DOTS than directly observed, short-course chemotherapy. The WHO-GTB has devised a complex and fairly comprehensive TB Control Policy Package that it recommends to, and helps implement with, national TB programs (NTP).[35] Its key components are listed in Table 16.2. The means by which TB cases are to be identified, registered, and treated are outlined in detail.

1. Case-finding is passive rather than active[58-61] (patients self-report when symptomatic, and the WHO-GTB has discouraged the use of mass screening with fluoroscopy or chest films).[62]
2. Diagnosis is based on smear microscopy of sputum[63] rather than on clinical diagnosis or radiography.
3. Drug regimens used in DOTS are variable but rely on standardized SCC for all smear-positive cases; doses are standardized, and a regular supply of first-line drugs is essential to DOTS ("essential anti-TB drugs" are held to include INH, RIF, pyrazinamide, streptomycin, ethambutol, and, in some areas, thiacetazone).

TABLE 16.2
Components of the WHO TB-Control "Policy Package"

- passive case-finding based on smear-microscopy
- standardized short-course chemotherapy for all smear-positive cases
- regular drug supply of "all essential anti-TB drugs"
- standardized monitoring and evaluation of program activities
- government commitment to a national TB program

Source: WHO, *Framework for Effective TB Control,* 1994. With permission.

4. A system of monitoring and evaluating NTP performance, based on standardized "cohort analysis" indicators, is also central to the WHO-GTB framework for effective TB control.
5. The package calls for high-level government commitment to DOTS-based TB control.

In recent years, financing for national TB programs, which has come, increasingly, from the World Bank, has often been made conditional upon demonstrated political commitment.[64,65]

One example of the efficacy of the DOTS strategy comes from Peru. After decades of poor program performance and dismal treatment outcomes,[66,67] the Peruvian NTP adopted, in 1991, the WHO's package with political commitment at the highest level and initiated a complete NTP reorganization along WHO-GTB recommended guidelines. Using a four-drug regimen with standardized doses (INH-RIF-PZA-EMB daily for 2 months, followed by biweekly INH-RIF), cure rates went from under 60% to well over 80% within 3 years of adoption (Table 16.3).

Although the strategy has some weaknesses (these will be discussed below), DOTS is clearly a major advance in TB control and could, if properly and rapidly implemented, improve treatment outcomes dramatically. Whether or not its implementation will affect the global pandemic remains to be seen, but a number of factors suggest that DOTS alone may be insufficient to affect incidence. First, as discussed below, many patients with active TB will not be detected by smear microscopy, a relatively insensitive means of diagnosing the disease.[69] Second, patients with a negative result on smear microscopy cannot, in the era of HIV, be considered noninfectious, as had previously been claimed.[70] Third, although chemoprophylaxis is used widely in the industrialized world in order to prevent disease among the latently infected, chemoprophylaxis does not currently figure on the list of WHO-GTB-endorsed interventions. Finally, as noted, only 12% of all patients with active TB are now being treated with DOTS.

Based on current trends in the uptake of DOTS, Murray and Salomon project 225 million new cases and 79 million deaths between 1998 and 2030. As they note, "Given the pace of uptake of DOTS, the heavy emphasis of WHO on smear-positive pulmonary cases only and the magnitude of the remaining problem, it is worth examining whether considerable gains against tuberculosis

TABLE 16.3
**Proportion of Patients Cured of all
Entering Treatment, Before and After
the Implementation of DOTS in Peru**

1980	57%
1991	74%
1994	86%
1998	91%

Source: National Tuberculosis Program, Peru, 1998.[68]

can be achieved through promotion of DOTS alone."[27] Thus, even if DOTS continues to be adopted at the current rate, which the WHO has termed "rapid," other tools are needed if TB incidence is to be reduced. (See the conclusion of this chapter for a consideration of complementary strategies for the control of TB in developing countries.)

IV. VACCINATION

BCG is an attenuated strain of *M. bovis* developed by Albert Calmette and Camille Guérin. Part of the WHO's Expanded Programme of Immunization, it is the world's most widely used vaccine, with over three billion doses administered since its introduction in 1921.[71] Although the vaccine's efficacy continues to be debated, one meta-analysis suggests an overall protective effect of 51%, with a 64% protective effect against tuberculous meningitis and a 78% protective effect against disseminated TB.[72] Because of BCG's efficacy in preventing death and severe disease among children, the WHO recommends universal BCG coverage at birth in high-prevalence countries. Each year, at this writing, approximately one million children receive BCG.[73] The duration of BCG's efficacy also has been a topic of debate, but duration-specific evidence suggests that protection may persist for up to 10 years after vaccination.[74]

There is now some evidence suggesting that BCG decreases the risk of MDR-TB disease among close contacts of infectious patients with MDR-TB,[75] and its potential benefits are being considered for high-exposure groups such as health workers.[76]

V. DIAGNOSIS IN RESOURCE-POOR SETTINGS

A. LATENT INFECTION

There is no highly sensitive test to diagnose quiescent infection with *M. tuberculosis*. Tuberculin skin testing, discussed elsewhere in this book, is not widely used in the Third World, in large part because TB control efforts have been directed to case finding and therapy of active disease. Yet the diagnosis of infection is critical to eradication efforts, since it is the sole means of identifying candidates for chemoprophylaxis. Even in settings with high rates of HIV coinfection, skin testing may be used to identify TB-infected individuals, since many such patients will not be anergic. Diagnosis of latent TB infection is critical among the HIV coinfected, since reactivation TB disease is perhaps an order of magnitude more likely in this population.[77] Skin testing is also critical to the diagnosis of TB infection and disease in children, and is discussed below.

In a number of areas, skin-test surveys to obtain estimates of the prevalence of infection in the population have been conducted in order to calculate annual risk of infection and estimate incidence of active TB.[78,79] But this method of estimating TB incidence was based on data from Europe during a period of TB decline, and its utility in estimating the burden of active disease in high-prevalence settings is debated. In rural Haiti, a survey of adults in one village revealed that 70% had indurations of greater than 15 mm upon challenge with PPD; 8 of 10 health professionals (physicians, nurses, and nurse assistants) serving this population were skin-test positive.[80]

B. PULMONARY DISEASE

Although smear microscopy is, at this writing, the most widely used means of diagnosing active TB in resource-poor countries, it, too, is an imperfect tool. TB has a pulmonary portal of entry but is a *systemic* infection that may affect any organ. Styblo et al. estimated that for every case of sputum smear-positive TB, there are 1.2 cases that are smear-negative or extrapulmonary.[81] That ratio is even more unfavorable among children with TB disease. In most series, the great majority of children with active tuberculosis are smear-negative. HIV has further complicated the picture by leading, in coinfected patients, to higher rates of disseminated and extrapulmonary disease, and also to lower rates of smear-positive cavitary disease among those with pulmonary TB.[82]

1. Smear Microscopy

Most smear microscopy is a variation of techniques developed over 100 years ago (see Chapter 4). The Ziehl-Neelsen stain is a "hot" stain requiring that a carbol-fuschin-stained specimen be steamed.[83] The Kinyoun modification is a "cold" method (the addition of a detergent to the carbol-fuschin reagent enhances penetration of the dye into organisms, obviating the need for heat).[84] Both stains require minimal technical capacity and can be used in difficult field conditions as long as quality control is assured.[85,86] But the sensitivity and specificity of these methods vary significantly, since the former depends on burden of disease and the latter depends on the local epidemiology of infection with acid-fast organisms.[87] Smear microscopy is expected to detect the most infectious patients, i.e., those with cavitary disease and a large bacillary load in the sputum.[88] But the overall sensitivity of smear microscopy in pulmonary TB is estimated to be between 22 and 65% — lower than culture of sputum.[89] The advent of HIV may further decrease the sensitivity of smear microscopy for detecting pulmonary TB. Several studies have shown that up to half of all patients subsequently shown to have culture-positive pulmonary TB had falsely negative smears.[90] It should be noted that, in settings with high rates of infection with *M. tuberculosis*, subsequent coinfection with HIV will increase the likelihood of reactivation disease, and that the clinical presentation is often similar to classic postprimary pulmonary TB, with apical involvement and cavitary lesions. Long and colleagues, working in Haiti, concluded that differences between the sensitivity of smear microscopy in TB patients with and without HIV coinfection "are small and do not significantly compromise the usefulness of sputum smears in developing countries."[91] Smith and coworkers, working in the U.S., argued that "positive acid-fast sputum smears are found as frequently in patients with, as in those without, HIV infection and pulmonary TB."[92] Thus, reliance on this diagnostic method alone will guarantee that some proportion of diseased individuals will be misclassified as nondiseased. Case-detection programs that rely exclusively on smear microscopy of sputum will necessarily miss a substantial number of cases. In TB-endemic regions, the presence of acid-fast bacilli in sputum or other clinical material usually signifies active TB. Among patients living with advanced HIV in the U.S., however, many patients found to have positive smears are ultimately shown to be infected with atypical mycobacteria.[93]

2. Culture

The recovery of *M. tuberculosis* in culture is also a surprisingly inexpensive means of diagnosis. A number of selective culture media are currently in wide use; Lowenstein-Jensen slants can be set up for as little as U.S. $0.80/slant.[94] Although this is considerably more expensive than three sputum smears, there are reasons to consider this technology even in resource-poor settings: culture is more sensitive in detecting most forms of TB and may be two to three times more sensitive than smear microscopy in diagnosing tuberculous meningitis, pleural TB, and peritoneal TB. In settings in which drug resistance has emerged, culture is the least expensive means of drug-susceptibility testing. Although susceptibility testing for pyrazinamide (PZA) is difficult, drug-susceptibility testing for many other first-line drugs has been more widely standardized and can be performed for as little as U.S. $2 per patient.[94] Quality control is critical and so drug-susceptibility testing is best performed in specialized laboratories.[95] Disadvantages of culture in resource-poor countries include costs as well as the need for a reliable source of electricity. Finally, *M. tuberculosis,* though not fastidious, is a slow-growing organism. In most laboratories, cultures are not declared negative until 60 days; results of susceptibility testing may take months to reach the appropriate clinicians.

3. Radiographic Methods

Radiographic methods, including chest films and fluoroscopy, have been used widely to diagnose TB.[96,97] Although these methods are more sensitive than smear microscopy, they are far less specific,

TABLE 16.4
Distribution of TB Cases Presented at the Clinique Bon Sauveur During 1993

Location	No. of Cases	Percentage of all Cases (%)
Pulmonary	318	77.8
Pulmonary plus extrapulmonary	24	5.9
Extrapulmonary	39	9.5
Lymphadenitis	24	5.9
Lymphadenitis/peritoneal	4	1.0
Peritoneal	2	0.5
Meningitis	2	0.5
Genitourinary	3	0.7
Skeletal	4	1.0
Disseminated/miliary	28	6.8
Total	409	100.0

Source: Lasante, Z., Harvard Medical School, Boston, 1998. With permission.

and have fallen out of favor given their high cost per case detected in the low-prevalence areas in which they have been primarily used.[98] Yet many diagnoses, especially those among children, are suggested by chest film. Furthermore, radiographic methods such as mass-miniature radiography (MMR) and fluorography may improve case-finding efforts. A recent review by Murray and Salomon suggests that continuous active case-finding by MMR could save 23 million lives over the next 3 decades.[27] It remains to be seen whether the introduction of such methods might be feasible in the high-prevalence regions in which they would, in principle, detect far greater numbers of cases of active disease.

C. EXTRAPULMONARY TB DISEASE

Extrapulmonary TB disease poses diagnostic dilemmas even in settings in which culture and a full range of invasive diagnostic procedures — from bone-marrow aspiration to stereotactic brain biopsy — are readily available. In settings with limited resources, these dilemmas are even more pointed. Our own experience in rural Haiti is instructive in this regard. Table 16.4 lists the distribution of all cases of TB diagnosed in our clinic in 1993. Even when many invasive diagnostic procedures are not available, a significant proportion — 22%, in our sample of 409 patients — of all cases had extrapulmonary involvement.

Experience in areas in which HIV and TB are co-endemic suggests that a greater proportion of future cases will be extrapulmonary.[99] As cell-mediated immunity wanes, disseminated TB comes to be the predominant form of disease among the coinfected. Furthermore, cavity formation becomes increasingly rare; smear microscopy, accordingly, is a less reliable tool for diagnosis of active disease.[77,82] This is particularly true in settings in which TB is epidemic and the leading cause of mortality among those living with HIV disease.[100]

D. TUBERCULOSIS IN CHILDREN

Tuberculosis in children likewise poses diagnostic difficulties wherever smear microscopy is held up as the gold standard, since this method is notoriously insensitive in detecting pediatric TB.[101,102] Skin testing, gastric aspirates, laryngeal swabs, and chest radiography are of greater utility. History of sustained exposure, often to a household contact with active pulmonary TB, is central to pediatric case finding.[103,104] Accordingly, even staunch advocates of passive case finding and reliance on smear microscopy recommend the use of other methods to diagnose TB among children.[105] In our experience in rural Haiti, the initiation of active case finding among household members of patients with active pulmonary disease trebled pediatric diagnoses in the space of less than a year.[80]

E. Novel Diagnostic Tools

Novel diagnostic tools (see Chapter 5) now available or currently in development have not been used in developing countries, the very settings in which they would have the greatest utility. Rhodamine-auramine stains permit more rapid evaluation of sputum smears than does Ziehl-Neelsen stains;[106] DNA amplification tests allow rapid detection of disease due to *M. tuberculosis*.[107] The polymerase chain reaction (PCR) can be used to detect the presence of mycobacteria in sputum within 5 hours.[108] On the other hand, numerous surveys suggest caution in relying on such methods in the examination of smear-negative samples, and the sensitivity of PCR is not well established in the examination of urine, CSF, gastric aspirates, and other fluids and tissues. The sensitivity and specificity of PCR and other nucleic acid amplification tests can vary, but two commercial assays recently tested demonstrated a sensitivity of 95.9% and a specificity of 99.6%.[109] PCR also can be used to differentiate mycobacteria at the genus, group, and species level.[110,111] The feasibility of using such tools in resource-poor countries remains to be evaluated, but the diagnostic yield will be far higher than in the low-prevalence, resource-rich countries in which they are already available.

VI. TREATMENT

A. Treatment of Active TB Disease

DOTS has become a cornerstone of global TB control; its primary therapeutic innovations are DOT and short-course chemotherapy (SCC). The justification for SCC and for the other key components of the DOTS strategy has been documented elsewhere,[112] but it is important to note here that the introduction of rifampin permitted the dramatic shortening of duration of therapy.[113,114] Field trials in East Africa, Singapore, and Hong Kong showed that SCC yields higher cure rates than conventional treatment, especially when treatment was fully supervised.[37,39,115-117] The most commonly used drugs are the first-line antituberculosis drugs (see Chapter 6). It should be noted that fixed-dose combinations of these drugs are available and preliminary studies suggest that such preparations, which are discussed below, may enhance adherence and decrease the possibility of inadvertent monotherapy.

Global surveillance suggests that most strains of *M. tuberculosis* implicated in disease remain susceptible to all antituberculous medications. But even when TB disease is due to pan-susceptible strains of *M. tuberculosis*, special circumstances may call for alterations in the duration of treatment. For example, prolongation of SCC is recommended for cases of HIV-associated tuberculosis, as well as for the treatment of TB of the bones, brain, or meninges.[118-124] Some would favor the addition of cycloserine, which has excellent central nervous system (CNS) penetration, to regimens used to treat TB of the central nervous system.[125] Drug-resistant TB also calls for alterations in therapy and is discussed more fully below.

B. Treatment of Latent TB Infection

Although some have argued that screening and prophylaxis should remain a low priority in developing countries, it is nonetheless clear that these interventions, when coupled with effective treatment of active disease, could have a significant impact on TB incidence. Murray and Salomon have recently argued that INH prophylaxis for patients diagnosed with HIV infection "could save nearly 1 million lives if 10% of the HIV-positive population were screened each year." They estimate that fully 36% of all deaths averted would be among the HIV-negative population because of reduced transmission,[27] a point echoed by others working in regions in which both *M. tuberculosis* and HIV are endemic.[126] Assuming susceptibility, among infecting strains, to INH, the impact of mass preventive therapy over a period of 32 years could be considerable, "even with only 33% treatment completion, this strategy would avert 42.6 million cases and 16.7 million deaths."[27]

VII. RESISTANCE TO ANTITUBERCULOUS MEDICATIONS

Resistance to antituberculous drugs has been known since their introduction more than 50 years ago.[127-129] Yet resistance to at least INH and RIF (by convention, the definition of MDR-TB) has only recently been recognized as a serious global problem, one that does not spare resource-poor regions.[24,30,130] "In developing countries," observed WHO in 1996, "people with multidrug-resistant TB usually die, because effective treatment is often impossible in poor settings."[131] Although it has in the recent past been persuasively argued that all energies should be directed to increasing the extension of DOTS (and, thus, of SCC), the emergence of *M. tuberculosis* resistant to first-line drugs has by now been documented in almost all settings in which modern chemotherapy has been introduced.[24] SCC will not cure MDR-TB.[132,133]

Although some have claimed that drug-resistant (DR) strains are somehow less virulent or less transmissible than drug-susceptible (DS) strains, there are to date few data to support these claims.[31] In a wide variety of settings in the industrialized countries, highly DR strains of TB have caused explosive institutional outbreaks in hospitals, prisons, and shelters. Many of these nosocomial outbreaks have been associated with HIV; they have been notable for high case-fatality rates among the immunosuppressed and for high rates of transmission to immunocompetent caregivers.[134-138] Significant foci of HIV-associated MDR-TB have also been reported in Argentina, the Ivory Coast, and South Africa.[130,139-141] These outbreaks led to the assumption that the emergence of MDR-TB was somehow necessarily related to deficient TB control programs in the context of an emerging HIV pandemic,[142-144] but it has since become clear that significant outbreaks of MDR-TB may readily occur where HIV prevalence is low. In an outbreak in urban Peru, for example, fewer than 2% of patients with MDR-TB were seropositive for HIV.[145] Reports from penal institutions in Russia, where rates of HIV coinfection are almost nil, indicate that one third to one half of patients with TB have MDR-TB.[146-149]

Because MDR-TB is not readily constrained by prison bars or hospital walls, the true impact of these institutional outbreaks is yet to be felt; thousands of active MDR-TB cases may signal tens of thousands of new infections with *M. tuberculosis* resistant to all first-line drugs. But studies of drug resistance among more representative patient samples are critical if we are to make projections that can influence global TB control policy. A recent survey of resistance to antituberculous drugs conducted by WHO and the International Union Against Tuberculosis and Lung Disease (IUATLD) revealed MDR-TB to be present in 34 of 35 countries surveyed. A number of MDR-TB "hot spots" were identified, several of them located in developing countries. The proportion of prevalent TB cases resistant to any of the four drugs tested (INH, RIF, EMB, and SM) was highest in the Dominican Republic, Peru, Bolivia, India (Delhi region), Sierra Leone, as well as in several countries in Eastern Europe, including the former Soviet Union.[24]

In conclusion, we see that, in some settings with excellent national TB programs (e.g., Peru) and in many with poor-quality TB programs (e.g., India), MDR-TB is already endemic and threatens to undermine recent gains in TB control. Once MDR-TB strains are well established in a population, SCC will fail to cure a growing proportion of patients with TB disease.[132,133] Furthermore, there is growing evidence that challenging drug-resistant strains of *M. tuberculosis* with SCC is a means of amplifying already existing resistance to first-line drugs; we have termed this the "amplifier effect of short-course chemotherapy."[13,150] It is not yet clear at what cut-off point universal SCC will lead to treatment failure in a significant proportion of patients and compromise DOTS program performance, but our own experience in Latin America suggests that this number is lower than might have been thought. New strategies are needed in all of the MDR-TB "hot spots" already identified.

TABLE 16.5
Attributes of DOTS-Plus Models

	ITRs	Standardized
Efficacy	Very high	Moderate–high
Cost	High	Moderate–high
Risk of amplification	Very low	Low–moderate
Toxicity	Moderate	Moderate
Technical capacity required	High	Moderate

Source: Farmer, P. E. et al., *Tuberculosis: A Comprehensive International Approach,* 2nd ed., Marcel Dekker, New York, 1999. With permission.

VIII. RESPONDING TO MDR-TB IN RESOURCE-POOR SETTINGS: "DOTS-PLUS"

Given the undisputed efficacy of the DOTS package in settings in which resistance to first-line drugs is rare, the concept of "DOTS-Plus" — complementary, DOT-based strategies to contain MDR-TB — has been advanced.[151,152] The WHO has recently issued preliminary DOTS-Plus protocols which are now to be tested in settings in which MDR-TB already accounts for significant morbidity and mortality.[153] Two DOTS-Plus models have been introduced: one is based on individualized treatment regimens (ITRs)[152] and the other on standardized MDR-TB regimens. Because ITRs are designed for each patient according to the drug-susceptibility pattern of the infecting isolate, such regimens tend to be more efficacious, and amplification of resistance is less likely.[154] Drawbacks of ITRs include labor-intensive and costly laboratory testing, nonstandardized dosing, and multiple adjustments of regimens during the course of therapy.[155] Although almost all of the second-line drugs are off patent, they remain significantly more expensive than first-line drugs.

Standardized "DOTS-Plus" treatment regimens could, in principle, also be used in the treatment of MDR-TB. If patients failing DOTS are presumed to have MDR-TB and drug-susceptibility testing is unavailable, they might be placed on an empiric retreatment regimen consisting of second-line drugs. Standardized MDR-TB regimens could be tailored to the local epidemiology of TB using population surveillance data. Regimens would be designed according to resistance patterns commonly encountered in an outbreak. Advantages of standardized MDR-TB regimens would arguably include lower cost and greater ease of administration, but the disadvantages are clear: there is ample reason to fear that use of such regimens without drug-susceptibility testing will result in a higher failure rate, since some patients will be inadvertently deprived of drugs to which they are susceptible, just as some will receive drugs to which their infecting strains are resistant. Features of these two approaches to MDR-TB control are reviewed in Table 16.5.

It should be noted that only ITRs have already been piloted. In Peru, this DOTS-Plus strategy has already been shown to lead to high cure rates among patients with highly DR disease and significant parenchymal destruction.[145] The second approach, based on standardized MDR-TB regimens, has yet to be tested, but the WHO intends to supervise pilot studies beginning this year.

IX. CHALLENGES AT THE START OF A NEW MILLENIUM

One of the great ironies of global TB control is that TB resources are concentrated in precisely those settings with the lowest burden of disease. Disparities of access seem to be growing. The advent of HIV, the emergence of drug-resistant TB, and the need for novel strategies are felt far more acutely in high-prevalence, resource-poor settings than in industrialized nations. If TB, which has no nonhuman reservoir, is ever to be eliminated, more aggressive TB control measures are urgently needed, as are the resources to fund them. Despite tremendous advances over the last decade, existing TB control strategies are inadequate. DOTS alone will not suffice to reduce TB incidence. "Even with high uptake of DOTS in the most favorable context," noted Murray and Salomon, "incidence and mortality from tuberculosis in the next 3 decades will be enormous."[27]

We may have found powerful weapons in the war against TB, but will need many more if we hope to diminish the global burden of TB. Although basic science research, which would serve those seeking to develop new vaccines and drugs effective against *M. tuberculosis,* has flagged in recent decades, a number of recent developments may produce new tools in the coming years.

A. VACCINE DEVELOPMENT

Vaccine development offers one of our best chances for improving TB control (see Chapter 15). Experiments attempting to modify the genome of *M. tuberculosis* in order to diminish strain virulence have shown limited success.[156] Attempts to create an auxotrophic mutant of *M. tuberculosis* may obviate the need for BCG; promising results have been shown in knock-out mice.[157] DNA vaccines, which would be formulated to code for few antigens and to not interfere with skin-test sensitivity, are also under development.[158-160]

B. CASE FINDING

The means by which TB cases are detected is again becoming the subject of debate in TB control. Should cases be actively sought through mass screening of populations or should they be registered passively when symptomatic patients seek care in centers equipped to diagnose TB? WHO has strongly recommended passive case finding (PCF)[161,162] because "active case finding (ACF) would be prohibitively expensive in most countries, and because population surveys typically find that four in five cases have already sought medical attention at the time of detection by mass screening," according to Dye et al.[29] In 1984, Styblo predicted that "mass indiscriminate radiography will have no place in any future tuberculosis control programme."[163] But confident claims about the case finding strategy appropriate for use in high-prevalence settings need to be questioned as long as TB remains such a significant cause of morbidity and mortality. This is likely true in some regions in which TB remains a ranking cause of mortality, and in certain congregate settings, such as homeless shelters and prisons. For example, Layton and colleagues, working in New York City during a time of resurgent TB, advocated universal "radiographic screening in correctional facilities where the inmate population changes rapidly and where tuberculosis and HIV infection are prevalent."[164] As noted earlier it is not possible to diagnose a large proportion of TB cases with smear microscopy alone. Thus, this method, though inexpensive, is not sufficient as long as TB-control policy is driven by clinical efficacy — the detection and cure of all cases of active TB. The analysis of Murray and Salomon suggests that ACF could reduce TB mortality by 25 to 33%. "Perhaps the time has come," they concluded, "for a critical reexamination of the costs, risks, and benefits of active screening." The same analysis suggests that continuous MMR screening could decrease TB incidence by 22%; TB mortality could be reduced by 29%.[165]

C. NEW DRUG DEVELOPMENT AND FIXED-DOSE COMBINATIONS

New drug development could reduce the need for prolonged courses of therapy. The advent of rifampin in the 1960s led to a significant reduction in the duration of chemotherapy for active TB. With the exception of rifapentine, a congener of rifampin, there have been no novel agents developed in years (the exception to this claim being the fluoroquinolones, serendipitously found to have activity against a wide array of mycobacteria).[166] Although certain drug companies have announced

---

TABLE 16.6
Advantages of Fixed-Dose Combinations

- Prevention of monotherapy
- Reduction in physician prescription error
- Simplification of procurement and prescribing practices
- Reduction in the number of tablets swallowed
- Reduction in patient confusion in self-administered chemotherapy

Source: Moulding, T., Dutt, A., and Reichman, L., *Ann. Intern. Med.,*
1999, 122(12):951–54. With permission.

---

plans to develop new drugs, progress has been slow. As Reichman has noted, "Most of the drug companies that publicly announced a quest for TB drugs at the time of the recent resurgence have been noticeably quiet. Few have even shown interest in developing such drugs."[167]

Therapy incorporating two or more drugs (the number of drugs depending on the relative cidal efficacy) to which the infecting isolate is fully susceptible is necessary in order to avoid the development of drug resistance in *M. tuberculosis.* One strategy to prevent inadvertent monotherapy is the use of antituberculous therapeutic agents in fixed-dose combinations (FDCs), in use since the introduction of isoniazid in 1952.[168] Although the WHO and IUATLD endorse the implementation of FDCs with proven bioavailability, only 25% of rifampin is presently used in such formulations.[169] Advantages of FDCs are listed in Table 16.6.[170]

D. RAPID DETECTION OF DRUG RESISTANCE

Rapid detection of drug resistance could avoid the inappropriate triage of patients likely to fail SCC to precisely such regimens. Among new technologies of obvious relevance are nucleic acid amplification tests and rapid genetic probes for resistance to rifampin and other first-line drugs. Tests based on such innovations would confer several advantages over conventional susceptibility testing, including a decrease in the turnaround time of test results and the possibility for automation.[171] In areas with a high prevalence of MDRTB, the identification of mutations in the *rpoB* gene, associated with resistance to rifampin, could serve as a surrogate marker for MDR-TB.[172] Techniques have been developed that can test for the presence of rifampin using PCR and a reverse hybridization assay with up to 97% sensitivity in less than 48 hours.[173] Riska and coworkers have recently developed a novel method to test for both INH and RIF resistance. The "Bronx Box" utilizes a bacteriophage to introduce the firefly luciferase gene into isolates of *M. tuberculosis,* which yields visible light in the presence of ATP and the exogenous substrate luciferin. Effective antituberculosis drugs will eliminate light production from susceptible isolates; resistant isolates will be unaffected. Results are analyzed using a light-tight box and a polaroid film cassette. This procedure can be completed within 3 days.[174] Such technologies could help triage patients with MDR-TB into up-front MDR-TB regimens that would lead to cure rather than to amplification of resistance through inappropriate empiric regimens.

X. CONCLUSIONS

The full characterization of the genome of *M. tuberculosis* reminds us that much has been accomplished, as does the decline of TB in much of the industrialized world. But the future of the global TB pandemic will be determined by the success of control measures in the high-prevalence areas in which resources are scarce. That TB could remain the world's leading infectious cause of adult deaths fully 50 years after the development of effective chemotherapy would no doubt surprise those who helped to develop these agents. The advent of HIV and of strains of *M. tuberculosis* resistant to all first-line drugs remind us of the need for new and more effective tools for the treatment and control of these persistent plagues. Applying these tools where the burden of disease is greatest will remain the central task of 21st century TB control.

REFERENCES

1. World Health Organization, Global tuberculosis control: WHO report 1999, Geneva, 1999.
2. World Health Organization, WHO report on the tuberculosis epidemic, Geneva, 1997, WHO/TB/97.224.
3. Sudre, P., ten Dam, G., and Kochi, A., Tuberculosis: a global overview of the situation today, *Bull. World Health Org.,* 1992, 70(2):149–59.
4. Kochi, A., The global tuberculosis situation and the new control strategy for the World Health Organization, *Tubercle,* 1991, 72:1–6.
5. Schulzer, M., Fitzgerald, J. M., Enarson, D. A., and Grzybowski, S., An estimate of the future size of the tuberculosis problem in sub-Saharan Africa resulting from HIV infection, *Tuberc. Lung Dis.,* 1992, 73:52–8.
6. Long, R., Scalcini, M., Manfreda, J., Carre, G., Philippe, E., Hershfield, E., Sekla, L., and Stackiw, W., Impact of human immunodeficiency virus type 1 on tuberculosis in rural Haiti, *Am. Rev. Respir. Dis.,* 1991 Jan., 143(1):69–73.
7. McKenna, M., McCray, E., and Onorato, I., The epidemiology of tuberculosis among foreign-born persons in the United States, 1986 to 1993, *N. Engl. J. Med.,* 1995, 332(16):1071–6.
8. Zuber, P. L., McKenna, M. T., Binkin, N. J., Onorato, I. M., and Castro, K. G., Long-term risk of tuberculosis among foreign-born persons in the United States, *JAMA,* 1997, 278(4):304–30.
9. Recommendations for prevention and control of tuberculosis among foreign-born persons, Report of the working group on tuberculosis among foreign-born persons, *Morbid. Mortal. World Rep.,* 1998, 47:1–49.
10. TB Prevention and Control, 1997 Annual Statistical Report, Division of Tuberculosis Prevention and Control, Bureau of Communicable Diseases, Massachusetts Department of Public Health.
11. Mitnick, C., Furin, J., Henry, C., and Ross, J., Tuberculosis among the foreign born in Massachusetts, 1982-1984: a reflection of social and economic disadvantage, *Int. J. Tuberc. Lung Dis.,* 1998, 2(9):S32–S40.
12. EuroTB (CESES/KNCV) and the national coordinators for tuberculosis surveillance in the WHO European Region, *Surveillance of Tuberculosis in Europe,* Report on tuberculosis cases notified in 1996, September 1998.
13. Farmer, P. E., Bayona, J., Becerra, M., Furin, J., Henry, C., Hiatt, H., Kim, J. Y., Mitnick, C. D., Nardell, E., and Shin, S., The dilemma of MDR-TB in the global era, *Int. J. Tuberc. Lung Dis.,* 1998, 2(11):869–76.
14. Stanford, J. L., Grange, J. M., and Pozniak, A., Is Africa lost? *Lancet,* 1991, 338:557–8.
15. Cantwell, M. and Binkin, N., Impact of HIV on tuberculosis in sub-Saharan Africa: a regional perspective, *Tuberc. Lung Dis.,* 3, 205–214, 1997.
16. Gaidamoniene, D., Butkiene, P., Davidaviciene, E., Sosnovskaja, A., Baravykiene, V., and Slapkauskaite, D., Tuberculosis trends in Lithuania, *Int. J. Tuberc. Lung Dis.,* 1998, 2(11):S241.
17. Program in Infectious Disease and Social Change, The Global Impact of Drug-Resistant Tuberculosis, Harvard Medical School, Boston, 1999.
18. Farmer, P. E., Cruel and unusual: drug-resistant tuberculosis as punishment, in Stern, V. and Jones, R., Eds., *Sentenced to Die? The problem of TB in prisons in east and central Europe and Central Asia,* London: Prison Reform International, 1999.
19. Narain, J. P., Raviglione, M. C., and Kochi, A., HIV-associated tuberculosis in developing countries: epidemiology and strategies for prevention, *Tuberc. Lung Dis.,* 1992 Dec, 73(6), 311–21.
20. Selwyn, P. A., Sckell, B. M., Alcabes, P., Friedland, G. H., Klein, R. S., and Schoenbaum, E. E., High risk of active tuberculosis in HIV-infected drug users with cutaneous anergy, *JAMA,* 1992, 268:504–9.
21. FitzGerald, J. M., Grzybowski, S., and Allen, E. A., The impact of human immunodeficiency virus infection on tuberculosis and its control, *Chest,* 1991, 100(1):191–200.

22. Cantwell, M. and Binkin, N., Impact of HIV on tuberculosis in sub-Saharan Africa: a regional perspective, *Tuberc. Lung Dis.*, 3, 205–214.

23. Farmer, P. E., Social inequalities and emerging infectious diseases, *Emerg. Infect. Dis.*, 1996, 2(4):259–269.

24. Pablos-Mendez, A., Raviglione, M. C., Laszlo, A., Binkin, N., Rieder, H. L., Bustreo, F., Cohn, D. L., Lambregts-van Weezenbeek, C. S. B., Kim, S. J., Chaulet, P., et al., Global surveillance for antituberculosis-drug resistance, 1994–1997, *N. Engl. J. Med.*, 1998, 338:1641–49.

25. Murray, C. J. L. and Lopez, A. D., Alternative projections of mortality and disability by cause 1990–2020: Global Burden of Disease Study, *Lancet*, 1997, 349:1498–504.

26. World Health Organization, TB: a crossroads, WHO Report on the Tuberculosis Epidemic, Geneva, 1998, WHO/TB/98.247.

27. Murray, C. J. L. and Salomon, J. A., Modeling the impact of global tuberculosis control strategies, *Proc. Natl. Acad. Sci.*, 1998, 95:13881–6.

28. Blower, S. M., Small, P. M., and Hopewell, P., Control strategies for tuberculosis epidemics: new models for old problems, *Science*, 1996, 273:497–500.

29. Dye, C., Garnett, G. P., Sleeman, K., and Williams, B. G., Prospects for worldwide tuberculosis control under WHO DOTS strategy, *Lancet*, 1998, 352:1886–91.

30. World Health Organization, Anti-tuberculosis drug resistance in the world: the WHO/IUATLD Global Project on Anti-Tuberculosis Drug Resistance Surveillance 1994–1997, Geneva, 1997, WHO/TB/97.229.

31. Farmer, P. E., Bayona, J., Becerra, M., Daily, J., Furin, J., Garcia, D., Kim, J. Y., Mitnick, C., Nardell, E., Raymonville, M., et al. Poverty, inequality, and drug resistance: meeting community needs, *Proc. Int. Union Against Tuberc. Lung Dis. N. Am. Reg. Conf.*, Feb 27 to Mar 2, 1997, 88–102.

32. Bifani, P., Plikaytis, B., Kapur, V., Stockbauer, K., Pan, X., Lutfey, M. L., Mogzaheh, S. L., Eisner, W., Daniel, T. M., Kaplan, M. H., et al., Origin and interstate spread of a New York City multidrug-resistant *Mycobacterium tuberculosis* clone family, *JAMA*, 1996, 275(6):452–7.

33. Timperi, R., Sloutsky, A., and Farmer, P. E., Global laboratory testing capacity for tuberculosis, *Int. J. Tuberc. Lung Dis.*, 1998, 2(11):S290–S291.

34. Murray, C. J. L., Social, economic and operational research on tuberculosis: recent studies and some priority questions, *Bull. Int. Union Against Tuberc. Lung Dis.*, 1991 Dec, 66(4):149–56 .

35. World Health Organization, WHO tuberculosis programme: framework for effective tuberculosis control, Geneva, 1994, WHO/TB/94.175.

36. Third East African/British Medical Research Council Study, Controlled clinical trial of four short-course regimens of chemotherapy for two durations in the treatment of pulmonary tuberculosis: second report, *Tubercle*, 1980, 61:59–69.

37. Cohn, D. L., Catlin, B. J., Peterson, F. N., Judson, F. N., and Sbarbaro, J. A., A 62-dose, 6-month therapy for pulmonary and extrapulmonary tuberculosis: a twice-weekly, directly-observed, and cost-effective regimen, *Ann. Int. Med.*, 1990, 112:407–15.

38. Hong Kong Chest Service/British Medical Research Council, Controlled trial of 4 three-times weekly regimens and a daily regimen all given for 6 months for pulmonary tuberculosis, Second report: the results up to 24 months, *Tubercle*, 1982, 63:89–98.

39. Snider, D. E., Graczyk, J., Bek, E., and Rogowski, J., Supervised six-months treatment of newly diagnosed pulmonary tuberculosis using isoniazid, rifampin, and pyrazinamide with and without streptomycin, *Am. Rev. Respir. Dis.*, 1984, 130:1091–4.

40. Singapore Tuberculosis Service/British Medical Research Council, Five-year follow-up of a clinical trial of three 6-month regimens of chemotherapy given intermittently in the continuation phase in the treatment of pulmonary tuberculosis, *Am. Rev. Respir. Dis.*, 1988, 137;1147–50.

41. Iseman, M. D. and Sbarbaro, J. A., Short-course chemotherapy of tuberculosis: Hail Britannia (and friends)! *Am. Rev. Respir. Dis.*, 1987, 136:697–98.

42. Murray, C. J. L., DeJonghe, E., Chum, H. J., Nyangulu, D. S., Salomao, A., and Styblo, K., Cost-effectiveness of chemotherapy for pulmonary tuberculosis in three sub-Saharan African countries, *Lancet*, 1991, 338:1305–8.

43. China Tuberculosis Control Collaboration, Results of directly observed short-course chemotherapy in 112,842 Chinese patients with smear-positive tuberculosis, *Lancet*, 1996, 347:358–62.

44. Raviglione, M. C., Dye, C., Schmidt, S., and Kochi, A., Assessment of worldwide tuberculosis control. WHO Global Surveillance and Monitoring Project, *Lancet,* 1997 Aug 30, 350(9078):624–9.

45. World Health Organization, The continually changing threat of infectious diseases, in *Investing in Health Research and Development,* Geneva, 1996.

46. Miles, S. H. and Maat, R. B., A successful supervised outpatient short-course tuberculosis treatment programme in an open refugee camp on the Thai-Cambodian border, *Am. Rev. Respir. Dis.,* 1984, 130:827–30.

47. Zhang, L. X. and Kan, G. Q., Tuberculosis control programme in Beijing, *Tuberc. Lung Dis.,* 1992, 73:162–66.

48. Iseman, M. D., Cohn, D. L., and Sbarbaro, J. A., Directly observed treatment of tuberculosis — we can't afford not to try it, *N. Engl. J. Med.,* 1993, 338:576–78.

49. Center for Disease Control and Prevention, Initial therapy for tuberculosis in the era of multidrug resistance, Recommendations of the Advisory Council for the Elimination of Tuberculosis, *Morbid. Mortal. Wkly. Rep.,* 1993, 42(RR7):1–8.

50. Frieden, T. R., Fujiwara, P. I., Washko, R. M., and Hamburg, M. A., Tuberculosis in New York City — turning the tide, *N. Engl. J. Med.,* 1995, 333:229–33.

51. Chaulk, C. P., Moore-Rice, K., Rizzo, R., and Chaisson, R. E., Eleven years of community-based directly observed therapy for tuberculosis, *JAMA,* 1995, 274:945–51.

52. Fox, W., The problem of self-administration of drugs with particular reference to pulmonary tuberculosis, *Tubercle,* 1958, 39:269–74.

53. Fox, W., Self-administration of medicaments: a review of published work and a study of the problems, *Bull. Int. Union Tuberc.,* 1961, 31:307–31.

54. Sbarbaro, J. A., The patient-physician relationship: compliance revisited, *Ann. Allergy,* 1990, 64:326–32.

55. Farmer, P. E., Robin, S., Ramilus, S. L., and Kim, J. Y., Tuberculosis, poverty, and "compliance:" lessons from rural Haiti, *Sem. Respir. Infect.,* 1991, 6:373–9.

56. Sumartojo, E., When tuberculosis treatment fails: a social behavioral account of patient adherence, *Am. Rev. Respir. Dis.,* 1993, 147:1311–20.

57. Farmer, P. E., Social scientists and the new tuberculosis, *Soc. Sci. Med.,* 1997, 44(3):347–58.

58. Banjeri, D. and Anderson, S., A sociological study of awareness of symptoms among persons with pulmonary tuberculosis, *Bull. World Health Org.,* 1963, 29:665–83.

59. Toman, K., *Tuberculosis Case-Finding and Chemotherapy,* Geneva, World Health Organization, 1979.

60. Shimao, T., *Tuberculosis Case-Finding,* Geneva, World Health Organization, 1982, WHO/TB/82.131.

61. Styblo, K., Epidemiology of tuberculosis, *VEB Gustav Fischer Verlag Jena,* 1984.

62. Garland, L. H., Studies on the accuracy of diagnostic procedures, *Am. J. Roentgenol. Radium Ther. Nucl. Med.,* 1959, 82:25–38.

63. Urbanczik, R., Present position of microscopy and of culture in diagnostic mycobacteriology, *Zbl. Bakt. Hyg.,* 1985, A260:81–87.

64. Weil, D., Drug supply — meeting a global need, in Porter, J. and McAdam, K. Eds., *Tuberculosis: Back to the Future,* Chichester, U.K., John Wiley & Sons, 1994, 124–149.

65. Chaulet, P., The supply of antituberculosis drugs and national drugs policies, *Tuberc. Lung Dis.,* 1992, 73:295–304.

66. Hopewell, P. C., Sanchez-Hernandez, M., Baron, R. B., and Ganter, B., Operational evaluation of treatment for tuberculosis. Results of a "standard" 12-month regimen in Peru, *Am. Rev. Respir. Dis.,* 1984 Mar, 129(3):439–43.

67. Hopewell, P. C., Ganter, B., Baron, R. B., and Sanchez-Hernandez, M., Operational evaluation of treatment for tuberculosis. Results of 8- and 12-month regimens in Peru, *Am. Rev. Respir. Dis.,* 1985, 132(4):737–41.

68. Ministerio de Salud, Tuberculosis en el Peru — Informe 1997, Lima, Peru: Ministerio de Salud, 1998.

69. Salfinger, M. and Pfyffer, G. E., The new diagnostic mycobacteriology laboratory, *Eur. J. Clin. Microbiol. Infect. Dis.,* 1994, 13(11):961–79.

70. DiPerri, G., Cade, G. P., Castelli, F., et al., Transmission of HIV-associated tuberculosis to health care workers, *Infect. Cont. Hosp. Epidemiol.,* 1993, 14:67–72.

71. Lotte, A., Wasz-Hockert, O., Poisson, N., Dumitrescu, N., Verron, M., and Couvet, E., BCG compli-
    cations. Estimates of the risks among vaccinated subjects and statistical analysis of their main
    characteristics, *Adv. Tuberc. Res.,* 1984, 21:107–93.
72. Colditz, G. A., Brewer, T. F., Berkey, C. S., Wilson, M. E., Burdick, E., Fineberg, H. V., and Mosteller,
    F., Efficacy of BCG vaccine in the prevention of tuberculosis. Meta-analysis of the published literature,
    JAMA, 1994, 271(9):698–702.
73. Young, D. B. and Duncan, K., Prospects for new interventions in the treatment and prevention of
    mycobacterial disease, *Ann. Rev. Microbiol.,* 1995, 49:641–73.
74. Colditz, G. A., Berkey, C. S., Mosteller, F., Brewer, T. F., Wilson, M. E., Burdick, E., and Fineberg,
    H. V., The efficacy of Bacillus Calmette-Guérin vaccination of newborns and infants in the prevention
    of tuberculosis: meta-analysis of the published literature, *Pediatrics,* 1995, 96(1):29–35.
75. Kritski, A. L., Ozorio-Marques, M. J., Rabahi, M. F., Silva-Vieira, M. A. M., Werneck-Barroso, E.,
    Carvalho, C. E. S., Noronha-Andrade, G., Bravo-de-Souza, R., Andrade, L. M., Gontijo, P. P., et al.,
    Transmission of tuberculosis to close contacts of patients with multidrug-resistant tuberculosis, *Am.
    J. Respir. Crit. Care Med.,* 1996, 153:331–5.
76. Jenney, A. W. and Spelman, D. W., In support of bacillus of Calmette and Guérin for healthcare
    workers, *Inf. Cont. Hosp. Epidemiol.,* 1998, 19:191–93.
77. Hopewell, P. C., Impact of human immunodeficiency virus infection on the epidemiology, clinical
    features, management, and control of tuberculosis, *Clin. Infect. Dis.,* 1992, 15:540–7.
78. Styblo, K., The relationship between the risk of tuberculous infection and the risk of developing
    infectious tuberculosis, *Bull. Int. Union Against Tuberc.,* 1985, 60:117–9.
79. Migliori, G. B., Borghesi, A., Spanevello, A., Eriki, P., Raviglione, M., Maciocco, G., Morandi, A.,
    Ballardini, L., and Neri, M., Risk of infection and estimated incidence of tuberculosis in northern
    Uganda, *Eur. Respir. J.,* 1994, 7(5):946–53.
80. Lasante, Z., Normes et Procedures du Traitement de la Tuberculose, Cange, Haiti, and Boston, MA:
    Program in Infectious Disease and Social Change, Harvard Medical School, Boston, 1998.
81. Murray, C. J. L., Styblo, K., and Rouillon, A., Tuberculosis, in Jamison, D. T., Mosley, W. H.,
    Measham, A. R., et al., Eds., *Disease Control Priorities in Developing Countries,* New York, Oxford
    University Press, 1993.
82. Jacobson, M. A., Mycobacterial diseases. Tuberculosis and disseminated *Mycobacterium avium* com-
    plex infection, in Sande, M. A. and Volberding, P. A., Eds., *The Medical Management of AIDS,* 3rd
    ed., Philadelphia, W.B. Saunders, 1992.
83. Bishop, P. J. and Neumann, G., The history of the Ziehl-Neelsen stain, *Tubercle,* 1970, 51(2):196–206.
84. Kinyoun, J. J., A note on the Uhlenhuths method for sputum examination, for tubercle bacilli, *Am. J.
    Pub. Health,* 1915, 5:867–70.
85. Baily, G. V. J., Savic, D., Gothi, G. D., Naidu, V. B., and Nair, S. S., Potential yield of pulmonary
    tuberculosis cases by direct microscopy of sputum in a district of South India, *Bull. World Health
    Org.,* 1967, 37:875–92.
86. Igupe, Y. A., Rieder, H. L., and Enarson, D. A., The yield of acid-fast bacilli from serial smears in
    routine microscopy laboratories in rural Tanzania, *Trans. R. Soc. Trop. Med. Hyg.,* 1996, 90(3):258–61.
87. Hall, G. H., The clinical application of Bayes' Theorem, *Lancet,* 1967, 2:555–57.
88. Hobby, G. L., Holman, A. P., Iseman, M. D., and Jones, J. M., Enumeration of tubercle bacilli in
    sputum of patients with pulmonary tuberculosis, *Antimicrob. Agents Chemother.,* 1973, 4(2):94–104.
89. Salfinger, M. and Pfyffer, G. E., The new diagnostic mycobacteriology laboratory, *Eur. J. Clin.
    Microbiol. Infect. Dis.,* 1994, 13(11):961–79.
90. Barnes, P. F., Bloch, A. B., Davidson, P. T., and Snider, Jr., D. E., Tuberculosis in patients with human
    immunodeficiency virus infection, *N. Engl. J. Med.,* 1991, 324(23):1644–50.
91. Long, R., Scalcini, M., Manfreda, J., Jean Baptiste, M., and Hershfield, E., The impact of HIV on
    the usefulness of sputum smears for the diagnosis of tuberculosis, *Am. J. Pub. Health,* 1991,
    81:1326–28.
92. Smith, R. L., Yew, K., Berkowitz, K. A., and Aranda, C. P., Factors affecting the yield of acid-fast
    sputum smears in patients with HIV and tuberculosis, *Chest,* 1994, 106:684–86.
93. Pitchenik, A. E. and Fertel, D., Tuberculosis and nontuberculous mycobacterial disease, *Med. Clin.
    N. Am.,* 1992, 76(1):121–71.

94. Heifets, L. B. and Cangelosi, G. A., Drug susceptibility testing of *Mycobacterium tuberculosis:* a neglected problem at the turn of the century, *Int. J. Tuberc. Lung Dis.,* 1999, 3(7):564–81.

95. Vareldzis, B. P., Grosset, J., de Kantor, I., et al., Drug-resistant tuberculosis: laboratory issues, World Health Organization recommendations, *Tuberc. Lung Dis.,* 1994, 75:1–7.

96. Krivinka, R., Drapela, J., Kubik, A., Dankova, D., Krivanek, J., Ruzha, J., Mikova, Z., and Hejdova, E., Epidemiological and clinical study of tuberculosis in the district of Kolin, Czechoslovakia, *Bull. World Health Org.,* 1974, 51:59–69.

97. Haygood, T. M. and Briggs, J. E., World War II military led the way in screening chest radiography, *Mil. Med.,* 1992, 157(3):113–6.

98. Garland, L. H., Studies on the accuracy of diagnostic procedures, *Am. J. Roentgenol. Radium Ther. Nucl. Med.,* 1959, 82:25–38.

99. Barnes, P. F., Bloch, A. B., Davidson, P. T., and Snider, Jr., D. E., Tuberculosis in patients with human immunodeficiency virus infection, *N. Engl. J. Med.,* 1991, 324(23):1644–50.

100. Harries, A. D., Maher, D., and Nunn, P., An approach to the problems of diagnosing and treating adult smear-negative pulmonary tuberculosis in high-HIV-prevanence settings in sub-Saharan Africa, *Bull. World Health Org.,* 1998, 76:651–62.

101. Kahn, E. A. and Starke, J. R., Diagnosis of tuberculosis in children: increased need for better methods, *Emerg. Infect. Dis.,* 1995, 1:115–23.

102. Starke, J. R. and Taylor-Watts, K. T., Tuberculosis in the pediatric population of Houston, Texas, *Pediatrics,* 1989, 84:839–55.

103. Jacobs, R. F. and Starke, J. R., Tuberculosis in children, *Med. Clin. N. Am.,* 1993, 77:1335–51.

104. Starke, J. R., Tuberculosis in children, *Prim. Care,* 1996, 23:861–81.

105. Crofton, J., Horne, N., and Miller, H., *Clinical Tuberculosis,* 2nd ed., London, MacMillian Education LTD, 1999.

106. Strumpf, I. J., Tsang, A. Y., and Sayre, J. W., Re-evaluation of sputum staining for the diagnosis of pulmonary tuberculosis, *Am. Rev. Respir. Dis.,* 1979, 119:599–602.

107. Cousins, D. V., Wilton, S. D., Francis, B. R., and Gow, B. L., Use of polymerase chain reaction for rapid diagnosis of tuberculosis, *J. Clin. Microbiol.,* 1992, 30(1):255–58.

108. Tan, M. F., Ng, W. C., Chan, S. H., and Tan, W. C., Comparative usefulness of PCR in the detection of *Mycobacterium tuberculosis* in different clinical specimens, *J. Med. Microbiol.,* 1997, 46:164–69.

109. Piersimoni, C., Callegaro, A., Nista, D., Bornigia, S., De Conti, F., Santini, G., and De Sio, G., Comparative evaluation of two commercial amplification assays for direct detection of *Mycobacterium tuberculosis* complex in respiratory specimens. *J. Clin. Microbiol.,* 1997, 35(1):193–96.

110. Böddinghaus, B., Rogall, T., Flohr, T., Blöcker, H., and Böttger, E., Detection and identification of mycobacteria by amplification of rRNA, *J. Clin. Micribiol.,* 1990, 28(8):1751–59.

111. Telenti, A., Marchesi, F., Balz, M., Bally, F., Böttger, E., and Bodmer, T., Rapid identification of mycobacteria to the species level by polymerase chain reaction and restriction enzyme analysis, *J. Clin. Microbiol.,* 1993, 31(2):175–78.

112. World Health Organization, Tuberculosis control: the DOTS strategy, Geneva, 1997, WHO/TB/97.228.

113. Nitti, V., Antituberculosis activity of rifampin, report of studies performed and in progress (1966–1971), *Chest,* 1972, 61:589–98.

114. Bates, J. H., Treatment of tuberculosis, *Adv. Intern. Med.,* 1975, 20:1–21.

115. Third East African/British Medical Research Council Study, Controlled clinical trial of four short-course regimens of chemotherapy for two durations in the treatment of pulmonary tuberculosis: second report, *Tubercle,* 1980, 61:59–69.

116. Hong Kong Chest Service/British Medical Research Council, Controlled trial of 4 three-times weekly regimens and a daily regimen all give for 6 months for pulmonary tuberculosis, second report: the results up to 24 months, *Tubercle,* 1982, 63:89–98.

117. Singapore Tuberculosis Service/British Medical Research Council, Five-year follow-up of a clinical trial of three 6-month regimens of chemotherapy given intermittently in the continuation phase in the treatment of pulmonary tuberculosis, *Am. Rev. Respir. Dis.,* 1988, 137:1147–50.

118. Perriens, J. H., St. Louis, M. E., Mukadi, Y. B., Brown, C., Prignot, J., Pouthier, F., Portaels, F., Willame, J. C., Mandala, J. K., Kaboto, M., et al., Pulmonary tuberculosis in HIV-infected patients in Zaire — a controlled trial of treatment for either 6 or 12 months, *N. Engl. J. Med.,* 1995, 332:779–84.

119. Pulido, F., Peña, J. M., Rubio, R., Moreno, S., González, J., Guijarro, C., Costa, J. R., and Vázquez, J. J., Relapse of tuberculosis after treatment in human immunodeficiency virus-infected patients, *Arch. Intern. Med.*, 1997, 157:227–32.

120. Rajeswari, R., Balasubramanian, R., Venkatesan, P., Sivasubramanian, S., Soundarapandian, S., Shanmugasundaram, T. K., and Prabhakar, R., Short-course chemotherapy in the treatment of Pott's paraplegia: report on five-year follow-up, *Int. J. Tuberc. Lung Dis.*, 1997, 1(2):152–8.

121. Moon, M. S., Kim, I., Woo, Y. K., and Park, Y. O., Conservative treatment of tuberculosis of the thoracic and lumbar spine in adults and children, *Int. Orthop.*, 1987, 11:315–22.

122. Griffiths, D. L., The treatment of tuberculosis of bone and joint, *Trans. R. Soc. Trop. Med. Hyg.*, 1978, 72(6):559–63.

123. Alarcón, F., Escalante, L., Pérez, Y., Banda, H., Chacón, G., and Dueñas, G., Tuberculous meningitis, short course of chemotherapy, *Arch. Neurol.*, 1990, 47:1313–17.

124. Goel, A., Pandya, S. K., and Satoskar, A. R., Whither short-course therapy for tuberculous meningitis? *Neurosurgery*, 1990, 27(3):418–21.

125. Erill, S., Cycloserine and tuberculous meningitis, *Lancet*, 1973, 2:1213.

126. Pape, J. W., Jean, S. S., Ho, J. L., Hafner, A., and Johnson, Jr., W. D., Effect of isoniazid prophylaxis on incidence of active tuberculosis and progression of HIV infection, *Lancet*, 1993, 342:268–72.

127. Crofton, J. and Mitchison, D., Streptomycin resistance in pulmonary tuberculosis, *Br. Med. J.*, 1948, 2:1009–15.

128. Canetti, G., Present aspects of bacterial resistance in tuberculosis, *Am. Rev. Respir. Dis.*, 1965, 92:687–903.

129. Public Health Service Cooperation Investigation, Prevalence of drug resistance in previously untreated patients, *Am. Rev. Respir. Dis.*, 1964, 89:327–36.

130. Cohn, D. L., Bustreo, F., and Raviglione, M. C., Drug-resistant tuberculosis: review of the worldwide situation and the WHO/IUATLD Global Surveillance Project, *Clin. Infect. Dis.*, 1997, 24:S121–S130.

131. World Health Organization, Groups at risk, WHO report on the tuberculosis epidemic, Geneva, 1996, WHO/TB/96.198

132. Manalo, F., Tan, F., Sbarbaro, J. A., and Iseman, M. D., Community-based short-course treatment of pulmonary tuberculosis in a developing nation, Initial report of an eight-month, largely intermittent regimen in a population with a high prevalence of drug resistance, *Am. Rev. Respir. Dis.*, 1990, 142:1301–5.

133. Shimao, T., Drug resistance in tuberculosis control, *Tubercle*, 1987, 68:5–15.

134. Beck-Sague, C., Dooley, S., Sutton, M., et al., Hospital outbreak of multidrug-resistant *Mycobacterium tuberculosis* infections: factors in transmission to staff and HIV-infected patients, *JAMA*, 1992, 268:1280–6.

135. Valway, S. E., Richards, S. B., Kovacovich, J., Greifinger, R. B., Crawford, J. T., and Dooley, S. W., Outbreak of multi-drug-resistant tuberculosis in a New York State prison, 1991, *Am. J. Epidemiol.*, 1994, 140(2):113–22.

136. Fujiwara, P., Cook, S., Rutherford, C., et al., A continuing survey of drug-resistant tuberculosis, New York City, April, 1994, *Arch. Intern. Med.*, 1997, 157:531–6.

137. Moore, M., Onorato, I. M., McCray, E., and Castro, K. G., Trends in drug-resistant tuberculosis in the United States, 1993–1996, *JAMA*, 1997 Sep 10, 278(10):833–7.

138. Bifani, P., Plikaytis, B., Kapur, V., Stockbauer, K., Pan, X., Lutfey, M. L., Mogzaheh, S. L., Eisner, W., Daniel, T. M., Kaplan, M. H., et al., Origin and interstate spread of a New York City multidrug-resistant *Mycobacterium tuberculosis* clone family, *JAMA*, 1996, 275(6):452–7.

139. Davies, G. R., Pillay, M., Sturm, A. W., and Wilkinson, D., Emergence of multi-drug resistant tuberculosis in rural South Africa, *Int. J. Tuberc. Lung Dis.*, 1998, 2(11):S327.

140. Aita, J., Barrera, L., Reniero, A., et al., Hospital transmission of multidrug-resistant *Mycobacterium tuberculosis* in Rosario, Argentina, *Medicina (Buenos Aires)*, 1996, 56:48–50.

141. Ritacco, V., Di Lonardo, M., Reniero, A., Ambroggi, M., Barrera, L., Dambrosi, A., Lopez, B., Isola, N., and de Kantor, I. N., Nosocomial spread of human immunodeficiency virus-related multidrug-resistant tuberculosis in Buenos Aires, *J. Infect. Dis.*, 1997, 176:637–42.

142. Crawford, J. T., Epidemiology of tuberculosis: the impact of HIV and multidrug-resistant strains, *Immunobiology*, 1994, 191:337–43.

143. Frieden, T., Fujiwara, E., Washko, R., and Hamburg, M., Tuberculosis in New York City: turning the tide, *N. Engl. J. Med.,* 1995, 333:229–33.

144. Brudney, K. and Dobkin, J., Resurgent tuberculosis in New York City: human immunodeficiency virus, homelessness, and the decline of tuberculosis control programs, *Am. Rev. Respir. Dis.,* 1991, 144:745–9.

145. Farmer, P. E., Bayona, J., Shin, S., Alvarez, L., Becerra, M., Nardell, E., Nuñez, C., Sanchez, E., Timperi, R., and Kim, J. Y., Preliminary results of community-based MDR-TB treatment in Lima, Peru, *Int. J. Tuberc. Lung Dis.,* 1998, 2(11):S371.

146. Coninx, R., Mathieu, C., Debacker, M., Mirzoev, F., Ismailov, A., and Jabrailov, I., Tuberculosis and prisons: implementing DOTS in a prison in Azerbaijan, *Int. J. Tuberc. Lung Dis.,* 1998, 2(11):S363–64.

147. Coninx, R., Mathieu, C., Debacker, M., Mirzoev, F., Ismaelov, A., de Haller, R., and Meddings, D. R., First-line tuberculosis therapy and drug-resistant *Mycobacterium tuberculosis* in prisons, *Lancet,* 1999, 353:969–73.

148. Habouzit, M., Drug resistance study inside the Georgian penitentiary system — I, *Int. J. Tuberc. Lung Dis.,* 1998, 2(11):S327.

149. Kimerling, M. E., Kluge, H., Vezhnina, N., Iacovazzi, T., Demeulenaere, T., Portaels, F., and Matthys, F., Inadequacy of the current WHO re-treatment regimen in a central Siberian prison: treatment failure and MDRTB, *Int. J. Tuberc. Lung Dis.,* 1999, 3(5):451–3.

150. Farmer, P. E., Managerial successes, clinical failures, *Int. J. Tuberc. Lung Dis.,* 1999, 3(5):365–67.

151. Farmer, P. E. and Kim, J. Y., Community-based approaches to the control of multidrug-resistant tuberculosis: introducing "DOTS-plus," *Br. Med. J.,* 1998, 317:671–4.

152. Farmer, P. E., Timperi, R., Mitnick, C., and Kim, J. Y., Responding to outbreaks of MDR-TB: introducing "DOTS-Plus," in Reichman, L. B. and Hershfield, E. S., Eds., *Tuberculosis: A Comprehensive International Approach,* 2nd ed., New York, Marcel Dekker, 1999.

153. World Health Organization, Report: basis for the development of an evidence-based case-management strategy for MDR TB within the WHO's DOTS strategy, Geneva, 1999, WHO/TB/99.260.

154. Program in Infectious Disease and Social Change, Community-based treatment and control of multidrug-resistant tuberculosis: a DOTS-Plus handbook, Program in Infectious Disease and Social Change, Harvard Medical School, Boston, 1999.

155. Iseman, M., Treatment of multidrug-resistant tuberculosis, *N. Engl. J. Med.,* 1993, 329(11):784–91.

156. Balasubramanian, V., Pavelka, Jr., M. S., Bardarov, S. S., Martin, J., Weisbrod, T. R., McAdam, R. A., Bloom, B. R., and Jacobs, Jr., W. R., Allelic exchange in *Mycobacterium tuberculosis* with long linear recombination substrates, *J. Bacteriol.,* 1996, 178(1):273–79.

157. Guleria, I., Teitelbaum, R., McAdam, R. A., Kalpana, G., Jacobs, Jr., W. R., and Bloom, B. R., Auxotrophic vaccines for tuberculosis, *Nat. Med.,* 1996, 2(3):334–37.

158. Lowrie, D. B., Tacson, R. E., Colston, M. J., and Silva, C. L., Towards a DNA vaccine against tuberculosis, *Vaccine,* 1994, 12:1537–40.

159. Orme, I., Progress in the development of new vaccines against tuberculosis, *Int. J. Tuberc. Lung Dis.,* 1997, 1:97–100.

160. Huygen, K., DNA vaccines: applications to tuberculosis, *Int. J. Tuberc. Lung Dis.,* 1998, 2:971–78.

161. Toman, K., Tuberculosis case-finding and chemotherapy: questions and answers, Geneva, World Health Organization, 1979.

162. Rieder, H. L., Case finding, in Reichman, L. B. and Hershfield, E. S., Eds., *Tuberculosis: A Comprehensive International Approach,* New York, Marcel Dekker, 1993, pp. 167–82.

163. Styblo, K., Epidemiology of tuberculosis, *VEB Gustav Fischer Verlag Jena,* 1984.

164. Layton, M. C., Henning, K. J., Alexander, T. A., Gooding, A. L., et al., Universal radiographic screening for tuberculosis among inmates upon admission to jail, *Am. J. Pub. Health,* 1997, 87:1335–37.

165. Murray, C. J. L. and Salomon, J. A., Modeling the impact of global tuberculosis control strategies, *Proc. Nat. Acad. Sci.,* 1998, 95:13881–6.

166. Cole, S. T. and Telenti, A., Drug resistance in *Mycobacterium tuberculosis, Eur. Respir. J.,* 1995, 20:S701–13.

167. Reichman, L. B., Tuberculosis elimination — what's to stop us? *Int. J. Tuberc. Lung Dis.,* 1997, 1(1):3–11.

168. Fox, W., Drug combinations and the bioavailability of rifampicin, *Tubercle,* 1990, 71:241–45.

169. Acocella, G., Human bioavailability studies, *Bull. Int. Union Against Tubercul. Lung Dis.,* 1989, 64(1):38–40.
170. Moulding, T., Dutt, A., and Reichman, L., Fixed-dose combinations of antituberculous medications to prevent drug resistance, *Ann. Intern. Med.,* 1995, 122(12):951–54.
171. Telenti, A., Genetics of drug resistance in tuberculosis, *Clin. Chest Med.,* 1997, 18(1):55–64.
172. Telenti, A., Imboden, P., Marchesi, M., Schmidheini, T., and Bodmer, T., Direct, automated detection of rifampin-resistant *Mycobacterium tuberculosis* by polymerase chain reaction and single-strand conformation polymorphism analysis, *Antimicrob. Agents Chemother.,* 1993, 37(10):2054–58.
173. De Beenhouwer, H., Lhiang, Z., Jannes, G., Mijs, W., Machtelinckx, L., Rossau, R., Traore, H., and Portaels, F., Rapid detection of rifampin resistance in sputum and biopsy specimens from tuberculosis patients by PCR and line probe assay, *Tuberc. Lung Dis.,* 1995, 76:425–30.
174. Riska, P. F., Su, Y., Bardarov, S., Freundlich, L., Sarkis, G., Hatfull, G., Carrière, C., Kumar, V., Chan, J., and Jacobs, Jr., W. R., Rapid film-based determination of antibiotic susceptibilities of *Mycobacterium tuberculosis* strains by using a luciferase reporter phage and the Bronx box, *J. Clin. Microbiol.,* 1999, 37(4):1144–49.

Index